EMERGENCY PUBLIC HEALTH

Preparedness and Response

Edited by

G. Bobby Kapur, MD, MPH
Associate Chief for Educational Affairs
Residency Program Director
Section of Emergency Medicine
Baylor College of Medicine
Houston, Texas

Jeffrey P. Smith, MD, MPH
Co-Director
Ronald Reagan Institute of Emergency Medicine
The George Washington University
Washington, DC

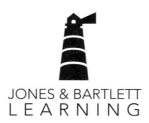

JONES & BARTLETT
LEARNING

World Headquarters
Jones & Bartlett Learning
40 Tall Pine Drive
Sudbury, MA 01776
978-443-5000
info@jblearning.com
www.jblearning.com

Jones & Bartlett Learning books and products are available through most bookstores and online booksellers. To contact Jones & Bartlett Learning directly, call 800-832-0034, fax 978-443-8000, or visit our website, www.jblearning.com.

Substantial discounts on bulk quantities of Jones & Bartlett Learning publications are available to corporations, professional associations, and other qualified organizations. For details and specific discount information, contact the special sales department at Jones & Bartlett Learning via the above contact information or send an email to specialsales@jblearning.com.

Production Credits
Publisher: Michael Brown
Associate Editor: Catie Heverling
Editorial Assistant: Teresa Reilly
Associate Production Editor: Kate Stein
Senior Marketing Manager: Sophie Fleck
Manufacturing and Inventory Control Supervisor: Amy Bacus
Composition: Achorn International
Art: diacriTech
Cover Design: Kristin E. Parker
Cover Image: FEMA/Andrea Booher
Printing and Binding: Malloy, Inc.
Cover Printing: Malloy, Inc.

Library of Congress Cataloging-in-Publication Data
Emergency public health : preparedness and response / edited by G. Bobby Kapur and Jeffrey P. Smith.
    p. ; cm.
  Includes bibliographical references and index.
  ISBN-13: 978-0-7637-5870-7 (pbk.)
  ISBN-10: 0-7637-5870-1 (pbk.)
  1. Disaster medicine—United States. 2. Disaster planning—United States. I. Kapur, G. Bobby. II. Smith, Jeffrey P.
  [DNLM: 1. Disaster Planning—United States. 2. Public Health—United States. 3. Civil Defense—United States. 4. Emergencies—United States. 5. Interinstitutional Relations—United States. 6. Public Policy—United States. WA 295 E543 2011]
  RA645.5.E4965 2011
  363.34'8—dc22
                          2010017338
6048
Printed in the United States of America
15 14 13 12   10 9 8 7 6 5 4 3 2

Dedication

For Jayne, Arjun, and Dylan. My strength and peace amidst all of life's complexities.

—G. BOBBY KAPUR

Contents

Preface ix

Foreword xiii

Contributors xv

About the Editors xix

Introduction 1

1 Public Health Security: Protecting Populations from Emergencies 3
G. Bobby Kapur and Jeffrey P. Smith

Section 1 **Government and Public Health Emergencies** 11

2 Government Capacity: Federal, State, and Local Agencies and
Responsibilities 13
Cedric Dark and Janice Blanchard

3 Public Health Law 31
Carl Hacker and Katherine Wingfield

4 National Response Plan 45
Mark E. A. Escott

5 Emerging Public Health Systems: Post-conflict and Post-disaster
         Settings   63
      C. James Holliman

Section 2   Private-Sector and Nongovernmental Organizations   81

6 Public–Private Partnerships During Emergencies   83
      Jennifer L. Chan and Christian Theodosis

7 Nongovernmental Organizations' Response to Crises   103
      Jeffrey P. Smith and Steven M. Anderscavage

8 Technology and Public Health Crises   131
      Ali Pourmand and Janelle Rios

Section 3   Public Health Tools During Emergencies   151

9 Epidemiological Studies   153
      Junaid A. Razzak and Uzma Rahim Khan

10 Surveillance and Monitoring   167
       Gregg Greenough and Satchit Balsari

11 Rapid Needs Assessment   185
       Hilarie H. Cranmer and Mary Pat McKay

Section 4   Infectious Diseases Emergencies   199

12 Contagious Diseases Epidemics   201
       Terry Mulligan and G. Bobby Kapur

13 Pandemic Influenza   227
       Terry Mulligan and G. Bobby Kapur

14 Emerging and Re-emerging Infectious Diseases   251
       Larissa May

Section 5   Terrorism   283

15 Bombing Events   285
G. Bobby Kapur

16 Biological Agents   305
L. Kristian Arnold

17 Chemical Agents   335
Katherine Douglass and Rodney Omron

18 Radiological Agents   357
Hamid Shokoohi, Mohammad Reza Soroush, and G. Bobby Kapur

Section 6   Natural Emergencies   377

19 Earthquakes   379
Christopher N. Mills

20 Hurricanes, Tsunamis, and Cyclones   403
Elizabeth DeVos

21 Extreme Temperature Emergencies: Heat Waves and Cold Storms   425
Joy Crook and Alexander Vu

Section 7   Industrial Emergencies   445

22 Hazardous Materials   447
Terry Mulligan

23 Nuclear Energy Reactors   473
Y. Veronica Pei and Angela Lee

Section 8   **Special Populations and Issues**   **491**

24   Mental Health Emergencies and Post-traumatic Stress Disorder   493
          Siddharth Ashvin Shah

25   Children and Public Health Emergencies   517
          Heather Machen

26   Public Health Emergencies and Substance Abuse   531
          Deborah Podus, Jane Carlisle Maxwell, and M. Douglas Anglin

          Index   545

Preface

After the SARS outbreak in 2003, Hurricane Katrina in 2005, and the Haitian earthquake in 2010, public health professionals, first responders, and medical providers questioned the effectiveness of preparedness and response activities for these large-scale emergencies, and almost everyone asked, "Is this the best we can do?" Recent domestic and international events have revealed the complex issues that arise from public health emergencies such as natural disasters, infectious disease epidemics, and terrorist events. Although international organizations, countries, or local governments may possess the emergency supplies and personnel for a region in crisis, on many occasions they are unable to deliver this assistance in a timely or coordinated manner. During an emergency, public health professionals face specific challenges: to conduct rapid needs assessments for matching resources with actual needs on the ground, to make critical decisions based on limited data, and to implement monitoring and surveillance techniques for tracking the results of the assistance. Recognizing these challenges and responding to public health crises with the appropriate knowledge and skills will increase the effectiveness of interventions made by public health and healthcare infrastructures.

The public health crises of the 21st century have demonstrated the need for enormous coordination among multiple entities for good outcomes. Historically, these preparedness and response activities have mostly been within the domain of local, state, and national government agencies. However, the private sector and nongovernmental organizations (NGOs) are playing larger roles in recent crises for multiple reasons. Often, the government may be limited in the immediate resources available to respond to an emergency or these agencies may not be able to provide assistance rapidly, and the private sector and NGOs may be able to deliver aid quickly through well-established formal and informal networks. In addition, as was seen in the 2010 Haitian earthquake, the government facilities may be disrupted or destroyed during the event, and other organizations are needed to fill the void left by the lack of government capacity. Once the government, private sector, and NGOs enter the emergency setting, communication and clarity of responsibilities are fundamental for stabilizing the affected community and for beginning relief efforts.

Although multiple books have been written on the topic of disaster medicine, this is the first book in the growing field of emergency public health. Unlike disaster medicine that focuses primarily on the medical treatment of specific conditions that occur during disasters, emergency public health encompasses the broad components of preparedness, response, and mitigation through a public health perspective for communities and nations that are at risk for large-scale emergencies. In addition, emergency public health explores the interactions and contributions of multiple sectors such as the government, non-governmental organizations, private enterprises, and individuals before, during, and after a public health emergency.

Most of the contributing authors in this book are emergency medicine physicians with public health degrees. These experts combine their public health and clinical experiences to give the reader a balance of both theory and practice on how to prepare and respond to public health emergencies. The book is divided into eight sections to address the breadth and depth of emergency public health:

1. Government and Public Health Emergencies
2. Private Sector and Nongovernmental Organizations
3. Public Health Tools during Emergencies
4. Infectious Diseases
5. Terrorism
6. Natural Disasters
7. Industrial Emergencies
8. Special Populations and Issues

The chapters are structured to provide the reader with a systematic and case-based approach to the topics. Each chapter begins with a detailed case study and then follows with historical perspectives to learn fom prior experiences. The chapter then provides valuable information on specific preparedness, response, and mitigation interventions. The chapter then reviews the case study to offer a detailed analysis. Each chapter concludes with a list of important on-line resources.

The primary objectives of this book are simple: to help improve how we prepare and respond to public health crises and to decrease the morbidity, mortality, and suffering of those individuals affected by large-scale emergencies. As public health professionals, first responders, and healthcare providers, we possess the obligation to achieve the highest level of public health security within the communities we serve.

G. BOBBY KAPUR
Houston, Texas

JEFFREY P. SMITH
Washington, DC

Foreword:
What Is Emergency Public Health?

The concept of emergency public health, while not new, is being defined and described in greater detail than in the past. In this book, the authors have focused on the nature of public health emergencies, as well as the role that various sectors have in responding to them. They describe tools that are common to public health, and identify some of the issues that are faced in preparing for and responding to public health emergencies. Defining emergency public health through the use of these examples provides a basis for understanding the concepts that are critical to the field—prevention, preparation, intervention, and recovery—as well as the critical need to take a multidisciplinary approach to public health emergencies.

In an environment in which we discuss public health emergencies, we need to discuss emergency public health as a specialty area within public health, much as environmental health, infectious disease, or injury prevention and control can be seen as public health specialty areas, and to provide a basis for its practice and research. Core competencies in emergency public health, currently under development, will take an all-hazard approach, and will cover the spectrum of prevention, protection, response and recovery, and will provide a foundation for advanced competencies in the specialty area of emergency public health. This multidisciplinary field will draw from the core values of the disciplines that contribute to it, and, at a minimum may serve the common mission of many of the disciplines: to improve health within the population. In addition, emergency public health can enhance the effectiveness with which health knowledge and technologies are applied in addressing public health emergencies. A core value of promoting equity in health will allow the field to decrease disparities in preventing, preparing for, intervening in, and recovering from public health emergencies.

For those who ask the question, "Why now? And why a new field of public health?" many of the answers are contained in the following chapters. The continued development of the science and practice of emergency public health through education, research and multidisciplinary collaboration is critical to ensuring health security, to responding to public health emergencies, and to ensuring that populations have access to prevention of, preparation for, intervention in and recovery from public health emergencies.

LINDA C. DEGUTIS, DRPH, MSN
Past President, American Public Health Association
Associate Professor of Emergency Medicine and Public Health
Yale University
New Haven, Connecticut

Contributors

Steven M. Anderscavage, DO, MPH
Fellow, International Emergency Medicine
Adjunct Instructor, Global Health
The George Washington University
Washington, DC

M. Douglas Anglin, PhD
Associate Director
Integrated Substance Abuse Programs
University of California at Los Angeles
Los Angeles, California

L. Kristian Arnold, MD, MPH, FACEP
ArLac Global Health Services
Lexington, Massachusettes

Satchit Balsari, MD, MPH
Instructor in Clinical Medicine, Division
    of Emergency Medicine
Weill Cornell Medical College
New York, New York
Fellow, Harvard Humanitarian Initiative,
    Harvard University
Cambridge, Massachusetts

Janice Blanchard, MD, MPH, PhD
Director of Health Policy Programs
Department of Emergency Medicine
The George Washington University
Washington, DC

Jennifer L. Chan, MD, MPH
Associate Faculty
Harvard Humanitarian Initiative
Cambridge, Massachusetts

Hilarie H. Cranmer, MD, MPH
Brigham and Women's Hospital
Harvard Medical School
Harvard School of Public Health
Harvard Humanitarian Incentive
Boston, Massachusetts

Joy Crook, MD, MPH
Instructor
Department of Emergency Medicine
John Hopkins School of Medicine
Baltimore, Maryland

Cedric Dark, MD, MPH
Department of Emergency Medicine
The George Washington University
Washington, DC

Elizabeth DeVos, MD, MPH, FACEP
Department of Emergency Medicine
The University of Florida College of
    Medicine—Jacksonville
Jacksonville, Florida

Katherine Douglass, MD, MPH
Assistant Professor
Department of Emergency Medicine
The George Washington University
Washington, DC

Mark E. A. Escott, MD, MPH
Assistant Professor/Assistant Director
Division of EMS and Disaster Medicine
Baylor College of Medicine
Houston, Texas
Instructor
Master's Degree in Homeland Security
    Program
Pennsylvania State University

Gregg Greenough, MD, MPH
Assistant Professor of Medicine
Harvard Medical School
Boston, Massachusetts
Research Director, Harvard Humanitarian
    Initiative
Harvard University
Cambridge, Massachusetts
Attending Physician, Division of
    Emergency Medicine
Brigham & Women's Hospital
Boston, Massachusetts

Carl Hacker, PhD, JD
School of Public Health
University of Texas
Houston, Texas

C. James Holliman, MD
Professor of Military and Emergency
    Medicine
Uniformed Services University of the
    Health Sciences
Bethesda, Maryland
Clinical Professor of Emergency Medicine
The George Washington University
Washington, DC

Uzma Rahim Khan, MBBS, MSc
Department of Emergency Medicine
Aga Khan University
Karachi, Pakistan

Angela Lee, MD, MPH
Department of Emergency Medicine
The George Washington University
Washington, DC

Heather Machen, MD, MPH
Attending Physician
Emergency Center
Texas Children's Hospital
Assistant Professor of Pediatrics
Baylor College of Medicine
Houston, Texas

Larissa May, MD, MSPH
Department of Emergency Medicine
The George Washington University
Washington, DC

Jane Carlisle Maxwell, PhD
University of Texas at Austin
Austin, Texas

Mary Pat McKay, MD, MPH
The George Washington University
Washington, DC

Christopher N. Mills, MD, MPH
Affiliate Clinical Instructor of Surgery
Division of Emergency Medicine
Stanford School of Medicine
Palo Alto, California

Terry Mulligan, DO, MPH
Director Emergency Medicine Residency
Co-director, Department of
    Emergency Medicine
Universitair Medisch Centrum Utrecht
Utrecht, The Netherlands
Assistant Professor of Emergency
    Medicine
Department of Emergency Medicine
University of Maryland School of
    Medicine
Baltimore, Maryland

Rodney Omron, MD, MPH
Clinical Assistant Professor
Department of Emergency Medicine
University of Michigan
Ann Arbor, Michigan

Y. Veronica Pei, MD, Med, MPH
Assistant Professor
Department of Emergency Medicine
University of Maryland School of
    Medicine
Baltimore, Maryland

Deborah Podus, PhD
UCLA Integrated Substance Abuse
    Programs
Associate Research Sociologist
University of California at Los Angeles
Los Angeles, California

Ali Pourmand, MD, MPH
Assistant Professor
The George Washington University
Washington, DC

Junaid A. Razzak, MD, PhD, FACEP
Associate Professor
Chair, Department of Emergency
    Medicine
Aga Khan University
Karachi, Pakistan

Janelle Rios, PhD
Public Health Consultant
Houston, Texas

Siddharth Ashvin Shah, MD, MPH
Greenleaf Intergrative Strategies, LLC
Arlington, Virginia

Hamid Shokoohi, MD, MPH, RDMS
Assistant Professor
Department of Emergency Medicine
The George Washington University
    Medical Center
Washington, DC

Mohammad Reza Soroush, MD
Janzaben Medical and Engineering Research
Tehran, Iran

Christian Theodosis, MD, MPH
Director of Global Health Programs
Emergency Medicine
University of Chicago
Chicago, Illinois

Alexander Vu, DO, MPH
John Hopkins School of Public Health
Baltimore, Maryland

Katherine Wingfield, JD, MPH
Center for Biosecurity and Public Health
    Preparedness
University of Texas School of Public
    Health
Houston, Texas

About the Editors

G. Bobby Kapur, MD, MPH, is the Associate Chief for Educational Affairs for the Section of Emergency Medicine at Baylor College of Medicine (BCM). Dr. Kapur developed and launched the new emergency medicine residency training program at BCM that began in July 2010, and he currently serves as the director of the residency program. Dr. Kapur also serves as the Director of Educational Affairs for the Emergency Center at Ben Taub General Hospital in Houston, Texas.

From 2005 to 2009, Dr. Kapur was the Director of the International Emergency Medicine and Global Public Health Fellowship Program for the Department of Emergency Medicine at The George Washington University. During this time, Dr. Kapur designed and taught one of the nation's first courses in emergency public health for law enforcement officials from local and national agencies. In addition, he developed and implemented emergency medicine and public health training programs for international physicians, nurses and primary healthcare workers.

Dr. Kapur's research has focused on the preparedness and response to terrorist bombing events. Collaborating with the Bureau of Alcohol, Tobacco, Firearms, and Explosives (ATF), he authored one of the most comprehensive assessments of bombing events in the United States, analyzing 20 years of ATF bombing data, and he has recently published a pre-hospital care algorithm for the management of bombing victims.

Dr. Kapur's projects have included establishing emergency medicine training programs in Beijing, New Delhi, and Kolkata. Dr. Kapur also provided leadership and oversight for a three-year program with the Emergency Medicine Association of Turkey to train nearly 2,500 physicians across Turkey in evidence-based medicine. He has also worked with partners globally on the development of emergency public health systems with an emphasis on low-cost, high-yield strategies.

Dr. Kapur has served as the Chair of the Section of International Emergency Medicine for the American College of Emergency Physicians and as Chair of the Committee of International Emergency Medicine for the Society of Academic Emergency Medicine.

Dr. Kapur earned his Bachelor of Arts degree in English Literature and Policy Studies from Rice University, his Doctor of Medicine degree with a concentration in medical ethics from Baylor College of Medicine, and his Master of Public Health in Global Health from Harvard University. Dr. Kapur completed his Emergency Medicine residency training at Yale University and his International Emergency Medicine fellowship at Harvard University and Brigham and Women's Hospital.

Jeffrey P. Smith, MD, MPH, earned his Doctor of Medicine degree from the University of Maryland, and his Master of Public Health degree from The George Washington University. In additon to serving as Co-Director of the Ronald Reagan Institute of Emergency Medicine at The George Washington University, Dr. Smith has also taught courses in emergency medicine.

Introduction

CHAPTER 1

Public Health Security: Protecting Populations from Emergencies

G. Bobby Kapur and Jeffrey P. Smith

PUBLIC HEALTH EMERGENCIES

Large-scale population crises continue to threaten communities in the United States and in other countries around the globe. The past few decades have seen an increasing number of both natural and deliberate events that have resulted in large numbers of injuries and deaths and billions of dollars of financial losses (see Figure 1-1). These public health emergencies not only have caused immediate devastation, but also have led to long-term periods of rebuilding and rehabilitation of the affected areas. Although nations frequently confront public health crises, critically important practices are not consistently being implemented during many of these events. Familiarity with and recurrence of public health emergencies has not necessarily led to improved outcomes.

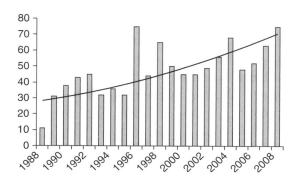

FIGURE 1-1   Number of Declared U.S. Disasters 1988–2008
Source: Data from FEMA. http://www.fema.gov/news/disaster_totals_annual.fema

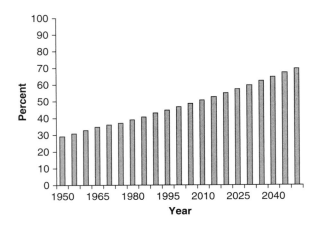

FIGURE 1-2   Current and Projected Percentage of Global Population Living in Urban Areas 1950–2050

Source: Data from UN World Urbanization Prospects: The 2007 Revision Population Database. http://esa.un.org/unup/index.asp?panel=1

Globalization is resulting in an increasing number of people living in urban areas. From 1950 to 2010, the share of the global population living in urban areas has expanded from 29 percent to more than 50 percent (see Figure 1-2). With increasingly larger numbers of people living in densely populated urban regions, the number of people who are vulnerable to public health risks and the magnitude of public health crises increases exponentially.[1,2]

Emergency public health differs from disaster medicine in that it involves more than just the management of specific hazards. The term "hazard" is used to describe the events that cause emergencies; these hazards can be natural (e.g., earthquakes, hurricanes, droughts), deliberate (e.g., bombing, chemical attack, biological attack), or accidental (e.g., nuclear plant malfunction). The scope of emergency public health addresses these hazards but additionally encompasses the following issues:

- Multiple sectors
- Public health tools applied during emergencies
- Resilience analysis
- Systemization of efforts

Multiple components of society are disrupted by public health emergencies: health, mental health, security, housing, food, and water. In addition, these events may threaten the political and economic stability of the community or the country. Large-scale crises will affect all sectors of the community, including the government, private sector, nongovernmental organizations (NGOs), and civilians.[3] Each of these sectors will collectively provide and utilize resources during a crisis, and, therefore, each of these sectors will possess a collective responsibility in a community's resilience to public health emergencies. By increasing the systemized surveillance, assessments, coordination, and communication among sectors and among levels of government jurisdictions, communities can achieve greater levels of protection from collapse in the event of a public health emergency.

A fundamental aspect of public health emergencies is their unpredictability. Even though they are unpredictable in terms of when and where they will strike, all public health emergencies progress through predictable stages: preparedness, response, and mitigation. Nevertheless, communities cannot prepare for every possible public health scenario that may occur. For this reason, communities must always maintain a range of preparedness regardless of the type of incident that may occur. Given the difficulty of preparing and responding to a large number and variability of potential public health emergencies, an "all hazards" approach can help protect a population by having available a continuous and minimum level of personnel, resources, and training that can address a broad scope of hazards.[4] Furthermore, the uncertainty regarding the timing and location of an incident will require communities to have baseline levels of capabilities to be able to respond effectively to public health crises.[4] Finally, to ensure mitigation, a community will need to apply lessons learned from prior events within the community and from other regions to implement measures to reduce vulnerability and decrease risks from future events.

HISTORICAL PERSPECTIVES

The past decade has seen a greater awareness for expanded and improved public health infrastructure to respond to increasing threats. In November 2000, the U.S. Congress passed the Public Health Threats and Emergencies Act of 2000 (P.L. 106-505), which was the first law to direct large amounts of resources toward public health preparedness for bioterrorism and other communicable disease outbreaks. The legislation authorized $540 million in fiscal year 2001 to improve public health agencies' response capabilities and capacities. The objective was to elevate state and local capacity and to meet the following goals:[5]

- Require the development of a fundamental set of public health capacities to be implemented by states and municipalities
- Establish a state grant program to evaluate their public health capacity

- Authorize increased funds for state and local planning and implementation of these capacity-building goals

In June 2002, the U.S. Congress passed the Public Health Security and Bioterrorism Preparedness and Response Act (P.L. 107-188) in response to the September 11, 2001, terrorist attacks and the anthrax attacks that occurred later in 2001. This legislation authorized even greater funding and provided new measures for the following purposes:[5]

- Improving public health capacity
- Upgrading health professionals' ability to recognize and treat diseases caused by bioterrorism
- Accelerating the development of new vaccines and other countermeasures
- Upgrading protections for water and food supplies
- Tracking and regulating the use of dangerous pathogens within the United States

Because of their specific focus on bioterrorism and communicable diseases, these legislative efforts did not address many aspects of emergency public health capacity building that will be required to respond to other public health hazards.

On May 23, 2005, the World Health Assembly unanimously passed the International Health Regulations (IHR). This legally binding international agreement emphasized the building and strengthening of national surveillance and response systems. The IHR contains a commitment from the World Health Organization (WHO) and its 193 member-states to improve capacity for disease prevention, detection, and response. It also provides recommendations to address national public health threats that have the possibility of escalating to global emergencies.[6] Fundamental changes include the following measures:

- Expanding reportable diseases beyond only cholera, plague, and yellow fever
- Improving notification processes
- Structuring contact points and communications among nations
- Strengthening surveillance and response capacities at the national level

Although the IHR advanced public health efforts at the national and global levels for communicable diseases, it remains a limited instrument and does not adopt an "all hazards" approach.

PUBLIC HEALTH SECURITY FRAMEWORK

Historically, public health security has been viewed narrowly as a domain encompassing infectious diseases and bioterrorism. In reality, the public health infrastruc-

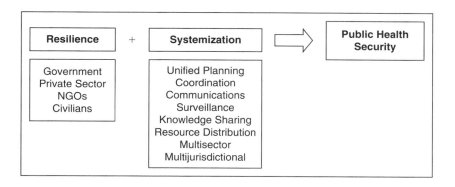

FIGURE 1-3 Public Health Security Framework

ture plays a critical role in ensuring a population's resilience to all hazards. In addition, specific systems criteria can determine whether a community will be able to provide protection to its residents from public health emergencies. The combination of resilience and systemization will lead to public health security for a population (see Figure 1-3).

Resilience Analysis Model

Resilience is a population's capacity to withstand adversity and to recovery quickly. A community's resilience to a public health crisis has traditionally been defined as the government's ability to provide personnel and resources to an affected group of people during a large-scale emergency. However, emerging studies and evaluations of communities during public health emergencies are revealing that multiple sectors contribute important functions to the preparedness and response to these large-scale crises.[7–9]

To analyze a community's resilience to public health emergencies, both actors and their contributions throughout the emergency cycle will provide valuable information on the level of resilience (see Table 1-1). In addition to the government, other key actors in public health emergencies include the private sector, NGOs, and civilian populations. Understanding their roles and contributions will allow public health professionals and policy makers to improve the community's capacity to provide public health security. Knowing the resources available from each actor during each stage of a potential emergency (preparedness, response, and mitigation) can optimize the collective protection of the population.

TABLE 1-1	**Resilience Analysis Model**		
Actors	**Stages of Public Health Emergency**		
	Preparedness	**Response**	**Mitigation**
Government	1. Training 2. Plans 3. Drills 4. Surveillance 5. Stockpiles	1. Personnel 2. Material supplies 3. Medical care 4. Security 5. Needs assessments	1. Return to normal activity 2. Design improvements 3. Technology advancements 4. Standards and regulations
Private sector	1. Contingency operations plans 2. Information backup 3. First-aid training	1. Evacuation 2. First aid 3. Material supplies	1. Return to normal activity 2. Design improvements 3. Technology advancements 4. Implementation of standards and regulations
Nongovernmental organizations	1. Training 2. Plans 3. Stockpiles	1. Personnel 2. Material supplies 3. First aid 4. Counseling 5. Family reunification 6. Food 7. Shelter 8. Clothing	1. Targeted stockpiles 2. Increased training
Civilian population	1. First-aid training 2. Emergency contacts 3. Home-preparedness kits	1. Evacuation 2. First aid 3. Counseling 4. Food 5. Shelter 6. Clothing	1. Return to normal activity 2. Housing modifications

Systemization

Although multiple actors provide capacity for public health emergencies, their resources and personnel alone cannot ensure public health security. Specific systems criteria must be established to unify the multisector and multijurisdictional capabilities that are deployed before, during, and after a large-scale crisis. The key systems components are summarized here:

- Unified planning
- Coordination
- Communications
- Knowledge sharing
- Surveillance
- Resource distribution

With this systemization of the actors and their capabilities, the available capacity can be more effectively and more quickly implemented during a sudden, large-scale event.

Unified planning allows sectors and government agencies the ability to plan and train together prior to an actual event. These interagency and multisector efforts offer various entities an opportunity to become familiar with one another's personnel and to become aware of all available resources. While conducting unified planning, the multiple actors can also develop plans on improved coordination among the responders. In 2005, Hurricane Katrina demonstrated that large-scale public health emergencies require enormous logistical planning and coordination to achieve effective results. The U.S. Government Accountability Office (GAO) found that there was inadequate delineation of responsibilities across agencies and jurisdictions to ensure effective outcomes.[10] In addition, resources were not shared and distributed among agencies that would have allowed for greater efficiency and more timely delivery of goods and services to the communities that were devastated by the storm.

Communications become vital for both knowledge sharing and surveillance. If different sectors or agencies have access to varying levels of information, then the public health infrastructure is at risk for a systemic breakdown. The September 11, 2001, terrorist attacks revealed the potential systems failures that may occur if the sectors do not possess shared communications. The New York Police Department (NYPD) and the New York Fire Department (NYFD) used separate radio communications channels. When it became evident that the World Trade Center towers were going to collapse, the NYPD officers in the helicopters who had knowledge of the threat posed by structural instability were not able to communicate evacuation information to the NYFD fire fighters in the buildings.[11] Hundreds of NYFD fire fighters lost their lives because of this lack of systemized communication and inability to share knowledge across jurisdictions.

CONCLUSION

Whether due to natural, deliberate, or accidental causes, public health emergencies continue to increase in the United States and other countries. As the global population becomes more urbanized, larger numbers of people living in densely populated "mega-cities" are exposed to public health hazards. If such an event does occur, the magnitude of its impact is likely to be enormous simply because of the large number of individuals exposed to the threat. Although recent U.S. and international laws have attempted to strengthen the public health infrastructure, these efforts have focused specifically on communicable disease threats and bioterrorism. A broader and more extensive public health security framework that includes resilience and systemization will assist federal, state, and local public health professionals, policy makers, responders, and public officials in protecting communities from public health emergencies. Collective multisector efforts will lead to collective public health security for populations.

NOTES

1. Uitto J. The geography of disaster vulnerability in megacities: A theoretical framework. *Applied Geography*. 1998;18(1):7–16.
2. Weichselgartner J. Disaster mitigation: The concept of vulnerability revisited. *Disaster Prevention and Management*. 2001;10(2):85–95.
3. Pan American Sanitary Bureau. *Health and hemispheric security*. Washington, DC: Pan American Health Organization; 2002.
4. Health Action in Crises Section of the WHO. *Risk reduction and emergency preparedness: WHO six-year strategy for the health sector and community capacity development*. Geneva, Switzerland: World Health Organization; 2007.
5. Frist B. Public health and national security: The critical role of increased federal support. *Health Affairs*. Nov./Dec. 2002;21(6):117–130.
6. Rodier G, Greenspan AL, Hughes JM, Heymann DL. Global public health security. *Emerging Infectious Diseases*. 2007;13(10):1447–1452.
7. McEntire DA, Fuller C, Johnston CW, Weber R. A comparison of disaster paradigms: The search for a holistic policy guide. *Public Administration Review*. 2002;62(3):267–281.
8. Pearce L. Disaster management and community planning, and public participation: How to achieve sustainable hazard mitigation. *Natural Hazards*. 2003;28:211–228.
9. Mason B. *Community disaster resilience*. Washington, DC: National Academies Press; 2006.
10. Woods WT. *Hurricane Katrina: Planning for and management of federal disaster recovery contracts*. Washington, DC: U.S. Government Accountability Office; April 10, 2006.
11. Dwyer J, Flynn K, Fessenden F. Fatal confusion: A troubled emergency response; 9/11 exposed deadly flaws in rescue plan. *New York Times*. July 7, 2002. Retrieved May 26, 2010, from www.nytimes.com/2002/07/07/nyregion/07EMER.html

SECTION 1

Government and Public Health Emergencies

Government Capacity: Federal, State, and Local Agencies and Responsibilities

Cedric Dark and Janice Blanchard

INTRODUCTION

The public health community, ranging from local, state, and federal levels of government, responds to a multitude of emergency events, both natural and human-made. Public health emergencies in recent memory have encompassed such natural incidents as disease outbreaks—for example, the H1N1 flu outbreak in 2009, the emergence of West Nile virus in the eastern United States in 1999, and the severe acute respiratory syndrome (SARS) outbreak in Asia in 2003—or environmental catastrophes like that seen during Hurricane Katrina in 2005. Human-made incidents that present public health emergencies can be either intentional (e.g., the Japanese subway Sarin incident of 1995) or unintentional (e.g., the massive power blackout in the northeastern United States in 2003).

While local and state officials deal with most public health emergencies initially, federal involvement is almost certain when the crisis is severe in scope. Legal authority for intervention in public health emergencies is left to the states and their localities under the Tenth Amendment to the U.S. Constitution. However, federal involvement in the day-to-day function of public health can be established through the Commerce Clause of the Constitution. Under these auspices, the federal government can engage in regulation of food security through the U.S. Department of Agriculture, air and water purity through the Environmental Protection Agency (EPA), pharmaceutical safety through the Food and Drug Administration (FDA), and many other spheres of influence.

Case Study

The immediate phase of any acute public health emergency (from the sentinel event up to the first 2 hours) requires first responders from the local community.[2] Consider, for instance, the attacks on the World Trade Center on September 11, 2001. The first few minutes of the crisis were marked by an overwhelming number of calls to the local 911 system. Immediate emergency response began with private firms and individuals already present within One World Trade Center (the North Tower). The first organized leadership on scene was the Fire Department of New York (FDNY) Battalion Chief, who arrived within 6 minutes of the crash of the first aircraft.[3] During the immediate phase, local incident command systems assumed authority for the developing crisis.

The intermediate phase (first 2 to 12 hours) of the response to a public health emergency remains the purview of local and perhaps state officials.[4] Toward the end of this phase, emergency response priorities should shift toward accepting and coordinating federal assistance. In the hours after the World Trade Center collapse, emergency response personnel from the Centers for Disease Control and Prevention (CDC) and the U.S. Department of Health and Human Services (DHHS) arrived on the scene, to the welcome relief of local officials.[5]

The third phase of an acute public health emergency is termed the extended phase and represents all events after 12 hours.[6] If the emergency is not contained and the emergency response concluding, preparations for extended federal operations occur at this time. Clearly, a large federal effort continued for months following the tragedy at the World Trade Center. Made immediately available was assistance from the CDC.[7] CDC personnel assisted with injury and disease surveillance, capacity assessment, emergency coordination, and provision of supplies. Later, the EPA undertook a significant public health action by declaring that air and water quality were suitable for individuals to return to New York's Financial District.[8] Many federal agencies may share a role during this extended phase of an emergency response.

Each of these phases involves federal, state, and local agencies in various roles and responsibilities. This chapter provides an overview of components of these roles by jurisdiction in responding to a public health emergency.

FEDERAL PREPAREDNESS AND RESPONSE _____

The federal government's role does not merely exist in the hours and days after a public health emergency occurs. According to the Institute of Medicine (IOM), the federal government fills six major roles in public health: (1) policy, (2) finance, (3) public health protection, (4) information gathering and dissemination, (5) capacity building, and (6) direct patient healthcare services.

Policy

The policy basis for public health derives from public health law; the vast majority of laws dealing with issues such as quarantine, disease reporting, or other aspects of public health are formulated at the state level. However, certain areas of law and regulation, including air and water purity, come from federal actions. Unfortunately, as many authorities have suggested, many public health laws are antiquated.[9] Multiple attempts aimed at modernizing these laws have been made, including the work of the Turning Point Initiative[10] and the Model State Emergency Health Powers Act.[11] At present, 38 states and the District of Columbia have enacted 66 bills or resolutions containing provisions of the Model State Emergency Health Powers Act. Continued action is necessary for the modernization of public health law.

Finance

In contrast to the perpetually cash-strapped state governments, the federal government possesses considerable resources to fund public health initiatives and to absorb the costs of mitigation and recovery from major public health emergencies. To demonstrate these disparate financial capacities, compare state and local budgets for public health with that of the federal government. It has been estimated that the average budget of state and local public health agencies was $6.9 million in recent years (based on some jurisdictions reporting data for fiscal year 2004, and others for fiscal year 2005).[12] This amounts to an average annual per capita expenditure for public health of $41. By comparison, federal funding for the public health components of the DHHS during fiscal year 2002 amounted to $41 billion, nearly $137 per capita.[13]

Public Health Protection

The federal responsibility for protecting the public's health comprises three major components: disease surveillance, maintenance of a national collective of laboratories, and management of threats. There currently exist multiple mechanisms by which the federal government monitors the prevalence and incidence of disease in the United States. The CDC maintains most of these disease surveillance networks, whose inputs come from data derived at the state or local level.

The Health Alert Network (HAN) is designed for two-way communication between the federal government and local agencies.[14] Currently, it transmits health alerts, health updates, and health advisories to more than 1 million recipients. Project BioSense, another CDC initiative, scans hospital emergency department and pharmacy data, thereby attempting to uncover diseases based on symptom patterns.[15] Uploads to the database are now electronic and occur as frequently as every 15 minutes.[16] While BioSense is intended to help detect spikes in disease incidence, it is no substitute for astute clinicians and, in fact, is dependent on physician diagnoses. However, because individuals who are affected by a public health emergency (consider the sporadic *Salmonella* outbreaks as examples) may not all present to the same healthcare provider, Project BioSense can help discover potential disease outbreaks spread across providers within a specific community.

These surveillance systems illustrate the fragmentation of the public health information network. To overcome this problem, the CDC is integrating these and other diverse monitoring systems into a single Public Health Information Network by utilizing the National Electronic Disease Surveillance System.[17,18] The CDC also operates the Epidemic Intelligence Exchange (Epi-X), which serves as a means of collaboration and intellectual exchange for public health providers at the local level.[19]

Additionally, the federal government assumes limited responsibility for emergency preparedness training for first responders and public health agents. Once a public health emergency has been identified, whether it is a natural event such as a disease outbreak or a human-made threat such as terrorism, the public health response becomes critical. Federal means by which emergencies may be mitigated are multiple and multidisciplinary. Under the disaster medical system, when a public health emergency arises, various health professionals from across the nation become temporary federal employees and can be deployed to the site of an incident.[20] Disaster Medical Assistance Teams (DMATs) include both medical professionals and paraprofessionals; a recent count identified 26 such teams, with formation of an additional 20 groups planned.[21] DMATs bring with them supplies sufficient to sustain a 72-hour mission.

Five national veterinary response teams, including veterinarians, technicians, pathologists, and other skilled staff, are available for deployment in the event that animals, either wild or domesticated, are involved in a public health emergency incident.[22] Ten regional mortuary response teams are available for situations in which casualties are expected to overwhelm local capabilities.[23] These teams can travel with completely portable morgues and assist with the recovery, identification, and burial of victims.

Additional response teams comprising the specialties of nursing and pharmacy are in development.[24] A strategic national stockpile (SNS) of pharmaceuticals and medical supplies is already available during public health emergencies, at the simple request of a state's governor.[25] Authorized in the Public Health Service Act, the SNS is designed to supplement and resupply local and state resources in the United States and its territories within a 12-hour time frame. The national stockpile also allows secondary pharmaceutical delivery, with medications being shipped directly from manufacturers if an initial stockpile package is insufficient to cover need.[26] Additional federal resources for protecting and preserving the public's health can be obtained from the U.S. Public Health Service Commissioned Officer Corps, a branch of the Uniformed Services capable of providing immediate relief and support for clinical, epidemiological, and mental health needs.[27]

Information Gathering and Dissemination

As described previously, the capacity of the federal government to collect and disseminate information rests mostly with the CDC. Through the HAN, Project BioSense, Epidemic Intelligence Exchange, the National Electronic Disease Surveillance System, and the Public Health Information Network, CDC is able, with certain limitations, to derive information from, and deliver critical information to, both state and local health agencies. At a practical level, the capacity at the local level tends to be the limiting factor in this communication process. There are at least 90,000 units of local government that require access to important information so that they can help quell outbreaks and other types of emergencies.[28] Many of these jurisdictions are relatively resource poor. Thus the ability of the federal government to improve the capacity of local governments to communicate and act remains paramount.

Capacity Building

The federal government's role with capacity building begins with individual providers and extends to hospitals and entire communities. Given that many public health officials are political appointees, their tenures in such positions are often limited. Therefore, intellectual capital is perpetually turning over and occasionally lost. The State Health Leadership Initiative, a program funded by the Robert Wood Johnson Foundation and operated by the National Governors Association, attempts to provide leadership skills to senior-level state health officials.[29] These skills are critical when a public health emergency arises.

At the institutional level, the Hospital Preparedness Program, which was established in 2002, keeps these community resources alert and prepared for natural and human-made disasters.[30] This prudently designed initiative fulfills a critical role because the initial waves of any emergency (as exemplified in the World Trade Center attacks) are likely to be felt at the local level first. The Cities Readiness Initiative is another CDC program geared toward ensuring that entire cities and towns are prepared to deliver medicines and medical supplies in the event of a public health emergency.[31,32] As of 2010, the program currently has 72 participating cities, and at least one site in each state (http://www.bt.cdc.gov/cri/).

The federal role for capacity building is, of course, limited by annual funding by Congress and the commitment of the executive branch in extending these appropriations to local public health agencies. Nevertheless, the hard-learned lessons of September 11, 2001 support the need for improved public health information and mitigation capacity.

Direct Services

The federal government maintains a limited role in the direct delivery of healthcare services. The bulk of direct healthcare services provided under the auspices of public health are typically relegated to the jurisdiction of states and local public health authorities.

Roles of Federal Agencies

In addition to DHHS, many different federal agencies or subagencies are available for response to a public health emergency. The Department of Homeland Security will most likely be involved if a human-made or terrorist activity is suspected. If a radiological agent is suspected to be present, response by the Department of Energy might be necessary to mitigate exposure and ensure adequate disposal of agents. Likewise, the Department of Justice, including the Federal Bureau of Investigation (FBI), may become involved in a federal law enforcement response. The EPA and U.S. Coast Guard may be needed for emergencies involving the air or water supply. The FDA and U.S. Department of Agriculture might take an active role in public health emergencies involving food or pharmaceutical supplies.

The CDC plays an important function specifically in the public health response to emergencies. The U.S. Congress authorized funding in 2002 for the Public Health Emergency Preparedness (PHEP) cooperative agreement to support public health preparedness in public health departments in all state, local, tribal, and territorial areas.[33] The CDC provides technical expertise for disease detection and investigation, public health laboratories, and response, including crisis communication. Utilizing well-established CDC relationships with regional public health departments is critical to the success of the PHEP. The CDC has established nine goals within the pre-event, event, and post-event phases of public health emergencies to facilitate coordination and response among various jurisdictions (see Table 2-1).

TABLE 2-1	CDC Goals During Public Health Emergencies	
		Prevent
Pre-event	Goal 1	Increase the use and development of interventions known to prevent human illness from chemical, biological, and radiological agents, and from naturally occurring health threats.
		Detect and Report
	Goal 2	Decrease the time needed to classify health events as terrorism or naturally occurring in partnership with other agencies.
	Goal 3	Decrease the time needed to detect and report chemical, biological, or radiological agents in tissue, food, or environmental samples that cause threats to the public health.
	Goal 4	Improve the timeliness and accuracy of communications regarding threats to the public's health.
Event		**Investigate**
	Goal 5	Decrease the time to identify causes, risk factors, and appropriate interventions for those affected by threats to the public's health.
		Control
	Goal 6	Decrease the time needed to provide countermeasures and health guidance to those affected by threats to the public health.
		Recover
	Goal 7	Decrease the time needed to restore health services and environmental safety to pre-event levels.
Post-event	Goal 8	Improve the long-term follow-up provided to those affected by threats to the public's health.
		Improve
	Goal 9	Decrease the time needed to implement recommendations from after-action reports following threats to the public's health.

Source: Centers for Disease Control and Prevention. Public health preparedness: Mobilizing state by state. Available at: http://www.bt.cdc.gov/publications/feb08phprep/background.asp. Accessed December 15, 2009.

The difficulty with having multiple agencies with different priorities and cultures interacting at a time of crisis can be a lack of unified leadership. It is important that personnel from multiple federal agencies cooperate as well as engage in frequent, quality communication to ensure seamless interaction during a public health emergency.

STATE PREPAREDNESS AND RESPONSE

While the federal government does provide the infrastructure that coordinates activities across state and local governments, day-to-day operations remain mainly under the jurisdiction of state and local governments.[34] States receive funds from a cooperative agreement between the CDC's Public Health Response and Preparedness for Bioterrorism Program and the Health Resources Services Administration's National Hospital Bioterrorism Preparedness Program.[35] Only a few local jurisdictions—large jurisdictions such as New York City, Chicago, Los Angeles, and Washington, D.C.—receive direct federal dollars. In most cases, funding trickles down to the local level through state agencies.

Organization of State Response

A state's public health response organizational structure can be centralized, decentralized, or a mixture of both approaches. In a centralized structure, the state has direct oversight over the local public health agencies. In a decentralized structure, the state employs a more loose oversight, with the primary responsibility for public health decisions being handled by local jurisdictions. There is no clear consensus as to whether one approach works better in terms of the effectiveness of the public health response.[36] Some argue that a decentralized approach allows for better coordination between local jurisdictions, hospitals, and emergency medical responders. Others suggest that a centralized approach allows for better coordination in case of mass-casualty events that require statewide efforts to respond to sudden surges in capacity.

Although a state's role in a public health emergency may vary depending on whether there is a centralized or decentralized system in place, some distinct responsibilities generally are assigned at the state level. States can request that a public health crises be declared a national emergency in the event that a major disaster overwhelms state and local capabilities and, in turn, poses a major public health threat to the affected community. Such a declaration can trigger support from federal agencies, such as the Federal Emergency Management Agency (FEMA), which can in turn provide states with needed support services and disaster relief funds. Federal agencies can also assist states through provision of surge support (such as through staffing provided by Medical Reserve Corps), patient evacuation, staffing of incident response coordination teams, and human support services.[37]

Governors also have the power to make use of the national pharmaceutical stockpile. In the event that an emergency causes a local or state pharmaceutical supply to be expended, local jurisdictions can appeal to a governor (or the mayor, in the case of Washington, D.C.) to ask the CDC to deploy the SNS for supplemental supply. Because state and local responses are often overlapping, depending on the individual jurisdictions, the state response will be discussed in more detail in context with the local response. For example, in some large cities, the primary public health response may actually occur at the city level. In other areas, these same responsibilities may instead be handled by the state agency.

LOCAL PREPAREDNESS AND RESPONSE

Although many strategic decisions to respond to a public health emergency are made on a federal level, it is at the local level that the response is implemented. Local jurisdictions are at the front line for identifying and carrying out federal implementation plans. Within local jurisdictions, many organizations are responsible for a unified public health response. In coordination with state and local public health agencies, local level response also involves emergency medical services (EMS), hospitals, law enforcement agencies, fire departments, and hospital associations as well as providers and local chapters of nonprofit disaster relief organizations, such as the Red Cross.

At the local level, there are several layers of response to a public health emergency. Although this response varies depending on the type of threat, in general it incorporates a number of key elements. Key components of public health preparedness include hazard analysis, emergency response planning, health surveillance, laboratory analysis, and consequence management.[38]

Hazard Analysis

Hazard analysis involves assessing which particular public health emergencies are most likely to occur within the community. This effort may involve identification of potential physical threats that exist in a community, such as the presence of nuclear plants, as well as formulation of a theoretical response to such threats based on the potential consequences. Local municipalities should also analyze their capacity to deal with such hazards, such as institutional capacity (beds, staff, pharmaceutical supply), surge capacity, and availability and analysis of existing disaster response plans.

Advance Response Planning

Advance response planning involves coordination of a number of agencies to develop a viable plan well ahead of any actual threat. Local public health agencies must engage with hospitals, emergency medical responders, law enforcement, fire, volunteer agencies (such as the Red Cross), and community-based organizations. Because the threat will always start locally, such agencies are at the forefront of ensuring that any needed state or federal resources be secured in an appropriate and timely manner. Although often a plan may exist within an individual institution, it should also provide a mechanism for cross-organizational coordination and linkages.

An effective preparedness plan should meet a number of goals. One such goal is a plan for adjustment for local surge. According to the U.S. Office of Inspector General, components necessary to deal with a medical surge include the ability to coordinate among various parties, supply of needed personnel through volunteer medical staff recruitment, supply of additional equipment resources, development of alternative sites of care and triage, and patient care guidelines. In developing an advance plan to address such a medical surge, localities should include a process to protect any medical volunteers involved in the surge from any subsequent legal action. Also, a system should be in place to help ease identification of available beds should the need for alternative care-delivery sites arise.[39]

A preparedness plan should also include an operational plan that can be adjusted to meet a variety of public health emergencies. This plan should delineate on-scene roles and responsibilities, recruitment of needed volunteers, and a system for communication with the public.[40] In addition, advance planning should include a mechanism to train first responders on their roles and responsibilities in the event of an emergency through periodic drills and updates. Such training should involve all levels of staff at a given institution.

Surveillance

Health surveillance is also a key function of the local public health agency. One of the earliest steps in local response is monitoring when a threat has occurred through an adequate surveillance system. This surveillance is particularly important for biologic terrorism events and infectious disease outbreaks; in both of these situations, there is likely to be a lag time between presentation of an initial case and recognition that a public health emergency is in progress. Surveillance is an active process that includes collection of specimens, analysis of those specimens, and interpretation of the results so that they can be used effectively in public health practice. Surveillance also encompasses a number of important public health functions, including determination of the extent of a public health emergency, recognition of the geographic magnitude of the emergency, detection of impending epidemics, evaluation of treatment and control measures, and facilitation of planning and research.[41]

Surveillance systems are categorized as being either passive, active, sentinel, or special systems. Passive reporting refers to the process in which an individual provider or hospital reports cases of a targeted disease of interest to a local or state public health agency, usually through a standardized form. For example, states use this approach for identifying sexually transmitted infections. Passive reporting is perhaps the simplest form of reporting, but has two distinct disadvantages: delays in reporting and underreporting, both of which occur because the system is often dependent on the individual provider or laboratory.[42]

Active surveillance involves outreach by phone or in person from public health officials to laboratories, hospitals, or providers, encouraging them to more closely track a disease of interest. Active surveillance is more timely and requires more resource expenditures on the part of the public health department that initiates the surveillance. The CDC has a number of surveillance programs in place, as described earlier, for local and state use in surveillance.

Sentinel surveillance evaluates a sample of the population to study trends in disease, such as microbial resistance for certain bacteria. This type of surveillance has the disadvantage that findings may not be generalizable to the larger population if a nonrepresentative sample is selected. Finally, other special systems may be set up to evaluate a public health emergency.[42]

An effective health information technology (HIT) infrastructure is crucial for effective surveillance. This infrastructure not only helps facilitate real-time data collection efforts at the local level, but also assists in rapid identification of an emerging public health threat at the federal level. The Institute of Medicine has called for establishment of a national health information infrastructure, which would link local and state public health agencies with federal components such as the CDC or other subagencies within DHHS. A true national health information infrastructure could also facilitate real-time reporting of individual-level cases in the population that could provide an early alert of an emerging public health illness, thereby extending the reach of disease surveillance into individual physicians' offices. Evidence already demonstrates the effectiveness of electronic reporting over traditional reporting. When a move from paper to electronic passive reporting occurs for disease surveillance, the delay decreases dramatically—falling from 35 days down to a single day.[43]

In a survey of local health departments around the time of the 2001 anthrax attacks, a mere 50 percent had full time Internet access. Approximately 20 percent of these departments had email access.[44] These data stress the fact that communication to and from the local and federal levels was compromised at the time of this major public health emergency.

Laboratory Analysis

Going hand-in-hand with adequate surveillance is the presence of a strong lab analysis component. Often lab analysis is a responsibility shared at both the local and state levels. A local jurisdiction may initially process lab specimens; however, in cases requiring specialized analysis, such jurisdictions may have to forward specimens to special statewide labs with expertise in a given area. Labs are often characterized as belonging at one of four levels:

- At the most basic level, a local lab may perform the first level of analysis— namely, general specimen characterization (e.g., a hospital lab's characterization of the H1N1 virus as influenza A).
- The second level involves more specific identification of an organism (e.g., local public health lab serotyping).
- Third-level labs can perform susceptibility testing (often state-specific labs).
- The most sophisticated labs exist at the federal level (the CDC and other federal labs such as the Department of Defense in the event of surge); they perform high-level analysis and help coordinate identification of threats across jurisdictions.[45]

Consequence Management

Once a public health emergency is identified through an effective surveillance system and the threat is characterized through laboratory analysis, the next stage of the public health response is consequence management. Consequence management encompasses a number of activities targeted at controlling a public health emergency and limiting any negative consequences associated with it. For example, it may include quarantining persons who are exposed to any disease with the potential for spread as well as the provision of treatment and vaccinations as needed. Such consequence management also involves federal-, state-, and local-level involvement. For example, although quarantine is usually initiated by a local authority, federal oversight is often involved when interstate travel is involved or if a local authority is unable to provide adequate control.[46]

In the provision of treatment and vaccinations, it is often critical that hospitals and local-level responders work together to pool needed resources and direct them to the areas of greatest need. Many hospitals and local agencies have established formal protocols and agreements to facilitate pooling of resources, thereby ensuring that the needed resources are made available quickly. Pharmaceuticals are one of the most common areas where resources are shared (such as through the national pharmaceutical stockpile system).[47] In addition to having an adequate supply, an organized system for distributing pharmaceuticals—or, in the case of H1N1, vaccines—should be in place in advance of any active public health threat. This plan should not only outline the operational details of how such medications or vaccines will be tracked, stored, and transported, but also specify which priority populations will receive the medications or vaccines and describe how to deal with vulnerable populations who may not have ready access to receipt of the medications.[48]

Risk communication is another critical function that should be addressed early in the consequence management phase and, as discussed, should be covered in any advance plan. Because public health emergencies often involve a great deal of uncertainty on the public's part, which might potentially lead to confusion and panic, having an effective risk communication strategy in place early is paramount.[49] Communication should take into consideration the needs of vulnerable populations and persons from diverse backgrounds (e.g., any messages should be made available in a number of languages and formats).

MITIGATION

Coordination across federal, state, and local jurisdictions is essential for preparing and responding to a public health emergency. This coordination of interactions may also be the most effective method to mitigate against the potential impacts of a large-scale public health crisis. In reality, the role of government in both routine public health and public health emergencies is a shared responsibility between all levels of government: local, state, and federal (see Table 2-2). By linking federal funding to specific state responsibilities (e.g., setting a minimum drinking age for alcoholic beverages), the federal government can influence public health policies in creative ways.[50] Such coordination efforts exist across all levels of response to a public health emergency, including coordination among response plans, in the surveillance and laboratory analysis period, in consequence management, and as part of risk communication.

In the case of the H1N1 outbreak of 2009, this coordination extended to the international realm, where surveillance across countries was critical. At the national level, the CDC was active in issuing surveillance and vaccination guidelines for local and state agencies and in coordinating broad public health education initiatives. The state or local

TABLE 2-2	Role of Federal, State, and Local Agencies in Public Health Emergencies		
	Federal Agencies	**State Agencies**	**Local Agencies**
Planning	Guidance to state and local jurisdictions on development of an emergency response plan Advance planning through programs such as the City Readiness Initiative	Development of statewide response plan Coordination of plans across local jurisdictions	Development of response plan for local jurisdictions (e.g., hospitals, public health departments) Coordination of plans across individual institutions and agencies
Surveillance	Operation of the National Electronic Disease Surveillance System Operation of Epidemic Intelligence Exchange (Epi-X) Special lab analysis, coordination of laboratory results across state and local jurisdictions	Lab analysis for specific serotyping Identification of impending threats across individual local jurisdictions through evaluation of trends or spikes in diagnoses (e.g., hospital flu cases)	Identification and diagnoses of public health emergencies (by first responders, providers) Submission of data about impending diagnoses through an effective health information technology infrastructure Initial general lab analysis; submission of specimens to local or state public health agencies
Consequence management	Development of guidelines for states Response to state declaration of federal emergency with supplies, man personnel for medical surge Coordination among states to assist with quarantine/containment within borders Coordination of pharmaceutical stockpile for collection of vaccines or medications, delivery of stockpile medications to state and local jurisdictions Preparation of guidelines for receipt of medications or vaccines Preparation for materials for risk communication	Preparation of a plan for local distibution of medications or vaccines Declaration of a federal emergency with subsequent activation of federal aid when needed (e.g., request for the National Guard or disaster assistance management team support) Activation of the national stockpile plan when local and state pharmaceutical resources are insufficient	Identification of populations at greatest need for treatment and vaccination Dissemination of medication or vaccines to at-need populations Containment measures to help prevent spread of illness (e.g., masks in local emergency departments) Tailoring of risk communication educational materials to specific populations within a locality

agencies then had to initiate distribution of flu vaccines, coordinate with providers for receipt of the vaccine supply, and initiate local provider agreements related to this supply.

CONCLUSION

The major area of need currently present for most local and state agencies is strengthening the public health infrastructure and community preparedness for mounting a response to an emergency. The federal government plays a key role, through its leadership and financing roles, in achieving these goals. Also, reformation of antiquated public health law remains necessary. However, the bulk of these activities fall within the purview of the states.

The challenges for the federal government include adequately supporting local efforts while avoiding overlapping roles. Additionally, delineation of a clear and rational command structure is required to balance the expertise and jurisdictions of various federal agencies as they interact with local and state officials.

INTERNET RESOURCES

National Emergency Management Association: Professional association of emergency management directors from all 50 states, 8 territories, and the District of Columbia
http://www.nemaweb.org

USA.gov: Resources for state and local officials for disasters and emergencies
http://www.usa.gov/Government/State_Local/Disasters.shtml

U.S. Computer Emergency Readiness Team: Government users
http://www.us-cert.gov/federal/

U.S. Department of Health and Human Services: *Public Health Emergency Response: A Guide for Leaders and Responders*
http://www.hhs.gov/disasters/press/newsroom/leadersguide/index.html

U.S. Disaster Management Interoperability Services: Enabling emergency information exchange
http://www.disasterhelp.gov/disastermanagement/

U.S. Federal Emergency Management Agency: Emergency managers and personnel
http://www.fema.gov/emergency/index.shtm

NOTES

1. United States Constitution, Article I, Section 8.
2. Centers for Disease Control and Prevention. *Public health emergency response guide for state, local, and tribal public health directors:* Version 1.0, p. 12. Available at: http://www.bt.cdc.gov/planning/pdf/cdcresponseguide.pdf. Accessed July 6, 2010.

3. *The 9/11 Commission Report*, p. 289. Available at: http://www.9-11commision.gov/report/911Report.pdf. Accessed July 6, 2010.

4. Centers for Disease Control and Prevention. *Public health emergency response guide for state, local, and tribal public health directors:* Version 1.0, p. 23. Available at: http://www.bt.cdc.gov/planning/pdf/cdcresponseguide.pdf. Accessed July 6, 2010.

5. Rosner D, Markowitz G. *Are we ready? Public health since 9/11.* Milbank Memorial Fund; 2006.

6. Centers for Disease Control and Prevention. *Public health emergency response guide for state, local, and tribal public health directors:* Version 1.0, p. 31. Available at: http://www.bt.cdc.gov/planning/pdf/cdcresponseguide.pdf. Accessed July 6, 2010.

7. Cruz MA, et al. The first 24 hours of the World Trade Center attacks of 2001: The Centers for Disease Control and Prevention emergency phase response. *Prehospital Disaster Medicine.* 2007;22(6):473–477.

8. Whitman C. Environmental Protection Agency press release. September 18, 2001. Available at: http://www.epa.gov/wtc/stories/headline_091801.htm. Accessed March 15, 2009.

9. Institute of Medicine. *The future of the public's health.* Washington, DC: National Academies Press; 2003.

10. Turning Point. Available at: http://www.turningpointprogram.org/. Accessed March 15, 2009.

11. The Model State Emergency Health Powers Act. Available at: http://www.publichealthlaw.net/ModelLaws/MSEHPA.php. Accessed March 15, 2009.

12. National Association of County and City Health Officials. *2005 national profile of local health departments.* July 2006.

13. Institute of Medicine. *The future of the public's health.* Washington, DC: National Academies Press; 2003.

14. Health Alert Network. Available at: http://www2a.cdc.gov/han/Index.asp. Accessed March 17, 2009.

15. U.S. Department of Health and Human Services. *Public health emergency response: A guide for leaders and responders.* August 2007.

16. BioSense. Available at: http://www.cdc.gov/BioSense/. Accessed March 17, 2009.

17. Public Health Information Network. Available at: http://www.cdc.gov/PHIN. Accessed March 17, 2009.

18. National Electronic Disease Surveillance System. Available at: http://www.cdc.gov/NEDSS. Accessed March 17, 2009.

19. Epidemic Intelligence Exchange. Available at: http://www.cdc.gov/epix. Accessed March 17, 2009.

20. Institute of Medicine. *The future of the public's health.* Washington, DC: National Academies Press; 2003.

21. U.S. Department of Health and Human Services. *Public health emergency response: A guide for leaders and responders.* August 2007, p. 29.

22. U.S. Department of Health and Human Services. *Public health emergency response: A guide for leaders and responders.* August 2007, p. 30.

23. U.S. Department of Health and Human Services. *Public health emergency response: A guide for leaders and responders.* August 2007, p. 30.

24. U.S. Department of Health and Human Services. *Public health emergency response: A guide for leaders and responders.* August 2007, p. 31.

25. Institute of Medicine. *The future of the public's health.* Washington, DC: National Academies Press; 2003.

26. Washington State Department of Health. Fact sheet: State role in national stockpile plan. Available at: http://www.doh.wa.gov/phepr/generalfactsheets/stockpileplan.doc. Accessed July 6, 2010.

27. U.S. Department of Health and Human Services. *Public health emergency response: A guide for leaders and responders.* August 2007, p. 28.

28. Institute of Medicine. *The future of the public's health.* Washington, DC: National Academies Press; 2003.

29. State Health Leadership Initiative. Available at: http://www.statepublichealth.org/. Accessed March 17, 2009.

30. Hospital Preparedness Program. Available at: http://www.hhs.gov/aspr/opeo/hpp/. Accessed March 17, 2009.

31. Cities Readiness Initiative. Available at: http://www.bt.cdc.gov/cri/. Accessed March 14, 2009.

32. U.S. Department of Health and Human Services. *Public health emergency response: A guide for leaders and responders.* August 2007, p. 24.

33. Centers for Disease Control and Prevention. *Public health preparedness: Mobilizing state by state.* February 2008, p. 7.

34. Garfield R. State preparedness for bioterrorism and public health emergencies. *The Commonwealth Fund Issue Brief.* July 2005.

35. Garfield R. State preparedness for bioterrorism and public health emergencies. *The Commonwealth Fund Issue Brief.* July 2005.

36. Wasserman J, Jacobson P, Lurie N, et al. *Organizing state and local public health departments for public health preparedness.* RAND Technical Report, 2006.

37. U.S. Department of Health and Human Services, Centers for Disease Control and Prevention. *Federal Public Health Emergency Law: Implications for state and local preparedness and response.* April 28, 2009.

38. Centers for Disease Control and Prevention. The public health response to biological and chemical terrorism. July 2001. Available at: http://emergency.cdc.gov/Documents/Planning/PlanningGuidance.PDF. Accessed July 6, 2010.

39. U.S. Office of Inspector General. *State and local pandemic influenza preparedness: Medical surge.* September 2009.

40. Centers for Disease Control and Prevention. *Public health emergency response guide for state, local, and tribal public health directors:.* Version 1.0, p. 12. Available at: http://www.bt.cdc.gov/planning/pdf/cdcresponseguide.pdf. Accessed July 6, 2010.

41. Epidemiology Program Office, Centers for Disease Control and Prevention. *Overview of public health surveillance.*

42. Program operations guidelines for STD prevention: Surveillance and data management. Available at: http://www.cdc.gov/STD/Program/surveillance/4-PGsurveillance.htm. Accessed July 6, 2010.

43. Institute of Medicine. *The future of the public's health.* Washington, DC: National Academies Press; 2003.

44. Brewin, B. Anthrax threat exposes IT's ills. *Computerworld 35*(43). October 22, 2001.

45. Centers for Disease Control and Prevention. The role of the laboratory: Public health and forensics. Available at: http://www2a.cdc.gov/phlp/docs/Pheldocs/2003_ForEpi/Presentations/ForEpi_LABslides.ppt. Accessed July 6, 2010.

46. U.S. Department of Health and Human Services, Centers for Disease Control and Prevention. *Federal Public Health Emergency Law: Implications for State and local preparedness and response.* April 28, 2009.

47. Grier R, Torres GW, Barerra SG, et al. *Hospitals' response to public health emergencies: Collaborative strategies.* Health Research and Educational Trust; 2006.

48. U.S. Department of Health and Human Services, Office of the Inspector General. *Local pandemic influenza preparedness: Vaccine and antiviral drug dispensing and distribution.* September 2009.

49. U.S. Department of Health and Human Services. Pandemic influenza plan. Available at: http://www.hhs.gov/pandemicflu/plan/sup10.html. Accessed July 6, 2010.

50. United States Code, Section 158 (a) (1).

CHAPTER 3

Public Health Law

Carl Hacker and Katherine Wingfield

> Public health as a profession does not exist but for law.
> —Anonymous

Case Study

Imagine that a major city in the United States is suddenly overtaken by an outbreak of smallpox. The citizens are scared, the hospitals are overwhelmed, and the city is burdened with the task of protecting the public's health and maintaining a sense of order. Assume that the Board of Health for this city votes, pursuant to a state statute, to require the vaccination of all residents in the city who have not previously been vaccinated against smallpox. Although many citizens are eagerly awaiting their vaccines, hoping to ward off actual disease, a small minority of citizens are afraid of the potential side effects and generally leery of decisions made by the medical establishment. One citizen in particular—an honest and upstanding member of the community—vehemently refuses to be vaccinated. He is brought to trial, and he argues persuasively that he sees vaccination, and particularly smallpox vaccination, as a means of contaminating his body with filth and disease.

Despite the best evidence produced by this citizen and his attorney, the court finds the man guilty and fines him a substantial amount of money for refusing to submit to vaccination. The case is appealed, but the verdict is upheld by both the state's Supreme Judicial Court and, ultimately, the Supreme Court of the United States. The U.S. Supreme Court notes that a community has a right, based on the principle of self-defense, to protect itself against an epidemic of disease that threatens the safety of its members. The Court upholds the right of the city to mandate vaccination against smallpox, declaring that states may limit individual liberty in the service of well-established public health interventions.

The year is 1905. More than 100 years later, this ruling will still be good law.

HISTORICAL PERSPECTIVES

The facts presented in the case study are based on an actual Supreme Court case in which the Court was asked to interpret whether a state had the power to compel a citizen to subject himself or herself to vaccination.[1] Although the holding by the U.S. Supreme Court in 1905 is still good law, some people might view the outcome as overly harsh today. They would note that the chance of dying from a smallpox vaccination is currently greater than the risk of contracting and dying from the actual disease. They would say our healthcare system is capable of handling outbreaks within a population. They would point out that even school-aged children, who are required to be vaccinated to attend school in most, if not all, states, can be exempt from vaccination for a variety of reasons. Indeed, many people may wonder whether we will ever need to rely on the ruling in that case again.

Unfortunately, in our world today, we face the probability that pandemics will occur, either through natural processes or as the result of intentionally evil acts. Practitioners whose job it is to protect the public's health can do so only if the laws support their efforts. This chapter addresses where law comes from and examines laws that directly relate to protecting the public's health, especially during times of public health emergencies.

PROTECTING THE PUBLIC'S HEALTH VERSUS THE PRACTICE OF MEDICINE

In the *practice of medicine*, when an individual seeks treatment from a physician and the physician agrees to treat the person, a *patient–physician* relationship is established. This relationship sets up several duties and expectations that are enforceable by courts. At the simplest level, the physician has a duty to provide an established standard of medical care, and the patient has a duty to pay for the services provided.

Over the past 50 years, who actually pays for this service has changed, making this relationship more complex. Physicians may also rely upon support from specialists and institutions. Most of these considerations are part of the business side of the relationship. Keep in mind that patients do not have to either seek medical help from a physician or heed the physician's advice. Physicians, in turn, need not offer medical help to all comers. Indeed, providers should limit their practice to areas where they have the requisite training and experience.

While physicians may owe a duty to their patients, they do not have a duty to treat the community at large. For instance, physicians in private practice know that individuals with elevated blood pressure are at increased risk of dying, but they have no duty to seek out and treat all individuals with elevated blood pressure. Furthermore, physicians in private practice may recognize that when habitats for mosquito populations increase, the risk of patients contracting an arbovirus increases, but they have no reason to reduce these mosquito habitats within the city.

By contrast, those who *practice public health* are concerned with the health of a community. Their "patient" is the community. Public health practitioners, therefore, are expected to identify and ameliorate behaviors and environments that place the health of the public at risk. How can this be done? If cigarette smoking is a hazard to the public's health, can practitioners ban smoking? Ban the sale of cigarettes? Ban the growing of tobacco? Which resources are available to accomplish these goals? If patients have an infectious disease that is contracted through airborne means, public health practitioners may want to isolate these patients until they are no longer contagious. Can they do this? Can they force patients to be vaccinated? Where would these practitioners get the *power* to do this? Where would they get the *money* to ensure that patients do, indeed, follow these steps?

Laws define the boundaries of what healthcare providers and public health professionals can do. This is true during both ordinary times and extraordinary times when the usual progression of health care is disrupted by natural pandemics or evildoers. Laws largely define expected kinds of behavior for given circumstances and the consequences that follow when a person fails to conform to these laws. This chapter describes the kinds of laws that a healthcare provider can expect to encounter. The number and kinds of laws are many and diverse, and we are limited in the detail that we can provide in a few pages. We especially note the origins of the power to make laws that affect the public's health and the limitations on the entities that operate under the authority of these laws. Law is not static. It evolves slowly, but it follows a reasoned progression, as legislatures and courts respond to new circumstances. We began this chapter by considering a relevant landmark case and will end with a reflection on the meaning of this case for our society today.

The set of healthcare providers who could respond to a sudden and perhaps widespread disruption to the public's health includes individuals from a variety of professions. Although the focus of this chapter is limited to the consideration of the laws that would influence how a physician might act, other professions might give heed to these principles by analogy. Several kinds of law are distinguished, including common law, statutory law, constitutional law, administrative law, and case law. Examples are then provided to illustrate how these kinds of laws are used to affect public health.

KINDS OF LAW AND THE PUBLIC'S HEALTH _____

Table 3-1 summarizes the various kinds of law relevant to public health, each of which is described in the following subsections.

Common Law

Common law is a large and ill-defined collection of principles, traditions, and precedents. Questions of common law are settled by *judges*, whose decisions are *recorded* for posterity. These recorded decisions form a *precedent* to be used in the future when similar issues come into litigation. For example, physicians and other healthcare providers are aware of the threat of a "malpractice" lawsuit. This is one of a group of lawsuits governed by *tort law*. Under common law, these cases have arisen when a physician had a duty to avoid harming a patient, and his or her breach of this duty led to a foreseeable injury (damage) to the patient. The remedy for this breach is to repair the damage sustained by the injured patient. Some states have tempered the redress available via this kind of common lawsuit through legislation. (See the section on statutory law.)

Issues that affect the public's health have also been settled through common law. For instance, suppose your neighbor has piled old tires next to your property. This pile of tires could provide a place for rats and mosquitoes to breed. Thus this situation could *unreasonably interfere* with your *use and enjoyment* of *your property*. Common law has established that this unreasonable interference is grounds for ordering your neighbor to remove the tires or pay you damages.

Statutory Law

Statutory law is law created by a sovereign body. Such a body can arise by "right" or by agreement. Examples of those who rule by "right" include monarchs, who acquire this right though conquest or birthright, and dictators, who exercise autocratic and dictatorial power. In the history of the United States, by contrast, the signers of the Mayflower Compact established a sovereign body by agreement. Before the settlers of Plymouth Colony disembarked from the Mayflower, they agreed in writing to "covenant and combine" themselves into a "civil Body Politick" and "promise all due Submission and Obedience" to those "Laws . . . as shall be thought most meet and convenient for the general Good of the Colony." This provision in the Mayflower Compact outlines the principle known as *police power*. Police power is the power of the state (namely, the *governed*) to place restraints on the *personal freedom* and *property rights* of individuals *to secure a common good*.

TABLE 3-1 Examples of Laws Relevant to Public Health Emergencies

Type of Law	Example in Public Health Emergency	Brief Description
Common law	Public/private nuisance	Prevents a person from maintaining an unhealthy condition on his property and from unreasonably interfering with another person's use and enjoyment of his property.
	Negligence	Requires a person to exercise the care that a reasonable person would exercise to prevent foreseeable harm.
Statutory law	National Emergencies Act	Prevents open-ended states of national emergency.
	Homeland Security Act of 2002	Created the U.S. Department of Homeland Security, which is charged with preventing terrorist attacks in the United States and responding to natural disasters.
	Emergency Medical Treatment and Active Labor Act	Requires participating hospitals to treat and stabilize patients with emergency conditions, regardless of the patients' ability to pay.
Constitutional law	U.S. Constitution, Article I, Section 8	Defines the powers of Congress, including the power to collect taxes, to provide for the common defense and general welfare of the United States, and to regulate commerce among the states.
	U.S. Constitution, Fourth Amendment	Prohibits unreasonable searches and seizures of persons or property.
Administrative law	Administrative Procedures Act	Details the way in which administrative agencies may propose and establish regulations.
	Code of Federal Regulations, Title 21	Provides regulations for food and drugs within the United States for various agencies, including the FDA. Many of these regulations are based on the Food, Drug, and Cosmetic Act.
Case law	United States v. Montoya De Hernandez, 473 U.S. 531 (1985)	Holds that a traveler may be detained at the U.S. border if customs agents, considering all the facts, reasonably believe that the traveler may be smuggling contraband.
	Jacobson v. Massachusetts, 197 U.S. 11 (1905)	Holds that states may limit individual liberty in the service of well-established public health interventions.
Ordinances	City of Houston, Texas, Ordinance No. 07-490, adopted 4/18/07 as Chapter 13 in the Code of Ordinances for Houston	Created an office of emergency management that is charged with establishing a disaster preparedness program for the city of Houston.

Under police power, the *common good* includes matters affecting health, safety, welfare, and morals. The police power of a state is large, bounded only by individual rights laid out in the bill of rights in a state's Constitution. The police power of a state is exercised through the *statutes* passed by its legislature. This is done after deliberation and agreement with the executive branch of a state government (i.e., the governor).

One way that a state exercises its police power is through the licensing of professionals. For example, to protect the public's health, a state can ensure that only those qualified to practice medicine are allowed to do so. The basis of this policy, which has been upheld by various state courts, is to assure the public of competent professionals. This can be done by establishing a Licensing Board (or a body with a related name). This Board is granted the authority by statute to define and review the requirements to practice medicine in the state and to discipline those persons who fail to uphold these qualifications.

Police power is also evident in state statutes that require individuals to be vaccinated. In the state of Texas, for instance, most vaccination laws relate to children. These laws essentially say that children must be vaccinated against various diseases, but allow exceptions if the vaccines would be harmful to the child or if the parent objects to vaccination for reasons of conscience, including religious belief.[2] Texas also has statutes that address vaccination for adults. Section 161.0102 of the Texas Health and Safety Code provides that "The department shall consult with public health departments and appropriate health care providers to identify adult immunizations that may be necessary to respond to or prepare for a disaster or public health emergency, terrorist attack, hostile military or paramilitary action, or extraordinary law enforcement emergency."[3] These vaccination statutes in Texas demonstrate the police power of the state to protect the public's health.

Constitutional Law

There are two forms of constitutional law in the United States: state constitutions and the federal (U.S.) Constitution. Each state has a constitution describing how laws are made in that state and the extent to which a legislature can act. State constitutions vary considerably in their length. Alabama's Constitution, for instance, contains more than 340,000 words, while Vermont's Constitution has slightly more than 10,000 words. The U.S. Constitution, by comparison, has approximately 7,000 words. The length of a state's Constitution may demonstrate how much authority or power the electorate wishes to entrust to the legislature. In addition to the individual state Constitutions, every state is bound by the provisions of the federal Constitution. The

U.S. Constitution specifies how laws are made by the federal government, which kinds of laws can be made, and the extent to which the Congress can impose the will of the majority on a minority.

How did the U.S. Constitution come to be? Every schoolchild knows that the United States of America began as 13 colonies of Great Britain located along the eastern seaboard of North America. Through a series of events largely related to taxation, these colonies declared their independence from the Crown on July 4, 1776. The War of American Independence continued until the surrender of Lord Cornwallis to George Washington at Yorktown, Virginia, on October 19, 1781. The American Revolution formally ended when the Paris Peace Treaty of 1783 was signed by representatives of the United States and Great Britain, and subsequently ratified by the Continental Congress and King George III.

Most states drafted constitutions shortly after the Declaration of Independence was signed. The Continental Congress also drafted and sent the *Articles of Confederation* to the states for ratification. This document was intended to become a constitution, laying out how these newly independent states would work together for a common good. Although not adopted by the states until March 1781 (approximately 7 months before Cornwallis's surrender at Yorktown!), the Articles of Confederation were used by the Continental Congress to manage the war.

The Articles of Confederation were useful for a time, but several of those who led the country during the war and shortly thereafter recognized various weaknesses and lobbied for changes that would create a central government with greater power. Disputes over taxes and the regulation of interstate commerce brought the inadequacies of the Articles of Confederation to the fore and led to a call for representatives to meet in Annapolis, Maryland, and finally in Philadelphia. Although the meeting was strongly opposed by some, a group of approximately 40 men from all the states except Rhode Island met in the State House in Philadelphia in May 1787 to discuss how to organize a confederation of states. By September 17, 1787, these men had drafted a Constitution, which was sent to the states for ratification. Following ratification by New Hampshire (the ninth state to ratify the document), the U.S. Constitution became effective.

The federal form of government created in Philadelphia provided that each state would retain the power to govern itself through its police powers and that the states would grant to the federal government specific and *enumerated* powers. These powers are listed in the 18 phrases in Article I, Section 8, of the Constitution, which lays out the powers granted to Congress by the people. An examination of this list shows no reference to "public health," but few can deny the pervasive presence of the federal government in matters affecting the public's health today. The seemingly all-encompassing presence of the federal government can be attributed to three powers granted to Congress: the power to tax, the power to spend, and the power "to regulate commerce . . . among the states." Recall that a state has the power to regulate matters affecting the public's health through its police power. Because regulating the public's health is not one of its specifically enumerated powers, the federal government, by contrast, must act largely through its spending powers and through the Commerce Clause.

Medicare is an example of a public health program that exists because of Congress's power to spend money to promote the general welfare. Congress raises money through taxes and then spends this money to fund programs that support the U.S. public. As a condition of receiving funds from Medicare or Medicaid, hospitals must comply with the provisions of the Emergency Medical Treatment and Active Labor Act (EMTALA).[4] This legislation has been criticized by many, particularly because it does not provide any methods of reimbursement for hospitals that provide emergency care to uninsured patients. However, because Congress has the power to spend money, it can fund programs such as Medicare and then condition receipt of the money on compliance with a program such as EMTALA.

While the state and the federal Constitutions outline the powers granted to state and federal governments, they also place limitations on government power, as stated in provisions such as the federal "Bill of Rights" found in the first 10 amendments to the U.S. Constitution. Some textbooks on public health and public health law declare that the states' power to regulate health comes from the Ninth Amendment. The purpose of this amendment, however, is to reinforce the relationship between the federal government and the states. In adopting the U.S. Constitution, the states gave to the federal government the enumerated powers listed in Article I, Section 8. At the same time, the states retained their police power to regulate within their boundaries matters affecting health, safety, welfare, and morals. It is this police power that truly gives states the authority to regulate public health.

Administrative Law

Administrative agencies are pervasive in the United States, and it is important to understand how these entities are created and how they carry out their responsibilities. The U.S. Food and Drug Administration (FDA), the U.S. Environmental Protection Agency (EPA), the Centers for Disease Control and Prevention (CDC), and the Occupational Safety and Health Administration (OSHA) are all examples of agencies. Each of these agencies has been charged with a specific set of tasks, and each has a direct role in affecting the public's health.

When the U.S. Congress or a state's legislature passes a statute dealing with the public's health, the makers of the law have neither the intention nor the time to administer the law on a day-to-day basis. To ensure that the law is properly applied and enforced, the legislators may create an administrative agency. If an appropriate agency already exists, the members of the legislature may simply assign the task of administering this law to the current "administrator" of the agency. The U.S. Constitution does not specifically mention or define the term "administrative agency," but references are made to "departments" in Articles I (legislative branch) and II (executive branch).

Although the U.S. Constitution establishes a system of checks and balances by separating the powers and duties of the three branches of government, an administrative agency will have varying degrees of each form of power—executive, legislative, and judicial. These powers allow the agency to carry out its functions and operations. This is not to say, however, that the principle of "checks and balances" does not apply to agencies. The powers and limits of agencies are, in fact, controlled through various mechanisms: The procedures used by an agency are laid out in the Administrative Procedure Act. Congress defines what an agency can do to enable legislation, and Congress provides a budget to fund the work.

Much of what an agency does is "fill in the details" of a statute. Suppose Congress wishes to provide nutritious food for certain groups of people whose level of income is such that they would benefit from this "entitlement." Congress could properly do this under its spending power. Members of the House of Representatives and the Senate would outline what they had in mind for this program, but leave the finer details to the agency. The agency given this job would study the problem, define what a "nutritious" food is, and publish a Notice of Proposed Rule Making in the *Federal Register*. Everyone who reads the *Federal Register* could then "comment" on the proposal. After reviewing these comments, the agency can publish its rule. This process of "notice and comment" fulfills the constitutional requirement of procedural due process and allows the agency to create a law, termed a rule, which will be published in the *Code of Federal Regulations*.

Case Law

Case law comes about in two ways. First, it may arise from a common lawsuit, as illustrated earlier in the medical malpractice example. Second, case law can arise when a court is asked to interpret the words of a regulation, statute, or the U.S. Constitution. For instance, the U.S. Supreme Court has been asked on numerous occasions to determine what qualifies as "speech" so as to assess whether specific words or actions should be protected under the First Amendment. Because the First Amendment does not define "speech" or list examples, the Supreme Court has frequently had to address this issue. The body of case law that has been created with respect to this issue serves as a reference for anyone who wishes to determine whether their words or actions might also qualify as "speech."

Ordinances

States may choose to distribute their authority to smaller jurisdictions such as municipalities. States that follow this route are termed *home rule* states. The requirements and conditions for a city or county to become a home rule jurisdiction are typically laid out in the state's constitution. Laws enacted by home rule jurisdictions are generally known as *ordinances* and must be heeded as any other law. If a group of citizens wishes to challenge the constitutionality of an ordinance, they must bring their case to the proper state or federal court.

Discussions involving public health issues at the local level require one to consider the particular ordinances in that jurisdiction. For instance, a city may pass an ordinance that prohibits smoking in all public places. This ordinance would outline what constitutes a "public place" and provide a penalty for violations. Such an ordinance would affect owners and operators of public places as well as citizens in this city.

LIMITATIONS ON THE POWER OF A LEGISLATIVE BODY

Although a legislature has the power to make laws, it is still limited in several ways. Recall that the states gave *enumerated powers* to the federal government. If a power is not specifically listed among those in Article I, Section 8 of the U.S. Constitution, the federal government arguably does not have that power. Further limitations on federal power were imposed during the first session of the U.S. Congress. Twelve amendments were sent to the states for ratification, and 10 were adopted. These 10 amendments, which are collectively known as the Bill of Rights, immediately restricted what the U.S. Congress could do to impose the will of the majority on a minority. In time, these and other amendments extended various rights to citizens of the states.

The story of the Bill of Rights is beyond this chapter, but the Fourth Amendment is particularly relevant to those who practice public health law. This amendment provides protection against unreasonable searches and seizures by government officials.[5] A considerable volume of case law exists that interprets the meaning of this amendment. Many cases have addressed the extent to which a person can be searched during a "police stop," while other cases have examined whether items such as garbage on a curb can be searched.

Those who practice public health should be familiar with a particular aspect of search and seizure known as the *administrative search*. Suppose that a fire marshal appears at the door of your hospital, announcing that she is prepared to inspect your facility to ensure compliance with the city's fire code (an ordinance promulgated under the city's police power). Can you refuse entry to the fire marshal or demand that she produce a "search warrant"? Of course, by the time the fire marshal finds a magistrate (defined by statute), shows probable cause, and returns with a search warrant, the element of surprise will be lost. You could have remedied any violations of the fire code. This cycle could be repeated, and the intent of the ordinance would be undermined.

To prevent this sort of subversive activity, the courts have authorized a procedure that still fulfills the intent of the Fourth Amendment.[6] A governmental officer is allowed to appear before a magistrate with a proposed inspection plan. For example, the fire marshal could present a list of hospitals listed at random and indicate that she will inspect the hospitals according to this list. This way the magistrate would be assured that certain classes of hospitals were not inappropriately being singled out.

ANALYSIS OF CASE STUDY

The case study that was presented at the beginning of this chapter is based on an actual Supreme Court case from 1905. The case of *Jacobson v. Massachusetts* arose after an outbreak of smallpox occurred in 1902. In response to the disease, the Cambridge Board of Health voted to require the vaccination of all residents who had not been vaccinated since March 1897. On March 15, 1902, Reverend Henning Jacobson refused to be vaccinated. He was convicted and fined $5. His conviction was upheld by both the trial courts and the Massachusetts Supreme Judicial Court. The defendant vehemently argued against vaccination: "We have on our statute book a law that compels . . . a man to offer up his body to pollution and filth and disease; that compels him to submit to a barbarous ceremonial of blood-poisoning, and virtually to say to a sick calf, 'Thou art my savior: in thee do I trust.'"[7]

Despite the objections of Reverend Jacobson, the U.S. Supreme Court upheld the right of the city of Cambridge, Massachusetts, to mandate vaccination against smallpox. The Court held that states may limit individual liberty in the service of well-established public health interventions. The Court noted that, "Upon the principle of self-defense, of paramount necessity, a community has the right to protect itself against an epidemic of disease which threatens the safety of its members."[8]

Over the years, other states have successfully relied on the *Jacobson* decision to support their own vaccination laws. Many of the cases have arisen as challenges to laws requiring children to be vaccinated before attending school, and the courts have uniformly upheld these laws.[9] Today, however, most states have provisions in their statutes to accommodate objections for medical reasons or for reasons of conscience, including religious beliefs.[10] The schools may then choose to exclude any unvaccinated children from attending school during an emergency or epidemic.[11] In this way, the statutes that exist today are less stringent than the laws that existed at the time of the *Jacobson* ruling, but the power of the state to make laws to protect the public health has remained unchanged. States still have the authority under their police powers to make laws that will affect the health of the people in that state, and they may limit individual liberty in an effort to protect the public health.

CONCLUSION

Widespread public health interventions do not simply happen at the whim of a particular hospital or university, and the authority to make laws and approve funding is not without limits. If it is to act, the federal government must make sure that it is acting under one of its enumerated powers, such as its power to spend money to provide for the general welfare. States, in contrast, must rely on their police powers to create laws that affect the health, safety, welfare, and morals of the citizens in the state. The enumerated powers of the federal government and the police powers of the state governments give these legislative bodies the ability to affect public health through law.

Although this chapter has provided only a brief overview of the types of laws that might be relevant for public health practitioners, we hope that we have at least conveyed the sense that public health as a profession exists only because of law. In turn, law is essential for prescribing the responsibilities and boundaries for those who would seek to affect public health.

INTERNET RESOURCES

Centers for Disease Control and Prevention, Public Health Law 101: www2a.cdc.gov/phlp/phl101/

Public Health Law and Policy: www.phlpnet.org

Public Health Law Association: www.phla.info

NOTES

1. *Jacobson v. Massachusetts*, 197 U.S. 11 (1905).
2. Tex. Health & Safety Code Ann. § 161.004 (2009); Tex. Educ. Code Ann. § 38.001 (2009).
3. Tex. Health & Safety Code Ann. § 161.0102 (2009).
4. 42 U.S.C. § 1395dd (2008).
5. The Fourth Amendment to the U.S. Constitution states: "The right of the people to be secure in their persons, houses, papers, and effects, against unreasonable searches and seizures, shall not be violated, and no Warrants shall issue, but upon probable cause, supported by Oath or affirmation, and particularly describing the place to be searched, and the persons or things to be seized."
6. In the case of *Nat'l Treasury Employees Union v. Von Raab*, the U.S. Supreme Court noted that "the traditional probable-cause standard may be unhelpful in analyzing the reasonableness of routine administrative functions, *Colorado v. Bertine*, 479 U.S. 367, 371; see also *O'Connor* v. *Ortega*, 480 U.S. at 723, especially where the Government seeks to *prevent* the development of hazardous conditions or to detect violations that rarely generate articulable grounds for searching any particular place or person. Cf. *Camara v. Municipal Court of San Francisco*, *supra*, at 535–536 (noting that building code inspections, unlike searches conducted pursuant to a criminal investigation, are designed 'to prevent even the unintentional development of conditions which are hazardous to public health and safety')." The Court found that "in certain limited circumstances, the Government's need to discover such latent or hidden conditions, or to prevent their development, is sufficiently compelling to justify the intrusion on privacy entailed by conducting such searches without any measure of individualized suspicion" (*Nat'l Treasury Employees Union v. Von Raab*, 489 U.S. 656, 668 (1989)).
7. Brief of the Defendant, *Commonwealth* v. *Jacobson*, 183 Mass. 242 (1903).
8. Supreme Court of the United States, *Jacobson v. Massachusetts*, 197 U.S. 11, 27 (1905).
9. See, for example, *New Braunfels v. Waldschmidt*, 207 S.W. 303 (1918), which denied children access to the public schools unless they submit to vaccination; and *Itz v. Penick*, 493 S.W.2d 506 (1973), which found that the Texas Education Code's requirement that school children be vaccinated, unless they qualify for an exception, is constitutional.
10. See, for example, Tex. Health & Safety Code Ann. § 161.004 (2009); Tex. Educ. Code Ann. § 38.001 (2009).
11. See, for example, Tex. Educ. Code Ann. § 38.001(f) (2009).

CHAPTER 4

National Response Plan

Mark E. A. Escott

INTRODUCTION

Scores of emergency events occur each day in the United States that encompass a large array of incident types and span varying levels of complexity. These incidents may range from simple car fires to massive forest fires, and from SWAT standoffs to large-scale terrorist attacks. With such a vast scope of operations under the umbrella of emergency response, a national system is critical to create an organized, flexible, and scalable system to address these public health emergencies.[1]

Previous iterations of a national plan for response led to bureaucratic documents that were not adaptable to different situations and that did not meet the needs of either state and local responders or other stakeholders. The development of the National Response Framework (NRF) represented a response to the shortcomings of previous versions. It is designed to take an "all hazards" approach, meaning that it is applicable at the local, state, and federal levels for all types of emergencies. This goal is achieved by creating engaged partnerships among stakeholders at all levels to increase the efficacy of the preparation, planning, response, and recovery stages. The NRF is also designed to be a living document, with changes expected based on experience with the evolving world of emergency management.[1]

Another key design feature of the NRF was its ability to address effectively the problem of constantly changing leaders with the responsibility of emergency management, including elected officials. The NRF encourages the role of emergency managers to be filled consistently within organizations and administrations while creating a structure that also accommodates novice leaders and officials. In support of the education of emergency management leaders at all levels, the Department of Homeland

Security (DHS) has made the NRF document and numerous supporting documents available online, along with online training programs maintained by DHS.[1]

Case Study

The initiation of a nationwide response plan occurred just prior to the landfall of Hurricane Andrew in August 1992. At that time, this natural disaster was the costliest hurricane on record in the twentieth century, with a death toll of 26 people, damage estimated to amount to $30 billion, 126,000 destroyed homes, and 180,000 people left homeless.[2,3] Unlike many storms in the past, whose damage had been concentrated in one area, Hurricane Andrew made landfall in the Bahamas, Florida, and Louisiana, causing devastation in each of those locations. In addition, it took on a northeasterly direction after making landfall in Morgan City, Louisiana, and caused catastrophic damage along the East Coast of the United States. The multiple-front disaster made application of federal resources difficult in the short term because of the need for disaster assessment and triage of the widespread areas affected by the hurricane.

There was also early criticism of the response effort made by the federal government under President George W. Bush because of the sluggishness of the response. A 3-day delay occurred until the full-scale federal response was initiated because the then-Governor of Florida, Lawton Chiles, did not make a formal request for federal aid at the time of Hurricane Andrew's landfall. There was further confusion because the initial request for help from the Army Reserves was denied because Governor Chiles had not yet mobilized the Florida National Guard units who had similar equipment, such as bulldozers.[4] These shortcomings of the initial attempt at a national response system as well as others motivated efforts to change the system to address these issues.

HISTORICAL PERSPECTIVES

The Federal Response Plan

The NRF has its roots in a 1992 document created shortly before Hurricane Andrew called the Federal Response Plan (FRP), which encompassed organization of a federal response among a number of federal agencies, including the Federal Emergency Management Agency (FEMA), as well as the American Red Cross.[5] This plan was developed as a "playbook" for the government in the event of a presidential federal disaster declaration, also known as a Stafford Act declaration.[6] This plan, therefore, addressed only the federal aspects of support to state agencies and largely consisted of laws and regulations related to the administrative aspects of disaster response. It was considered a part of the library of emergency management, which outlined a portion of the federal role in public health emergencies (see Figure 4-1).[2,3]

The FRP also established various "annexes" to the base plan, which continue to be part of the current version of the NRF. These annexes provide details surrounding the mission and specific roles of lead agencies for elements of critical functions in emergency management; there are 15 Emergency Support Function (ESF) Annexes, 7 Support Annexes, a Recovery Function Annex, and Incident Annexes. The ESFs describe the functions of federal agencies that are providing support to state and local stakeholders in terms of defining the scope of the particular ESF and assigning responsibilities of specific federal agencies in lead and support roles within the ESF. They also define the methods of official activation of the ESF and regional response coordination, and they specify the immediate and ongoing response actions that are necessary in the event of activation. In addition, the documents clarify local and state responsibilities when the primary responsible party is not the federal government.[5]

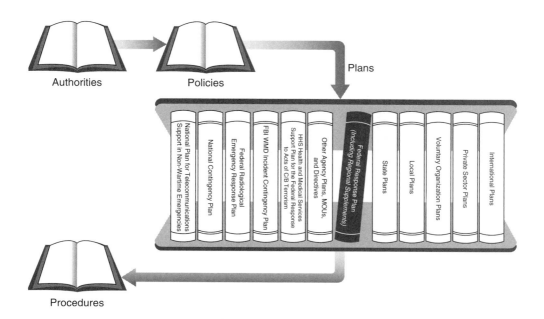

FIGURE 4-1   Federal Response Plan's Role
Source: FEMA. *Federal Response Plan.* Washington, DC: April 1992.

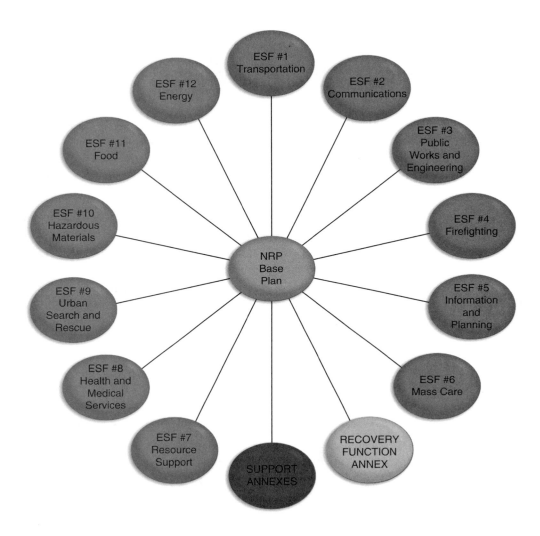

FIGURE 4-2 National Response Plan Emergency Support Functions and Annexes

Support Annexes were also initiated in the FRP and carried over to the current version of the NRF. Similar to the ESF Annexes, these documents define missions and responsibilities of support operations (see Figure 4-2). These support functions include the following areas:

- Community relations
- Congressional affairs

- Donations management
- Financial management
- Logistics management
- Occupational safety and health
- Public affairs

Incident Annexes, such as the one entitled "Terrorism," are threat-specific plans that define the scope, roles, and responsibilities of federal agencies in the event of a specific Stafford Act event. Also involved in the FRP was the "Recovery Function Annex," which discusses the federal role as well as nonfederal aspects of mitigation and recovery. It outlines the development of strategies and prioritization of recovery efforts. This annex also deals with a number of critical federal programs, including the National Flood Insurance Program (NFIP), which helps communities mitigate their losses from floods and retrofit existing structures to be in compliance with updated guidelines.[5]

The National Response Plan

The National Response Plan was developed in 2004 in reaction to the terrorist attacks on September 11, 2001, and mandated by the Homeland Security Act of 2002 and the Homeland Security Presidential Directive 5 (HSPD-5). It represented an effort to create a common method of emergency planning among all emergency management stakeholders. Its creation marked the first time there was a concerted effort to develop a common strategy in planning, response, recovery, and mitigation by local, state, and federal governments as well as community stakeholders and non-governmental organizations (NGOs).[7]

The NRP was based on the common operating structure of the National Incident Management System (NIMS), which provides a common language and design for the response phase of emergency operations at the local, state, and federal levels. It has also been adopted by NGOs including hospitals, schools, transportation companies, energy suppliers, and other elements of critical infrastructure.[4] The NRP established a number of new programs, including the National Response Coordination Center (NRCC), the Joint Field Office (JFO), the Homeland Security Operations Center (HSOC), and the Interagency Incident Management Group (IIMG), to administer the new plan managed by the Department of Homeland Security under then-Secretary Tom Ridge. The plan was signed by 32 cabinet secretaries, federal administrators, and leaders of private response organizations to symbolize its cooperative design.[7]

Much as the FRP had been tested immediately following its implementation in 1992, a major test of the new system occurred with the 2005 hurricane season. During this hectic period, the United States was presented with a new definition of catastrophic damage when Hurricane Katrina struck New Orleans (and much of the rest of the Gulf Coast), followed shortly thereafter by Hurricane Ike's landfall in Galveston, Texas. These two hurricanes served up a "one-two punch" to two of the nation's most vulnerable cities and taught Americans yet another hard lesson about redefining the scope of emergency management. The NRP was revised in 2006, but the criticisms of its scope and implementation did not cease. Further revisions recommended from the emergency management community resulted in the current NRF, which reflects the need for more operational guidelines for all stakeholders.[1]

PREPAREDNESS

The National Response Framework was created in a bottom-up design, such that a great deal of responsibility for preparation and planning is placed on local communities, businesses, NGOs, and individual households. It places the responsibility for funding, development, and implementation on these groups while providing the foundation upon which to build these emergency management plans. This philosophy has to do with lessons learned from Hurricane Katrina, when many individual families were found to lack an emergency plan and failed to heed warnings to evacuate or had not made arrangements to obtain transportation to do so. There was a lack of planning for care of pets, care for family members with limited mobility, food and water rations, and continuity of medication supplies. Organizing resources to fulfill these responsibilities is best suited for individual households and communities, because the scale of complexity makes it difficult for governmental units to adequately address these issues in an emergency response.

Community leaders and local organizations that provide critical infrastructure also have an obligation to prepare by development of comprehensive vulnerability assessments. From these assessments, they derive emergency response plans (ERPs) to act as a detailed playbook within the NRF and NIMS. A significant aspect of planning and preparedness hinges on the effective application of vulnerability assessments in the community. The National Infrastructure Protection Plan (NIPP) outlines the national plan for development of infrastructure protection to ensure the uninterrupted availability of critical infrastructure and key resources (CIKR; see Figure 4-3).[8]

Various stakeholders may use a number of methods to complete their assessment of vulnerability of the CIKR as well as individual, community, or system-wide vulnerabilities. One of these approaches is a systems-based strategy to identify components of infrastructure vulnerability, including communications, water, transportation, information technology, energy, as well as interdependencies between these components.

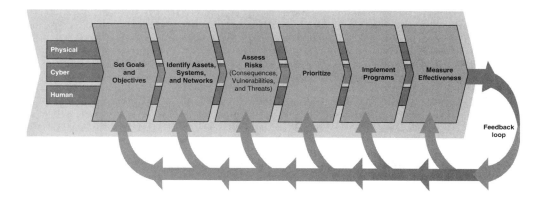

FIGURE 4-3 Continuous Assessment and Protection of Critical Infrastructure and Key Resources

Source: From Department of Homeland Security. *National Infrastructure Protection Plan.* Washington, DC 2009. Available at: http://www.dhs.gov/xlibrary/assets/NIPP_Plan.pdf. Accessed February 2010.

This method was modeled by the Department of Energy and provides a comprehensive base assessment of vulnerability.[9] Other models of vulnerability assessment include threat-based assessment based on specific threats, such as those identified in the "national planning scenarios."[10] These techniques may also be used in combination.

Once the vulnerabilities are assessed, they must be prioritized based on consequences as well as frequency or likelihood, and planning must be undertaken to mitigate these vulnerabilities. This planning often takes the form of ERPs, which are developed by stakeholders in compliance with NIMS to preplan for "all hazards" contingences and both to address vulnerabilities and define roles and responsibilities in the event of activation of the ERP. Following mitigation efforts, ongoing reassessment of risk potential must occur to ensure that attention is maintained to areas of risk.

National Preparedness Guidelines

The *National Preparedness Guidelines* (NPG)—a document whose development was mandated by HSPD-8—outlines a common strategy for U.S. preparedness activities. At the NPG core is the "National Preparedness Vision," which acts as a credo for national preplanning that can be embraced by all stakeholders:[11]

> A nation prepared with coordinated capabilities to prevent, protect against, respond to, and recover from all hazards in a way that balances risk with resources and need.

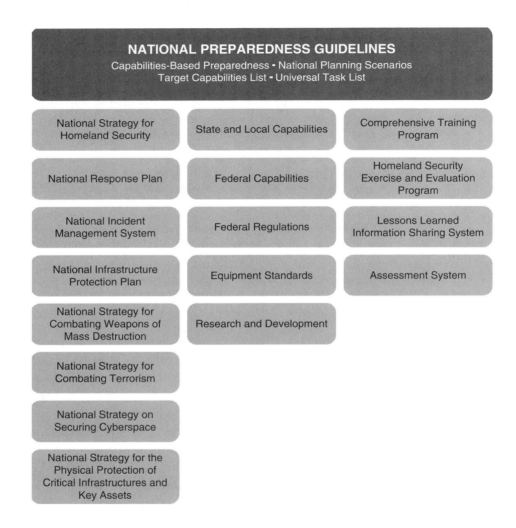

FIGURE 4-4   National Preparedness Guidelines in Context
Source: From Department of Homeland Security. *National Preparedness Guidelines.* Washington, DC: 2007. Available at: http://www.dhs.gov/xlibrary/assets/National_Preparedness_Guidelines.pdf. Accessed February 2010.

These guidelines provide focus and continuity of policy for a number of other federal and state programs and organize them under one overarching guideline to create a risk-based, "all hazards," and capability-based approach to preparedness (see Figure 4-4).[11]

The capability-based approach helps to further focus stakeholders on specific missions to preparedness. These capability areas are divided into five divisions:

- Common mission area
- Prevent mission area
- Respond mission area
- Protect mission area
- Recover mission area

The common mission areas include features such as communications, risk management, and intelligence, which are factors applicable to all of the other mission areas. The remainder of the mission areas define a "target capabilities list" (TCL)—that is, necessary functional capabilities of local, state, and federal governments needed to respond effectively to a disaster (see Figure 4-5).[11]

There is further elaboration and guidance of these individual TCLs through a "universal task list" that provides linkage to the "national planning scenarios." The national planning scenarios were designed to help public health personnel develop more highly detailed plans regarding preparedness and planning by placing a focus on a minimal number of the most catastrophic circumstances with a reasonable possibility of occurring. Among these scenarios are the following:[10]

1. Nuclear detonation: 10-kiloton improvised nuclear device
2. Biological attack: aerosol anthrax
3. Biological disease outbreak—pandemic influenza
4. Biological attack: plague
5. Chemical attack: blister agent
6. Chemical attack: toxic industrial chemicals
7. Chemical attack: nerve agent
8. Chemical attack: chlorine tank explosion
9. Natural disaster: major earthquake
10. Natural disaster: major hurricane
11. Radiological attack: radiological dispersal devices
12. Explosives attack: bombing using improvised explosive device
13. Biological attack: food contamination
14. Biological attack: foreign animal disease (foot and mouth disease)
15. Cyberattack

The selection of these scenarios was purposely limited to create a broad spectrum of disaster situational readiness (rather than developers creating an extensive list that is likely to result in unnecessary redundancies in planning). While the spectrum is limited, stakeholders are encouraged to develop incident-specific plans for their particular region of responsibility to enable an effective response to the incident.

- Communications
- Community Preparedness and Participation
- Planning
- Risk Management
- Intelligence/Information Sharing and Dissemination

Common Mission Area

- CBRNE Detection
- Information Gathering and Recognition of Indicators and Warnings
- Intelligence Analysis and Production
- Counter-Terror Investigations and Law Enforcement

Prevent Mission Area

- Animal Health Emergency Support
- Citizen Evacuation and Shelter-in-Place
- Critical Resource Logistics and Distribution
- EOC Management
- Environmental Health
- Fatality Management
- Fire Incident Response Support
- Isolation and Quarantine
- Mass Care (Sheltering, Feeding, and Related Services)
- Mass Prophylaxis
- Medical Supplies Management and Distribution
- Medical Surge
- On-site Incident Management
- Emergency Public Safety and Security Response
- Responder Safety and Health
- Emergency Triage and Pre-Hospital Treatment
- Search and Rescue (Land based)
- Volunteer Management and Donations
- WMD/HazMat Response and Decontamination

Respond Mission Area

- Critical Infrastructure Protection
- Epidemiological Surveillance and Investigation
- Food and Agriculture Safety and Defense
- Laboratory Testing

Protect Mission Area

- Economic and Community Recovery
- Restoration of Lifelines
- Structural Damage Assessment

Recover Mission Area

FIGURE 4-5 Target Capabilities

Source: Data from Department of Homeland Security. *National Preparedness Guidelines.* Washington, DC: 2007. Available at: http://www.dhs.gov/xlibrary/assets/National_Preparedness_Guidelines.pdf. Accessed February 2010.

Once plans are developed in regard to "all hazards" and specific threats, there must be appropriate assessment of personnel and physical capabilities to carry out these plans. Where there are deficiencies, capability improvements must be made through partnerships, acquisition of equipment, and training. Following these improvements, regular and comprehensive tests of these plans must be performed involving all levels of response. These exercises must be of sufficient complexity to evaluate common weak points in emergency response plans effectively. For example, these weaknesses may include interoperability of communications, activations of other responders at the state and federal levels, and activation of NGOs and private contractors to supply equipment and supplies. Following effective testing of the plans as well as actual response activities, there must be a systematic evaluation of the time-liness and efficacy of the simulated or actual response. This preparedness cycle has the common goal of building response capability (see Figure 4-6). As an evolving cycle, it must be constantly reassessed to ensure that readiness is maintained despite

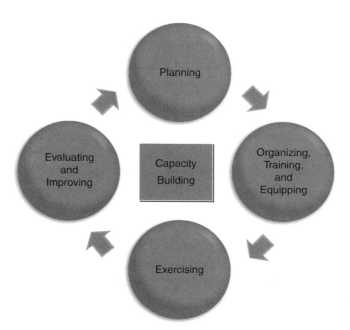

FIGURE 4-6 National Response Framework Preparedness Cycle
Source: Adapted from Department of Homeland Security. *National Response Framework*. Washington, DC: 2008. Available at: http://www.fema.gov/pdf/emergency/nrf/nrf-core.pdf. Accessed February 2010.

changes in response capabilities such as relocating equipment, changing contractors, and competing interests for resources.[11]

RESPONSE

The preparedness phase of the NRF is intimately associated with response, with the understanding that a critical aspect of response is the cycle of capacity building. In the response phase, the NRF identifies four critical elements necessary to limit loss, save lives, and aid in recovery.

The first key action is the development of "situational awareness," a concept that varies depending on the type of incident, but is defined by the ability to detect an incident and gain intelligence about the scope of the incident. In addition to gaining information, this information must be shared among members of the community through partnerships developed in the preparation phase. This engagement is most often organized through emergency operation centers (EOCs) at the local, state, and federal levels, as well as in private organizations and NGOs. Communication between these stakeholders and individual EOCs is critical to develop and maintain situational awareness. Public health emergencies are not always as obvious as an explosion or earthquake, and, therefore, situational awareness includes an element of detection. Situational awareness is an active process of monitoring elements of CIKR, illness patterns, terrorist suspect behaviors, and numerous other elements to ensure that an incident is detected in a timely fashion. It is also critical that standard reporting mechanisms are used across all layers of responders and that timely analysis of the reports occurs to ensure optimized response to the information. The federal government has developed the National Operations Center (NOC) to act as the reporting hub for intelligence that relates to the NRF, including information from state-level operations centers.[1]

Lack of information sharing was a critical weakness discovered during the terrorist attacks that occurred on September 11, 2001, when essential information about known hijackings was not shared among other stakeholders in real time. More than 8 years later, on Christmas Day 2009, an attempted detonation of an explosive device on a Detroit-bound plane from Amsterdam was not shared in real time with other airliners, echoing the lack of communication noted with the 2001 terrorist incidents. To be successful at real-time information sharing, established communication systems must exist at all levels, as well as among experts who are able to interpret the incoming information, screen it for credibility, and distribute it to other stakeholders in a timely fashion. As technology has progressed, emergency managers have found that timely information to aid in situational awareness is often found on the television, on the

Internet, or through social networking mechanisms. While these information sources are not traditional and are not always subject to scrutiny, they remain a potential valuable source for pertinent information. State operation centers, as well as the NOC, are also responsible for disseminating the information to appropriate state and federal agencies, which are in turn responsible for response and coordination (see Figure 4-7). The NOC provides coordination and maintains the coordinated operating vision for the NRCC, the FBI's Strategic Information and Operations Center (SIOC), the National Counterterrorism Center (NCTC), and the National Military Command Center (NMCC).

The next key response action is the "activation and deployment of resources and capabilities,"[1] which is described in great detail in the NIMS. These guidelines focus on establishing a common operating system with common organizational management that makes it scalable beyond local response to include state and federal response within the same structure. After initiation of a NIMS response, the incident command, unified command, or even area command is charged with activating necessary resources, personnel, and capabilities based on an incident action plan and perhaps preplanned responses. At the local level, much of the routine resource activation is based on the preplanned response structure for specific types of incidents, such as structure fires,

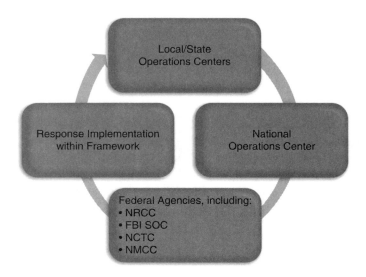

FIGURE 4-7   Information Sharing and Situational Awareness
Source: Data from Department of Homeland Security. *National Response Framework.* Washington, DC: 2008. Available at: http://www.fema.gov/pdf/emergency/nrf/nrf-core.pdf. Accessed February 2010.

multiple-vehicle crashes, and hazardous materials leaks. These preplanned responses include calls for automatic or routine mutual aid that allow assets and personnel to respond within or outside their normal territory of operation by simply being dispatched. Other mutual aid agreements or implementation of contractual arrangements usually require specific requests according to a previously agreed activation mechanism. In development of mutual aid agreements, care must be taken to address the essential aspects of these agreements (see Figure 4-8).[1]

Certain public health emergencies may require the activation of local, state, and federal EOCs. In some regions, EOCs are staffed 24 hours a day by dedicated experts from stakeholder agencies. More commonly, these centers will need to be formally activated and organizational leadership assigned to operate the center. EOCs do not provide direct incident management, but instead help to maintain a larger-scale situational awareness and to provide logistical support to the incident command.[1]

Less commonly, state-level resources may be needed to augment the response and recovery in situations that go beyond the capabilities of local government and local resources. Additional capabilities from the state are often able to address successfully the majority of public health emergencies that exceed the capabilities of the local response. Because these relationships are less often implemented, however, greater care must be taken to ensure that there is clear understanding regarding the procedure for making official requests for aid. In addition to resources and capabilities, the state's governor can provide assistance by suspending various regulations to allow for a more timely and effective response, such as allowing for emergency credentialing of medical personnel and lifting regulations regarding bed limitations or treatment areas

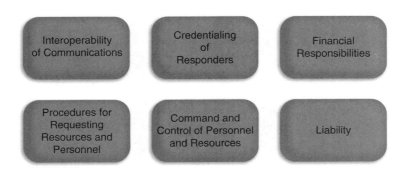

FIGURE 4-8   Key Components of Mutual Aid Agreements
Source: Data from Department of Homeland Security. *National Response Framework.* Washington, DC: 2008. Available at http://www.fema.gov/pdf/emergency/nrf/nrf-core.pdf. Accessed February 2010.

of healthcare facilities. The governor may also activate members of the National Guard who are "under State Active Duty or Title 32 status."[1] These units are often used to supplement local law enforcement in disaster-stricken areas, but may also be called upon to handle specific functions such as communications, logistics, medical support, and engineering.[1]

States may also activate an Emergency Management Assistance Compact (EMAC)—that is, an agreement between states to provide mutual aid to one another. When the resources and capabilities needed to handle the incident go beyond those that are available at the state and interstate levels, a request for federal assistance is needed. There are some circumstances outlined in the NRF that allow federal resources to respond without a state request or a presidential Stafford Act declaration. Prior to the governor requesting an "emergency declaration" or "presidential major disaster declaration," the state must activate its emergency response plan and coordinate its actions with FEMA to ensure that appropriate damage assessments have been performed. The FEMA regional administrator must be involved with this evaluation and notification

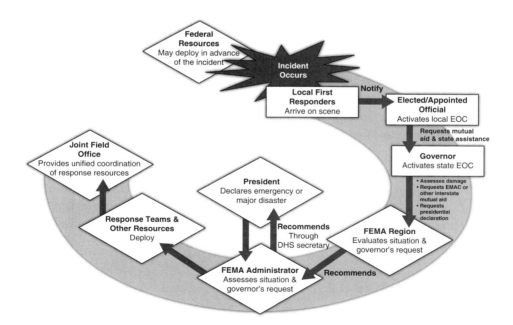

FIGURE 4-9   Information Sharing and Situational Awareness
Source: FEMA. *Overview of Stafford Act Support to States.* Available at: http://www.fema.gov/pdf/emergency/nrf/nrf-stafford.pdf. Accessed February 2010.

process to ensure that the situation is beyond the capabilities and resources of the local and state response system.[1]

The NRF encourages the activation of EOCs at the local and state levels in advance of an expected event to allow for pre-positioning of resources in the state or region. In some circumstances, the governor may request, or the president may unilaterally declare, a disaster or major disaster prior to the event (see Figure 4-9). The pre-activation and pre-positioning is done in an effort to provide more timely response from all levels of responders so as to limit loss of life and property as well as to expedite recovery.[1]

Following the response phase, all levels of government must demobilize responders and return them to their readiness status as soon as possible following mission completion. Some of the greatest benefits of state and federal disaster declarations are the aid available during the recovery phase. The recovery phase in the event of a federal disaster declaration is administered by the JFO. A multitude of federal programs are available to help individuals, businesses, local governments, and responders return to normal function through grants, insurance programs, and mitigation efforts.

CONCLUSION

The past two decades have introduced the United States to new levels of disaster and have exposed weaknesses in the systems of response. The National Response Framework has created a complex, yet manageable system that is adaptable to numerous types of public health emergencies. Its scalability and applicability to federal, state, and local governments as well as to private organizations and NGOs have helped to ensure that a common disaster "language" is spoken in the United States. These common origins, the development of more clearly defined systems of communication, and the formation of community-engaged partnerships will improve the nation's ability to respond to an emergency public health event. The living nature of this system ensures that as the United States is exposed to new types and scales of public health emergencies, the country can adapt for future system improvement.

INTERNET RESOURCES

National Response Framework: www.fema.gov/emergency/nrf

National Infrastructure Protection Plan: http://www.dhs.gov/files/programs/editorial_0827.shtm

National Preparedness Guidelines: http://www.dhs.gov/files/publications/gc_1189788256647 .shtm

National Planning Scenarios: http://cees.tamiu.edu/covertheborder/TOOLS/NationalPlanningSen
.pdf

Incident Annexes: http://www.fema.gov/emergency/nrf/incidentannexes.htm

Emergency Management Institute NRF Training: http://training.fema.gov/nrfres.asp

NOTES

1. Department of Homeland Security. *National Response Framework*. Washington, DC: Department of Homeland Security; 2008. Available at: http://www.fema.gov/pdf/emergency/nrf/nrf-core.pdf. Accessed February 2010.
2. National Hurricane Center. *Hurricane Andrew 16–28 August, 1992*. Miami, FL: National Hurricane Center; 1993, Addendum 2005.
3. *USA Today*. August 26, 2004. Available at: http://www.usatoday.com/weather/hurricane/2004-08-26-charley-fema_x.htm. Accessed February 12, 2010.
4. Hurricane Andrew: Breakdown seen in U.S. storm aid. The *New York Times*. August 29, 1992. Available at: http://www.nytimes.com/1992/08/29/us/hurricane-andrew-breakdown-seen-in-us-storm-aid.html?pagewanted=1. Accessed February 10, 2010.
5. Federal Emergency Management Agency. *Federal response plan*. Washington, DC: Federal Emergency Management Agency; 1992.
6. Federal Emergency Management Agency. Robert T. Stafford Disaster Relief and Emergency Assistance Act, as amended, and Related Authorities. FEMA 592. Washington, DC: Federal Emergency Management Agency; June 2007. Available at: http://www.fema.gov/pdf/about/stafford_act.pdf. Accessed February 2010.
7. Department of Homeland Security. *National response plan*. Washington, DC: Department of Homeland Security; 2004.
8. Department of Homeland Security. *National infrastructure protection plan*. Washington, DC: Department of Homeland Security; 2009. Available at: http://www.dhs.gov/xlibrary/assets/NIPP_Plan.pdf. Accessed February 2010.
9. Department of Energy. *Vulnerability assessment methodology, electric power infrastructure*. Washington, DC: Department of Energy; 2002.
10. Department of Homeland Security. *National planning scenarios: Executive summaries*, Version 20.2; Washington, DC: Department of Homeland Security; 2005.
11. Department of Homeland Security. *National preparedness guidelines*. Washington, DC: Department of Homeland Security; 2007. Available at: http://www.dhs.gov/xlibrary/assets/National_Preparedness_Guidelines.pdf. Accessed February 2010.

CHAPTER 5

Emerging Public Health Systems: Post-conflict and Post-disaster Settings

C. James Holliman

INTRODUCTION

Development of effective public health systems in countries emerging from armed conflict or large-scale disasters involves dealing with a number of difficult challenges. International responsibility to assist these countries is essential because of the possibility of widespread public health emergencies originating from poor governance and ineffective healthcare systems. Public health training programs need to include instruction on the unique aspects of post-conflict and post-disaster settings. This chapter highlights Afghanistan as an illustration of the complex and numerous factors that need to be considered when implementing public health systems in post-conflict and post-disaster states. Although the obstacles, challenges, and strategies to developing a public health system in Afghanistan are multifactorial and extensive, similar evaluations and efforts can be applied to other countries even if they possess fewer specific issues.

Case Study: Afghanistan

Afghanistan can be considered to represent the absolute worst-case scenario for a public health system operation in a post-conflict setting. In fact, the application of the term "post-conflict" to Afghanistan may not be considered accurate given that ongoing armed conflict has continued in this country ever since the defeat and expulsion of the Taliban government in 2001 (this same terminology quandary also applies to a number of other countries, including Iraq, Sudan, and the Democratic Republic of the Congo). The intersection of a number of calamities has resulted in Afghanistan having some of the worst health indices ever recorded (see Table 5-1).[1] Many of these factors have included natural disasters, and, therefore, Afghanistan can be regarded as both a post-conflict *and* a post-disaster setting. Armed conflict, through its contribution to deforestation and damage to agricultural systems, makes the country that has already suffered from the military destruction also more susceptible to disasters such as landslides, avalanches, and floods.

BACKGROUND

Historical Perspectives

Afghanistan suffered a number of destructive invasions over the centuries and emerged as an independent country only in the early twentieth century. Even though it possessed a number of natural resources, the country never fully utilized these resources mostly because the government refused to allow the construction of railroads; thus the national economy was never robust. Consequently, healthcare systems and facilities were not adequately financed or developed.

The country's major current woes can be considered to have started in 1978, when a violent overthrow of the government occurred, which was then followed by the Soviet invasion in 1979. War between the Soviets and the Afghan resistance devastated much of the country. The Soviets left in 1989, but the various resistance

TABLE 5-1 Comparison of Health Indices in Afghanistan and the United States		
	Afghanistan	**United States**
Births attended by skilled health personnel (%)	18.9	100
Maternal mortality ratio (per 100,000 live births)	1800	11
Infant mortality (per 1,000 live births)	129	7
Under age 5 mortality (per 1,000 live births)	191	8
Life expectancy (years)	42	78
Physician density (per 10,000 population)	2	26

Source: Data from World Health Organization (http://www.who.int/whosis/en/index.html) and the author.

groups continued full-scale warfare, initially against the communist Afghan government, and then after its fall, against one another. Ultimately, the Taliban conquered much of the country, and armed conflicts continued between its forces and residual resistance groups. October 2001 brought the U.S. invasion to oust the Taliban and Al-Qaeda, which was largely completed by December 2001. Because Taliban supporters found sanctuaries in Pakistan, resurgence of the Taliban since 2001 has resulted in continued armed conflict until the present throughout the country, but particularly in the southern and border provinces.

Obstacles to Public Health System Development

The healthcare system reconstruction situation in Afghanistan contains many factors similar to other nations' "post-conflict" situations; however, Afghanistan probably represents the most challenging predicament ever faced by public health system planners. In fact, some object to the use of the term "reconstruction" when discussing the Afghan situation, given that many "core" aspects of a national healthcare and public health system never existed and have to be created de novo rather than being "reconstructed."[2] The following factors make the overall Afghanistan reconstruction efforts and public health system development problematic.

Security

Afghanistan faces an ongoing and dangerous security situation, with large areas of the country affected by suicide bombers, improvised explosive devices, direct attacks by heavily armed paramilitary units, landmines, and criminal activities that include an extensive trade in opiate narcotics and kidnappings for ransom. One critical security-related issue is the direct targeting of healthcare facilities and personnel, teachers, and other aid workers by the Taliban. A number of facilities have been bombed and a number of personnel murdered simply for attempting to provide health care or education.[3]

Infrastructure

Due to the many years of indiscriminate warfare, many of the core elements of Afghanistan's infrastructure have been damaged or outright destroyed, including healthcare and education facilities. In addition, the country has a poor road network and a complete absence of railways. Even after multilateral development efforts, Afghanistan possesses an unreliable electric power supply in most parts of the country and lacks telephone landlines across much of the nation. There is also little access to clean and safe water in most areas. In fact, even though most health facilities in Kabul are served by deep wells, much of this water is contaminated. Contributing to this water contamination, of course, are the ineffective sewage systems in most regions.

Education

The breakdown in the education system in Afghanistan for many decades has led to low literacy rates and a small number of skilled and professional individuals to fill basic and advanced roles in society. This problem is magnified by the almost complete neglect of education for females during the Taliban's reign. In addition, during Taliban rule, there existed few educational standards or accountability at higher education institutions. Prior to Taliban rule, the Soviet communist dominance of the education systems in the 1970s and 1980s resulted in limitations in business and banking systems. Another primary obstacle to education and an educated class in Afghanistan has been the phenomenon of "brain drain," with numerous professionals immigrating to other countries to escape the warfare and poor living conditions. The population also uses two languages (Dari and Pashto) throughout the country, requiring many courses and educational materials to be translated into both languages, and there is little knowledge of the English language.

Economy

Afghanistan's economic system is debilitated, with few international companies investing in the country and very few resources available to help local companies expand or become successful. Without effective infrastructure or education, industries are unable to be productive. In addition, large numbers of internally displaced refugees and returning refugees from Iran and Pakistan have placed a strain on the fragile economy and added to high levels of unemployment. Furthermore, most of the surrounding countries also have relatively poor economies and cannot serve as stable trading partners.

Governance

The Afghan national government is largely dependent on outside funding from nongovernmental organizations (NGOs), the United Nations, other international organizations, and other countries. Poor coordination of efforts among government branches and external organizations exists, and many of the resources being brought into the country are not being effectively used or reaching target populations. In addition, corruption is widespread in the government and among police, often driven by many of the remaining regional leaders or "warlords." The lack of an effective judiciary hampers government effectiveness. Salaries of most government workers are too low to maintain a reasonable standard of living, and the government often is unable to recruit talented individuals. Therefore, many of the government's basic functions do not occur, such as recording of vital statistics (e.g., births, deaths), and government data are still not uniformly reliable across the country.

Geography, Climate, and Culture

Afghanistan's geography and climate provide difficult challenges for development. The country's landscape includes an arid south and a mountainous northeast, with limited sources of fresh water in large areas. This geography has been further destroyed through extensive deforestation and deliberate destruction of agricultural and irrigation systems during the years of warfare. Also, the country has faced prolonged multiyear droughts in the last decade, and severe winter storms with heavy snowfall and resulting avalanches.

Culturally, a history of tribal and ethnic rivalries has been continued and exacerbated by the practice of carrying on "blood feuds" that can persist from generation to generation. Regions with heavy tribal influences still greatly limit the activities of females.

Public Health Systems Challenges

As a result of the many obstacles present in Afghanistan, the country's public health and medical systems face specific challenges for development. Public health professionals within a post-conflict or post-disaster country as well as those individuals from other nations assisting these efforts need to be aware of these challenges to design programs and policies that address these needs.

Today, minimal integration of healthcare services among the Afghan National Army (ANA), the Afghan National Police (ANP), and the Ministry of Public Health (MoPH) exists. Each of these entities has developed separate healthcare delivery facilities that do not consistently take care of the constituents of the others, and the current situation has led to the inefficient nonsharing of staffing and supplies. Even though a multiple-ministry memorandum of agreement was signed in 2006 denoting that the ministries would support full integration of the healthcare system, various rivalries, prejudices, and "territorialism" by some of the staff of each ministry have so far prevented appropriate integration of the Afghan healthcare system.

The current limitations in Afghanistan related to the infrastructure, trained healthcare personnel, and finances are recognized by all outside parties as barriers to the development of parallel and independent healthcare systems for the ANA, ANP, and the MoPH (which is primarily responsible for health care for all Afghan citizens who are not members or beneficiaries of the ANA and ANP). Because of the high birth rates in Afghanistan, each ANA or ANP member has an average of six to eight family member dependents. The ANA and ANP each numbered close to 80,000 as of mid-2008. Thus, together with their dependents, these groups account for a significant proportion of the Afghan population.

Infrastructure

Many of the large, tertiary healthcare facilities in Afghanistan have been damaged. Furthermore, large numbers of local or rural clinics, including some that had been constructed in the past few years, have been damaged or destroyed by floods, landslides, avalanches, or conflicts, and have not been completely repaired or rebuilt due to administrative, financial, or security issues. The country also has a limited number of functioning medical laboratories due to lack of reagents, equipment, and trained technicians. In addition, there is minimal capacity to operate, repair, or maintain sophisticated biomedical equipment. Afghanistan has little or no prehospital care system in most regions, has limited capabilities to deal with trauma patients, and has no referral system for high-acuity trauma cases.

Most of Afghanistan lacks pathology services, which precludes using autopsies to determine causes of death and hampers data collection on morbidity and mortality statistics. There are fewer than five trained pathologists in the entire country, and none of the MoPH hospitals have a functional pathology laboratory.

Finally, most people in Afghanistan have little or no access to allied health services, including optometry, occupational therapy, physical therapy, respiratory therapy, and dentistry. Moreover, they have access to only poor-quality prescription medications that are subjected to minimal government oversight or regulation.

Education

Oversight of medical education programs occurs through two different ministries: the Ministry of Public Health (MoPH) and the Ministry of Higher Education (MoHE). Another ministry ("Martyrs and Disabled") has oversight for the care and education of disabled and handicapped individuals.

Afghanistan does not have a sufficient number of qualified and experienced faculty for the training programs at Kabul Medical University, the other six medical schools, the allied health training centers, and the various residency programs. In addition, no residency training programs exist in the fields of emergency medicine, anesthesiology, preventive medicine, or occupational medicine. Most of the other residency training programs do not have a sufficient number of trainees to graduate general or specialist physicians.

The country also lacks appropriate and effective medical and nursing certification and recertification exams and processes, and this lack of oversight has led to a poor level of knowledge and skills by many healthcare providers, including ambulance attendants, technicians, nurses, and physicians. For those with baseline training and skills, no well-organized and regularly conducted continuing medical education programs exist for healthcare personnel, and these providers have difficulty practicing updated, evidence-based medicine.

Governance

With a weak central government and the regional leadership often ruled by provincial "warlords," Afghan government capacity has been limited in its ability to provide for the medical and public health needs of the Afghan people. The government possesses minimal centralized and updated information on the geographic locations and staffing of all healthcare facilities in the country. The MoPH does not have an accurate and current listing of its own facilities, and collection of data on location and staffing of ANA and ANP facilities has been limited by security concerns.

These coordination and operations issues are further exacerbated by the lack of well-trained senior- and middle-level management personnel for these healthcare institutions. They are worsened even further by the absence of a reliable medical logistics system for supplies. This is particularly problematic for MoPH hospital and clinic laboratories, most of which are nonfunctional due to lack of a funding stream to support the purchase of reagents. Because of these minimal resources, both personnel and financial, the MoPH has been placed in the position of functioning primarily as a contract manager. It contracts with NGOs by using external funding to provide most of the direct healthcare delivery programs that in other countries would be provided by the national Ministry of (Public) Health. Even these reconstruction programs and efforts are hampered by poor coordination among the various NGOs, agencies, and military forces involved with these programs.[4,5]

Because multiple, acute public health and healthcare needs are always on the agenda, the Afghan government has very little capacity for effective and coordinated planning for future disasters and pandemics. In addition, government-operated healthcare facilities have scant physician coverage in the afternoons and evenings because most of the physicians conduct their private medical practices during these time periods to supplement their low government salaries.

POST-CONFLICT AND POST-DISASTER PUBLIC HEALTH SYSTEMS DEVELOPMENT

Multiple public health components within a country emerging from a conflict or disaster setting will need to be implemented in a stepwise manner to serve as the basis of an effective and sustainable public health system. These core components include surveillance systems, data management, effective intervention strategies, public health education, and coordination of efforts. Continuing to focus on Afghanistan, this section analyzes public health development initiatives that can be applied as a framework in other settings.

Public Health Surveillance

The primary purposes of a public health surveillance system are to collect data on the health status and/or risk factors for disease in a population and to analyze, interpret, and utilize the data in a manner that will lead to prevention and control of disease. The current status of public health surveillance plans, initiatives, and active programs in Afghanistan is significantly limited.[6] In general, health surveillance varies widely by province and district or by NGO mandate and interest.

In many areas, surveillance is focused on just disease-specific health concerns, especially vaccine-preventable conditions and avian influenza (AI).[7] Communicable diseases cause more than 50 percent of all morbidity and mortality in Afghanistan. Most of these conditions are preventable with basic public health measures and by immunizations. Establishment of potable water, sanitation systems, environmental pollution controls, and education on safe injections, blood transfusion, and basic hygiene would go far to limit the adverse health impacts of many environmental conditions.[8]

The recent reestablishment of the Afghan Public Health Institute (APHI) as an implementation arm of the MoPH will help in the development of public health surveillance in this country as the APHI matures over time. The *National Strategy for Reconstruction* and the *Afghanistan National Development Strategy*—two extensive, nationally adopted policy documents—include health surveillance activities and acknowledge the importance of public health surveillance. These plans encompass activities to calendar year 2020, and they contain specific target indicators to be attained by the year 2010 (such as "malaria mortality will be reduced by 80 percent").

The Afghan MoPH has developed a Disease Early Warning System (DEWS) based on the World Health Organization's (WHO) "communicable disease cluster" program. This project began in 2002 with attempts to integrate public health surveillance at the basic health center (BHC) and comprehensive health center (CHC) levels as "sentinel sites." The project calls for more than 400 sites that track through a provincial Centers for Disease Control and Prevention (CDC) officer to a central office at the MoPH. The extension of the DEWS to all 400 sites has not yet occurred, due to the many challenges and obstacles cited earlier, but DEWS has been able to identify a few outbreaks of meningitis and polio for which MoPH response teams were sent. At a conference in 2008, it was reported that DEWS detected 165 disease outbreaks in 2007. Tuberculosis, malaria, and leishmaniasis are the three main diseases monitored by DEWS.

Four or five regional centers for health surveillance would be useful to develop (for example, one at each of the four regional ANA hospitals) around Afghanistan, with training and staffing to be fully functional in all aspects of civilian and military public health, including surveillance and outbreak response. After the regional centers are trained by APHI with outside assistance, APHI needs to begin training provincial-level public health and surveillance personnel and, eventually, extend training and surveillance to the district level. Utilizing the logistical and communications infrastructure that is being developed by the ANA at the regional level will be a major step in the correct direction. Coordination between the military and civilian sectors will be required to begin this process, and complete integration should be the goal at the regional level.

The currently available information on population mental health status is abysmal, and is clearly in need of a surveillance system. The incidence of violence and abuse directed at females, depression, and suicide seem very high but are probably underreported, and the problems of child abuse and depression go almost completely unreported in Afghanistan. Initiation of social changes to deal effectively with these problems and identification of the factors involved in these behaviors are imperative and research needs to be applied to assist with these changes. The lack of psychiatry services (there is only one 50-bed psychiatry hospital with only one fully trained psychiatrist for the whole country at this time) has contributed to the lack of information on population mental health. Mental health system infrastructure and capacity need to be built for mental health surveillance information to be able to be acted upon.

Within the MoPH, future contractual obligations for the participating NGOs need to routinely include capacity for surveillance activities (both disease-specific activities and those conducted in general health areas), and an independent accountability process needs to be in place to assure NGO compliance. As the Afghan economy and national government finances improve, eventual phasing out of the NGO contract work now done and assignment of this work directly to the offices or subministries of the MoPH should be a long-term goal. Surveillance information on displaced and nomadic populations (which number several million people in Afghanistan) is sparse and needs to be researched and communicated to the MoPH. Specific contracted survey teams will be needed to handle this task.

Key Lessons

Emerging public health surveillance systems should initially be implemented by using available health infrastructure and reliable data from NGOs. These systems should then be expanded to the regional and local levels, with a concerted effort being made to include at-risk and vulnerable populations (e.g., women, children, elderly, and minority groups).

Public Health Statistics and Data Management

There are no established historical public health data in the ANA. Instead, most information on the general status of health in Afghanistan has been derived from a WHO/United Nations Children's Emergency Fund (UNICEF)/MoPH "cluster survey" performed in 2004. This survey formed the basis for health status documentation used in national follow-on planning after the development of the Basic Package of Health Services (BPHS; discussed in the next section) and Essential Package of Hospital Services (EPHS; also discussed in the next section). Importantly, the survey collected data on only 20 of the 34 Afghan provinces and failed to incorporate data from the ANA and the ANP as well as information from the more isolated and remote areas of the country.

A follow-up survey in 2006 conducted by Johns Hopkins University's Bloomberg School of Public Health and the Indian Institute of Health Management Research sampled healthcare facilities in 29 of the 34 Afghan provinces and showed some modest improvements in measured indices.[7] Other health surveillance information has come from limited case reports and two health surveys, one on tuberculosis skin testing in 2002 and another in 2006 that included skin testing and the clinical status of 1,600 adults presenting for employment to the coalition forces. There have also been some sporadic NGO-driven public health "needs assessment" documents published on Afghanistan.

The Afghan MoPH currently does have active reporting programs for tuberculosis, HIV/AIDS, malaria, and avian influenza, but these programs suffer from multiple deficiencies, such as inconsistency, lack of oversight of reporting, and lack of computerization. Although reporting requirements for acute respiratory illness (ARI) and acute watery diarrhea exist, the actual compliance in reporting these data from MoPH facilities varies. Viral hemorrhagic fever and cholera reporting is tracked by UNICEF in its district-level facilities and routed to the MoPH. There appears to be a lack of clearly identified case definitions and little acceptance and use of the passive reporting system, which is also hampered by poor communication systems and the remoteness of some reporting facilities.

A vaccine-preventable surveillance program has been implemented in Afghanistan as part of the National Solidarity Project (NSP). The Expanded Program on Immunization (EPI) has existed since 2003, and national and provincial EPI teams oversee this vaccination program. Polio, measles, and diphtheria cases are screened for by syndromic surveillance; under the direction of UNICEF and the MoPH, these data are tabulated and vaccine delivery is given accordingly. Outreach teams from the district vaccination sites attempt to cover the more rural areas, but in the remote far north and in the chaotic south there is less coverage. Additionally, rates of vaccine coverage are believed to be over-reported due to issues with corruption, incompetence, and security. Polio continues to be a problem in Afghanistan in spite of a high reported vaccination rate.

MoPH reports that it has invested heavily in the development of a routine Health Management Information System (HMIS), which was created under the auspices of the U.S. Agency for International Development (USAID) REACH (Rural Expansion of Healthcare) program. Starting early in 2003, a computerized system was proposed, allowing data entry and analysis at the provincial and/or NGO level. A protocol has reportedly been set up to allow for the aggregation of computerized data from lower levels at the provincial and national levels and the rapid distribution of analysis copies to all lower levels. Reporting from the provinces to the national level is required on a quarterly basis. Full implementation of the HMIS has been delayed due to a combination of problems, particularly staffing issues in the MoPH, lack of landline phone cables, and the unreliable electric power supply throughout the country.

The main purpose for any health surveillance system is to provide data on which to base public health action. Robust data systems have the potential not only to be used for assessing the health status of the country and provinces, but also to be used and integrated with national logistics and financial systems. The creation of a culture of data-driven health care that can be measured and tracked utilizing full implementation of the HMIS will require the active involvement of the leadership of the MoPH, ANA, and ANP. The MoPH needs to be the lead agency in health policy development in the government of Afghanistan. The APHI needs to be empowered to take the lead in implementing public health directives of the MoPH, much like the CDC acts as the implementing arm of the U.S. Department of Health and Human Services (HHS). Health surveillance needs to be centralized under the APHI. The ANA and ANP need to be incorporated into the health surveillance system. In particular, leaders within each organization with a strong interest in public health need to be identified and charged with making this happen and maintaining ongoing cooperative interaction.

A system of vital records needs to be established under the APHI. Nationally standardized birth and death certificates must be developed and should be maintained at the provincial—if not district—level. Monthly reporting should be mandatory to the APHI using a standard report format (yet to be developed). ANA and ANP reports all must feed into the MoPH/APHI system and could enter at either the regional or national level.

Key Lessons

Emerging public health systems will need to be built upon a foundation of data-driven implementation of initiatives. Standardized reporting of public health data will help collate and analyze the information being collected. Much of modern public health statistics and data management systems depend on information technology systems, and countries emerging from conflicts or disasters will need technical and professional assistance in these areas.

Public Health Services and Interventions

One relatively unique aspect of Afghan healthcare planning was the Afghan government's endorsement of the Basic Package of Health Services (BPHS) in 2003 (updated in 2005).[9] The BPHS specifically lists the (limited) health services that will be provided for all Afghan citizens by the government (a constitutionally mandated provision), and it takes into account the existing limitations of financing, personnel, and infrastructure. In 2005, the Afghan government also endorsed the Essential Package of Hospital Services (EPHS), which very specifically identifies the number of people to be served, and the clinical services, personnel, equipment, facility size and structure, and medications that will be available at each level of the Afghan healthcare system.[10] There are seven levels (proceeding from more basic to advanced care and "covering" an increasingly larger number of people):

- Health post (staffed by a single community healthcare worker)
- Basic health center (BHC)
- Comprehensive health center (CHC)
- District hospital
- Provincial hospital
- Regional hospital
- National or specialty hospitals (almost all of which are in the capital city of Kabul)

The BHCs and CHCs are supposed to directly supervise the activities of the community health workers and receive regular reports from them on the local health situation. Some of the community health workers are illiterate, but picture forms have been devised for them so they can still submit regular community health status reports.

A national commission has been appointed to develop a technical response, a risk communication strategy, and financial assessments of a control program for avian influenza. A national influenza pandemic preparedness and response plan is in place, although it is not extensive enough to adequately address the situation, nor has it been coordinated with the ANA and the ANP. No ANA plan exists yet for handling an outbreak of avian influenza. Within the MoPH and Ministry of Agriculture (MoA), all animal and suspected human outbreaks can be detected and rapidly diagnosed at this time only with the assistance of the U.S. Naval Medical Research Unit (NAMRU-3) based in Cairo, Egypt. A system for transporting specimens to international reference laboratories (including NAMRU-3) for diagnostic confirmation has been established and tested. An active surveillance system is in development for pandemic avian influenza (and epidemic influenza), with influenza-like illness (ILI) and acute respiratory illnesses (ARI) hospitalizations being tracked and reported. This system is apparently functioning in 15 of 34 Afghan provinces. The active case finding is limited to the UNICEF/WHO/MoPH vaccination centers providing the infrastructure, and outreach into the rural areas has been sporadic and limited to date. Three provinces in the north of Afghanistan have had avian influenza noted in the poultry population, and have active surveillance in the animal population as well, led by MoA working with international experts and veterinarians to set up animal surveillance. NAMRU-3 has some active research in animal and human surveillance, but these investigations are not performed in concert with the governance programs. Of note, the WHO considers Afghanistan to be high risk for avian influenza based on the fact that the country is in the migratory pathway for a number of bird species and on the common practice in rural areas of keeping poultry within the family home.

Afghanistan has established a national tuberculosis (TB) control program as part of the BPHS. Through its REACH program, the rural arm of the BPHS is currently administered by the Management Sciences for Health (MSH) agency and overseen by the Office of Rural Recovery and Development under the MoPH. TB control as part of the national health plan is administered by WHO and MoPH; this function has been contracted out to local and national NGOs to perform the delivery of TB-related services using directly observed therapy—short course (DOTS). Three provinces are covered directly by the MoPH and appear to have greater success and case finding in the public health and TB control aspects. This program has primarily been a passive surveillance system relying on case identification and has clearly been rudimentary in case finding, with detection rates of less than 20 percent, compared with more than 85 percent success in therapy with DOTS. However, follow-up and end-of-therapy sputum cultures and chest x-rays are not routinely performed due to lack of capacity. The NGOs are under contractual agreement to perform this function with MoPH oversight; however, it is estimated that only 13 provinces are fully functional at this time, with a Kabul-centric distribution of services.

Although Afghanistan has a national HIV/AIDS control program, no comprehensive systematic data regarding the prevalence of HIV/AIDS or other sexually transmitted diseases in the country are currently available. A recent report cited only a few hundred confirmed cases in the entire country, but this report is assumed to be inaccurate due to very low testing rates. Sero-prevalence rates are derived from testing of blood samples several years ago at the Central Blood Bank and the Voluntary Counseling and Testing Centre in Kabul. Lack of a reliable supply of test reagents has kept most clinics from being able to perform serologic and other screening tests on most of their patients. Many international public health officials fear that the incidence of HIV/AIDS may be much higher than in adjacent countries due to the interlocking problems of high rates of injection drug use (fueled by the fact that Afghanistan produces more than 90 percent of the world's supply of opium), low rates of barrier contraception, and lack of prescreening for blood transfusions.

One of the main initiatives in Afghanistan for reconstruction relies on the work of provincial reconstruction teams (PRTs). These teams are under the military authority of the International Security Assistance Force; currently, there are 23 PRTs striving to rebuild the Afghan infrastructure (13 under U.S. leadership and the others headed by other lead nations). Each PRT includes a combination of military and civilian personnel who are responsible for carrying out reconstruction and development projects (such as building schools and digging wells) in consultation with local leaders. Most of the PRTs have not emphasized or focused on medical-related reconstruction projects. Assignment of personnel trained in public health to each PRT would clearly be useful in terms of providing more coordination of MoPH-approved public health programs and could improve health surveillance reporting. In addition, PRTs have their own security forces, so they are capable of operating in areas considered unsafe for civilians, and their outreach efforts could extend health surveillance into the areas not currently well served due to security issues.

Key Lessons

Emerging public health systems initially may need to focus interventions and strategies on known public health risks until up-to-date data become available. These may be public health risk factors that were considered to be a high priority prior to the crisis and still persist post-crisis, such as malaria, TB, or diarrheal diseases. In addition, new public health emergencies, such as a communicable disease outbreak or an earthquake, will need to be addressed with international assistance until local capacity and resources are fully functioning.

Public Health Education

Long-term, embedded mentors and trainers for the ANA and ANP healthcare leaders and personnel have been very successful and well received by the mentees to date. These trainers have helped with logistics support, hospital capacity building, medical/and nursing education, combat medic training, and combat casualty care. The lessons learned from this extensive mentoring program can be used to provide policy and guidance for further nation-building and health diplomacy projects. The development of a similar civilian-oriented system of mentorship, perhaps led by the U.S. Department of Health and Human Services (DHHS) and CDC, should be similarly effective in developing personnel skill and capacity in the MoPH. The educational venue of choice in Afghanistan is mentorship, rather than a didactically based learning modality. Literacy issues aside, training and hands-on mentorship are the most viable and best-accepted modes of education for the populace and seem to be the most effective way forward. Doctrine, policy, and further nation-building activities should be structured around this type of learning/educational process.

The training program for combat medics for the ANA has produced several thousand graduates to date. The curriculum of this program has focused on combat casualty care but has not included public health education. The addition of information on public health, prevention, and health surveillance to the medic curriculum would have a number of major benefits. It would foster general public health measures within the ANA and lay the groundwork for emergence of public healthcare workers in the future, especially if additional training of exceptional students leads to development of a public health worker degree or certification. Some of the medics' public health knowledge would be of direct use in their dealing with disasters.

Similarly, there is a need for development of public health courses that will educate Afghan military and civilian physicians. Both short courses (perhaps two weeks) for generalist physicians and longer courses for those who want to specialize as public health officers could be offered (one such "refresher" course for Afghan physicians in practice was completed in 2008). The need for this physician education in public health is particularly applicable to Afghanistan because of the poor quality of medical school education during the Taliban years, when coverage of public health in the curriculum was very sparse. Improving the content and amount of public health information in the curriculum is already under way at Kabul Medical University (the "flagship" medical university for the country) for its medical, nursing, and dental students.

Key Lessons

Emerging public health systems will need to tailor education programs to allow professionals providing public health assistance or direct medical care to balance both their professional demands and their education goals. Public health education can consist of a combination of direct mentoring and short courses. In addition, allied public health and medical professionals, such as nurses and paramedics, should receive public health training because they serve as frontline medical and public health providers. Public health components should be incorporated into healthcare teaching curriculums that will also be revised in the post-crisis era.

CONCLUSION

Afghanistan is an example of a post-conflict and post-disaster state, and multiple interrelated development processes need to occur to bring about improvements in its public health system. These same development processes need to be considered when conducting public health planning for other post-conflict and post-disaster countries. The major public health system development components needed for countries emerging from large-scale crises are summarized here:

- Fix the medical logistics supply system. This step is a prerequisite to having functional clinical laboratories and the ability to perform diagnostic clinical tests, particularly those related to infectious diseases.
- Perform the political maneuvering needed to bring about full integration of various healthcare agencies involved in public health within the government, and establish a single entity to assume leadership for public health.
- Develop and provide all necessary training programs for healthcare personnel who will be responsible for public health. This training should include public health training for students, training of healthcare workers at each "level" of the healthcare system, and leadership and administrative training for public health officials. In addition, provide education programs in basic public health measures for the general population.
- Train personnel and provide the equipment needed for biomedical equipment repair and maintenance. This training allows extended function of the clinical laboratories and directly helps with the entire healthcare delivery and public health surveillance systems.

- Expand infrastructure components to include improved communication systems, laboratory facilities, and emergency response teams.
- Support parallel systems development improvements in sanitation, water supply, food supply, and the economy, with the eventual goal of the national government operating the public health and healthcare system and supporting it entirely through its national funding and its national personnel.

As in many post-conflict and post-disaster regions, there is a generalized absence of depth of training, knowledge, and understanding of public health systems throughout the Afghan healthcare system. For many complicated reasons, including unreliable communications, lack of middle management capacity, and corruption, the focus of Afghan health care—both civilian and military—is currently on curative medicine and not on public health and prevention. For preventive medicine to be effectively enacted, two major changes will be required: (1) The curative healthcare system will need to mature and (2) a cultural shift to emphasize prevention at all levels of the government and by the population will need to occur. While this chapter has focused on Afghanistan, most of the very same problems and considerations noted here apply to many other countries facing similar challenges. The acronyms for a number of the national organizations will, of course, be different, but the public health functions they will need to carry out and the order of priority for their implementation will be the same as for Afghanistan.

INTERNET RESOURCES

Afghanistan Ministry of Higher Education: www.mohe.gov.af

Afghanistan Ministry of Public Health: www.moph.gov.af

Afghanistan National Development Strategy (ANDS): www.ands.gov.af

Center for Disaster and Humanitarian Assistance Medicine (CDHAM): www.cdham.org

Disease Control Priorities Project: www.dcp2.org

United Nations, *Index of Public Health Programs*: http://esa.un.org/subindex/pgViewSites
.asp?termCode=TF

United States Agency for International Development (USAID), *Health*: http://www.usaid.gov/
our_work/global_health/#

United States Institute of Peace (USIP), *Post-conflict Health Reconstruction*: http://www.usip
.org/resources/post-conflict-health-reconstruction

World Health Organization, *Public Health Mapping and GIS Programme*: http://www.who.int/
health_mapping/en/

NOTES

1. Personal communications: Dr. S. M. Amin Fatimie (Afghan Minister of Public Health), Dr. Faizullah Kakar (Deputy Minister of Public Health), Dr. Jawad Mohfleh (MoPH officer): March 2007, July 2007, January 2008.

2. Holliman CJ, Courniotes C, Amundson D, et al. *Program management plan: Afghan National Security Forces Healthcare Sector Reachback Project: Planning document for healthcare system improvement and integration for the Afghan National Security Forces.* Bethesda, MD: Center for Disaster and Humanitarian Assistance Medicine; February 7, 2008.

3. Bricknell MCM, Thompson D. Roles for international military medical services in stability operations (security sector reform). *Journal of the Royal Army Medical Corps.* 2007;153(2):95–98.

4. Sabri B, Siddiqi S, Ahmed AM, Kakar FK, Perrot J. Towards sustainable delivery of health services in Afghanistan: Options for the future. *Bulletin of the World Health Organization.* 2007; 85(9):712–719.

5. Sharp TW, Burkle FM Jr., Vaughn AF, Chotani R, Brennan RJ. Challenges and opportunities for humanitarian relief in Afghanistan. *Clinical Infectious Disease.* 2002;34(5):S215–S228.

6. Waldman R, Strong L, Wali A. Afghanistan's health system since 2001: Condition improved, prognosis cautiously optimistic. *Afghanistan Research and Evaluation Unit Briefing Paper Series.* 2006;1–21.

7. Peters DH, Noor AA, Singh LP, et al. A balanced scorecard for health services in Afghanistan. *Bulletin of the World Health Organization.* 2007;85(2):146–151.

8. Thompson D. The role of medical diplomacy in stabilizing Afghanistan. *Defense Horizons.* 2008;63:1–8.

9. Basic Package of Health Services. Ministry of Public Health, Government of Afghanistan. 2005.

10. Essential Package of Hospital Services. Ministry of Public Health, Government of Afghanistan. 2006.

SECTION 2

Private-Sector and Nongovernmental Organizations

Public–Private Partnerships During Emergencies

Jennifer L. Chan and Christian Theodosis

INTRODUCTION

A public health emergency arises when an acute cataclysmic event occurs of sufficient magnitude to overwhelm the capacity of routinely available local resources to solve key problems. In these situations, resources and assistance external to the event are needed to ensure the security, health, and basic needs of the population. For the purposes of this chapter, two types of public health emergencies are distinguished: (1) natural disasters and (2) complex humanitarian emergencies. Disasters, whether natural or human-made, are often sudden and unplanned. Disasters have increased since 1987, with a more than twofold increase occurring in the past 30 years.[1] In 2006, there were 427 disasters reported to the Center for Research on the Epidemiology of Disasters (CRED) EM-DAT database. These disasters killed 23,000 people and affected 143 million. More than half of the disasters (55 percent) were floods and are suggestive of a growing impact of climate change. Forty-four percent of all disasters occurred in Asia.[2] The U.S. Agency for International Development's (USAID) Office of Foreign Disaster Assistance has responded to an increasing number of disasters throughout the past decade (see Figure 6-1).[2–7]

Complex emergencies are defined by the United Nations (UN) as "a humanitarian crisis in a country, region, or society where there is total or considerable breakdown of authority resulting from internal or external conflict and which requires an international response that goes beyond the mandate or capacity of any single and/or ongoing UN country program."[8] Although the number of complex emergencies has

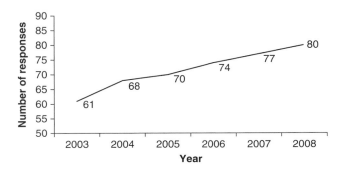

FIGURE 6-1   Number of USAID Disaster Responses 2003–2008

declined in recent years, the increasing severity and prolonged duration of each complex emergency has a longstanding impact.

In natural disasters or complex humanitarian emergencies, governmental agencies may directly execute a response strategy or they may contract with interstate actors (i.e., UN agencies) and nongovernmental organizations (NGOs), which accept responsibility for direct implementation of emergency response for support and services. In most scenarios, both public and private agencies are involved. The effectiveness of the technical approach in real time frequently depends on how well the lead governmental agencies perform their planning and coordinating functions.

This chapter describes the confluence of interests among the public and private actors in the setting of disasters and humanitarian emergencies. The frequency of these events continues to rise, along with the demands for improvement in disaster response performance. Demands from multiple stakeholders to improve efficiency and accountability and the growth of new global markets have led to the forging of new partnerships between public and private actors during emergencies.

The Asian tsunami of 2004—one of the largest natural disasters and humanitarian emergencies in recent history—brought about many public–private partnerships (PPPs). A case study of this emergency will describe PPPs' role in that response and the future roles that these organizations can play in disaster preparedness and mitigation. Emerging trends from accumulated experience among PPPs will be discussed, focusing on lessons learned from these efforts. These partnerships have engendered controversies around their effectiveness and potential for harm, with an ongoing debate among multiple stakeholders focusing on their value.

Case Study

On December 26, 2004, a 9.1-magnitude earthquake struck the Indian Ocean west of Indonesia, sending a series of large tsunami across the region. Four countries—Indonesia, Thailand, Sri Lanka, and India—were severely affected by these phenomena, and approximately 225,000 people were killed in 11 countries. The Asian tsunami is considered the largest natural disaster in recorded history. Sri Lanka, Indonesia, and the Maldives declared a state of emergency. Governments, UN agencies, NGOs, and organizations from the private sector from all around the world responded to the disaster.

According to the Tsunami Evaluation Coalition, more than $14 billion was donated from the international community for emergency relief and reconstruction.[9] Although the Asian tsunami did not constitute the largest official response to a natural disaster, it was the largest private-sector response. Individuals gave cash and in-kind donations to NGOs. Corporations donated cash and in-kind contributions to governments, UN agencies, and NGOs. For-profit companies also created partnerships with public and UN institutions.

In the wake of this disaster, a number of questions arose: Which types of public–private partnerships emerged during the 2004 Asian tsunami disaster response? What may have influenced private for-profit organizations to engage in these partnerships? Do companies and corporations have resources that benefit disaster and humanitarian response? What are the challenges that public and private organizations face in these new partnerships? And what are the proposed solutions?

HISTORICAL PERSPECTIVES

Although public–private partnerships are a new and often debated topic in the disaster response environment, PPPs are more established in the development sector.[10] The UN facilitates PPPs in many of its agencies. Currently, the UN has 62 PPPs in its Population and Women program and an additional 61 projects through its Children's Health Program. (www.un.org/partnerships/population_and_woman.html and www.un.org/partnerships/childrens_health.html). The World Health Organization (WHO) fosters partnerships focusing on pharmaceutical and vaccine programs. For example, Merck & Co. has partnered with the WHO Tobacco Free Initiative by providing staffing and technical expertise.[11] The UN Global Compact, a public–private initiative under the UN functions as a policy platform for businesses. More than 5,100 corporate agencies are involved in 130 countries. Businesses participating in the Global Compact will guide their strategies and business activities along principles related to human rights, labor, anticorruption, and the environment.

The U.S. President's Emergency Plan for AIDS relief (PEPFAR) participates in PPPs with multiple pharmaceutical companies, such as Bristol-Myers Squibb, GlaxoSmithKline, and Merck & Co. These organizations partner to assist in providing access to pediatric HIV medications and services.[12] The 2004 Asian tsunami sparked an increase in disaster and humanitarian PPPs. Prior to this event, there were a small but constant number of PPPs. In the aftermath of this disaster, the number of partnerships increased twofold to tenfold and has remained elevated compared to pre-tsunami levels.[13]

Politically and Economically Fragile Settings

A fundamental and recurring theme is that disasters and complex humanitarian emergencies are especially challenging to manage and mitigate when the financial or political strength of the partners is compromised. Hence the problem: Populations in developed countries, though far less vulnerable to such incidents, are far better protected against disasters. Political instability can likewise have serious negative repercussions on PPPs. When conditions deteriorate politically, governing structures can become significantly eroded or splintered into competing autonomous factions. In these cases, it can be unclear which "public" actors could or should be engaged as partners at all.

State Actors (Governments)

States are obligated to provide essential services in times of public health emergencies, consistent with international norms (e.g., conventions, treaties, declarations). Many governments in economically and politically stable countries have developed detailed and mandatory emergency systems, many of them integrated across both the public and the private sectors.[14] An example is the existence, at a minimum, of an organized defensive national military, which could respond to and resolve significant public health emergencies. Many states have detailed emergency plans that address the need to defend the territory against hostile invaders, landslides, hurricanes, epidemic diseases, and fires. In the United States, the Federal Emergency Management Administration (FEMA), in cooperation with state agencies, is tasked with providing assistance during domestic emergencies. In response to Hurricane Katrina, federal and state agencies coordinated and provided assistance in cooperation with the American Red Cross.[15]

In some contexts, the appropriate resources needed to address affected societies will exceed those available to the government whose population is directly affected by the crisis. In the aftermath of the Asian tsunami, the government of Indonesia sought the international assistance of NGOs, UN agencies, governments, and private organizations because it was unable to meet its obligations without assistance. Emergencies—and especially those with political dimensions—can occur with sufficient scale and duration to cause a state to fail. As a result, failed states or governments may be unwilling or entirely unable to ensure the safety of the population. The complex emergency in Darfur, Sudan, is one such example where the state is complicit in causing the crisis and exacerbates its human cost. When a state fails, the international community and institutions step forward to ensure public safety and temporarily assume roles of quasi-sovereign public agencies. This phenomenon significantly changes the types of PPPs that are possible.[16]

Public Actors (United Nations Institutions)

Intergovernmental networks—particularly the UN Security Council, United Nations High Commission of Refugees (UNHCR), and the Office of Coordination of Humanitarian Affairs (OCHA)—provide peacekeeping activities and coordination, and facilitate assistance during emergencies, particularly in the setting of a complex humanitarian crisis. These networks and authority structures influence the effectiveness of emergency responses and take on particular prominence when emergencies occur in settings where state governments are either unable or unwilling to ensure the population's basic safety.[14]

Private Actors

Private actors include nonprofit organizations, NGOs (including faith-based organizations, foundations, and academic institutions), and for-profit organizations (companies and corporations). Theoretically, the distinction between public actors and the private sector is relatively straightforward:

- Governments, including their domestic subdivisions and interstate unions, are public agencies and are mandated to ensure public safety.
- The private sector includes private for-profit firms, whose mandates must align with the interests of governing boards and shareholders (in the case of publicly traded firms).

In practice, this distinction is less obvious as many private firms (nonprofit organizations and for-profit businesses) are often active partners with governments and intergovernmental actors in providing essential services.

Nongovernmental organizations provide the bulk of humanitarian assistance and play a significant role in emergency response. International NGOs (e.g., Save the Children and Doctors Without Borders), national and local NGOs, and the Red Cross and Red Crescent Societies make up this group of stakeholders. National Red Cross and Red Crescent organizations (e.g., American Red Cross, Norwegian Red Cross) respond to national disasters and are guided by humanitarian values and international humanitarian law. NGOs are commonly the operational arms of many PPPs, and they frequently share stakes with both "public" and "private" interests. Legally, these entities are private nonprofit organizations that may serve the public interest, but their mandate for doing so often remains linked to a relationship with a governmental or intergovernmental actor.

The primary lens through which this chapter views partnerships is between private-sector enterprises and public agencies. Although not considered a partnership, a large degree of private-sector participation in disaster response takes the form of cash and in-kind donations. Less commonly, some businesses engage directly in emergency response; they are referred to as single-company engagements and often are involved in partnerships with governments directly.[13] IBM's Worldwide Crisis Response Team is one such example.

PREPAREDNESS AND RESPONSE

Mandates

Because the destabilizing effects of a public health emergency necessitate, by definition, resource mobilization beyond the direct control of the local authorities, establishing an ordered hierarchy of successive mandates for emergency intervention becomes crucial. In theory, mandates for agencies in domestic emergencies are relatively clear. Moreover, if an emergency occurs that requires substantial nonlocal inputs but not more than are available in the country where the emergency has occurred, it is a fairly straightforward matter to establish which levels of government should be held to account for success or failure.[17] In theory, each sovereign nation bears ultimate responsibility to plan for and ensure public safety; in practice, this feat has proved less easy to achieve during real-time crises.[18]

Increasing Demands for Capacity and Resources

From the 1980s to 2006, humanitarian assistance expenditure increased from $2 billion to nearly $9 billion.[19] Much of this increase was due to complex humanitarian emergencies and natural disasters. The Asian tsunami represented a notable variation in this trend, as it was one of the largest official and private responses ever. Prolonged complex humanitarian emergencies and the increasing size and frequency of natural disasters have created increasing stress among humanitarian agencies, as they have struggled to adequately respond to these incidents with limited resources.[19] To fill this gap, private funders and private for-profit organizations have responded to this increased demand for resources. Funding in the form of private contributions and corporate philanthropy has increased, as have overall emergency public health expenditures. According to OCHA, there was a 21 percent increase in private contributions, totaling 35 percent of overall expenditures, from 2001 to 2005.[13]

Calls for Accountability, Efficiency, and Technical Expertise

Some previous emergency relief interventions have left both responders and donors disappointed with the quality of responses (for example, in Rwanda and following Hurricane Katrina), prompting a growing number of stakeholders to call for accountability in the disaster response environment. The UN has proposed humanitarian reform and use of a cluster approach, which aims to coordinate key disaster responders. Interaction—the name of a coalition of U.S. humanitarian organizations—has come together to define principles of accountability. Many have also sought the experiences of the business sector to tackle the recognized need for metrics, efficiency, and accountability in responses to crises.

In addition, demand for technical expertise as a vehicle to improve efficiency and accuracy is growing. Accurate assessments improve the understanding of what is necessary at each phase of the response and how many resources are required for affected populations. These assessments require technical experts with special skills. To ensure accountability to beneficiaries and donors, technical experts are also needed for monitoring and evaluation of relief programs. Expertise in logistics, communication technology, and program management can improve the efficiency of operations, and for-profit companies have the potential to fulfill this need.[20]

Incentives for Private-Sector Engagement

Incentives for for-profit engagement in public health emergencies vary by company, emergency, and sector of involvement. Partnerships have been more commonly found in natural disaster settings. Companies and corporations tend to shy away from complex emergencies due to the common coexistence of insecurity and political ties that they may find themselves bound to.[13]

Indeed, Binder and Witte's research on business engagement in humanitarian relief found that many for-profit companies prefer partnerships rather than direct company engagement in disaster response. This preference arises because traditional emergency responders are recognized as being more familiar with complicated and often insecure disaster environments. Binder and Witte describe incentives for for-profit companies that engage in relief efforts as follows:[13]

- Growing sense of corporate social responsibility, which includes staff motivation
- Benefits of "positive branding"
- Business intelligence
- Pure willingness to do good

Corporate social responsibility has grown over the past decade, especially with the rise of global companies and corporations. Company philanthropic activities stem not only from employee interests, but also from shareholders, customers, and the global corporate partners.[10,13] These multifaceted interests lend themselves to the "positive branding" phenomenon. In turn, this positive visibility helps retain the companies' key staff as well as helps maintain relationships and business opportunities with existing and future customers.[13,21]

Moreover, rapidly emerging markets in Asia and India are highly susceptible to large-scale emergencies. Given this fact, companies have an incentive to build relationships with disaster responders, if only so that they can better understand how to protect their business ventures—and, therefore, their profits—in these volatile environments.[13,22] For example, in Bangladesh, Motorola partnered with CARE and a local telecommunications organization providing remote radio technology to facilitate communication between at-risk flood communities and CARE staff.[22] This is one example of a for-profit firm's expansion strategy providing an incentive to participate in humanitarian activities.

Principles of Partnerships

Many private companies and corporations interested in engaging in PPPs are challenged with finding common principles of partnership and practice with public actors in emergency response. This challenge is particularly relevant in humanitarian emergencies of conflict and war. The Global Compact recognizes the challenges of business engagement in these settings and has taken steps to create business principles that adhere to 10 core principles (see Table 6-1). The Global Compact asks compa-

TABLE 6-1   United Nations Global Compact: Ten Principles

Human Rights

Principle 1: Businesses should support and respect the protection of internationally proclaimed human rights.

Principle 2: Businesses should make sure that they are not complicit in human rights abuses.

Labor Standards

Principle 3: Businesses should uphold the freedom of association and the effective recognition of the right to collective bargaining.

Principle 4: Businesses should seek to eliminate all forms of forced and compulsory labor.

Principle 5: Businesses should support the effective abolition of child labor.

Principle 6: Businesses should seek to eliminate discrimination with respect to employment and occupations.

Environment

Principle 7: Businesses should support a precautionary approach to environmental challenges.

Principle 8: Businesses should undertake initiatives to promote greater environmental responsibility.

Principle 9: Businesses should encourage the development and diffusion of environmentally friendly technologies.

Anticorruption

Principle 10: Businesses should work against corruption in all its forms, including extortion and bribery.

Source: Adapted from United Nations Global Compact. *The ten principles.* Available at: http://www.unglobalcompact.org/AbouttheGC/TheTENPrinciples/index.html. Accessed June 11, 2009.

nies to commit to these principles related to human rights, labor standards, the environment, and anticorruption. These commitments set the stage for a common approach to guide preparedness and planning in emergencies.

A variety of PPPs have emerged with varying organizational structures. Logistics, telecommunications, and applied technologies appear to predominate in these types of partnerships.[13] PPPs can be described as taking one of two forms: noncommercial PPP or for-profit PPP. Similar to Binder and Witte's description of business engagement, private actors with noncommercial interests are often engaged in single-company partnerships with government, partnerships with UN agencies, and partnerships with coordinating bodies that engage with public actors.[13]

Single-Company Public–Private Partnerships

IBM is an example of a for-profit company that has engaged in nonprofit single-company PPPs. As of 2006, the IBM Crisis Response team had responded to more than 70 events in 40 countries, including the civil war in Rwanda, the conflict in Kosovo, Hurricane Katrina, and the Asian tsunami of 2004. The team's goals are to restore communication systems after emergencies to facilitate real-time decision making for immediate response. The company also assists in the coordination and collaboration among stakeholders using IBM technology and in the development of innovative, flexible, and interoperable communication technology.[23]

In the wake of the Asian tsunami, IBM created multiple communication systems with the aim of fulfilling the goals outlined above. Partnering with the Indonesian, Indian, Sri Lankan, and Thai governments, IBM offered communication services and consultations to national disaster authorities. The Sistem Informasi Manajemen Bencona Aceh (SIMBA) provided administrative and logistical systems management, as well as registration systems and damage assessments.[24] The Secure Wireless Infrastructure System (SWIS) had a wide range of wireless coverage and technology to withstand high demand for data transfer. It facilitated official government communications from Aceh to Jakarta. The IBM Crisis Response team also participates in partnerships with UN agencies and NGOs.

Private Sector/United Nations Partnerships

Microsoft has partnered with the United Nations High Commissioner for Refugees (UNHCR) since 1999 by helping displaced individuals establish their status as refugees using mobile registration systems.[10] Establishing refugee status enables a displaced person to access health care and other social services. In 1999, Microsoft and UNHCR started the Kosovar Refugee Registration Project with 35 Microsoft volunteers, and Microsoft provided novel technology to expedite the refugee registration process. The company has continued to improve its registration kits, which have now been tested in nine countries.

In addition to donating almost $3 million in cash and in-kind donations for disaster response during the Sichuan earthquake in 2008, Coca-Cola partnered with the United Nations Development Programme (UNDP) and the Ministry of Water Resources of the Chinese government to provide clean drinking water immediately after the earthquake.[25] According to the Coca-Cola Web site, "Our system is in a unique position to provide assistance during and after natural disasters. Because we have such a large distribution network, we can deliver necessities to some communities that are not easily accessible."[26]

Meta-initiatives

Binder and Witte's term "meta-initiative" best describes collaborative organizations of business partners that are emerging to provide disaster and humanitarian assistance.

> Meta-initiatives involve companies and other actors joining forces to enhance coordination in humanitarian relief work and to share lessons learned. . . . Meta-initiatives are designed to facilitate more effective industry-wide action in humanitarian relief, to avoid duplication of effort and to take advantage of economies of scale.[13]

The Disaster Resource Network (DRN) and the Fritz Institute are examples of meta-initiatives that coordinate companies interested in responding to natural disasters and complex humanitarian emergencies.

DRN is a meta-initiative of engineering and construction businesses that collaborates with UN logistics agencies and governments to provide disaster assistance and disaster mitigation. This initiative was created in response to the 2001 Gujarat earthquake in India by the World Economic Forum members to provide a focal point and mechanism for coordination of businesses interested in providing assistance in disasters.[27]

In response to the 2004 tsunami, DRN partnered with the UN Logistic Centre and the Sri Lankan Air Force to provide 7,400 tons of relief supplies to the region by leveraging its experience in airport logistics.[28] In the same year, DRN facilitated the deployment of two emergency response teams: New York City Medics and Medical Action Network emergency teams.[28] Direct medical care was provided via mobile clinics with medical kits supplied by the healthcare supply company Henry Schein, Inc.

The Fritz Institute provides support for a group of 40 business organizations that are interested in participating in disaster response through supply chain management. Created in 2005 to help achieve the goal of improving logistics and supply chain management, the Institute has brought together corporations and traditional humanitarian actors to learn from one another through training and certification programs.[29]

MITIGATION

Mitigation is defined as "all actions to reduce the impact of a disaster that can be taken prior to its occurrence, including preparedness and long-term risk reduction measures."[30] Successful mitigation requires identification of hazards so as to assess latent vulnerabilities and identify measures that reduce risks by minimizing the impact of disasters when they do occur or by decreasing the probability of an occurrence. Mitigation strategies may entail any of five basic types of interventions:[17]

- Engineering and construction measures
- Physical planning measures
- Economic measures
- Management and institutional measures
- Societal measures

Successful strategies generally require a long-term approach and several of these types of interventions. Studies on the effectiveness of PPPs reveal that the partnerships most likely to be successful are those that are sustained over time and those that produce standby capacity that can be activated quickly after a public health emergency occurs.[13]

The aim of mitigation strategies is to reduce losses in the event of a future occurrence of a hazard. The primary goal is to reduce the risk of death and injury to the population. Secondary goals include reducing damage and economic losses inflicted on the public-sector infrastructure and reducing private-sector losses given that they are likely to affect the community as whole.

Measures to reduce risk can be either active or passive. Passive measures include government regulations designed to mitigate disasters by requiring compliance with building codes, land-use restrictions, or compulsory insurance, for example. In these cases, governments interact separately with the public and with private corporations, focusing on each as subjects of regulation. Inability to benefit from PPPs may be a limitation of passive strategies. Passive strategies are also likely to fail when (1) no enforceable system of control exists, (2) the affected community denies the legitimacy of the regulation or the governing authority, or (3) economic issues prevent compliance.

Active risk reduction strategies promote mitigation efforts by offering incentives for desired performance objectives such as economic assistance to obtain safer building materials, subsidies on safety equipment, and education and training programs. When successful, PPPs are able to leverage the production of diverse outputs (e.g., building materials, scholarships) to ensure a well-coordinated and highly effective emergency management system. This approach can be effective when large budgets, skilled personnel, and extensive administration are available.[14]

Critical to the current conversation is the reality that businesses and public actors, in the right conditions, have substantial and potentially complementary resource portfolios. The challenge is to determine which features of those portfolios support successes and minimize risks. Potential prototypes of this idea are DHL's partnership with governments to assist in air transport and logistics during disasters and Microsoft's ongoing partnership with UNHCR to facilitate registration of affected refugees. Growing corporate social responsibility among businesses and the increasing need for technical expertise by traditional disaster responders are key motivators for pursuing these kinds of partnerships. The challenges are reflected in cross-cutting themes:

- Economic and political stability are needed to support realization of potential advantages.
- There is a need for coordination that requires subordination of some actors' decision-making latitude.
- Harmonizing the interests and capacities of various actors is complex and challenging but potentially rewarding.

A number of emerging issues related to formation of successful and robust PPPs have yet to be resolved. Notably, either business or humanitarian quandaries may lead to friction between those organizations participating in PPPs and among the various disaster and humanitarian responders to an incident.

Private-Sector Quandaries

Private-sector engagement in disasters and complex emergencies, whether for commercial or noncommercial purposes, invariably exposes companies to potential risks and benefits.[13] The specific risks and benefits for noncommercial engagements hinge on the potential of the partnership to improve or diminish the company's brand, staff morale, and regional business knowledge. When companies engage in partnerships on a commercial basis, they may evaluate the potential for risk and benefit in monetary terms. By comparison, noncommercial engagement may confer fewer tangible benefits to the core business in the mind of corporate managers and shareholders, and it poses obvious risks in terms of reputation, financial costs, and safety. These concerns may explain why companies tend to favor partnerships with well-established NGOs working in development activities or even natural disasters, as opposed to intervening in complex emergencies where the political risks may outweigh any potential benefits.

At the same time, examples exist where noncommercial investments have ultimately brought significant commercial value to companies in the long term. Specifically, companies may be able to leverage knowledge gained from noncommercial engagements to benefit other commercial operating units of the business.[13] Naturally, which investments are likely to return value to the company is a reasonable question that any for-profit business might ask. If a company is able to serve both its shareholders and its desire to do good deeds and to retain staff, then perhaps it should follow this path, all the while recognizing these actions as distinct from classical "humanitarian action." Determining which options to pursue and which methods are most likely to result in success are emerging issues that businesses face both internally and in relation to partners in the public and quasi-public realms.

Humanitarian Quandaries

Much has been written about the friction between the "humanitarian principles" of NGOs and the market motives characteristic of traditional businesses. It remains true that principled action is critically important and that market motives can neither replace nor co-opt humanitarian action. At the same time, recognition is growing of the need for professionalized operations in disaster and humanitarian settings on the part of all actors. In addition, the need for broad coordination between actors, regardless of their core principles, is well documented. The emerging challenge might now be described as how best to integrate the work of various actors with varying interests, principles, and skill sets so as to realize benefits for all stakeholders.

In the setting of a complex emergency, "humanitarian" action has distinct advantages over business action in terms of legitimacy and legal authority, as established by the Geneva Conventions.[30] This advantage does not prohibit businesses from serving a role in a crisis. Nevertheless, businesses are unlikely to be seen as credible leaders of programmatic and policy direction in these settings. Instead, humanitarian actors are in the best position to take leading roles early in a crisis, such as in assessing needs, setting goals, and determining the best methods for collaboration. Importantly, they do so impartially, neutrally, and independently, consistent with their mandate. Where appropriate, they may choose to contract with private-sector partners to fill gaps in essential services.

A more challenging question is how humanitarian organizations should interact with existing businesses in settings where gray markets exist but legitimate governments do not. For example, an international telecommunications company provides infrastructure for several humanitarian and relief agencies operating in the Darfur region of Sudan. Many have argued that international businesses should withdraw from Sudan, because their presence supports the government in Khartoum. Similar problems have arisen elsewhere, in locales where the legitimacy of the governing regime was questionable. For example, an oil company operating in Myanmar made substantial investments in free access to health care, claiming 43,000 beneficiaries from this donation. An associated 4.5 percent drop in infant mortality and significant reductions in deaths associated with malaria were reported. The argument has been made that if these "responsible" companies simply leave, then others might replace them, arguably without the same social commitments.[31]

Humanitarian actors, unlike for-profit businesses, have clear authority to operate independently of governmental authority. Indeed, humanitarian actors are often required to serve de facto governmental roles when legitimate sovereign authority is lacking. Businesses, however, have no such independent legal authority, as they are generally subjects of governing authority rather than independent actors. Therefore, humanitarian actors generally cannot enforce compliance with humanitarian mandates/strategy. An emerging challenge is how to encourage businesses to cooperate with the quasi-public authority of humanitarian actors when no consequences for refusal and few incentives for collaboration remain.

Long-Term Solutions

Humanitarian intervention is understood to be a temporary solution. Over time, it is hoped, public health conditions will improve, emergencies will be resolved, and stability will return (or be established). Predictably, natural disasters are resolved more quickly than complex emergencies: Wars often last many years, whereas mudslides may be acutely cataclysmic but most of the underlying society returns to normal function relatively quickly.[16] In either case, the need to take stock of lessons learned and improve mitigation efforts remains.

Both humanitarian and business actors have stakes in the resolution of disasters and the establishment of lasting peace. In the context of humanitarian action, the emergence of stable governance and business activity means humanitarian actors can withdraw to other areas where their skills are acutely needed. In the case of business actors, stable peace means they can prioritize and optimize the performance of their central strengths. In either case, a clear lesson learned so far is that a longer-term planning horizon is required to maximize effectiveness. This is true for both businesses and humanitarian actors. Long-term planning is especially important with regard to mitigation efforts. PPPs that produce standby capacity are particularly desirable because they improve both future acute responses and current frameworks for the discipline, as reflected in the growth of meta-initiatives.[13]

Post-conflict settings are especially challenging. They are not amenable to either classical "development" or "humanitarian" approaches. In addition, some businesses, at least in their noncommercial forms, tend not to work in post-conflict settings.

Instead, they prefer to work in acute disaster settings where "challenges are easier to understand" or in stable "development" settings, where the rule of law and the role of business are relatively well established. Post-conflict settings are where businesses stand to gain more if their partnerships are successful at assisting the consolidation of peace. In addition, post-conflict settings are more likely to open options for lasting peace and, therefore, are more likely to serve the interests of investors in emerging markets. This environment may be favorable to businesses, but not necessarily to humanitarian actors.

ANALYSIS OF CASE STUDY

After the initial impact of the 2004 Asian tsunami, the private sector responded to the need for resources, technical expertise, and accountability. Governments, UN agencies, NGOs and private actors mobilized throughout the world to provide a disaster response. While the majority of private donations came from individuals and company in-kind contributions, a number of PPPs emerged and changed the landscape of response in public health emergencies. IBM's single-company engagement with the governments of Sri Lanka, Thailand, and Indonesia provided information communication technology. Deutsche Post World Net, in collaboration with the DRN meta-initiative, mobilized its air logistics expertise, thereby enabling the government of Sri Lanka to receive and distribute tons of relief materials arriving from around the world.

During the response, PPP challenges arose primarily around common principles of engagement, coordination, and efficiency. Organizations preparing for the next disaster have stepped forward to address these challenges. The World Economic Forum and UN have established guiding principles for PPPs. The Business Roundtable Partnership for Disaster Response, which was formed after the 2004 Asian tsunami, has brought together more than 160 companies to improve the appropriateness and efficiency of private-sector collaborations with disaster organizations. This meta-initiative has established an emergency protocol outlining how businesses should communicate with U.S. government agencies and the American Red Cross during U.S. national disasters.

CONCLUSION

Public–private partnerships have emerged as stakeholders in public health emergency response, preparedness, and mitigation. While for-profit private-sector engagement in emergency response primarily takes the form of cash and in-kind donations, single-company PPPs, PPPs with UN agencies, and meta-initiatives do exist. PPPs can play a crucial role in providing needed resources and technical support while fulfilling private-sector interests related to corporate social responsibility and, sometimes, long-term business investments.

The 2004 Asian tsunami was a catalyst for PPPs, but it also revealed ongoing challenges of aligning partnership principles and coordination. The ongoing debate around PPPs' role in conflict-related disasters and post-conflict space continues. Humanitarian actors and businesses will need to define their roles further. These more clearly defined roles will, in turn, become more important in complex emergencies where impartiality, neutrality, and independence are valued highly by disaster responders, but ongoing needs for efficiency and technical expertise are also well recognized.

INTERNET RESOURCES

Fritz Institute: http://www.fritzinstitute.org

Sphere Project, Humanitarian Charter and Minimum Standards in Disaster Response: http://www.sphereproject.org/

World Bank, public–private partnerships in infrastructure: http://web.worldbank.org/WBSITE/EXTERNAL/WBI/WBIPROGRAMS/PPPILP/0,,menuPK:461142~pagePK:64156143~piPK:64154155~theSitePK:461102,00.html

United Nations, Global Compact: http://www.unglobalcompact.org/

U.S. Agency for International Development, global partnerships: http://www.usaid.gov/our_work/global_partnerships/

World Economic Forum, Disaster Resource Network: http://www.weforum.org/en/initiatives/drn/index.htm

World Health Organization, partnerships management: http://www.who.int/management/partnerships/en/

NOTES

1. Hoyois P, Below R, Sheuren J, et al. *Annual disaster statistical review: Numbers and trends 2006.* Brussels: Center for Research on the Epidemiology of Disasters (CRED); 2007.
2. U.S. Office of Foreign Disaster Assistance. *Annual report for fiscal year 2008.* Washington, DC: U.S. Office of Foreign Disaster Assistance; 2008.
3. U.S. Office of Foreign Disaster Assistance. *Annual report for fiscal year 2007.* Washington, DC: U.S. Office of Foreign Disaster Assistance; 2007.
4. U.S. Office of Foreign Disaster Assistance. *Annual report for fiscal year 2006.* Washington, DC: U.S. Office of Foreign Disaster Assistance; 2006.
5. U.S. Office of Foreign Disaster Assistance. *Annual report for fiscal year 2005.* Washington, DC: U.S. Office of Foreign Disaster Assistance; 2005.

6. U.S. Office of Foreign Disaster Assistance. *Annual report for fiscal year 2004*. Washington, DC: U.S. Office of Foreign Disaster Assistance; 2004.

7. U.S. Office of Foreign Disaster Assistance. *Annual report for fiscal year 2003*. Washington, DC: U.S. Office of Foreign Disaster Assistance; 2003.

8. Burkle FM. Lessons learnt and future expectations of complex emergencies. *British Medical Journal*. 1999;319(7207):422–426.

9. Flint M, Goyder H. *Funding the tsunami response: A synthesis of findings*. London: Tsunami Evaluation Coalition; 2006.

10. Paul R, McKinsey K. "Fotola": Microsoft and UNHCR team up to better protect refugees. Available at: http://www.unhcr.org/cgi-bin/texis/vtx/partners/opendoc.htm?tbl=PARTNERS& id=4444dd522. Accessed June 11, 2009.

11. World Health Organization. 1999 annual report from WHO's Tobacco Free Initiative. 1999. Available at: http://www.who.int/ncd/mip2000/documents/annual_tfi_en.pdf.

12. Health partnerships: Developing world—2008. Available at: http://www.ifpma.org/index .php?id=628. Accessed June 11, 2009.

13. Binder A, Witte JM. *Business engagement in humanitarian relief: Key trends and policy implications*. London: Overseas Development Institute; 2007.

14. U.S. Department of Homeland Security. *National response framework*. Washington, DC: U.S. Department of Homeland Security; 2008.

15. U.S. Government and Accountability Office. *National response framework: FEMA needs policies and procedures to better integrate non-federal stakeholders in the revision process: Report to Congressional committees*. Washington, DC: U.S. Department of Homeland Security; 2008.

16. Noji EK. *Public health consequences of disasters*. New York: Oxford University Press; 1997.

17. Davis I. *Learning from disaster recovery: Guidance for decision makers*. United Nations International Strategy for Disaster Reduction Secretariat; 2007. Available at: www.unisdr.org/eng/ about_isdr/isdr-publications/irp/Learning-From-Disaster-Recovery.pdf.

18. Abiew F. *The evolution of the doctrine and practice of humanitarian intervention*. The Hague: Kluwer Law International; 1999.

19. Development Initiatives. *Global humanitarian assistance*. United Kingdom: Development Initiatives; 2007, p. 208.

20. Strategic philanthropy for humanitarian relief: Lynn Fritz: Mobilizing business expertise for measurable gain in humanitarian relief. *Global Giving Matters*. 2005:2.

21. Deutsche Post DHL. Sustainability. Available at: http://www.dp-dhl.de/dp-dhl?tab=1&skin= hi&check=yes&lang=de_EN&xmlFile=2002216. Accessed June 11, 2009.

22. Motorola. Motorola and CARE Bangladesh celebrate inauguration of radio communications system [press release]. November 24, 2004.

23. Woodworth B. IBM Crisis Response Team. *Disaster Response Coordination*. 2008:2–31.

24. IBM. Southern Asia tsunami: IBM response final report: March 28, 2005. Available at: www .935.ibm.com/services/us/bcrs/pdf/rp_2005-03-28_tsunami.pdf. Accessed June 14, 2009.

25. UNDP joins emergency relief efforts in Sichuan earthquake. Available at: http://www.undp .org.cn/modules.php?op=modload&name=News&file=article&catid=14&topic=12&sid=4297 &mode=thread&order=0&thold=0. Accessed June 11, 2009.

26. The Coca Cola Company. Sustainability: Disaster relief. Available at: http://www.thecoca-cola company.com/citizenship/disaster_relief.html. Accessed June 11, 2009.

27. Thomas A, Fritz L. Disaster Relief, Inc. *Harvard Business Review*. 2006;8(11):114–126.

28. World Economic Forum. Disaster Resource Network: Highlights of response efforts 2005–2007. Available at: http://www2.weforum.org/en/initiatives/drn/ResponsesandProjects/index.html. Accessed June 11, 2009.

29. New "Corporations for Humanity" initiative mobilizes and expands corporate support for global humanitarian relief; Fritz Institute leverages corporate expertise and resources for long-term improvement in the delivery of aid. *Business Wire*. December 13, 2005. Available at: http://findarticles.com/p/articles/mi_m0EIN/is_2005_Dec_13/ai_n15932217/. Accessed June 11, 2009.

30. Coburn AW, Spence RJS, Pomonis A. *Disaster mitigation*. United Nations Development Programme; 1994.

31. Morrison J. Report of the informal consultation with the institution investor and business communities. United Nations Global Compact; 2007. Available at: www.unglobalcompact.org/NewsAndEvents/articles_and_papers/ResponsibleInvestmentinWeakxConflictProneStates.pdf. Accessed June 11, 2009.

CHAPTER 7

Nongovernmental Organizations' Response to Crises

Jeffrey P. Smith and Steven M. Anderscavage

INTRODUCTION

Although there is some debate about the exact definition, the term "nongovernmental organization" (NGO) refers to a legally constituted organization created by a group of persons with no participation or representation of any government. This term encompasses a broad category of organizations that can operate at a local, provincial, regional, national, or global level. Unlike the term "intergovernmental organization" (IGO), which refers to an entity such as the United Nations and is legally defined, NGO is a term in general use but does not have a legal definition. Currently, the accepted criteria for defining an NGO as an entity depend on the location of its headquarters, its membership, its funding sources, and the content of its programs. By definition, an NGO must not engage in criminal activity.

Until the early 1990s, in academic, media, and political discussions, the term NGO was reserved for national NGOs; regional or global bodies were specifically referred to as international NGOs (INGOs). During that period, the overwhelming majority of local and provincial NGOs never engaged in transnational activities. Although national NGOs did engage in transnational development and humanitarian activities, they rarely participated in international political discourse. Currently, there are several million NGOs in operation around the world, and the vast majority of them are national in nature. For example, of the 1 to 2 million NGOs operating in India, most have local or national agendas. More than 40,000 NGOs work internationally.[1]

There are two general classifications of NGOs: those that are operational and those that focus on advocacy issues.[2] Operational NGOs, which include most NGOs involved in emergency public health issues, focus on relief efforts and/or the design and implementation of development-related projects. Advocacy NGOs, by comparison, concentrate on the defense or promotion of a specific cause.

This chapter discusses the role of NGOs in response to public health emergencies. Their history, classification, code of conduct, funding, interaction with governments, and roles in disasters and complex humanitarian emergencies will be reviewed. The activities of NGOs in the areas of preparedness, mitigation, response, and recovery in crises are emphasized throughout the chapter.

Case Study

Hurricane Katrina made landfall in southeast Louisiana during the early morning of August 29, 2005, as a Category 3 storm with sustained maximal winds of 125 miles per hour. The combination of the storm surge, heavy rainfall, and breached levees resulted in flooding that affected 80 percent of the city of New Orleans. Despite evacuation measures, approximately 60,000 people remained in the city, many of whom were impoverished African Americans. Within 24 hours, it was clear that a major disaster was unfolding, which would eventually result in the largest humanitarian crisis in the history of the United States. Property damage caused by the storm and its aftermath put the total cost of the storm at $81.2 billion; at least 1,836 lives were lost, with hundreds more missing. U.S. Department of Homeland Security Secretary Michael Chertoff at the time referred to Hurricane Katrina as probably the worst catastrophe, or set of catastrophes, the United States had ever faced.

In the days, weeks, and months following the event, global news coverage of the storm's aftermath dominated the media. Viewers were bombarded with vivid images of the devastation, including flooding, large-scale destruction, stranded and displaced populations, disruption of communities, and shortages of vital community services including public health and essential medical services. The local and federal governments drew much criticism for their lack of preparedness for and inadequate response to this crisis. Due to the large impact of the storm, aid to the region came from numerous domestic NGOs, several international NGOs, and foreign governments. In fact, NGOs provided more than $3 billion in aid to the region, which was primarily devoted to response and short-term recovery efforts and, to a lesser extent, to longer-term programs.[3]

What is the role of NGOs in disaster preparedness and response? Specifically, which types of activities did domestic and international NGOs provide in the aftermath of Katrina? How do NGOs integrate into the National Incident Management System (NIMS)? Who provides their funding, and what are the requirements of funders? What are the challenges facing NGOs in disaster response? How can the activities of NGOs mitigate against the devastating impact of another major disaster to the region?

HISTORICAL PERSPECTIVES

National NGOs date back to the colonial period. In their early days, they primarily represented local civil organizations that addressed social and advocacy issues outside of government operations. By 1914, there were an estimated 1,083 NGOs in existence.[4]

International NGOs have a history dating back to the mid-1800s and were important in the antislavery and women's suffrage movements.[5] Prior to 1854, approximately 6 international NGOs were in existence. At the turn of the twentieth century, the number of NGOs grew to roughly 160. By 1945, more than 1,000 international NGOs had been formed. One of the most recognizable and longstanding NGOs, the International Committee for the Red Cross (ICRC), was established in 1863. Based on the founders' observations of poorly treated war casualties, this organization's initial goal was to improve the treatment of wounded soldiers. The American Red Cross was founded several years after the establishment of the ICRC and continues to be a vital member of the NGO community.

The term "nongovernmental organization" came into popular use in 1945 with the establishment of the United Nations (UN) organization, for which provisions in the UN Charter defined the consultative role between intergovernmental specialized agencies and international private organizations.[6] Since then, the number of NGOs has grown exponentially. At the UN, international NGOs include virtually all private bodies not founded by international treaty that are independent of government control and not seeking to challenge governments as a political party. Today there are more than 3,200 NGOs with varying levels of consultative status with the UN.[7]

Over the last 50 years, globalization has helped to fuel the rise of NGOs, many of which have been formed to address social issues that could not be adequately addressed by local, regional, or national governments. Both domestic and international NGOs have been established to provide developmental aid and humanitarian assistance. This rapid increase in the number of NGOs reflects global awareness of issues related to sustainable development and the desire of persons to address social inequities in a global fashion. In addition, there is increased grassroots awareness that the care of persons who are victims of a natural disaster, conflict, or complex humanitarian emergencies cannot always be fully accomplished by government agencies alone.

The vital role of NGOs as significant players in sustainable development was further supported in 1992 by Agenda 21, a UN-run program that serves as a blueprint for sustainable development in the twenty-first century.[8] Agenda 21 is designed to guide the actions of the UN, governments, and major groups (i.e., NGOs) in their activities that affect the environment at the local, national, and global levels. The program includes measures to combat poverty, change consumption patterns, and promote health and sustainable settlement patterns. This program was adopted by 178 governments during the UN Conference on Environment and Development (Earth Summit), held in Rio de Janeiro on June 14, 1992.

Overview of NGOs

As noted earlier, there has been an exponential increase in the NGO population, which now number in the millions globally, over the past several decades. Thousands of NGOs provide crisis relief within this sector, which is dominated by mega-NGOs such as CARE, Oxfam, Red Cross, Save the Children, World Vision, and Medecins sans Frontieres (MSF). Despite the existence of these major organizations, most of the NGOs working in the relief arena remain more community-based or regionally oriented organizations.

NGOs play an important role in public health crises and interact with many other entities involved in response. In public health emergency response, a complex relationship exists among overriding themes and various entities including the Red Cross, international organizations, and national programs (see Figure 7-1).

The structure of NGOs varies considerably: They can be global hierarchies with either a relatively strong central authority or a more loosely federated arrangement. Alternatively, they may be based in a single country. Owing to improved communications and networking, more locally based groups (referred to as grassroots or community-based organizations) have the potential to achieve global outreach. In the majority of cases, there is no significant difference between an NGO and a private voluntary organization (PVO), but the NGO label carries a more neutral connotation and has greater applicability to a diverse range of activities. In contrast, PVO suggests moral approval of its membership or a limited range of groups and implies a more exclusionary hierarchy. Typically, NGOs do not include professional associations, businesses, or foundations.

The general organization of NGOs varies widely. Each NGO is differentiated and governed largely by its charter. Four basic models are possible:[9]

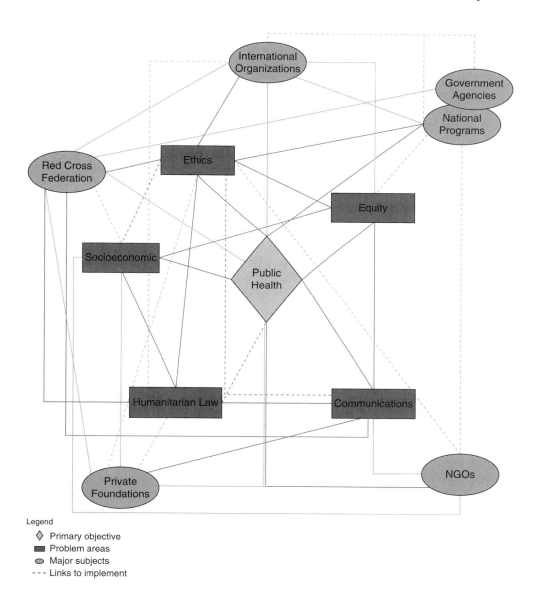

FIGURE 7-1 The Complex Interaction of the Entities and Their Challenges (Problems) in the Delivery of Public Health

- The NGO works internationally with headquarters in one country (e.g., International Medical Corp [IMC], International Red Cross and Red Crescent [IRC]).
- The NGO has many national chapters with independent field organizations (e.g., World Vision International [WVI]).
- The NGO creates national or multinational fundraising offices that raise and pool their funds through single field organizations, which are in turn staffed and managed by indigenous staff (e.g., WVI).
- The NGO works only through indigenous local organizations with no independent operational capacity in the field (e.g., Oxfam).

As mentioned earlier, there are two general classifications of NGOs: those that are operational and those that focus on advocacy issues. Operational NGOs, which include most NGOs involved in emergency public health issues, concentrate on relief efforts, the design and implementation of development-related projects, or both. Advocacy NGOs defend or promote a specific cause. Once NGOs decide to influence public policy, they typically may organize in broad coalitions for this purpose. Coalitions may take the form of umbrella NGOs, networks, or caucuses.[10] Other types of NGOs may be characterized by their mission or scope of services (i.e., disaster relief, technical assistance), their geographic outreach (i.e., international), their membership (i.e., faith based), or their autonomy (i.e., government operated, quasi-autonomous). A plethora of acronyms have emerged to describe these types, and many NGOs may demonstrate several of these characteristics (see Table 7-1).[10]

Operational NGOs mobilize resources in the form of financial donations, materials, and/or volunteer labor in an effort to sustain their projects and programs. This process often requires a sophisticated and multidimensional administrative and operational institution with strong organizational and motivational skills. An excellent example of such an NGO is AmeriCares, a global health and disaster relief NGO based in Stamford, Connecticut, which both provides emergency relief services and supports sustainable developmental projects globally. Most of the resources used to finance projects come through donations from industry and individuals, volunteer and subsidized labor, governmental and institutional grants, and in-kind support from international and community-based NGOs. AmeriCares takes on the role of a catalyst by conveying resources of different forms and amounts into viable projects in impoverished countries.

The devastating earthquake in Haiti in January 2010 highlights the evolving scope of services provided through AmeriCares. As the healthcare situation in Haiti transitioned from acute relief efforts to rebuilding a healthcare system that has the capacity to manage acute and chronic medical conditions, AmeriCares increased its

TABLE 7-1   Characteristics of Nongovernmental Organizations

Classification

Operational: design and implement relief efforts and/or development-related projects

Advocacy: defend or promote a specific cause

Alternative Terms

Private voluntary organization (PVO)

Non-state actor (NSA)

Grassroots organization

Transnational social movement organization

Community-based organization

Faith-based organization

Civil organization

Types

International NGO (e.g., Oxfam): INGO

Civil society organizations (faith-based, academia): CSO

Donor organized NGO (e.g., Amnesty International): DONGO

Environmental NGO (e.g., Greenpeace): ENGO

Government-operated NGO (e.g., Kenya Democracy Project): GONGO

Quasi-autonomous NGO (e.g., International Organization for Standardization): QUANGO

Grassroots organization (e.g., Idealist.org): GSO

Market advocacy NGO (e.g., ActionAid International, Care International): MANGO

Source: Data from World Bank. Criteria defining NGO. Available at: http://docs.lib.duke.edu/igo/guides/ngo/define.htm. Accessed February 2010.

commitment to the country from $15 million to $50 million in recognition of the tremendous health care needs and through the generous outpouring of support from donors, medical product manufacturers, and distributors. Like other well-funded NGOs, this NGO, which has both experienced headquarters staff and appropriate in-country staff, has the flexibility and community connections to expand and execute its programs quickly based on resources and need.[11]

Nongovernmental organizations have developed and expanded greatly since the advent of post–Cold War globalization. They have gained strength, popularity, and momentum. Thanks to their flexibility to respond rapidly to crises, including complex humanitarian situations, NGOs have solidified their role in the national and global emergency response network. In fact, their role and impact will likely continue to increase as the number of disasters continues to climb. According to the Centre of Research on the Epidemiology of Disasters, fewer than 50 disasters were reported in 1950. By 2008, that number had risen to approximately 450 disasters (see Figure 7-2). This near-exponential rise in the number of disasters over the past several decades

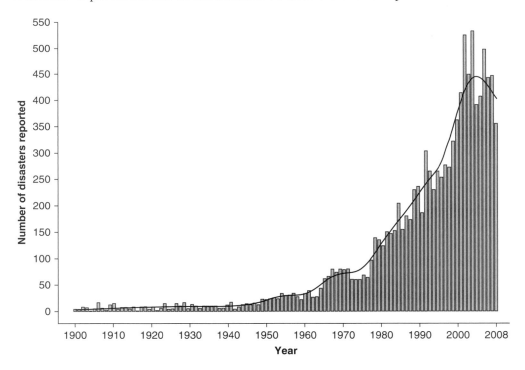

FIGURE 7-2   The Exponential Rise in Number of Disasters over the Past 50 Years
Source: From EM-DAT, The OFDA/CRED International Disaster Database, 2009.

pales when compared to the growth of NGOs during this same time period; their numbers increased from the thousands to more than 5 million.[12]

Advantages of NGOs include the facts that they are smaller than governmental organizations and that the vast majority are independent of direct government influence. With a less rigid hierarchy, significant flexibility, and more authority for field staff who need to adjust operations to a changing environment, NGOs' structure is more like that of businesses.

Although most NGOs are completely independent from governments, the relationship between the American Red Cross and the U.S. federal government is unique. The American Red Cross is an independent entity that is organized and exists as a nonprofit, tax-exempt, charitable institution pursuant to a charter granted to it by the U.S. Congress. Unlike other congressionally chartered organizations, the Red Cross maintains a special relationship with the federal government. It has the legal status of "a federal instrumentality,"[13] due to its charter requirements to carry out responsibilities delegated to it by the federal government including fulfilling provisions of the Geneva Conventions, blood banking, and maintaining a system of domestic and international disaster relief with mandated responsibilities under the National Response Plan coordinated by the Federal Emergency Management Agency (FEMA).

Code of Conduct

With the growing prominence of the nonprofit sector, NGO accountability has become an emerging issue of concern in recent years. NGOs need to be accountable to their internal stakeholders (e.g., staff, board of directors), donors, partners, beneficiaries, those entities that NGOs' activities affect (e.g., businesses, communities, government, other NGOs), and civil society at large. The nature of the various stakeholders involved and the degree of accountability to each stakeholder makes the issue of NGO accountability very complex and challenges NGOs to clarify and balance their responsibilities vis-à-vis their different stakeholders.

NGO accountability covers issues such as organizational management, project implementation, financial management, participation, and information disclosure, all of which have been addressed in various codes of conduct. In addition to setting core values and guiding principles, NGOs' codes of conduct typically provide for instituting strong oversight boards that are independent from management and establishing conflict of interest policies and whistleblower protection policies. Many organizations face major challenges related to implementing and maintaining these codes. As nonbinding and rather generic, loosely defined instruments, codes of conduct often remain ineffective because they do not include clear mechanisms for their implementation and compliance.[14] Transparency, accountability, and legitimacy are closely intertwined notions. The legitimacy of each NGO is tied to its accountability to its constituency and the public at large, the transparency of its processes, its adherence to its mission, and its effectiveness in fulfilling its mandate. Various tools have been developed to promote NGO accountability—namely, regulating instruments such as certification or rating systems, self-assessments, independent evaluations, financial and social audits, disclosure of financial statements, and annual reports and participation processes.

According to a 2006 UN dossier on NGO accountability, the legitimate authorities to which NGOs should be primarily accountable include those they affect who have less power.[15] The code of conduct for NGOs involved in disaster relief and other forms of humanitarian relief is not a single nonbinding doctrine or document, but rather includes several similar guidelines. For example, a code of conduct in disaster relief has been developed by the International Federation of Red Cross and Red Crescent Societies and the International Committee of the Red Cross and sponsored by numerous NGOs. Table 7-2 provides a 10-point summary of this code of conduct.[16]

Other standards guiding NGOs' activities include InterAction's *Private Voluntary Organization Standards*[17] and Sphere Project's *Minimum Standards in Disaster Response*.[18] The Sphere Project, which was funded by multiple donors and represents the most comprehensive review to date, resulted in a set of recommendations and programs to help ensure NGO work meets certain standards and complies with ethics considerations. The Sphere Project addresses key humanitarian issues including the imperative to provide services to those in need.

Funding

NGOs have multiple sources of funding including private donations, corporate donations (e.g., money, goods, services), grants, other NGOs, intergovernmental organizations (e.g., United Nations), bilateral or multilateral development organizations (e.g., USAID), and governments. Government funding is typically allocated in the form of "cost-recovery fees" to the NGO for participating in certain government programs (e.g., emergency housing, blood banking, immunizations). Large NGOs can have an annual budget in the hundreds of millions of dollars. For example, the American Red Cross has an annual budget of more than $4 billion, the International Committee of the Red Cross has an annual budget of approximately $235 million, and the American Association of Retired Persons (AARP) has an annual budget exceeding $575 million.

TABLE 7-2   Code of Conduct for NGOs in Disaster Relief

1. The first priority is the humanitarian imperative (the right to receive humanitarian assistance, unimpeded access to affected populations).

2. Aid is given regardless of race, creed, or nationality and is prioritized based on need alone.

3. Aid will not be used as a tool to support a particular political or religious standpoint.

4. NGOs will act independently of governments and not act as instruments of government foreign policy.

5. Culture, structures, and customs of communities and countries will be respected.

6. Disaster response will attempt to strengthen local capacities (staff, materials, companies, local NGOs), when possible.

7. Intended beneficiaries should be involved in the design, management, and implementation of assistance programs, when possible.

8. Relief efforts should not only meet basic needs but also should strive to reduce future vulnerabilities to disaster (mitigation).

9. NGOs will be accountable to their partners, both the populations who need assistance and the donors who wish to assist, in a responsible and transparent manner.

10. NGOs will recognize disaster victims as dignified people and not hopeless individuals in their organization's information, publicity, and advertising activities.

Source: Global Development Research Center. Available at http://www.gdrc.org/ngo/codesofconduct/ifrc-codeconduct.html. Accessed February 2010.

Although the term "nongovernmental" implies independence from governments, many large NGOs depend heavily on governments for financial support. Oxfam, a famine-relief organization, receives 25 percent of its donations from the British government and the European Union; World Vision collected $55 million worth of goods from the U.S. government; and Medecins sans Frontieres (MSF) receives more than 40 percent of its funding from governmental sources.[19] Despite its close relationship with the U.S. federal government, the American Red Cross does not receive federal funding on a regular basis to carry out its services and programs. Instead, it obtains its financial support in the form of voluntary public contributions and cost-recovery charges for some of its services, such as the provision of blood and blood products and health and safety training courses. Under limited circumstances, however, it sometimes becomes necessary for the American Red Cross to seek appropriations for certain programs when the funding requirements exceed those supported by the charitable public.

Funding and fundraising are critical to the success of any NGO. Although NGOs, especially those working in the relief and development areas, ideally should target those populations with the greatest needs, donors' wishes and government initiatives can certainly influence NGOs' program designs and project initiatives. Critics from all sides have suggested that because NGOs must rely on outside funding, they are, by their very nature, obligated to "serve the funding masters." Some argue that even if the charter of an NGO states its commitment to impartiality, it will feel obligated to provide services in accordance with the wishes of the funding source.

An excellent example of how funding can be used to influence the agenda of NGOs is the political drama that has played out over the last few decades regarding U.S. funding of NGOs that provide family planning services in other countries. In 1984, at the UN population conference in Mexico, then-President Ronald Reagan announced that the United States would not provide funds to any organization that so much as mentioned abortion-related services to its clients, even if the funds would not be used to fund such services. This policy became known as the "Mexico City Policy" or the "Global Gag Rule."[20] Many NGOs involved with women's health found that they had to choose between providing women with comprehensive family planning advice and receiving U.S. funding. The clear parallel between the U.S. domestic debates on reproductive rights and the affected funding of NGOs can be seen in the fact that the gag rule was reversed by President Bill Clinton, then reinstated by President George W. Bush, only to be reversed again by President Barack Obama in June 2009.

PREPAREDNESS, RESPONSE, AND RECOVERY

NGOs are involved in all levels of emergency public health response, yet their greatest contributions to date have come mostly in the areas of response and recovery. Planning, response, recovery, and mitigation are not linear processes with clear transitions from planning to recovery, and NGOs involved in crises can contribute simultaneously to the various phases in this "disaster cycle." In the United States, the integration of NGOs in planning and preparedness at local and state levels is not well defined, and this integration is only just beginning at the national level, based on the federal government's aftermath analysis and recommendations related to its response to Hurricane Katrina.[21] It is clear that NGO–government coordination is not adequate. While it is certainly acknowledged that NGOs are essential to emergency preparedness and response, there are still many unanswered questions about which roles they should play in these areas.

The aftermath of a major disaster is not simply the restoration of infrastructure such as roads, utilities, and buildings, but rather comprises a long process of restoring individual and community functioning. Human recovery includes restoring social and daily routines and support networks that foster physical and mental health and promote well-being.[22,23] In many instances, NGOs' activities remain on the periphery of the recovery efforts because policies to support essential recovery services and engage NGOs have not been formally incorporated into planning at state and local levels. Recovery is a very long process: It may take years to fully rebuild the infrastructure, and perhaps even longer to restore communities. For example, it is estimated that long-term recovery and reconstruction in the wake of Hurricane Katrina will take approximately 11 years given that the immediate recovery took 60 weeks.[24] Both government and private industry will need ongoing assistance from the NGO community to complete this recovery. InterAction, an alliance of more than 150 NGOs involved in disaster and humanitarian assistance, and the United Way (another NGO) are participating in long-term recovery committees that will engage NGOs in appropriate recovery efforts.

The response and recovery efforts provided by NGOs in crises are substantial— for example, totaling more than $3 billion in the aftermath of Hurricane Katrina and far more in relation to the Haiti earthquake of 2010. NGO efforts include everything from immediate services to both short- and long-term recovery services. These efforts may be focused on nutrition, housing, transportation, relocation, supply acquisition and distribution, restoring primary and secondary education, providing medical services for acute and chronic services, rebuilding components of the healthcare system, reuniting missing persons with their family and communities, and many other components of humanitarian recovery, including job recovery, reestablishing essential community services, and much needed financial assistance.

As with any crisis, ongoing dialogue must occur between the levels of government, community organizations, and NGOs to determine what the needs are and who will provide which services with how much funding and for how long. Development of a recovery-specific National Incident Management System (NIMS) could provide detailed parameters regarding how government and NGOs should coordinate recovery services and how those activities should be structured and financed. Ideally, this recovery-specific plan could include a defined model that operationalizes the phases of recovery; identifies target capabilities, key roles, and responsibilities for each phase; allows for coordination between phases; and provides fiscal support structures in the short and long terms. NGOs should be part of the design of such a recovery plan.

NGOs and Disasters

Disasters have been defined as a series of catastrophic events that overwhelm a community's capacity to respond adequately, resulting in threats to both the public health and the environment. Partnerships between the local authorities, governmental agencies, international organizations (e.g., UN), and NGOs are much needed to maximize coordination, avoid unnecessary redundancy, and reduce the waste of resources that have been witnessed many times in responses to disasters in the past. This multisector approach to disasters requires the transparent interaction of professionals among participating organizations.

For domestic disasters, the National Response Framework (NRF), which became effective in March 2008 and replaced the National Response Plan (NRP), establishes a comprehensive "all hazards" approach to enhance the ability of the United States to manage domestic incidents.[25] These incidents may include natural disasters, mass-casualty incidents, disease outbreaks, terrorism, and mass immigration. The NRF plan incorporates and integrates best practices and procedures into a unified structure from a variety of incident management disciplines, including homeland security, emergency management, law enforcement, firefighting, public works, public health, responder and recovery staff, health and safety staff, emergency medical services, and the private sector. It describes how the federal government should coordinate its activities with state, local, and tribal governments and the private sector, including NGOs, during incidents. The framework has been signed by 29 federal agencies, the American Red Cross, national voluntary organizations that are active in disaster response (i.e., NGOs), and the Corporation for National and Community Service.

Disaster response is organized under the Incident Command System (ICS) structure and NIMS, which allows for interoperability and compatibility among federal, state, and local capabilities. The NRF is an "all hazards" framework built on the template of the NIMS. NIMS was developed to enable responders from different jurisdictions and disciplines to work together more smoothly while responding to natural disasters and emergencies, including acts of terrorism.[26] Selective implementation through the activation of one or more of the NRF elements allows maximum flexibility to meet the unique operational and information-sharing requirements of any situation and enables effective interaction among various federal, state, local, tribal, private-sector, and other nongovernmental entities.

The NRF brings together a wealth of resources, including people, supplies, equipment, and funding. It organizes a response into 15 emergency support functions (ESFs), each of which is handled by a lead agency and various support agencies. Of the 15 ESFs, 3 functions highlight areas where the government and NGOs can work together: ESF 6 (mass care, housing, and human service), ESF 8 (public health and medical services), and ESF 14 (community recovery, mitigation, and economic stabilization). For example, the ESF 6 function is implemented by 17 federal agencies (including the Departments of Interior, Housing, Labor, Agriculture, and Treasury), one public–private partnership (Corporation for National and Community Service), and private voluntary organizations (i.e., NGOs), which are involved in response, recovery, and mitigation efforts. The American Red Cross functions as the primary NGO under ESF 6 in coordinating the use of federal mass-care resources in the context of incidents of national significance.

The typical cycle for an NGO in disaster response would be to do an initial assessment; agree, when possible, to respond with assistance; and develop a project design targeting beneficiaries. Fundraising, establishing agreements to work with local organizations including local NGOs, establishing field offices, and procuring materials are all key elements for success. Implementation, project monitoring, reporting, and evaluation are critical. As the immediate crisis subsides, some NGOs will leave the area, while others will stay and more NGOs will come to work on sustainable development programs. NGOs with established relationships in the disaster region have a unique advantage because they have firsthand observation and knowledge; understand the local environment and community organizations; have strong community ties; may have fluency with the dialect; know the local health and medical issues, religious practices, and clan and tribe relationships; and may have direct access to local leaders.

One of many examples of how NGOs can improve the disaster environment is by implementing a health surveillance system with the ultimate goal of reducing communicable disease transmission. NGOs provided essential services in the aftermath of the tsunami that hit Southeast Asia in December 2004. Sri Lanka was the second most severely hit country, suffering a partial or total destruction of all buildings located within 2 kilometers of the coastline in 13 of the 25 districts of the country. The number of casualties exceeded 31,000; more than 23,000 people were wounded, and there were more than 500,000 internally displaced persons (IDPs).

According to the World Health Organization (WHO), the risk for the spread of communicable disease was high in Sri Lanka in the aftermath of the tsunami, with threats including cholera, typhoid, shigellosis, hepatitis A, dengue fever, malaria, scrub typhus, leptospirosis, acute lower tract respiratory infections, measles, meningitis, and tuberculosis.[27] District health authorities from the public health department in the Eastern Province of Sri Lanka combined efforts with the Italian Red Cross and Oxfam to set up communicable disease surveillance. Outbreaks of scabies and acute hepatitis occurred. NGOs assisted local officials with surveillance, early identification, treatment, and isolation of infected individuals and community public health education. Implementation of rapid containment strategies successfully avoided the spread of communicable diseases in the many settings of poor personal hygiene. Additionally, coordination between the divisional health authorities and NGOs increased accountability and strengthened the relationship with the host country. This kind of "good governance," which works toward the reduction of the impact of disasters, can exist only where there is participation of the various stakeholders, including the vulnerable community, the state, the civil society, volunteers, NGOs, and other partners involved with relief and development.

NGOs and Complex Humanitarian Emergencies: War and Conflict

The term "complex humanitarian emergency" (CHE) refers to a humanitarian crisis where there is total breakdown of authority requiring international assistance that exceeds the capacity of any single agency. These situations typically occur in areas of war or internal civil conflict. Over the past 20 years, CHEs have occurred in many countries, including Bosnia, Afghanistan, Sudan, Rwanda, Uganda, the Palestinian Territories, and Ethiopia, to name a few.

The main entities involved in providing humanitarian assistance include UN agencies, NGOs, the various Red Cross organizations, governmental organizations, and donors. Minor players in these humanitarian emergencies include the military, academic and research institutions, private contractors, and the news media. Most of these entities are involved during the crisis and in the immediate post-crisis period; some play roles in the long process of post-conflict rehabilitation and recovery. Although the military is often visible in the reporting of these emergencies, their personnel are not involved in the majority of CHEs. When they do step in, they are typically involved only during the actual crisis and the immediate post-crisis period.

Principles guiding NGOs involved with emergency humanitarian action, as stated in the International Committee of the Red Cross's mission statement and upheld by the Geneva Convention, include humanity (saving lives and alleviating suffering wherever it is found), impartiality (implementation of actions solely on the basis of need), neutrality (not favoring any side in an armed conflict), and independence (the autonomy of humanitarian objectives from political, economic, military, or other objectives). The post–Cold War era during the final decades of the twentieth century brought high visibility to humanitarian assistance in areas of conflict. The nature of war changed considerably during this period, with more wars occurring within states than between states. More than 90 percent of casualties in these conflicts are civilians. Characteristics of these prolonged civil conflicts include poorly disciplined soldiers (militias), human rights abuses, high levels of violence and murder, mutilation, and lack of protection for civilians, refugees, and aid workers. Women and children are frequently victims of intimidation, and child soldiers are common. Humanitarian NGOs are active in addressing the consequences of these conflicts, including the disruption of social networks, malnutrition, population displacements of refugees and IPDs (80 percent of whom are women and children), disruption of public health and essential health services, and disruption and destruction of vital infrastructure.

Over the past 30 years, NGOs have played a significant role in providing humanitarian relief to the affected populations and supporting sustainable recovery following these kinds of conflicts. NGOs typically focus on key sectors including health care, shelter, food and nutrition, water and sanitation, and security and protection. Loretz identifies four areas where NGOs apply themselves to war and conflict:[29]

- To mitigate the consequences of armed conflict (the breakdown of public health and health infrastructure including health services, sanitation facilities, and food and shelter) by providing immediate delivery of relief assistance and more delayed sustainable project development
- To research the effects of war
- To educate the public and decision makers about the impact of war on health and the environment
- To advocate for changes in global attitudes and policies toward war

Additionally, NGOs may play a role in direct conflict resolution and provide assistance in monitoring elections. NGO humanitarian assistance is often the major means for populations in conflict areas to sustain themselves.[30]

Health as a Bridge for Peace (HBP) is a multidimensional policy and planning framework that supports health workers in delivering health programs in conflict and post-conflict situations and, at the same time, contributes to peace building.[31] It is defined as the integration of peace-building concerns, concepts, principles, strategies, and practices into health relief and health-sector development. NGOs, with their non-governmental and non-military affiliations in conflict zones, are optimal champions of the concept of health and relief services as one component of achieving peace. The HBP framework was formally accepted by the 51st World Health Assembly in May

1998 as a feature of the "Health for All in the 21st Century" strategy. In achieving the primary goal of health for societies prone to and affected by war, health professionals recognize their responsibilities to create opportunities for peace. In the last three decades, the tie between health and peace has found expression through a series of different players. During the years of the war in El Salvador, for example, UNICEF repeatedly organized temporary ceasefires to allow vaccinations and essential public health services for children.[31]

Despite the often critical role that NGOs play in maintaining the safety of populations in war areas, they are not governed by the same uniform code of ethics that govern military personnel in regard to their dealings with noncombatants. In one notable case, the failure of adequate and effective NGO relief efforts in Goma, Democratic Republic of Congo, resulted in thousands of unnecessary deaths and led to several major reviews of humanitarian NGOs' conduct. The most comprehensive of these reviews was the Sphere Project, which was funded by multiple donors and resulted in a set of recommendations and programs to help ensure NGOs abide by work standards and ethics. The Sphere Project addresses humanitarian issues and provides training to NGO personnel in the protection of human rights and the desire to denounce those who violate them as well as the humanitarian imperative to provide services for those in need. Accordingly, a humanitarian charter was promulgated that calls upon agencies to recognize the right to life with dignity, the distinction between combatants and noncombatants and the principle of nonrefoulment (protection of refugees from returning to areas where there lives and well-being are threatened). These issues are based on aspects of international humanitarian law embodied in the Geneva Convention and two additional protocols (A and B) established in 1977.[32]

Numerous NGOs have become involved in CHEs, including such well-recognized NGOs as Medecins sans Frontieres, Physicians for Human Rights, International Medical Core, CARE, Oxfam, Save the Children, and International Physicians for the Prevention of Nuclear War. All of these groups are actively involved in conflict zones and/or participate in advocacy against conflict.

- CARE was founded after World War II. It provides emergency aid to survivors as part of emergency relief efforts that are complemented by post-conflict rehabilitation and capacity-building programs focusing on basic structures for health, nutrition, and sanitation.[34]
- International Medical Corps is a humanitarian NGO established by physicians and nurses in 1984 to provide primary and mental health care, nutritional ser-

vices, and emergency relief. It is engaged in healthcare training and capacity-building activities in 40 countries affected by war, poverty, and disaster.[35]

- Medecins sans Frontieres is an NGO formed by physicians, who refuse to be co-opted by governments, that delivers healthcare services to endangered populations. Their volunteerism and life-saving efforts were major factors in MSF's winning the Nobel Prize for Peace in 1999.[36]
- The International Committee of the Red Cross (ICRC), founded in 1860, delivers assistance based on need in areas of conflict, maintains neutrality, and provides medical access to both sides of the conflict, allowing ICRC to cross sides without harm and without payment. The ICRC assumes guaranteed protection from aggression when carrying out its work, which is supported by international treaties.[37]
- Save the Children is a global federation of more than 100 organizations that operate in more than 100 countries and has programs to help war-affected children to meet the United Nations' Millennium Development Goals. Save the Children promotes the concept of schools as zones of peace, reintegration of child soldiers into society, and preventing forced recruitment.[38]

Challenges Facing NGOs

A number of challenges face NGOs that become involved with public health emergencies. As an overarching mandate, their goal is to provide the most appropriate services or supplies to the people with the greatest need at the right time. This is a laudable goal, but one that is often difficult to achieve in practice. Effective emergency response requires access at multiple levels:

- Access to the best available information about the crisis (populations affected by the crisis, coordinated response plan, governmental response plan, NGO response)
- Access to the vulnerable populations
- Access to the appropriate supplies
- Access to adequate funding

Given that accurate information about a crisis situation is often limited initially and the NGOs have a mandate to respond based on both their charter and the expectations of their funders, their response will inevitably involve some degree of duplication of services, wasted resources, and inappropriate allocation of resources and personnel. Additionally, NGOs may overcommit their resources and overextend their capacity to the detriment of the relief efforts. In some cases, the response may be so focused on immediate relief efforts that sustainable development is hampered.

Another challenge for NGOs involved in relief and development is their struggle between the functionalist ideals of sending aid where it is needed most (independent of the influence of political agendas) and the realist considerations of focusing on projects where there may be political will and funding opportunities to address the issues at hand. Some evidence suggests that an NGO's funding sources and the willingness of intended recipient governments to accept aid significantly affect the NGO's level of response in instances of humanitarian crisis.[38] Conversely, strong negative political sentiment coupled with difficult access to certain populations in need may discourage or dampen an NGO response. Labonte refers to a "humanitarian marketplace" in which both donors and NGOs care more about the bottom line of delivery than their stated mission to deliver aid to the most vulnerable populations.[39] Competition among relief organizations to respond quickly can lead to greater waste and inappropriate allocation of scarce resources. In the worst-case scenario, such as in the setting of complex humanitarian emergencies, an ill-planned donor response can aggravate a fragile situation, exacerbate conflict, and magnify the crisis.[40]

The common practice of staffing field operations with expatriate staff is always a sensitive and challenging issue. NGOs are responsible to their charter, their board of directors, their funders, and the recipient clients for delivering services in the most effective way. Having key program personnel from the home base working in the field allows NGOs to monitor and account for delivery of these essential services to the target population. It is justifiable to use expatriate staff in the formative stages of the project, when communities may be more receptive to initiatives by expatriate "authorities," to build the confidence of the donor in the short term and when local skills are not available. But as the NGO's involvement matures from a focus on relief to a focus on development, the principles of grassroots development—such as participation, capacity building, and sustainable approaches with local partners—require different forms of management. Part of the management goal is to shift field management operations to local staff and ultimately give local management personnel overall control of field operations. While it may have been the case that local skills were not available a few years ago, it is no longer a reasonable argument[41] and local recruitment efforts should be able to identify capable individuals. Although expatriates may be good at ensuring accountability to donors, reports in the literature indicate that expatriate staff are expensive, have a high turnover, require a higher standard of living, undervalue local staff knowledge, have limited cultural awareness, may not be effective in actually transferring skills to local managers, and are not as effective at building community links.[42]

MITIGATION

Mitigation can be defined as any action taken before, during, or after a public health emergency to minimize its impact or potential impact. Mitigation activities range from physical measures, such as flood defenses or building reinforcements, to non-structural measures, such as mitigation and preparedness training, land-use regulation, legislation, public awareness raising, and capacity building, especially with the most vulnerable populations.

There are two main reasons why NGOs should become involved in public health emergency mitigation and preparedness. First, emergencies triggered by natural hazards (e.g., cyclones, droughts, earthquakes, and floods) pose a major threat to sustainable development. During these incidents, communities and regions may experience significant structural and environmental damage; disruption of businesses, schools, and community activities; and relocation of community members vital to the re-building of the area. Second, poor and socially disadvantaged people, whom NGOs support through their development programs, are usually the most vulnerable to such disasters.[43] For example, Hurricane Mitch in October 1998 was particularly significant in its massive impact on Central America's development, including 9,200 lives lost and economic losses totaling $5 billion.[44] As in most disasters, the socially disadvantaged population suffered the greatest impact.

Overall, research shows that a focus on disaster mitigation has not become fully established as a part of NGO activities—either those involved in relief efforts or those focused on sustainable development, or both.[45] Thinking about disasters and vulnerability is beginning to penetrate NGO consciousness at the policy level, but these concepts are not being translated to the operational level, where disaster risk-reduction activity tends to be sporadic, poorly integrated with development planning, and largely unsupported by institutional structures and systems. While external barriers to mainstreaming disaster mitigation exist in NGOs—in particular, limited interest among donors—some of the problem is internal and reflects limited understanding and limited time to embark on new initiatives. When a series of 60 relief and development NGOs were examined, only 3 were found to have formal preparedness and mitigation policies.[46]

At the country project level, there is a lack of hazard risk assessment in NGO program plans. Most NGOs' operational and funding guidelines have little to say about disaster mitigation preparedness and provide only limited practical guidance on planning and implementing projects. Program officers have considerable leeway in applying guidelines, thereby making them influential players within NGOs, especially development NGOs. They may also have great influence over the development of country plans, project approval, and, in some cases, choice of local partners. In a study that conducted semi-structured interviews among program officers in these NGOs, researchers found that these officers could play a major role in promoting disaster mitigation, but they typically have very heavy workloads and are generally too busy with their ongoing concerns to integrate the concepts of mitigation.

In the development NGO community, there has been a shift in attitude away from the old view of disasters as one-off events and toward an awareness that development processes can influence the impact of disasters. Emergency units and advisory teams have grown in both the relief and development areas. The concept of risk-hazard analysis and risk reduction is becoming increasingly less marginalized to the emergency relief arena, and development departments are becoming more comfortable with incorporating mitigation into sustainable action plans aimed at creating greater community resilience for the next crises.[46]

CASE STUDY ANALYSIS

Hurricane Katrina changed the landscape in terms of the involvement of voluntary organizations, NGOs, and the private sector in disaster response. The immense size of the area struck by the hurricane required resources and capabilities beyond the usual government programs. The massive evacuation in advance of the hurricane created an extraordinary demand for shelters, medicine, food, and temporary housing. Katrina proved to be a "perfect storm"—one that was exacerbated by a lack of preparation, timely coordination, and response by local, state, and federal governments. The devastation of this event, coupled with the 24-hour media coverage of the ongoing disaster, spurred NGOs, including international NGOs, to respond quickly to the area. By most official accounts, nonprofits and NGOs played a substantial relief role in response to Katrina. In many areas hit by this disaster, NGOs provided the quickest relief.

NGO response to this disaster had many components. Relief efforts at the administrative level included coordinating agencies, transportation agents, freight forwarders, health personnel, food allocation, fundraising and budgeting, and volunteer service coordination. Housing, food, essential public health and health services, location of missing persons, and relocating families and communities were merely some of the myriad services provided by NGOs. As important as their specific relief efforts were, NGOs also put a compassionate face on disaster relief. Where the U.S. government failed administratively, NGOs filled the gaps.

The number of volunteer, nonprofit, faith-based, and private-sector entities that aided in the Hurricane Katrina relief effort was truly extraordinary. Nearly every national, regional, and local charitable organization in the United States, and many from abroad, contributed aid to the victims of the storm. Trained volunteers from member organizations of the National Volunteer Organizations Active in Disaster (NVOAD), the American Red Cross, Medical Reserve Corps (MRC), and Community Emergency Response Team (CERT), as well as untrained volunteers from across the United States, deployed to Louisiana, Mississippi, and Alabama.

Faith-based organizations also provided extraordinary services. For example, more than 9,000 Southern Baptist Convention of the North American Mission Board volunteers from 41 states served in Texas, Louisiana, Mississippi, Alabama, and Georgia. These volunteers ran mobile kitchens and recovery sites. Many smaller, faith-based organizations, such as the Set Free Indeed Ministry in Baton Rouge, Louisiana, brought comfort and offered shelter to the survivors. They used their facilities and volunteers to distribute donated supplies to displaced persons and to meet their immediate needs. Another NGO, the National Center for Missing and Exploited Children, helped successfully reunite more than 5,000 children with their families.

While providing relief in New Orleans, NGOs reported numerous problems in their interactions with government officials. Government officials did not know where they needed help, which resources were available, and which resources were scarce, and they delayed in communicating important information to the NGOs. Unfortunately, there was not a formal governmental plan for integrating NGOs, volunteer organizations, and private industry into the overall disaster response effort, so duplication of services and ineffective use of these much-needed resources occurred. More often than not, NGOs successfully contributed to the relief effort despite the government-imposed obstacles and with almost no government support or direction. Time and again, government agencies failed to effectively coordinate relief operations with NGOs. Often, government agencies failed to match relief needs with NGO and private-sector capabilities. Even when agencies matched nongovernmental aid with an identified need, there were problems moving goods, equipment, and people into the disaster area. For example, the government relief effort was unprepared to meet the fundamental food, housing, and operational needs of the surge volunteer force.

The destruction from Hurricane Katrina was so significant and the initial government response so inadequate that a number of large international NGOs violated their own charters and made the unprecedented decision to respond with aid within the

United States. Oxfam America, for example, stated that responding to Katrina was a major shift in its organizational policy.[47] The International Rescue Committee's president stated that IRC responded at the request of the Baton Rouge Area Foundation (the largest community foundation in Louisiana), which said that the hurricane was a "Banda Aceh–type" crisis, and it wanted an NGO experienced in responding to that type of disaster situation. At least four other international NGOs were contacted by local organizations in the devastated area to ask for the help that they were not getting from government agencies or the American Red Cross. Multiple international NGOs responded to Katrina in the area of emergency health and public health assistance (see Table 7-3).[47]

The long-term recovery from Katrina is far from over. In Louisiana, 70,000 persons are still displaced and 4,800 residents remain in FEMA trailers. Daily routines and community activities continue to be disrupted in some of the affected areas. The

TABLE 7-3   Examples of NGOs Providing Emergency Public Health and Essential Health Disaster Relief for the First Time in the United States During Hurricane Katrina

NGO	Focus
American Refugee Committee	Health care, shelter repair, legal aid, community development services, repatriation assistance
CARE USA	Women's needs, sanitation, environmental protection, emergency relief
Interchurch Medical Assistance	Emergency aid, health, and development
International Medical Corps	Primary health care, women's health, disaster response, AIDS, mental health
Islamic Relief	Education, training, sanitation, income generation, orphan support, nutrition, emergency relief
Jewish Health Care International	Health care, immigrant health, disaster response
Project HOPE	Infectious disease, women's and children's health, health professional education, humanitarian assistance
Save the Children	Economic opportunities, education, emergencies and protection, health
U.S. Fund for UNICEF	Early childhood development, immunization and malnutrition, girls' education, child protection, HIV/AIDS
World Relief	Disaster response, maternal and child health

Source: Eikenberry A, Arroyave V, Cooper T. Administrative failure and the international NGO response to Hurricane Katrina. *Public Administration Review.* 2007;12:160–170.

resulting decline over time in relationships between residents and community organizations has fueled the long-term psychological impact of the disaster. More than 5 years have passed since the hurricane, and recovery continues. It is estimated that it will take more than 11 years for the region to fully recover from this disaster. There remains a lack of adequate resources and expertise (governmental and nongovernmental) to cover longer-term complex services such as job training, child care, substance abuse treatment, and rehabilitations services. NGOs will be part of this human recovery, and NGOs' roles in this endeavor must be better defined and supported by state and federal policy.

CONCLUSION

Nongovernmental organizations represent a very diverse group of organizations, none of which permits any participation or representation of any government as part of its operations. In the area of emergency public health crises, such as disasters and humanitarian emergencies, NGOs tend to be involved in operational activities focusing on relief efforts or sustainable development, or both. Globalization has helped fuel the rise of NGOs, and many have been formed to address social issues that could not be adequately addressed by local, regional, or national governments.

Advantages of NGOs are that they are much smaller than governmental organizations, have a less rigid hierarchy, possess significant flexibility, and confer more authority on field staff so that they can respond to a changing environment. In the areas of relief, humanitarian assistance, and sustainable development, NGOs face many challenges in providing the most appropriate services to the populations in need. These challenges include responding rapidly in an environment typically characterized by limited data, satisfying funders, working with other NGOs in a noncompetitive manner, accessing vulnerable populations, reducing waste and duplication of services, meeting community commitments, and maximizing the presence of local field staff to enhance capacity building and sustainable development. Although there are no binding codes of conduct regulating NGOs, self-regulation should occur and be based on such codes and standards as the Red Cross and Crescent's code of conduct, InterAction's private voluntary organization standards, and the Sphere Project's minimum standards in disaster response.

NGOs depend on funding that may come from a variety of sources, including private donations, corporate sponsors, grants, other NGOs, development organizations, and governments. Ideally, funding should be directed toward well-designed initiatives aimed at the most appropriate beneficiaries and the funding source should not dictate the scope and activities of the NGO's programs.

NGOs play an important role in providing key services in both disasters and complex humanitarian emergencies. Because they provide important services during a multifaceted response by governments, local authorities, international agencies and organizations, and private industry, NGOs must communicate and collaborate with all parties to ensure best use of resources and optimal outcomes with relief and sustainable development initiatives. As part of their essential role in these events, NGOs must continue to advocate for response, recovery, and mitigation efforts for the most vulnerable populations.

INTERNET RESOURCES

AlertNet, *Alerting Humanitarians to Emergencies:* http://www.alertnet.org

NGO Watch: http://www.globalgovernancewatch.org/ngo_watch/

International Strategy for Disaster Reduction (ISDR): http://www.unisdr.org

Prevention Web: http://www.preventionweb.net

Relief Web: http://www.reliefweb.int

Sphere Project, Humanitarian Charter and Minimum Standards in Disaster Response: http://www.sphereproject.org/

United Nations, Department of Economic and Social Affairs NGO Branch: http://www.un.org/esa/coordination/ngo/

World Health Organization, Global Health Workforce Alliance: http://www.who.int/workforcealliance/en/

NOTES

1. Edwards M, Hulme D (eds.). *Nongovernmental organizations: Performance and accountability: Beyond the magic bullet.* London: Earthscan; 1995.
2. Willetts P. What is a nongovernmental organization. In *UNESCO encyclopaedia of life support systems: Section 1. Institutional and infrastructure resource issues.* Available at: http://www.staff.city.ac.uk/p.willetts/CS-NTWKS/NGO-ART.HTM. Accessed February 2010.
3. Smith, S. Rebuilding social welfare services after Katrina: Challenges and opportunities. In Boris E, Steuerle E (eds.), *After Katrina: Public expectation and charities' response.* Washington, DC: Urban Institute. Available at: http://www.urban.org/url. Accessed February 2010.
4. Davies TR. The rise and fall of transnational civil society: The evolution of international nongovernmental organizations since 1939. In Charnovitz S, *Two centuries of participation: NGOs and international governance. Michigan Journal of International Law.* Winter 1997.
5. Davies TR. The Possibilities of transnational activism: The campaign for disarmament between the two world wars. In Charnovitz S, *Two centuries of participation: NGOs and international governance. Michigan Journal of International Law.* Winter 1997.

6. Charter of the United Nations: Chapter X. Available at: http://www.un.org/aboutun/charter/chapt10.htm. Accessed February 2010.

7. Consultative relationship between the United Nations and nongovernmental organizations. Available at: http://www.un.org/documents/ecosoc/res/1996/eres1996-31.htm. Accessed February 2010.

8. Agenda 21: Chapter 27. Strengthening the role of nongovernmental organizations: partners for sustainable development, Earth Summit, 1992. Available at: http://habitat.igc.org/agenda21/a21-27.htm. Accessed February 2010.

9. Anheier H. *Nonprofit organizations: Theory, management, policy*. New York: Routledge; 2005.

10. World Bank. Criteria defining NGO. Available at: http://docs.lib.duke.edu/igo/guides/ngo/define.htm. Accessed February 2010.

11. AmeriCares. Mission and activities. Available at: http://www.americares.org/whatwedo/model.html. Accessed February 2010.

12. Simon M, Stone D (eds.). *Global knowledge networks and international development: Bridges across boundaries*. New York: Routledge; 2005, pp. 104–121.

13. Congressional Charter of the American National Red Cross. Available at: http://www.redcross.org/www-files/Documents/Governance/charter.pdf. Accessed February 2010.

14. Edwards M, Hulme D (eds.). *Nongovernmental organizations: Performance and accountability: Beyond the magic bullet*. London: Earthscan; 1995, pp. 54–74.

15. The NGO accountability debate. Available at: http://www.un-ngls.org/IMG/pdf/launch_report_pdf.pdf. Accessed February 2010.

16. Code of conduct for NGOs in disaster relief. Available at: http://www.gdrc.org/ngo/codesofconduct/ifrc-codeconduct.html. Accessed February 2010.

17. InterAction's PVO standards. Available at: http://www.interaction.org/document/interactions-pvo-standards. Accessed February 2010.

18. Sphere Project's humanitarian charter and minimum standards in disaster response. Available at: http://www.savethechildren.org/publications/technical-resources/emergency-health-and-nutrition/general/The-Sphere-Project-Handbook.pdf. Accessed February 2010.

19. Edwards M, Hulme D. Too close for comfort? The impact of official aid on nongovernmental organizations. *World Development*. 1996;24(6):961–973.

20. Mexico City policy. Available at: http://www.usaid.gov/press/releases/2009/pr090126.html. Accessed February 2010.

21. The federal response to Hurricane Katrina: Lessons learned. 2006, pp. 51–63. Available at: http://library.stmarytx.edu/acadlib/edocs/katrinawh.pdf. Accessed February 2010.

22. Waugh R, Barbee J, et al. Mental health and recovery in the Gold Coast after Hurricanes Katrina and Rita. *Journal of the American Medical Association*. 2006;296(5):585–588.

23. Kessler R, Galea S, Gruber N, et al. Trends in mental illness and suicidality after Hurricane Katrina. *Molecular Psychiatry*. 2008;13(4):374–384.

24. Cutter S, Emrich C, et al. The long road home: Race, class and recovery from Hurricane Katrina. *Environment: Science and Policy for Sustainable Development*. 2006;48(2):8–20.

25. National Response Framework. 2008. Available at: http://www.dhs.gov/files/programs/editorial_0566.shtm. Accessed February 2010.

26. National Incident Management System. 2008. Available at: http://www.fema.gov/pdf/emergency/nims/NIMS_core.pdf. Accessed February 2010.

27. World Health Organization. Situational report on Sri Lanka. Available at: http://www.who
    .int/hac/crises/lka/en/. Accessed February 2010.

28. Anderson M. *Humanitarian NGOs in conflict intervention: Managing global chaos.* Washington,
    DC: U.S. Institute of Peace; 1990.

29. Baeryswil E. ICRC experience in Kosovo. *Refugee Survey Quarterly.* 2001;20:130–134.

30. Gutlove P. *Health as a Bridge for Peace: Briefing manual.* Cambridge, MA: Institute for Resource
    and Security Studies; 2000. Available at: http://irss-usa.org/pages/documents/HBPbriefmanual
    .pdf.

31. Children as Zones of Peace. Available at: http://www.unicef.org/sowc96/14zones.htm. Ac-
    cessed February 2010.

32. Waldman R. The roles of humanitarian assistance organizations. In Levy B, Sidel V (eds.), *War
    and public health,* 2nd ed. New York: Oxford University Press; 2008, pp. 369–380.

33. CARE. Available at: http://www.care.org/. Accessed February 2010.

34. International Medical Corps. Available at: http://www.imcworldwide.org. Accessed February
    2010.

35. Medecins sans Frontieres. Available at: http://www.msf.org/. Accessed February 2010.

36. International Red Cross. Available at: http://www.ifrc.org. Accessed February 2010.

37. Save the Children. Available at: http://www.savethechildren.org. Accessed February 2010.

38. White J, Darville S. Where to help: An analysis of NGO response to humanitarian crises. All
    Academic Research; 2006. Presented at the Annual Midwest Political Science Association
    National Conference, Chicago, IL, April 2006.

39. Labonte MT. How universal? Principles of humanitarian action and NGO realities. Paper pre-
    pared for the 2005 Annual Meeting of the International Studies Association, Honolulu, HI, and
    the panel entitled, "Universality: Is It in Jeopardy?"; 2005.

40. Minear L. Humanitarian aid and intervention: The challenges of integration. Informing the
    integration debate with recent experience. *Ethics and International Affairs.* 2004;18(2):53–59.

41. Mukasa S. Are expatriate staff necessary in international development NGOs? A case study of
    an international NGO in Uganda. *CVO International Working Paper.* 2008;4.

42. Dichter T. Issues critical to a shift in responsibilities between US PVOs and Southern NGOs.
    Washington, DC: USAID; 1989.

43. Blaikie P, Cannon T, Davis I, Wisner B. *At risk: Natural hazards, people's vulnerability and disas-
    ters.* London: Routledge, 1994.

44. Munich R. Annual review of natural catastrophes. Munich Reinsurance; 1998.

45. Twigg J, Steiner D, Myers M, Benson C. NGO natural disaster mitigation and preparedness
    projects: A study of international development and relief NGOs based in the UK. 2000.
    Available at: www.redcross.org.uk/dmp.

46. Twigg J, Steiner D. Mainstreaming disaster mitigation: Challenges to organizational learning
    in NGOs. *Development in Practice.* 2002;8(12):473–480.

47. Eikenberry A, Arroyave V, Cooper T. Administrative failure and the international NGO
    response to Hurricane Katrina. *Public Administration Review.* 2007;12:160–170.

CHAPTER 8

Technology and Public Health Crises

Ali Pourmand and Janelle Rios

INTRODUCTION

Technology—a word derived from the Greek *technología*, meaning the "study" of "craft"—encompasses a broad spectrum of machines, techniques, and systems. These generally include communications, information technology,[1] clinical diagnostics and imaging systems, laboratory systems, biosurveillance, patient tracking technology, computerized physician order entry systems, and geographic information systems (GIS).

Information technology (IT)—including computers, networking systems, and mobile devices—is rapidly coming to influence every aspect of public health and medical practice.[2] The recent innovations and advances in this field such as mobile devices and wireless technology can strengthen and support public health professionals in all aspects of public health emergencies. For example, by utilizing various modeling programs for natural events such as hurricanes or earthquakes, IT can help planners and responders focus on available resources in the preparedness for, response to, and recovery from such large-scale emergencies.

Information technology has made enormous strides in the past three decades. This development would not have been possible without ongoing innovations in microprocessing and handheld devices. When compared with the 1989 Loma Prieta, California, earthquake, the 2010 Haiti earthquake vividly shows us how advances in IT can affect preparedness, response, and mitigation. Many of the response improvements can easily be attributed to the variety of laptops, mobile devices, networking protocols, and wireless communications now available to public health professionals and medical providers.

Emergency management is the combination of knowledge, skills, and abilities to manage a complex response effectively within organizations and between organizations, at a local, regional, national, and even international level. Emergency management is defined by basic principles and stages such as prevention, preparedness, response, and mitigation. Emergency information systems gather data regarding an emergency during the multiple stages through which it unfolds; this information then plays a critical role in facilitating effective emergency management. Emergency information systems are characterized by a complex interaction among various components of computer hardware, software, handheld devices, and mobile phones for the data collection, transfer, and retrieval of information.[3]

Case Study

On August 23, 2005, Hurricane Katrina began as a tropical depression. Two days later, it made landfall in Florida as a Category 1 hurricane. Over the next 48 hours, the storm grew in intensity, achieving its maximum strength as a Category 5 hurricane on August 26. The National Weather Service and the National Hurricane Center predicted that it would make landfall for a second time along the coasts of Louisiana and Mississippi, causing extensive damage. Utilizing a disaster database and prediction models, New Orleans and surrounding areas were thought to be the most vulnerable regions. Based on this information and at the request of Louisiana Governor Kathleen Blanco, a national emergency was declared by President George W. Bush. National Guard troops were deployed and an unprecedented amount of water and food was positioned throughout the areas.[4] Despite days of advanced warning, one of the most extensive mandatory evacuations of a major city was ordered only 19 hours prior to the hurricane's landfall.

On August 29, 2005, Hurricane Katrina struck land near Buras-Triumph, Louisiana, as a Category 3 hurricane, with winds up to 125 miles per hour, and traveled along a path approximately 120 miles wide.[5] It crossed through southeastern Louisiana and maintained Category 3 force winds into Mississippi. The magnitude of the storm, coupled with an inadequate response, contributed to massive destruction and loss of human life. Katrina is now recognized as one of the top five deadliest storms in the history of the United States, causing more than 1,000 storm-related deaths. The destruction and loss of life were most vivid in New Orleans, where several portions of the city are below sea level and more than 80 percent of the city flooded. The Army Corps of Engineers had predicted that the levees that protected the areas below sea level of the city would not survive a direct blow from a hurricane, and they did not.

Over the days following Hurricane Katrina, public health and rescue personnel faced tremendous challenges. Communication networks failed, transportation routes proved difficult to navigate, and health information transfer was impossible. In fact, simply locating survivors was nearly impossible in the face of flooded streets and destroyed road signs. Although technology provided significant benefits in the planning and response to Katrina, better use of technological advances could have better aided in the preparation and response to the many challenges posed by Hurricane Katrina.

HISTORICAL PERSPECTIVES

The history of information processing started more than 5,000 years ago, when Abacus invented a counting device that was used for solving arithmetical problems in the days before calculators and computers. Later, the first calculator was reported in Egypt in the thirteenth century. More than 800 years of human development passed until the creation of personal computers, laptops, mobile devices, routers, hubs, satellites, and other devices that have made a tremendous impact on IT and its application.

Comparing the Hurricane Katrina incident with the 2010 Haiti earthquake allows us to see how information systems have changed during the last five years. Hurricane Katrina made landfall on August 29, 2005. The federal officials deployed their plan 3 days earlier but were unable to provide the testing mission for 3 weeks.[6] The Haiti earthquake, which was not preceded by any warning signs, occurred January 12, 2010. The critical coordination centers, landlines, and a satellite telecommunications system were disrupted. It took 2 days to restore Haiti's cellular communication and install 40 satellite terminals for basic communications, with a short-term plan to deploy 60 other terminals to facilitate broadband connections. Technology also facilitated donations to this devastated area: Cellular-phone users donated tens of millions of dollars just through text messaging within the first week following the event.[7]

In the last few years, emergency response and crisis management have greatly benefited from major investments in sophisticated information technology. Recent deliberate emergencies, such as the terrorist attacks on the World Trade Center and Pentagon in 2001, and natural public health crises, such as Hurricane Katrina, have shown that modern society is still far from being able to make rapid, adequate responses to major public health emergencies. As a consequence of these and other devastating events, significant efforts are now being made to design various emergency information systems that can support and improve the outcomes at multiple organizational levels and interorganizational levels. Such initiatives are being developed for all jurisdictions of government, including municipal, state, and federal levels. Independent of the scale of the emergency or crisis, these systems are designed to provide improved situational awareness and improved coordination and information sharing so as to support actions by a range of emergency responders. To accomplish such a task, information systems must address the needs within strategic emergency management organizations as well as provide support for the time-critical work being conducted by the first responders.

Public Health Informatics

Public health informatics is the application of computer science and information technology to public health. It is a field that studies how to best utilize resources and that develops technology to optimize the storage, retrieval, and use of information in the public health arena. Public health informatics has been formally defined as "the systematic application of information and computer science and technology to public health practice, research, and learning."[8]

Information and communication technology play important roles when public health practice attempts to overcome the limitations of time and distance to communicate, exchange information, analyze data, and facilitate teamwork. The application of technology creates changes and challenges within organizations. It also plays a critical role in improving communication and crisis management in multiple ways: decision making, knowledge management, coordination, and optimal utilization of resources.[9]

Different technologies assist public health professionals during emergencies. For example, telecommunication is technology that is used to establish communication over a distance, whereas information technology is used to store, process, and analyze data entered into the system. The convergence of telecommunication and information technology has resulted in information and communication technology (ICT)—a general term used to describe a large number of different technologies and their applications. ICT is employed in various emergency management information systems that provide strategic support to public health organizations during crises.[10]

IT has brought new challenges to public health communication, such as the need to provide an IT structure for emergency crisis management and the need to design information systems that support emergency crisis management. The ambiguity and unpredictable nature of disasters make designing information systems geared toward these incidents difficult. However, failure to design a robust infrastructure can ultimately affect the functionality of IT systems in crisis management during public health emergencies.

PREPAREDNESS

The public health objectives in emergencies have multiple components that aim to decrease unnecessary morbidity and mortality as well as create an infrastructure to minimize the future impact of these crises.[11] The first step is to recognize the parameters of the public health emergency and to make accurate predictions of public health threats. These predictions are possible only if the responders have immediate access to previously collected pre-emergency data for the affected area. The collection of such information will give the public health professionals an opportunity to prepare for the public health hazards efficiently and effectively.[12] Public health information systems include the ability to collect and exchange epidemiological information. During the preparedness stage, these systems include those supporting biosurveillance, outbreak management, electronic laboratory reporting, and health information exchange.

Biosurveillance

Biosurveillance is an epidemiologic practice that utilizes information systems to monitor selected health data and provides appropriate analysis and interpretation so as to provide an early warning of potential health threats, early detection of health events, and awareness of patterns of disease progression.[13] According to Wagner et al., biosurveillance is "a process that detects disease . . . and characterizes outbreaks of disease" by systematically collecting and analyzing data.[14] In the United States, the Centers for Disease Control and Prevention (CDC) has had a nationwide program to improve sharing of information among local, state, and federal agencies in place since late 2007. BioSense is a real-time biosurveillance tool that can identify, track, and manage signs and symptoms of potential disease outbreaks using data transmission, data analysis, data reporting, and public health response. This program was initially created as a Web-based program to facilitate access by local or state health departments and the federal government.[15]

An important component of biosurveillance is syndromic surveillance, defined by the International Society for Disease Surveillance (ISDS) as the "ongoing, systematic collection, analysis, and interpretation of health-related data essential to the planning, implementation, and evaluation of public health practice, [and] closely integrated with the timely dissemination of these data to those responsible for the prevention and control of diseases, injuries, and other health problems."[16] The goal of syndromic surveillance is the *early* detection of outbreaks, *before* disease is confirmed, so that response efforts can be mobilized.[17] With this goal in mind, several syndromic surveillance systems are in use around the United States, including the Electronic Surveillance System for the Early Notification of Community-Based Epidemics (ESSENCE), Real-time Outbreak and Disease Surveillance (RODS), Syndrome Reporting Information System (SYRIS), BioSense, RedVat, and Argus-1. These systems collect data from a variety of sources, such as 911 calls, over-the-counter medication sales reports, calls to poison control centers and nurse hotlines, work and school absentee reports, and reports describing chief complaints from clinics and emergency department visitors, among others.[18]

Limitations to these systems exist. Some require a manual approach to data collection and sharing; others, although automated, share data in batches rather than in real time. Furthermore, none of these systems is used on a global basis. In fact, in response to the severe but limited 2004 outbreak of H5N1 influenza in Asia, the World Health Organization (WHO) expressed concern that the global community was "inadequately prepared to respond to an influenza pandemic" due to an insufficient response capacity "ranging from vaccine manufacturing to the sensitivity of surveillance systems, the number of hospital beds, the affordability of diagnostic tests, and the supply of respirators and face masks."[19]

With these limitations in mind, researchers are working to create better syndromic surveillance systems. For example, Ortiz et al. recently described a sentinel surveillance system that collects severe influenza outcomes as a primary measure.[20] However, not all syndromic surveillance systems are highly technical, and some researchers have recently described low-tech surveillance methods that can be effectively used in low-income countries.[21]

Outbreak Management

Outbreak management defines a system that includes an outbreak control team (OCT) that initiates detection of a potential outbreak, attempts to control the source and transmission of communicable diseases, and provides links to other components of the outbreak management system.[22] The CDC provides the Outbreak Management Program, which consists of a variety of measures designed to minimize the impact of disease outbreaks. This U.S. government agency offers at least three applications in outbreak management that provide for data collection and transmission, analysis, and reporting (see Table 8-1).

TABLE 8-1	Public Health Informatics Applications Provided by the CDC		
Application	**Function**	**Focus**	**Platform**
Epi Info	• Develop questionnaire or form • Customize data entry process • Data analysis • Create epidemiologic statistics, tables, graphs, and maps	Outbreak management	Microsoft Windows
Countermeasure Response Administration (CRA)	• Custom event creation and configuration • Collection of information • Management of multiple simultaneous events	Outbreak management	Web-based
Outbreak Management System (OMS)	• Capture of data on demographics, case investigations, laboratory results, countermeasures, exposures, and relationships between persons, animals, other organisms, events, travel, vehicles, objects, organizations, and locations • Case follow-up • Contact tracing • Data import, export, and analysis	Outbreak management	Web-based
BioSense	• Data transmission • Data analysis • Data reporting • Public health response	Biosurveillance	Web-based

Electronic Laboratory Reporting

Electronic laboratory reporting (ELR) is the electronic transfer of laboratory data for public health monitoring; it emphasizes the importance of the adoption and implementation of uniform standards from clinical laboratories for public health uses.[23] Basically, ELR is an automated transmission of laboratory results between a laboratory information system and the local public health department. The result of this communication will enhance and strengthen state and local disease surveillance capacity and promote public health by providing a mechanism for collecting and managing laboratory data.[23,24]

Health Information Exchange

Health information exchange (HIE) is defined as the coordination, communication, and transmission of healthcare-related information among organizations via electronic devices. The benefits of this communication and transmission include the ability to identify key data points more easily, to detect events early, and to provide a timely response.[25] Ideally, these tools and skills will identify risks earlier during a public health emergency, thereby enabling responders to prevent unnecessary morbidity, mortality, and economic loss resulting directly from a crisis. In addition, HIE can mitigate morbidity, mortality, and economic loss directly attributable to the mismanagement of emergency relief efforts.[26]

RESPONSE

Information technology allows public health and medical responders to improve their assessment, communication, and transmission of data during an emergency. Data user friendliness is often considered a necessary step for successful implementation. Additionally, some other factors help providers deal better with information: data portability, simplicity, and flexibility.[27] The goal of technology in the response stage is to enhance the fit between the tasks the user wishes to perform and the possibilities offered by the technology. Ideally, data should be user friendly, ensuring that all personnel understand the basic concept underlying the data and have immediate access to the information they need. Data systems should be designed so they can be easily taught, requiring a minimal amount of training of users. Familiarity with and use of technology and data systems should be incorporated by personnel into everyday tasks to ensure functional familiarity during public health crises.[28]

Application Factor

The application of IT during a public health crisis can be divided into four components: collection, storage, dissemination, and management of information. The IT system architecture can be centralized or distributed.

In a centralized architecture, a stand-alone server is dedicated for processing all user functions and the control panels, associated power supplies, input, output, and reader control modules for each access device are located in a central location. Through a centralized architecture, it becomes possible to manage all resources—including replacements, repairs, and upgrades—in a seamless manner with minimal impact on the users. An additional advantage of such a centralized approach is the ability to monitor and control access of personnel to this central location. This type of restriction limits the accessibility to the critical data communication circuits between the door access control panels and the control modules. With a centralized system, a provider can troubleshoot the electronic components at a single location and all data are stored on the servers, which generally have greater security controls. The biggest challenge with a centralized architecture is traffic congestion on the network. This obstacle occurs when many clients attempt to access the same server, causing an overload of the system.

Distributed IT architectures allow each individual's node to allocate, reallocate, and deallocate communication; there is no single centralized controller. For these reasons, distributed applications have different features. They are more likely to avoid the problem of congestion during peak user times, have no single points of failure or attack, and allow multiple alternative routes for service. However, distributed architectures have more complicated designs and can be difficult to service because each service person must know the exact location of the remotely installed control modules.[29,30]

Application challenges related to emergency information systems include designing programs that increase ease of data access, information sharing, and communication during a public health emergency. Planning, development, architecture, and application selection will pose challenging tasks for emergency informatics designers. Emergency informatics and public health informatics need tools to assist and facilitate communications during emergencies. Some of these tools will be utilized only during certain stages of a crisis; others will be used during all stages of the incident. The ability to develop decision-making tools to be used either before or after an emergency will depend on having available common shared information.

Databases

A database is a collection of structured data items that are stored, controlled, and managed as a single unit. Databases come in different forms and follow several different models, but are generally a very effective way for storing and retrieving data as well as for transferring and sharing data. When categorized information is updated or changed, databases generate reliable updates, backup, and recovery plans, which provide safeguards against the possibility of losing valuable data. Databases that provide descriptive data about disaster-affected areas and vulnerable communities can be generated, designed, and developed with the use of computer hardware, information software, and telecommunication technology. Similarly, the utility of many epidemiological tools, such as public health surveillance systems, simulation models, decision-making tools, and training tools for disasters, depend on good databases.[26,31]

Information Retrieval Systems

Information retrieval (IR) systems cover a broad spectrum of activities that allow the user to search for relevant information from a collection of unstructured documents. They differ from structured databases in that IR systems can be used for managing unstructured data that cannot be fit neatly into a uniformly formatted database. This information can be obtained from text, pictures, audio, video, and Web-based or other online resources.[32]

Localization and Directional Systems

Global Positioning Systems

Global positioning systems (GPS) are tools based on a global navigation system that provides crucial information at the time of public health emergencies. GPS will generate a geographical positioning and navigation system that can provide reliable routing in a chaotic situation. This ability is not limited to ground rescue: GPS also can provide information in aviation and maritime rescue operations. GPS gives public health officials and emergency providers critical information regarding the exact locations of transportation routes, buildings, hospitals, and police and fire departments as well as accurate estimates of the time needed to reach these facilities.[33]

Geographical Information Systems

Geographical information systems (GIS) enable the user to organize data based on a geographical area, and they permit the user to access data based on spatial or geographic coordinates. GIS includes a database that captures, stores, and analyzes data and provides for the retrieval or manipulation of information based on a given location on a geographically referenced map. When a natural disaster occurs, GIS facilitates all phases of the disaster response, including planning, mitigation, preparedness, response, and recovery. In the preparedness stage, it serves as a valuable tool for allocation of resources such as fire stations, paramedics, evacuation routes, and storage facilities. In the response phase, GIS can be incorporated with global positioning systems in a disaster area to help with rescue operations. In addition, GIS in combination with GPS can be used to map each location where damage has occurred and to assess the type and extent of the damage; it can then be combined with other data to develop an action plan for reconstruction.[34]

Wireless Technology

Wireless technology offers organizations and users many benefits, such as portability, flexibility, increased productivity, and lower installation costs. Such technology plays a critical role in information sharing during emergency responses.[35] Wireless technology refers to transmissions of data across geographical areas without using cables or wires. The advantages associated with this method of data transfer include enhanced mobility and flexibility, increased bandwidth for digital radio-transmission, increased efficiency, and reduced wiring costs.[36]

The traditional method of communication is to establish a local area network (LAN)—that is, a network to share resources including files, printers, data, or other applications through a centralized architecture, albeit over a relatively limited geographic area. By comparison, a wide area network (WAN) or metro area network (MAN) provides the same abilities but functions over a larger geographic area (see Table 8-2).

One of the disadvantages of wireless networks relates to security concerns. Anyone with the right equipment in physical proximity to the network might be able to capture network traffic, gather unprotected passwords, and launch an attack on the computers that are part of the network. Therefore, any information transported across a network must be encrypted to ensure that it remains private and secure.

Personal Digital Assistants

A personal digital assistant (PDA) is a handheld device that can provide access to the Internet through a wireless network. These types of devices can assist first responders by providing a variety of capabilities that will enhance the opportunity for information sharing during an emergency crisis: word processing, GPS, database access, camera, video, audio recording, and telephone service.[37] One of the advantages of PDAs is that users typically are very familiar with these devices because they may use them on a daily basis and, therefore, do not need training. With PDAs, emergency responders can easily carry contacts information and knowledge databases such as pharmaceutical information—a valuable function given that responders usually do not have remote access to books at an emergency site.

TABLE 8-2   Comparison of Different Network Types

Network	Design	Characteristic
LAN	Local area network	• Connects networking devices within a relatively small geographic area • Uses the TCP/IP network protocol • Provides higher data-transfer rates • Relies on inexpensive equipment
WAN	Wide area network	• Covers a large distance for communication between computers • Uses different protocols (ATM, X.25, and Frame Relay) • Provides a lower data-transfer rate than a LAN • Relies on expensive equipment
MAN	Metropolitan area network	• Falls in the middle between a LAN and a WAN • Covers a larger physical area than a LAN but a smaller area than a WAN, such as a city • Provides moderate data-transfer rates • Relies on moderately expensive equipment
CAN	Campus area network	• Interconnects multiple LANs throughout a limited geographical area • Covers a smaller area than a MAN, such as a university campus or a corporate campus • Provides moderate to high data-transfer rates • Relies on moderately expensive equipment
WLAN	Wireless local area network	• Is a LAN based on wireless network technology • Unlike LAN, no wires are used, and radio signals are the medium for communication • Provides higher data-transfer rates than a LAN • Relies on expensive equipment

PDAs were very useful to first responders in the immediate aftermath of the 2010 Haiti earthquake. Applications such as GPS and texting allowed responders to estimate distances and times needed to get to specific locations and text messages to incident commanders and responders alerting them of road conditions, scene safety, and needed equipment and supplies. Using PDAs, information can be updated in real time and subsequently influence additional response efforts.

Diagnostic Technology

During a bioterrorist crisis or a communicable disease epidemic, separating actively ill individuals from healthy ones in the community will be vital for providing scarce resources directly to those in need. In the 1920s, a positive diagnosis of the flu was based on symptoms observed by the physician or complaints from the patient. Today, an accurate diagnosis can be obtained very quickly. Modern-day testing for the presence of influenza virus in patients can be classified into the following technology types:

- Viral isolation in cell culture
- Serology
- Immunofluorescence assays (IFA)
- Nucleic acid testing using polymerase chain reaction (PCR)
- Direct antigen tests

Viral culture is considered the so-called gold standard for virus identification because of its accuracy. This method, however, is labor intensive and takes from 3 to 7 days to complete, though the wait can be as little as 2 days if a shell-vial technique is used. Serological testing is available at only a limited number of laboratories and requires paired acute sera (collected within 4 days of illness onset) and convalescent sera (collected 2 weeks after illness onset). This method takes 2 weeks or more to yield and is used primarily for research purposes.

Immunofluorescence assays involve fluorescent antibody staining. Such tests are widely available in hospital laboratories, and results are obtained quickly, within 2 to 4 hours. Although immunofluorescence technology can distinguish between influenza types A and B, it cannot readily identify different influenza A subtypes.

Real-time reverse transcriptase-PCR (rRT-PCR) is a type of nucleic acid amplification test. It is highly sensitive, but it is not widely available and care must be taken to use an rRT-PCR assay designed to identify specifically the H1N1 influenza virus (if that is the suspected pathogen).

Direct antigen tests detect viral nucleoprotein antigens.[38] A fairly new technology, they have been categorized as a type of rapid influenza diagnostic test (RIDT). RIDTs are widely available via commercial vendors, and they can detect influenza virus in 30 minutes or less. Some RIDTs are simple enough to be performed outside of the laboratory. However, false negatives are a limitation to this group of diagnostic tests.[39]

MITIGATION

In the twenty-first century, technology has been crucial to mitigating loss of life and suffering during public health crises. Early warning systems and satellite technology have allowed for early detection of natural disasters such as hurricanes and tsunamis. Although the forces of nature remain unpredictable, modeling by supercomputers allows experts to predict the path of a storm with more certainty and to give advanced warning to threatened populations. These prediction models allow public health officials to deploy rapidly supplies and response personnel prior to the arrival of the potential catastrophe. National emergency response orders can be executed, and the evacuation of vulnerable populations, if necessary, can be achieved more quickly.

Once a public health emergency has occurred, the proper application of technology is again critical to mitigation. Communication is always one of the biggest challenges during these events. The advent of satellite and mobile phones has allowed rescue workers to communicate more easily while in the field. Geocoding, which is the translation of street addresses to GPS coordinates, allows rescue workers to navigate in conditions where street signs are swept away and normal landmarks are destroyed.[40] Moreover, GPS-enabled laptops and map plotters are able to identify adverse road conditions, power outages, and supply storage locations during a crisis.

The U.S. federal government is encouraging the development and use of new technology in other areas of public health. For example, on December 30, 2009, the Health Information Technology for Economic and Clinical Health (HITECH) Act was passed by the U.S. Congress. This law is intended to increase the "meaningful" use of electronic health records. It may be the first step toward a nationwide, private, and secure electronic health information system.[41]

Public Health Mitigation and Technology: Rapid Vaccine Development

The first case of novel H1N1 was confirmed by laboratory testing on April 15, 2009, and the second case on April 17. It was clear that the virus was being transmitted from person to person. With this information, a cascade of official reactions ensued, and vaccine development began quickly and in earnest. The first step was to prepare a virus reference strain, also called a vaccine virus.[26] To do so, the novel H1N1 virus was combined with another virus that readily grows in chicken eggs. The goal was to create a new virus strain with the same immunologic properties as novel H1N1 that would grow in eggs, the conventional method of producing vaccines. The newly created virus reference strain was used to create a master virus seed, commonly called seed stock.[42] Seed stock was also created using a new technology, reverse genetics. Although a decision had not yet been made to create a 2009 H1N1 vaccine, the seed stocks were sent to vaccine manufacturers in late May 2009. The next steps included pilot lot production, clinical testing, and dosage formulation.

On July 29, 2009, the CDC's Advisory Committee on Immunization Practices (ACIP) announced that vaccine production for novel H1N1 was recommended. However, production problems slowed progress. The virus grew but failed to thrive in eggs, and many manufacturers did not recognize how low their yields were until a potency test became available in August 2009. Potency tests determine how many vaccine doses are produced per egg.[43] The first doses of H1N1 vaccine were shipped to physicians in early October 2009.[44] According to the CDC between 39 million and 80 million cases of H1N1 flu occurred in 2009, and between 7,880 and 16,460 deaths from this cause occurred between April and December 2009.[45]

CASE ANALYSIS

The tragedy of Hurricane Katrina provided many opportunities to apply current technologies to public crisis management and to identify areas where current technology falls short. In particular, it highlighted the incompatibility of communications and hospital information management systems between local, state, and federal levels.

One of the most important failures in the response to Katrina involved communication. Hurricane Katrina disabled most of the means of communication on which the response teams depended. A federal investigation of the response to this natural disaster noted that massive inoperability of communications limited command, control, and situational awareness. In the immediate aftermath of the storm, landlines and cell phones became inoperable, leaving local, federal, and state responders with only satellite phones or radios for communication.

Many areas had no communication at all, which meant that coordinated efforts became impossible. FEMA deployed several of its Mobile Emergency Response System (MERS) units near the command centers in the three states that were affected by the hurricane. These command and control units are equipped with satellite, video and telephone connections. During the storm and immediately following, they were the only means of communication in many areas.

Prior to Hurricane Katrina's landfall on the Gulf Coast, some medical facilities were evacuated, but others were not. Once the storm passed, it became apparent that all hospitalized patients needed to be moved. In addition, newly injured or ill patients provided various challenges for responders. First, there was no access to the patients' medical history, including their medications and prior conditions. This lack of information forced providers to treat victims based on what they saw and, if the patient was alert, what a patient could remember. Once treated, those who needed to be transferred to medical centers required a transfer of medical records detailing the treatment rendered. The inability to make these transfers emphasized the need for a medical information repository or some way (such as a biochip or readable card) to store medical information.

Geocoding was used extensively in the early days of the public health response to Hurricane Katrina. Because so many street signs were underwater, the Coast Guard would call in addresses to a group of volunteers from the Geological Society of America. They would provide longitude and latitude coordinates that enabled the rescuers to locate survivors. In addition, other geocoders mapped out working cell phone towers in Mississippi, enabling workers to know in which areas they would have communication.

CONCLUSION

Information technology serves a crucial role in all aspects of public health emergencies. This role affects both the preparation and the response to crises by decreasing morbidity and mortality during and after the event. Effective and efficient public health crisis response requires a sophisticated IT infrastructure whose design and utilization enable responders to properly collect, share, process, and retrieve data. The hierarchies of all organizations involved in a rescue effort need to interact closely. Such coordination of efforts will remain a challenge in the future, but secure IT can facilitate information sharing and optimal utilization of data.

ACKNOWLEDGMENTS

The authors would like to express special appreciation to Griffin Davis, Rich Clive, and Rob Brown for their assistance with the chapter.

INTERNET RESOURCES

Centers for Disease Control and Prevention, emergency preparedness and response surveillance: http://emergency.cdc.gov/episurv/

Healthcare Information Technology Standards Panel: http://www.hitsp.org

National Association for Public Health Information Technology: http://www.naphit.org

Partners in Information Access for the Public Health Workforce: http://phpartners.org

U.S. Health Resources and Services Administration, health information technology: http://www.hrsa.gov/healthit

U.S. National Library of Medicine, health services research and public health information programs: http://www.nlm.nih.gov/hsrph.html

World Health Organization, public health mapping and GIS: http://www.who.int/health_mapping/en/

NOTES

1. Agency for Healthcare Research and Quality. Health information technology. Available at: http://healthit.ahrq.gov/portal/server.pt?open=512&objID=1135&mode=2&pid=DA_1003919&cid=DA_1003703&p_path=/DA_1003922&pos=). Accessed November 2009.
2. Chen H, Nicogossian A, Olsson S. Electronic health. *International Journal of Telemedicine Application*. 2009; Article ID 308710.
3. The Katrina effect on American preparedness. Available at: http://wagner.nyu.edu/performance/files/Post-Katrina%20preparedness.pdf. Accessed October 2009.
4. Congressional Reports. H. Rpt. 109-377: *A failure of initiative: Final report of the Select Bipartisan Committee to Investigate the Preparation for and Response to Hurricane Katrina.*
5. Centers for Disease Control and Prevention. Public health response to hurricanes Katrina and Rita—United States, 2005. *Morbidity and Mortality Weekly Report.* 2006;55(9):229–231.
6. Lawson S. Haiti earthquake: Technology comes to the rescue in Haiti. *MacWorld News.* 2010. Available at: http://www.macworld.co.uk/digitallifestyle/news/index.cfm?newsid=28341. Accessed July 2010.
7. Inspector General, Department of Defense. Report on the effects of Hurricane Katrina on the Defense Information Systems Agency continuity of operations and test facility (Report No. D-2007-031) Available at: http://www.dodig.mil/Audit/reports/FY07/07-031.pdf. Accessed December 2009.
8. Yasnoff WA, O'Carroll PW, Koo D, Linkins RW, Kilbourne EM. Public health informatics: Improving and transforming public health in the information age. *Journal of Public Health Management and Practice.* 2000;6(6):67–75.
9. Rinkineva K. *The role of information technology in crisis management.* The 14th EINIRAS Conference 30.9.-1.10. 2004.
10. Landgren J. Shared use of information technology in emergency response work: Results from a field experiment. *Proceedings of the Second International ISCRAM Conference*, Carle B, Van de Walle, B (eds.). Brussels, Belgium; April 2005.
11. Sever MS, Vanholder R, Lameire N. Management of crush-related injuries after disasters. *New England Journal of Medicine.* 2006;354(10):1052–1063.

12. The Katrina effect on American preparedness. Available at: http://wagner.nyu.edu/performance/files/Post-Katrina%20preparedness.pdf. Accessed October 2009.

13. Fleischauer A, Diaz P. Biosurveillance: A definition, scope and description of current capability for a national strategy. *Advances in Disease Surveillance.* 2008;5:175.

14. Wagner M, Moore A, Aryel R. *Handbook of biosurveillance.* Burlington, MA: Elsevier Academic Press; 2006.

15. Centers for Disease Control and Prevention. BioSense. Available at: http://www.cdc.gov/biosense/subtopic/background/index.html. Accessed October 2009.

16. International Society for Disease Surveillance. Definition of syndromic surveillance. Available at: http://isds.wikispaces.com/message/view/home/1710637. Accessed January 2010.

17. Sosin DM. Syndromic surveillance: The case for skillful investment. *Biosecurity and Bioterrorism: Biodefense Strategy, Practice, and Science.* 2003;1(4):247–253.

18. Calcote JC, Gaddis KB, Phipps JA, Herbold JR. Syndromic surveillance in Texas: a brief overview of current activities. *TPHA Journal.* 2009;61(4);22–24.

19. World Health Organization. WHO consultation on priority public health interventions before and during an influenza pandemic. Geneva; March 16–18, 2004 (cited April 22, 2007). Available at: http://www.who.int/csr/disease/avian_influenza/final.pdf. Accessed January 2010.

20. Ortiz JR, Sotomayor V, Uez OC, Oliva O, Bettels D, McCarron M, et al. Strategy to enhance influenza surveillance worldwide. *Emerging Infectious Diseases.* August 2009. Available at: http://www.cdc.gov/EID/content/15/8/1271.htm. Accessed January 2010.

21. May L, Chretien JP, Pavlin JA. Beyond traditional surveillance: Applying syndromic surveillance to developing settings—opportunities and challenges. *BMC Public Health* 2009;9:242.

22. Disease surveillance and outbreak management. Available at: http://www.who.int/water_sanitation_health/hygiene/ships/en/gssanitation9.pdf. Accessed October 2009.

23. Overhage JM, Suico J, McDonald CJ. Electronic laboratory reporting: Barriers, solutions and findings. *Public Health Management and Practice.* 2001;7(6):60–66.

24. Pinner RW, Jernigan DB, Sutliff SM. Electronic laboratory-based reporting for public health. *Military Medicine.* 2000;165(7 suppl 2):20–24.

25. Agency for Healthcare Research and Quality (AHRQ). Evolution of state health information exchange: A study of vision, strategy, and progress. Available at: http://www.avalerehealth.net/research/docs/State_based_Health_Information_Exchange_Final_Report.pdf. Accessed October 2009.

26. Mathew D. Information technology and public health management of disasters: A model for South Asian countries. *Prehospital and Disaster Medicine.* 2004;20(1):54–60.

27. Rinkineva, K. *The role of information technology in crisis management.* The 14th EINIRAS Conference 30.9.-1.10. 2004. Available at: http://www.einiras.net/conf/conferences/conferences_helsinki2004.cfm. Accessed October 2009.

28. Stead WW, Miller RA, Musen MA, Hersh WR. Integration and beyond: Linking information from disparate sources and into workflow. *Journal of the American Medical Informatics Association.* 2000;7(2):135–145.

29. Staes CJ, Xu W, LeFevre SD, Price RC. A case for using grid architecture for state public health informatics: The Utah perspective. *BMC Medical Informatics and Decision Making.* 2009;9:32.

30. Arnold JL, Levine BN. Information-sharing in out-of-hospital disaster response: The future role of information technology. *Prehospital Disaster Medicine*. 2004;19(3):201–207.

31. Patoli A. Role of telemedicine in disaster management. *eHealth International Journal*. Available at: http://www.ehealthinternational.org/vol2num2/Vol2Num2p34.pdf. Accessed December 2009.

32. Hersh WR. *Information retrieval: A health and biomedical perspective* (2nd ed.). New York: Springer; 2003.

33. Nakajima Y, Shiina H, Yamane S, Ishida T, Yamaki H. *Disaster evacuation guide: Using a massively multiagent server and GPS Mobile phones*. Presentation at 2007 International Symposium on Applications and the Internet (SAINT'07); 2007.

34. Johnson R. *GIS technology for disasters and emergency management*. ESRI white paper. May 2000. Available at: http://www.esri.com/library/whitepapers/pdfs/disastermgmt.pdf. Accessed October 2009.

35. Li YC. Constructing a disaster medical resource information center and database. In: Chiu WT (ed.), *International Symposium on Recent Advances in Disaster Prevention*. Taipei, Taiwan: National Institute of Injury Prevention; 2002, pp. D49–D54.

36. Stephenson R, Anderson PS. Disasters and the information technology revolution. *Disasters*. 1997;21:305–334.

37. Garshnek V, Burkle F. Applications of telemedicine and telecommunications to disaster medicine historical and future perspectives. *Journal of the American Medical Informatics Association*. 1999;6(1):26–37.

38. Centers for Disease Control and Prevention. Interim recommendations for clinical use of influenza diagnostic testing during the 2009–2010 influenza season. Available at: www.cdc.gov/h1n1flu/diagnostic_testing_clinicians_qa.htm. Accessed January 2010.

39. Centers for Disease Control and Prevention. Interim recommendations for clinical use of influenza diagnostic testing during the 2009–2010 influenza season. Available at: http://www.cdc.gov/h1n1flu/diagnostic_testing_clinicians_qa.htm#c. Accessed January 2010.

40. Walton M. "Geocoding" used to locate Katrina survivors. *CNN Special Report*. November 10, 2005.

41. Blumenthal D. Launching HITECH. *New England Journal of Medicine*. 2010;362(5):305–310.

42. U.S. Department of Health and Human Services. 2009 H1N1 vaccine development activities. Available at: www.medicalcountermeasures.gov/BARDA/MCM/panflu/factsheet.aspx. Accessed February 2010.

43. Pollack A, McNeil DG Jr. A nation battling flu, and short vaccine supplies. *New York Times*. October 25, 2009. Available at: www.nytimes.com/2009/10/26/health/26flu.html?scp=1&sq=A%20nation%20battling%20flu,%20and%20short%20vaccine%20supplies&st=cse. Accessed February 2010.

44. McNeil DG Jr. "Bumpy" start seen for swine flu vaccine plan. *New York Times*. September 25, 2009. Available at: www.nytimes.com/2009/09/26/health/research/26flu.html?_r=1. Accessed February 2010.

45. Centers for Disease Control and Prevention. CDC estimates of 2009 H1N1 influenza cases, hospitalizations and deaths in the United States, April–December 12, 2009. January 15, 2010. Available at: www.cdc.gov/h1n1flu/estimates_2009_h1n1.htm. Accessed January 2010.

SECTION 3

Public Health Tools During Emergencies

CHAPTER 9

Epidemiological Studies

Junaid A. Razzak and Uzma Rahim Khan

EPIDEMIOLOGY

Epidemiology is defined as the study of the distribution and determination of health-related states or events in specific populations. This field also includes the application of these investigations in an attempt to control health problems. It helps planners to focus on the main problems of a *community* rather than of *individual patients*, and to identify measures for improving the health of the community as a whole.

EPIDEMIOLOGICAL STUDIES

Epidemiology allows public health professionals to learn more about the effects that emergencies have on the health of affected populations. Case-series, cross-sectional, case-control, and cohort studies are commonly used in public health emergencies (see Table 9-1). In contrast, ecological and correlation studies have rarely been used to assess emergencies because the unit of analysis is an aggregate of individuals and information is collected on a population rather than on individual members.[1]

Case-series studies have been useful to identify the clinical features and specialized treatment of specific types of injuries. However, they usually include a single hospital sample whose members may not be representative of the full spectrum of injuries for the event, and they do not address the variety of outcomes experienced during the disaster, including less severe injuries treated outside the hospital setting.

Cross-sectional surveys are an efficient way to collect information about behaviors during and after disasters, the precise location of individuals during the event, and the diversity of outcomes experienced during the event, including less-severe

TABLE 9-1 Role of Epidemiological Studies in Public Health Emergencies		
Type of Epidemiological Study	**Data Collected**	**Limitations**
Case series: sequence of case reports with common elements such as similar clinical features and suspected common exposures	• Clinical features • Specialized treatment of specific types of injuries	• Lack of generalizations • Nonreporting of less severe injuries treated outside the hospital setting
Cross-sectional: study of several individuals at one point in time, focusing information on health status, health-related behaviors, and other exposure factors	• Frequencies of mortality and morbidity • Behaviors during and after emergencies • Diversity of outcomes experienced during the event	• Absence of population counts • Poor sampling methods leading to nonrepresentative samples • Bias from selective survival, population movement, and recall
Case control: study of individuals in whom a disease has already occurred to find out whether these individuals have been exposed to a particular risk factor	• Risk factors	• Bias due to selection of cases and controls
Cohort study: study of a group exposed to a particular factor and another group not exposed to this factor, who are followed over time to determine the occurrence of disease	• Estimate incidence and magnitude of risk • Short- and long-term and direct and indirect health effects • Emergency-related outcomes	• Identification of a defined cohort • Logistics of long-term data collection • Loss to follow-up

injuries treated outside the hospital setting. Limitations of cross-sectional studies of disasters include poor sampling methods leading to nonrepresentative samples and bias from selective survival, population movement, and recall.

Retrospective studies involving victims or healthcare workers involved in a disaster may include only a small percentage of the victims (35 to 40 percent), and they may not report the disaster events accurately. These shortcomings can reduce the internal and external validities of emergency public health epidemiological studies.

However, if collection of data in real time occurs, patient reliability and response rates may be more accurate. Confounding factors that potentially could be introduced into such a study by use of proxy measurements also are reduced. If primary care workers or emergency personnel (prehospital care or emergency department professionals) are able to record the medical data in real time, there will be no need to use proxy measurements; by comparison, such proxies are often used in retrospective studies to collect research data.

Case-control studies are an efficient design for estimating specific risks, and their use for examining disaster-related outcomes has increased during the last decade. Cases can be collected from multiple sources of data, including existing records or surveys. Controls should be sampled from the same population from which the cases arose (e.g., controls from the community). Finding a representative control group is the most complicated feature of the case-control design because of the difficulty in defining a base population for a disaster. Matching can be used to control for confounding factors that might be difficult to measure at the population level, such as location within a building. For example, Roces et al. matched injured cases to uninjured family members to estimate the risk of mortality associated with such factors as building type and being inside a building compared with being outside a building in an earthquake.[2] In reality, family members are likely to be in the same structures and to be located together.

The ideal epidemiological design is the cohort study. In emergency public health studies, follow-up can be substantially shortened if only direct consequences are examined; accounting for injuries after extrication or during post-disaster activities could lead to a lengthier study process. Some loss to follow-up of the cohort may occur because of death, relocation, and missing contact information. Cohort studies are rarely conducted in the setting of emergency-related injuries because of the difficulties in identifying a defined cohort. Part of the problem is that researchers cannot define when and where an emergency will occur and, therefore, must necessarily rely on retrospective cohorts.

Epidemiological studies have also introduced public health emergency statistics and analysis into assessment of quality of life indicators. Some examples include restricted-activity days, number of days for which the ability to work was lost, number of days hospitalized with disabilities, and disability adjusted life-years (DALY). Most of the DALYs attributable to emergencies occur immediately at the time of the incident, such as in cases involving burns, drowning, suffocation, or fractures. Numerous questions arise after a large-scale emergency has resolved—for example, the number of disabilities and deaths that might have been prevented through improved search and rescue operations, the importance of time to interventions in reducing DALY losses, and the assessment of the effectiveness of external search and rescue assistance teams and temporary facilities. Refining the existing methodology and developing quantitative indicators to estimate both direct and indirect losses and costs due to public health emergencies should be a research priority.[3]

EPIDEMIOLOGY IN PUBLIC HEALTH EMERGENCIES

The basic epidemiological approach in large-scale emergency settings is no different from that used in any standard epidemiological investigation. Specifically, researchers describe the adverse health effects of natural and human-caused public health emergencies and the factors that contribute to those effects (Table 9-2). However, the difference lies in the importance of gathering data and making decisions in a short period of time.

The three fundamental phases of public health emergencies are preparedness, response, and rehabilitation. Each of these phases is characterized by predictable patterns of health indicators and expected public health responses.[4] If these patterns are addressed with appropriate management responses, a decline in morbidity and mortality and a shortening of the duration of each epidemiological phase will result.

TABLE 9-2   Application of Epidemiology in Public Health Emergencies
Rapid needs assessment (vulnerability and hazard assessment)
Demographic studies of population size and structure, death, disease, nutrition, and immunization (outbreak investigation)
Public health monitoring and information systems management (surveillance and action-oriented information systems)
Research methodologies
Injury and disease profiles
Disease-control strategies for well-defined problems
Needs of special populations
Assessment of the use and distribution of health services
Etiologic research on morbidity and mortality
Development of long-term epidemiological studies of the affected populations

Epidemiology in the Preparedness Phase

Epidemiological preparation and planning before an event includes collecting information on infrastructure, institutional knowledge and capabilities, training, and prediction models. In short, all these activities will lead to risk reduction. Having current and continuously updated epidemiological data on the capacities of the various components of public health systems in a community will allow public health professionals and policy makers to direct resources appropriately (Table 9-3). In addition, the data from the preparedness phase can ensure plans are developed that respond to actual threats and serve actual at-risk populations rather than to hypothetical situations. The goals of this phase are as follows:

- Developing baseline data for assessing the needs of affected populations and matching available resources to needs
- Preparing for training resources
- Planning for contingencies
- Evaluating program effectiveness

Strong community linkages are essential to a public health organization's overall preparedness for emergencies and are key to achieving these goals.

TABLE 9-3 **Epidemiological Studies During the Preparedness Phase of Public Health Emergencies**	
Study Questions	**Study Design/Information Source**
• Size and distribution of the population area	• Surveys (demographic health survey)
• Major communication lines and topography	• Observation
• Distribution and services provided by health facilities	• Mapping
• Surveillance and prevention strategies	• Interviews
• Identification of groups at the highest risk (displaced groups, specific age groups, low-income groups)	• Focus groups
• Estimation of the number of people needing assistance	• Media reports
• Determination of baseline parameters to monitor the impact of planning and future response	

Epidemiology in the Response Phase

Carrying out epidemiological investigations in the middle of a public health emergency may be viewed as an unnecessary endeavor when many people require immediate and direct assistance. In reality, contingency response and relief programs can be implemented and managed more effectively if decisions are based on epidemiological findings. The goals of the response phase are outlined here:

- Rapid assessment of health and medical needs during the emergency situation
- Understanding of the effects of current and forecasted weather conditions
- Continuous monitoring of the health problems faced by the affected population
- Knowledge of available resources
- Implementation of disease control strategies
- Evaluation of the use and distribution of health services

The epidemiological information gathered through study during this phase can be used to direct ongoing response activities and provide feedback for mitigation efforts.

Collecting data in "real time" during an active public health emergency is challenging, but recent technological innovations can certainly assist these efforts (Table 9-4). Computer hardware and software databases are now able to collect data rapidly under highly adverse conditions, and this information can be analyzed rapidly to provide timely intelligence on morbidity and mortality to public health decision makers. In addition, this technology makes it possible to model or simulate complex public health emergencies for planning and drills. Moreover, information technology facilitates disease telemonitoring that will help in monitoring the spread of disease in the affected area and help in determining necessary interventions. Geographic information systems (GIS) also serve an important role in effective community hazard and vulnerability analysis.[5]

Surveillance systems are another important target of epidemiological studies of public health emergencies. These systems are intended to ensure that the number of casualties can be reduced and the cases that do occur can be treated promptly and effectively.[6] Surveillance data on health events are analyzed, transformed, and disseminated to decision makers for policy development and action.

The media, including the Internet, radio, and television, can be used for collecting and disseminating emergency surveillance data. Without question, media coverage plays an important role in the epidemiology of an emergency. It should also be considered a potential intervention strategy, an indirect exposure, or an effect modifier. The ability of a society to use the media to provide warnings and forecasts, motivate volunteers, and raise funds can play a crucial role in limiting the short-term effects of emergencies. However, just as the media can limit primary exposures, so they can be contributors to secondary, psychologically driven, health outcomes.[6]

TABLE 9-4   Checklist for Planning and Implementing a Survey in a Public Health Emergency

1. Which population is to be assessed (e.g., country, region, ethnic group)?

2. What is the smallest unit to be assessed (e.g., camp, village, district)?

3. Is there a need to analyze subgroups (e.g., by gender, age, ethnicity)?

4. Which sampling methods will be used (e.g., systematic, cluster)?

5. Which personnel, equipment, transport, number of teams, and resources will be needed?

6. Workload: How many subjects (clusters) per day per team?

7. Has a training schedule for field workers been prepared?

8. Who will conduct the training? Where?

9. Who will supervise the teams during the survey?

10. Are computers and operators available?

11. Who is responsible for the logistics (e.g., transport, equipment, accommodation, information for target population)?

12. Who is responsible for report writing and interpretation of findings?

13. Who is the target audience?

14. What is the target date?

15. Who is responsible for taking action on the report's findings?

Local response capability and infrastructure management must be strengthened to reduce mortality and morbidity in the first hours and days following an emergency because external assistance teams are unlikely to arrive within the scope of one or two days. Table 9-5 outlines ways that epidemiological studies can facilitate achieving the goals of the response phase for a public health emergency.

Epidemiology in the Rehabilitation Phase

By collecting mortality and morbidity data in real time, critical information about the health needs of a vulnerable population can be applied to mitigation efforts and the rehabilitation phase. This phase is characterized by a prolonged period that may take months or years to complete. The primary endpoint is returning the affected community back to pre-emergency baseline levels of functioning for most parameters such as health,

TABLE 9-5   Epidemiological Studies During the Response Phase of Public Health Emergencies

Study Questions	Study Design/Information Source
• Assessment of physical condition of health, transport, and communications facilities by competent technicians and engineers	• Aerial observation
• Status of relief activities: food, shelter, and protective clothing	• Cross-sectional surveys
• Total number of casualties	• Observation
• Number of people requiring immediate treatment	• Mapping
• Number of people requiring continued care after emergency treatment	• Interviews
• Prevalence or incidence of adverse health outcomes (injuries, death)	• Focus groups
• Development of a registry of adverse health outcomes	• Review of census, situation reports
• Disease outbreaks and the major disease risks in the affected area	• Reports from the community/relief workers and media
• Number of people requiring evacuation	• Screening
• Availability of essential health supplies and personnel	• Regular reporting from existing facilities
• Needed supplies and repairs to local medical facilities	• Case-control studies that can identify risk factors, eliminate confounding factors, and study the interactions of multiple factors
• Characterization of the population at risk and/or exposed to the emergency (e.g., size, location, susceptibility, and age distribution)	
• Estimation of the exposure to the emergency (e.g., being in an area affected by an earthquake, flood, heat wave, or war)	
• Exposure to physical or psychological stressors	
• Location and number of people who have moved away from their homes	
• Estimates of the number of unaccounted deaths and missing people	

TABLE 9-6	Epidemiological Studies During the Rehabilitation Phase of Public Health Emergencies
Study Questions	**Study Design/Information Source**
• Short- and long-term, direct and indirect health effects, effect modifiers (e.g., building infrastructure, living conditions, communication systems including the media and the Internet) • Identification of a control (not exposed) population • Incidence and magnitude of risk • Identification of risk factors for death and injury • Planning strategies to reduce impact-related morbidity and mortality • Evaluation of the effectiveness of various types of assistance and the long-term effects of the emergency	• Longitudinal studies to measure changes over time • Population-based surveys • Ongoing health information system data collection • Cohort studies with sufficient follow-up for long-term consequences

housing, transportation, and communications. Epidemiological studies are easier to conduct during this phase because the pressures of an ongoing public health emergency are no longer constraining data collection. The goals of this phase are as follows:

- To estimate incidence and magnitude of risk
- To determine short- and long-term direct and indirect health effects and effect modifiers
- To identify risk factors for death and injury
- To plan strategies that reduce impact-related morbidity
- To evaluate the effectiveness of various types of assistance and long-term effects after the response phase of an emergency

Directing reconstruction efforts so as to restore the public health infrastructure to pre-emergency conditions is the key to achieving these goals. Table 9-6 outlines the types of epidemiological studies undertaken as part of this effort.

CHALLENGES OF EPIDEMIOLOGICAL STUDIES IN PUBLIC HEALTH EMERGENCIES

Data are often ephemeral in an emergency. As time passes on, populations change in terms of their exposure to and effects experienced from the public health emergency.

In addition, individuals and officials are often more willing to share information in the immediate aftermath of an emergency than later, during the rehabilitation phase. In sudden-onset events, the researcher usually cannot select the location where the data collection will occur, and the number of variables that can be controlled is often limited. The unexpected nature of public health emergencies also leads to retrospective data collection. These retrospective data, in turn, create difficulties in making before-and-after comparisons of the community affected by the emergency situation. For example, many of the affected individuals may be displaced from their homes or may be in the area only temporarily as visitors, whereas others may have been in the area only to assist with the emergency response (assigned or volunteer responders). These individuals may prove difficult to identify and locate after the immediate crisis has passed. Over time, recall bias also becomes a problem.

Some researchers have found that preliminary assessment of needs by drawing a representative sample of the affected population may be the preferable approach.[7] However, obtaining a truly representative sample of adequate size may be difficult due to the vastness of the affected area, poor connectivity to the disrupted communities, and the limited time available with the team. Data gathering may also be hindered by poor communications, reliance on secondary sources for information, lack of expert personnel, loss of preexisting data during the emergency, and loss of street signs and landmarks due to destruction of the geographical area. Many local physicians, public health, and nearly all other professionals who remain in the local setting will confront personal problems with loss of family, friends, and property, and these personal challenges will affect their ability to respond effectively during the crisis situation. In addition, healthcare workers involved in a public health emergency may be assisting only a small percentage of the victims, and they may not report the emergency events accurately. These factors and the destruction of the healthcare facilities make the epidemiological assessment and the management of the public health emergency even more complex.[8]

Frequently, a lack of an organized effort for gathering data by governmental organizations and a lack of coordination with the separate efforts of nongovernmental organizations (NGOs) are observed during an emergency situation. The shortage of available information from NGOs and the reluctance of NGOs to share data on their activities has been reported following sudden-onset emergencies due to natural hazards.[9]

All of these shortcomings can reduce the internal and external validities of emergency epidemiological studies. Table 9-7 summarizes these challenges.

In an emergency situation, rigorous epidemiological approaches may not produce data quickly enough to aid responders. Nevertheless, an immediate need for quantitative data with which to manage emergencies does exist. Record keeping sometimes

TABLE 9-7   Epidemiological Challenges in Emergencies
Unexpected nature of public health emergencies
Retrospective data collection
Recall bias
Representative sample size
Poor communication
Secondary sources of information
Lack of expert personnel/deaths of local physicians and professionals
Loss of preexisting data
Loss of street signs and landmarks
Lack of coordination

may be abandoned in favor of patient care under the pressure to provide life-saving assistance to a large number of victims. In these situations, because abstraction of historical data is highly time-consuming, decisions may be made based on data that are received from hasty assessments and quick estimates made at times of crisis, rather than being based on concrete data. In other words, health decisions made during emergencies are often based on insufficient, or even false, information. Clearly, there is a need for reliable and early data collection to assist in making correct decisions.

Research on responses to public health emergencies has, for the most part, used qualitative methods. Generally, this material has come from interviews, sometimes supplemented by government documents, private organizations' reports, emergency department logs, after-action critiques, media, and other sources of information. It may then be coded for quantification and analysis. Examples of information that may be coded include the existence of an emergency plan, number or proportion of casualties transported by ambulance, hospital notifications, number of casualties received or admitted, injury or illness severity, and damage to hospital systems. Some reports provide quantitative estimates, albeit often without documentation of methodology. The statistics identified in these reports include such variables as number of casualties, number of patients rescued by other survivors, and number of patients transported by ambulance. Furthermore, although mean values are reported, measures of variation (e.g., standard deviation or 95 percent confidence intervals) are often lacking in the analysis part of these studies.

Behavioral health consequences are prominent after emergencies but are understudied in epidemiologic investigations.[10] Notably lacking are studies that examine mitigation, preparedness, response, and recovery variables with respect to their outcomes in terms of morbidity and mortality. Another limitation of the existing literature is that many of the research reports are not published in peer-reviewed journals, but rather appear in reports published by government agencies or academic institutions. Finally, some of the more useful case studies are outdated, and significant changes in public health and emergency medical systems have occurred since their publication. Although these studies need to be validated with more recent data, some case studies and anecdotal reports suggest that problems identified by these earlier systematic studies may still be major obstacles to effective response. Because of these limitations, research on public health emergencies is not likely to meet with the expectations of those who think of research in terms of randomized, double-blind, clinical studies, or even the less rigorous observational case-control or cohort studies.

ACTION VERSUS RESEARCH: ETHICS OF RESEARCH

Progress in medical care and disease prevention depends on an understanding not only of physiological and pathological processes, but also of the social, cultural, economic, and other environmental determinants of health, including the effects of the healthcare system and other social institutions. Producing this broad understanding requires performing research involving human subjects. Such research should be carried out only by, or strictly supervised by, suitably qualified and experienced investigators under accepted ethical guidelines. All research involving human subjects should be conducted in accordance with three basic ethical principles: respect for persons, beneficence, and justice. Researchers and ethicists generally agree that these principles, which in the abstract have equal moral force, guide the conscientious preparation of proposals for scientific studies.

The emerging best practice for research conducted during a public health emergency, such as population studies of outbreaks of disease or of disaster relief efforts, is to establish the basic research design for various categories of research before the public health emergency actually occurs. Among other benefits, this preparation permits prior ethical review of the major features of the research design. When prior review has not occurred, a review should be conducted as quickly as possible. A further question to be raised in this context focuses on how much knowledge is needed before action can be taken. Within NGOs, tension often exists between researchers and program managers: The former, who are typically more detached and analytical, want to understand the situation as fully as possible before intervening, and the latter, who are typically much closer to communities, are keen to get involved with a minimum of delay.

Challenges associated with allocating facilities and resources to people with different kinds of disabilities and rehabilitation needs in the face of time, personnel, and equipment shortages present everyone with ethical dilemmas, including many persons who have not had the benefit of training and guidance in how to make decisions in emergency situations.[8] One can see how this consideration might also apply to emergency mitigation and preparedness work, where the methodological difficulties in obtaining good data on costs and benefits of interventions add strength to the argument for rapid engagement without waiting for the data. Exploiting or abusing emergency survivors for inexpensive or easy research should never be tolerated. Perhaps not everything can be measured or calculated.

INTERNET RESOURCES

Centers for Disease Control and Prevention: Disaster Epidemiology
www.cdc.gov/nceh/hsb/disaster/

Centers for Disease Control and Prevention: Principles of Epidemiology in Public Health Practice
http://www.ihs.gov/medicalprograms/portlandinjury/pdfs/principlesofepidemiologyinpublichealth practice.pdf

Centers for Public Health Preparedness: National network of academic institutions collaborating with state and local public health departments and community partners
http://preparedness.asph.org/cphp/

National Institutes of Health: Division of International Epidemiology and Population Studies
http://www.fic.nih.gov/about/dieps.htm

World Health Organization: Technical guidelines for health action in crises
http://www.who.int/hac/techguidance/en/

World Health Organization: Epidemiology
http://www.who.int/topics/epidemiology/en/

NOTES

1. Ramirez M, Peek-Asa C. Epidemiology of traumatic injuries from earthquakes. *Epidemiology Review*. 2005;27:47–55.
2. Roces MC, White ME, Dayrit MM, Durkin ME. Risk factors for injuries due to the 1990 earthquake in Luzon, Philippines. *Bulletin of the World Health Organization*. 1992;70(4): 509–514.

3. de Ville de Goyet C, Zapata Marti R, Osorio C. Natural disaster mitigation and relief. In: *Disease control priorities in developing countries* (2nd ed.). New York: Oxford University Press; 2006, pp. 1147–1162.

4. Burkholder BT, Toole MJ. Evolution of complex disasters. *Lancet.* 1995;346(8981):1012–1015.

5. Mathew D. Information technology and public health management of disasters: A model for South Asian countries. *Prehospital Disaster Medicine.* 2005;20(1):54–60.

6. Dominici F, Levy JI, Louis TA. Methodological challenges and contributions in disaster epidemiology. *Epidemiology Review.* 2005;27:9–12.

7. Chadda RK, Malhotra A, Kaw N, Singh J, Sethi H. Mental health problems following the 2005 earthquake in Kashmir: Findings of community-run clinics. *Prehospital Disaster Medicine.* 2007;22(6):541–545; discussion: 546.

8. Raissi GR. Earthquakes and rehabilitation needs: Experiences from Bam, Iran. *Journal of Spinal Cord Medicine.* 2007;30(4):369–372.

9. von Schreeb J, Riddez L, Samnegard H, Rosling H. Foreign field hospitals in the recent sudden-onset disasters in Iran, Haiti, Indonesia, and Pakistan. *Prehospital Disaster Medicine.* 2008;23(2):144–151; discussion: 152–153.

10. Shultz JM, Russell J, Espinel Z. Epidemiology of tropical cyclones: The dynamics of disaster, disease, and development. *Epidemiology Review.* 2005;27:21–35.

CHAPTER 10

Surveillance and Monitoring

Gregg Greenough and Satchit Balsari

INTRODUCTION

Emergency managers and providers consider establishing surveillance to be one of the top 10 priorities in an emergency response.[1] Surveillance is variously described as an iterative systematic collection of data, usually a set of specific public health outcome indicators of interest to public health planners, programmers, and policy makers, collected through a networked system and regularly analyzed and disseminated to these key stakeholders. Surveillance information provides a consistent means for not only recognizing and characterizing events of public health concern as they arise, but also for monitoring events as they evolve and are addressed. Therefore, the surveillance process incorporates both functions for prevention and control and links public health practice to public health action. Surveillance may be active or passive, household or facility based, depending on its intended purpose, the needs of the population under surveillance, and the degree to which the event constitutes a public health emergency and a need for immediate response. Surveillance and monitoring methods should be simple, easily understood by and acceptable to all stakeholders, flexible enough to take new public health concerns into account, and specific to the type of humanitarian crisis at hand.

Surveillance systems established during emergencies should either draw on the framework of established surveillance systems (where they exist) or, if created de novo, provide a foundation for a more robust and sustainable surveillance mechanism in a rebuilt health information system once the public health crisis has passed.

Case Study

Surveillance is one of the critical actions that should occur early in any public health emergency response. In August 2005, Hurricane Katrina's devastation of the Gulf Coast triggered the largest mass population displacement in U.S. history. Nearly 50,000 evacuees fled to Louisiana shelters, most operated and staffed by the American Red Cross (ARC). Shelter populations varied in size from a handful of families in rural church social halls to several dozens and hundreds in school buildings to several thousand individuals in civic auditoriums and sports arenas.

Regardless of the shelter size, local, state, and federal public health officials were concerned about venues of high population density (numbers of individuals per square meter of space), given the likelihood for overcrowding and high shelter resident to sanitary facility ratio and the potential for airborne and waterborne disease outbreaks. Although initial rapid assessments indicated that communicable diseases among the evacuee population were less of an immediate concern than noncommunicable diseases, the potential of such an outbreak certainly existed.[2] Other epidemiological and demographic data suggested that noncommunicable health indicators unique to this largely urban and socioeconomically disadvantaged population—notably, chronic disease (e.g., coronary artery disease, hypertension, diabetes, chronic obstructive pulmonary disease), access to health care and medications, mental health, and injury—should be considered for surveillance given that acute exacerbations of chronic disease could also overwhelm sheltering operations.[3] By mid-September 2005, the Centers for Disease Control and Prevention (CDC), in collaboration with the Louisiana Red Cross branch, the Louisiana Department of Health and Hospitals, Office of Public Health, and the U.S. Public Health Service had established a basic shelter-based surveillance system at 489 evacuation centers (ECs) that tracked symptoms of communicable and noncommunicable disease potential.[4]

Because ECs provided first-aid care only (and were not equipped with diagnostic laboratory capacity), shelter health managers defined potential cases based on syndromes. For instance, diarrheal illness was defined as three or more watery stools per day and differentiated as bloody or nonbloody. Flu-like illness was defined as fever with either sore throat or cough. Besides airborne and waterborne communicable disease, the surveillance instrument elucidated skin infections, conjunctivitis, and injury as well as preexisting or newly diagnosed chronic diseases, substance abuse, and mental health problems (Figure 10-1). Thus this particular surveillance instrument took into account the unique characteristics of the population of interest.

American Red Cross

Hurricane Katrina Emergency Disease Surveillance

Shelter Name: _____ Phone: _____

Current Shelter Census: _____ FAX: _____

Point of Contact: _____ EMail: _____

For the past 24 hour period from 12:00 am to 11:59 pm: _____ Number of patients treated in past 24 hour period: _____

date (mm/dd/yy)

Count each person receiving medical attention only once, according to their most severe symptom (chief complaint):

Symptom category	Total # patients evaluated or treated	# Patients referred to another facility for care
Epidemic Disease Potential		
Fever >100.4°F (38°C) ALONE without localizing symptoms/signs		
Bloody diarrhea		
Watery diarrhea (3 or more watery bowel movements per day) with or without vomitting		
Vomiting only (One episode or more)		
Flu-like or other severe respiratory infection (e.g., fever and either cough or sore throat)		
Rash (circle: measles, rubella, chickenpox/varicella, skin infections, other)		
Scabies, lice, or other infestation		
Wound infection		
Conjunctivitis (pink eye)		
Other (suspected tuberculosis or hemoptysis, whooping cough, meningitis/encephalitis, jaundice/hepatitis,etc) Please specify:		
Mental Health/Psychological Problems		
Any pre-existing psychiatric disorder (major depression, anxiety, depression, bipolar disorder, schizophrenia)		
New psychiatric disorder since hurricane (post traumatic stress disorder, disorientation, dementia, confusion, out of control behavior, threats to self or others, loss of touch with reality)		
Drug/alcohol substance abuse or withdrawal		
Injury/Chronic Disease/Other		
Self inflicted injury		
Injury – Intentional (circle: violence, sexual assault)		
Injury – Unintentional (accidents)		
Dehydration		
Heat related injury (not dehydration)		
Diabetes Mellitus		
Asthma/COPD		
High blood pressure and other cardiovascular diseases		
Sexually Transmitted Disease/HIV		

Number of deaths within the past 24 hours _____

Do you need assistance with or additional resources for:

	Yes	No		Yes	No
Physician staffing	☐	☐	Nurse staffing	☐	☐
Pharmacist staffing	☐	☐	Mental Health staffing	☐	☐
Sanitation/Environmental Health	☐	☐	Medications/Drugs/Medical supplies	☐	☐

Additional Comments/Concerns: _____

THE FORM SHOULD BE TRANSMITTED DAILY. (FAX 225-216-2337)

If you do not have access to a fax, please call us at 225-216-2313 to provide the information by phone, or if you have any difficulties, questions or comments.

Rev: 9/9/2005 - final

FIGURE 10-1 Hurricane Katrina Louisiana Shelter Surveillance Form

Source: U.S. Centers for Disease Control and Prevention.

Health managers faxed, emailed, or phoned the data on the completed forms on a daily basis to a central reporting center at ARC Louisiana headquarters in Baton Rouge for analysis and rapid identification. Using CDC-developed software for surveillance indicators—the Early Aberration Reporting System (EARS)[5]—each indicator posted a cumulative sum score (CUSUM) that served

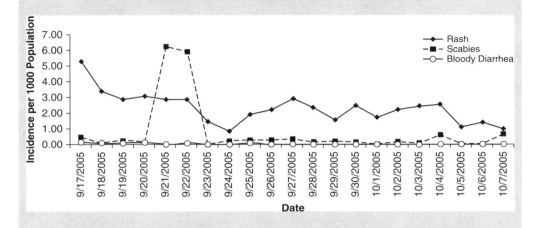

FIGURE 10-2   Hurricane Katrina Louisiana Shelter Surveillance for Select Diseases, 2005
Source: U.S. Centers for Disease Control and Prevention.

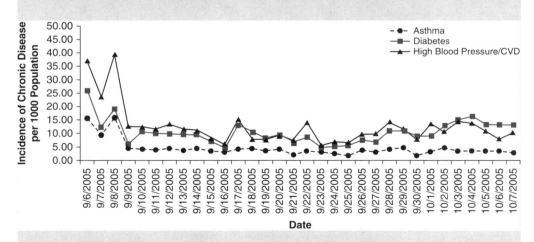

FIGURE 10-3   Hurricane Katrina Louisiana Shelter Surveillance for Chronic Disease, 2005
Source: U.S. Centers for Disease Control and Prevention.

as the "threshold" for further investigation. The CUSUM technique, as a sequential statistical method for detecting a shift in baseline, is more sensitive for moderate changes in health event rates and can be adjusted when the structure or size of the population changes.[6]

Although no airborne or waterborne outbreaks occurred at the ECs, a scabies infestation cluster was identified during the week of September 20, 2005 (Figure 10-2), and subsequently investigated and managed by local public health providers. As might be expected, patients with chronic diseases visited EC health posts early in the displacement period (Figure 10-3), reflecting the fact that the act of rapid evacuation with no other sheltering alternative meant they

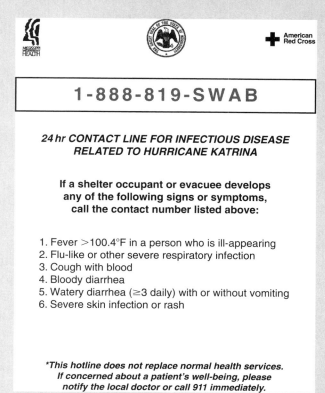

FIGURE 10-4   Hurricane Katrina Mississippi Case Definition Form for Shelter Health Managers

Source: The Working Group on the American Red Cross Public Health Response to Hurricane Katrina.

were likely to be without prescribed medications, without access to their regular health providers, and often without access to health insurance.[3]

ARC volunteers in Mississippi initiated an alternative surveillance mechanism in the aftermath of Hurricane Katrina, working with the Mississippi Department of Health (MDH), a cadre of public health academics, trained shelter health managers, and educated evacuees on communicable disease case definitions (Figure 10-4) at each of the 43 ARC-managed shelters in the state. They then instituted a toll-free telephone hotline through which cases could be identified, investigated by the team, and referred as needed. While 37 percent of 93 cases were referred for further evaluation, no outbreaks of communicable diseases occurred. This simple, flexible, inexpensive, proactive, and rapid response model not only provided much-needed surveillance for shelter venues likely to be out of the public health safety net, but also raised public health awareness in medical providers and evacuees and reassured providers that public health support was readily available to them.[7]

HISTORICAL PERSPECTIVES

Traditionally surveillance mechanisms involved a network of health services delivery actors, trained to detect changes in defined health events (indicators), usually rises in death rates or communicable disease cases. If, during their analysis, a certain threshold for an event was crossed, the actors would "sound the alarm" to those who should respond—typically agents within ministries of health at the national or district level with appropriate technical support from the World Health Organization (WHO) or other international support agencies as needed.[8] Surveillance evolved from the public health science of epidemiology: In this discipline's parlance, an epidemic exists when the observed number of cases of a given disease exceeds what is expected and is associated with a common or propagated source of infection. Over time, surveillance has become the informative process by which public health officials can make this comparison between observed and expected cases in the population.

With the recognition that complex emergencies generate an equally complex and multidisciplinary response, humanitarian stakeholders have moved surveillance beyond its communicable disease outbreak role. Today, surveillance is designed to monitor responses to particular interventions, inform public health programs, evaluate resource use, track noncommunicable diseases and injuries, recognize early signs of bioterrorism, and engage in program quality improvement, to name a few. In any application, surveillance defines itself as a trending mechanism of information.

The first globally focused communicable disease surveillance began in 1948 for influenza viruses. This system rapidly expanded to include a long list of reportable common communicable and rare noncommunicable diseases in developed countries where established health information systems could sustain them. By the latter quarter of the twentieth century, when large refugee and internally displaced population movements in developing countries necessitated a systematic vigilance for outbreaks of endemic diseases (particularly among persons who were not immune to those diseases), implementing surveillance became a humanitarian necessity. For instance, the active surveillance system for 73,000 Bhutanese refugees displaced to Nepal in 1991 identified that the leading causes of death were measles, diarrhea, and acute respiratory infections, and subsequently informed what we have come to learn as essential program interventions in the early phase of a humanitarian crisis: measles vaccination, vitamin A supplementation, and diarrhea and acute respiratory infection control using oral rehydration therapy and early antibiotic therapy, respectively. By identifying these target interventions, the surveillance system reduced high mortality rates over a period of several months.[9]

Surveillance also identified and tracked the most lethal infectious disease outbreak in a displaced population in recent history: The high crude mortality rates from the infections with *Vibrio cholera* 01 (and later *Shigella dysenteriae*) that swept through the massive Rwandan refugee population that crossed into Goma, Zaire, in July 1994 bordered on apocalyptic.[10] A rigorous daily surveillance system initiated by humanitarian nongovernmental organizations (NGOs) followed crude death and death from diarrhea rates in nearly 800,000 refugees, along with the effects of a rapid NGO response consisting of treatment, water, and sanitation interventions. Crude mortality rate peaked at 25 to 30 deaths per 10,000 per day, then quickly declined to 5 to 8 deaths per 10,000 per day by the second month. Since this incident, the international community—especially donor governments, the United Nations (UN) operational agencies, NGOs, and affected ministries of health—have come to expect surveillance mechanisms during crises to routinely trend crude mortality rates, mortality rates in children (younger than 5 years), malnutrition, and cause-specific mortality rates in light of relief interventions.

The lethality of the Goma outbreak provided the momentum to establish humanitarian practice standards among a major consensus of stakeholders. The resultant Sphere guidelines (a manual that establishes humanitarian response best practices) mandated surveillance as a standard for health and nutrition information systems in humanitarian crises.[11] Humanitarian actors further realized the need to train and professionalize providers on evidence-based practice, skillfully designing and implementing such data-generating activities as surveillance in a timely and informative fashion.

For present-day suddenly displaced populations with marginal access to a full range of health services, the focus of surveillance activities remains communicable diseases, particularly high-impact morbidity and mortality events (i.e., diseases with high epidemic potential) such as diarrheal illness (often nonspeciated), acute respiratory infections (frequently differentiated between upper and lower respiratory infections), measles, malaria, and meningococcal meningitis. Other endemic communicable diseases such as typhoid, dengue, rabies, neonatal tetanus, HIV/AIDS, and tuberculosis are also considered as geographically dictated. Acute and chronic malnutrition—indicated by weight-for-height ratios and height-for-age ratios below two standard deviations of the mean—is often a contributing factor to mortality from these preventable infectious diseases and, therefore, is included in the form of "nutritional surveillance." The rationale for selecting this initial group of indicators derives from the risk of mortality they pose to the most vulnerable of humanitarian populations, notably children younger than age 5 years, immunocompromised persons, malnourished persons, and larger populations lacking herd immunity for vaccine-preventable diseases. Maternal death, neonatal death (a live-born infant death younger than 28 days old), and trauma/injury (intentional and unintentional) are often included early in surveillance programs during emergencies.

To conduct surveillance for communicable diseases through networks of healthcare facilities, providers identify cases using standardized case definitions, as facility diagnostic capacity (i.e., microscopy or rapid diagnostic testing for malaria) may be nonexistent during emergencies. If a case meets the clinical case definition, it is considered "suspect." If, in addition, other clinical or epidemiologic evidence is identified, the case is termed "probable." If it can be identified through laboratory tests regardless of clinical signs or symptoms, it is called "confirmed." Some examples of case definitions follow:

- Diarrhea: three or more loose or watery stools per 24-hour period, with or without dehydration
- Measles: maculopapular rash and cough, coryza, or red eyes
- Acute (lower) respiratory infection in children: cough or increased work of breathing and respiration rate of more than 50 breaths per minute (for infants aged 2 to 12 months) or more than 40 breaths per minute (for children aged 1 to 5 years)
- Meningitis: sudden onset of fever (greater than 100.4°F/38°C) and either stiff neck, altered level of consciousness, or petechial/purpuric rash

Cholera, as the etiology of a diarrheal case, would be suspected if severe dehydration or death from diarrhea resulted; would be considered probable if it occurred among other similar cases; and would be confirmed by isolation of *V. cholerae* from a stool sample. A list of commonly used case definitions and reporting forms can be found in the WHO's *Communicable Disease Control in Emergencies* field manual, which was last updated in 2005.[12]

Public health emergencies that precipitate sudden or prolonged food insecurity (e.g., famines, collective losses of livelihood from conflicts or natural disasters) require surveillance for acute or chronic malnutrition. Nutritional surveillance is typically based at health facilities capable of monitoring growth and, therefore, following a cohort of children younger than age 5 years. In this type of surveillance, weight-for-height ratios (for acute malnutrition), height-for-age ratios (indicator of chronic malnutrition), and kilocalorie/day intake are linked to not only other health and demographic indicators, but also measures of household food distribution and access. By 2005, WHO had modified the conceptual framework suggested by McNabb et al.,[13] establishing through consensus the six core activities of surveillance: detection, registration, confirmation, reporting, analysis, and feedback (Figure 10-5). Four functions—communications, training, supervision (for quality assurance), and resource acquisition—support these six core activities. Health providers at surveillance sites must be trained in case definition and recognition, and communication networks must exist for data streams (reporting) to reach trained and supervised data managers, who analyze the information and send it on to decision makers at the programmatic level. Critically, the activities that bring this analysis to light in real time—surveillance—are inextricably linked to public health action at the policy and decision levels of local and national governments and, in the case of emerging infectious diseases and terrorism events, regional and global actors.

The emergence of severe acute respiratory distress syndrome (SARS) in March 2003 highlighted the fundamental need for shared information across global surveillance networks. This disease spread rapidly across borders (through personal travel), appeared to be readily transmissible, had nonspecific symptoms, and was associated with a high case-fatality rate. Given those characteristics, the need for rapid detection and containment and the identification of measures for prevention and control were immediate and international.

The transborder, transcontinental spread of established infectious disease and the prospect of emerging infectious diseases remain the primary concerns of international surveillance efforts. To this end, WHO maintains the Global Alert and Response (GAR) program, which provides technical support to signatory countries for strengthening their respective surveillance mechanisms and public health preparedness efforts. In accordance with the 2005 International Health Regulations, state parties are obligated, under defined criteria, to notify WHO of "events that may constitute a public health emergency of international concern."[14] The document

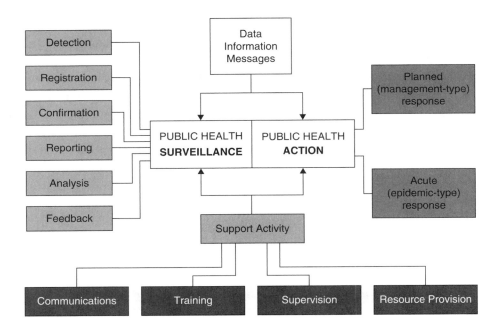

FIGURE 10-5   WHO Framework for Surveillance
Source: World Health Organization.

further elaborates the conditions by which such public health information must be shared in a timely fashion.

PREPAREDNESS AND RESPONSE

The prospect of bioterrorism events, emerging infectious diseases such as SARS and influenza A subtype H1N1, mass chemical or radiation exposure, mass gatherings,[15] and natural disasters or conflicts generating massive population movements or the cataclysmic devastation of a country's socioeconomic and governing structures—all signal the need for preparedness through surveillance mechanisms.

Ideally, a country will have a functioning surveillance and vital registration system in place prior to the occurrence of a disaster or conflict. A vital data registration system that systematically records births, deaths, and in- and out-migrations is critical to establishing a baseline estimation of the population chosen for surveillance. Unfortunately, resource-poor health ministries rarely have the capacity to sustain or manage these systems while at the same time often being located in countries prone to disaster- and conflict-generated public health emergencies. On occasions when public health emergencies have occurred in these countries, the international community, led by WHO (often with assistance from international governmental agencies) and working through the large international humanitarian relief agencies, will assist the specific ministry of health in constructing or fortifying its surveillance system.

Regardless of whether a surveillance system is constructed (or rebuilt) in the pre-emergency, immediate aftermath, or post-emergency phase, all such efforts share similar qualities, common data sources, and comparable indicators. For instance, surveillance systems should be simple, flexible (adaptable to changes in focus as an emergency evolves and resolves), easily understood by all stakeholders (public health practitioners and policy makers, international and local communities), and readily accessible (preferably through the Internet, fax, email, or SMS [short message service] text). These qualities enhance the speed of data collection, analysis, and dissemination.

Data sources are typically health facility or household based, depending on the indicators of interest. Facility-based surveillance sites are usually hospitals and/or clinics, but other facilities of interest may include factories, ports of entry such as airports or other customs stations, or places where large populations tend to gather. In general, the choice of surveillance sites is dictated by the place where an individual with a specific disease entity would likely present himself or herself. Household-based sites may be needed if the population of interest cannot access health facilities due to lack of transportation or finances. For example, in a rural district of Zimbabwe where access to healthcare facilities is limited, a water and sanitation NGO relied on a network of community volunteers in villages throughout the district to periodically report syndromically defined diarrheal incidence during the cholera outbreak of 2008–2009. Community-perceived "blips" above baseline were investigated and reported to the ministry of health and WHO officials in the country's capital.[16]

Comparable emergency indicators typically include high mortality communicable disease incidence; crude, pediatric (younger than age 5 years), and cause-specific mortality rates; acute and chronic malnutrition and food security; and program specific impact markers (e.g., immunization coverage, health system function). As the emergency transitions to a post-emergency development phase, the surveillance system will expand to include demographic information; other group mortality (maternal, infant); morbidity from noncommunicable disease and injury (e.g., traffic accidents, sexual and nonsexual violence); morbidity from additional, less rapidly fatal communicable diseases (e.g., HIV, TB, sexually transmitted diseases); mental health; and livelihoods.

In constructing a surveillance system, one must take into account the "disease profile" of a place—namely, the air-, water-, and vector-borne endemic diseases likely to emerge above baseline with environmental disruption and subsequent degree of exposure. For example, in the surveillance system established following the January 2010 Haiti earthquake, malaria and dengue—both endemic in Haiti—were included, especially given that the rainy season was fast approaching and would increase vector (mosquito) activity.

Surveillance systems that are constructed and implemented during crises tend to be active systems—that is, they require trained providers to actively record (and possibly investigate) cases into the system. Ministry of health administrative personnel regularly solicit data logs from providers at regular intervals. In contrast, passive systems, which tend to be ongoing concerns in post- and pre-disaster phases, rely on the initiative of the provider to bring cases to the system. As a result, passive systems, while cheaper and less labor-intensive over the long run, are less detailed and complete than active systems. As a consequence, passive systems tend to be less sensitive to changes in indicators from baseline and, in general, less representative of the population under surveillance. Deaths from a specific cause may go unreported in a passive system due to a cultural need to dispose of a body quickly; unless a monitor observes a mass burial, talks to grave diggers, and interviews village leaders, cause-specific mortality rates may be falsely low and an opportunity for life-saving intervention missed as a result.

The choice of sites for a surveillance network depends on whether the population under surveillance is the whole population, a representative sample of that population, or a specific population that might frequent only a certain site. Universal surveillance systems favor entire populations or whole segments of populations and, like active systems, are demonstrably more representative for a given indicator. Sentinel surveillance implies the use of specialized sites that are linked to indicators of specific interest: A voluntary testing center for HIV or a prenatal clinic, for instance, would be most appropriate for capturing increases in the transmission of HIV; a clinic at a major airport with international routes would be a logical sentinel site for identifying passengers with flu-like illnesses returning from abroad. GeoSentinel is an example of a network of global travel medicine clinics that opt-in as sentinel sites for patients presenting with travel-related illnesses. While the data they collect are less representative of the entire population than the data collected at universal sites, sentinel sites provide higher-quality, more complete, and more timely data on high-risk populations.

Multiple examples of surveillance networks exist, each with specific objective functions and health areas of concern. The rise in global networks reflects the boundary-ignorant quality of emerging infectious diseases and the irreversible trajectory of international travel. WHO's Global Alert and Response Network (GAR) supports individual states' surveillance efforts, links surveillance information across member states, and manages surveillance databases to ensure a timely coordinated and collaborative global response. Government surveillance information networks also play a critical role in sharing real time outbreak information: Public Health Agency of Canada's Centre for Emergency Preparedness and Response, the United Kingdom's Health Protection Agency, the U.S. Centers for Disease Control and Prevention (CDC), and the European Centre for Disease Prevention and Control (ECDC), to name a few, all contribute to this effort. The policy consequences of the terrorist attacks on September 11, 2001, in the United States included shifting public health resources to biological and chemical terror event surveillance at U.S. federal and state levels. That said, local surveillance systems—whether in the developing world or the developed world—continue to serve as the fundamental first line of defense for identifying changes in the baseline of a population's health. The global networks depend on local systems' ability to function iteratively and sustainably.

The boom in rapid communications technology and information management has significantly enhanced surveillance networks' ability to gather and disseminate information. ECDC's *Eurosurveillance*, an open-source journal, CDC's *Morbidity and Mortality Weekly Report*, and WHO's *Weekly Epidemiologic Record* are salient examples of timely peer-reviewed, quality surveillance analysis for programmatic and public awareness purposes. Canada's Global Public Health Intelligence Network (GPHIN) monitors global media sources, Web sites, and newsfeeds for infectious disease outbreaks, including foodborne and waterborne diseases; events with the potential for bioterrorism exposure; and health outcomes of natural disasters. CDC's National Electronic Disease Surveillance System (NEDSS) maintains an Internet-based cyber-infrastructure for the exchange of surveillance data from state and local partners.

Taken together, communications technology and the refining of digital information management have exponentially improved the speed and efficiency of the entire surveillance process. Data collected at sentinel sites can be immediately SMS-texted from mobile phones directly into easily managed, readily familiar database programs such as Microsoft Excel. Many cell phones come equipped with global positioning systems (GPS) capable of "tagging" specific surveillance data with a spatial characteristic (coordinates of latitude and longitude) at a moment in time. This additional geospatial information can be readily analyzed and presented in an animated format, graphically depicting an outbreak as it develops over time and place. Maps also provide rapid, user-friendly "analysis" for policy makers and decision makers, answering questions about whether the new events arise in a *geographically significant* pattern (e.g., in a cluster perhaps) in addition to the more traditional temporal and orders of magnitude pattern changes. When these data are combined as a time–space scan statistic in the analysis, public health officials can craft a more targeted response—equipping specific health facilities with antibiotics or initiating local vector control measures, for example—with greater confidence and a clearer mandate.

Beyond the established surveillance networks, public health experts are gleaning infectious disease information from such nontraditional sources as local observers and news informants through rapid mobile communications such as SMS, blogs, and Twitter feeds. Health Map, an independent organization supported by Google, uses automated text processing to gather outbreak information from unsolicited crowd sources as well as official sources. While reliability and information quality remain a challenge with this approach, the open, user-friendly manner of data collection has brought a new public awareness and engagement at the local level that can only benefit the surveillance process and improve response.

ANALYSIS OF CASE STUDY

Both CDC and WHO have published detailed guidelines for the evaluation of surveillance systems.[17] These recommendations take into account the qualities, design, degree of stakeholder engagement, and costs of the system, in addition to the technical components. Multiple factors, individually or in combination, can disrupt the trending of even basic morbidity and mortality indicators.

Perhaps the greatest challenge to any surveillance system, however, is sustaining it. Stakeholders—donor governments, operational UN agencies, field-level NGO personnel, ministry of health, and local data collectors—must all have a sufficient level of "buy-in" to consistently maintain a flow of communication to and from field sites. Lack of feedback to field personnel, loss of morale, arduous reporting demands, and lack of training can be significant factors leading to the failure of surveillance systems over time. Insecure environments may limit access to sites or the ability of surveillance sites to function. The rote, manual method of collecting data slows down the process; incomplete data can leave critical gaps in the analysis.

Surveillance systems have limitations, of course. Because not all cases with a given indicator will necessarily have access to the surveillance network, surveillance systems will not be able to capture every morbidity event and, therefore, cannot provide incidence or prevalence rates of an event in a population. Depending on how the surveillance system is designed, it may not be able to explain reasons for changes in indicators (i.e., why are children younger than age 5 years dying of diarrheal illness in this population?), without links to other data sources (e.g., the quality and quantity of water, access to sanitation, hygiene). Likewise, surveillance may not be able to explain the reasons for improvement or failure of a given program or initiative.

The shelter-based Hurricane Katrina example discussed earlier in this chapter illustrates the typical challenges and limitations involved in establishing and maintaining surveillance systems in public health emergencies. Compliance from harried shelter health managers tasked with daily surveillance reporting over several weeks was nominal: On average, CDC received reports from 23 percent (range: 3 to 49 percent) of the surveillance sites daily. As a result, only an average of one third (range: 4 to 64 percent) of the shelter site population was under surveillance each day. Also, even though shelter health managers had been trained to gather surveillance data, the majority were unable to identify diseases with outbreak potential in another study,[18] indicating a general lack of public health understanding in a displaced population.

CONCLUSION

Although today's surveillance systems, with their integration of mobile technology, sophisticated analysis software, and Internet access, look very different from the traditional paper-based surveys of the last century, their objectives remain the same: early recognition of changes in baseline epidemiological characteristics of disease in a population to trigger and guide an appropriate emergency public health response. Intuitively, earlier recognition should translate into better mitigation and response strategies. This quest for speed has driven the explosive rise in the use of new technology to promote crowd sourcing, real-time data integration, and live feedback. As the ease of use, acceptance, and dependence on new data-gathering methods grow, a paradigm shift may occur in how passive data reporting is perceived. While technology may, indeed, make it easy for a larger number of agents to serve as event reporters (especially through open crowd-sourcing platforms), researchers may— probably for the first time—face the prospect of having too much data. Mining for statistical "gold" in this influx of live data streaming into surveillance platforms, ensuring strict adherence to epidemiological definitions, sustaining stakeholder engagement and a focus on local events in real time, and validating the authenticity of the users and data, while simultaneously maintaining the relevance of potentially large data sets to local programming and policy needs, may be the challenges for the surveillance efforts of the coming decade.

INTERNET RESOURCES

Health Map: http://healthmap.org

WHO Global Alert & Response network: http://www.who.int/csr/outbreaknetwork/en/

Global Public Health Intelligence Network (GPHIN): http://www.phac-aspc.gc.ca/media/nr-rp/2004/2004_gphin-rmispbk-eng.php

Health Protection Agency (United Kingdom): http://www.hpa.org.uk/HPA/

GeoSentinel: http://www.istm.org/geosentinel/main.html

NOTES

1. Medecins sans Frontiere. *Refugee health in emergency situations.* London: Macmillan; 1997.
2. Working Group on the American Red Cross Public Health Response to Hurricane Katrina. *American Red Cross and public health: The response to Hurricane Katrina and beyond.* Cambridge, MA: Harvard Humanitarian Initiative; March 2006.
3. Greenough PG, Lappi MD, Hsu EB, et al. Burden of disease and health status among Hurricane Katrina–displaced persons in shelters: A population-based cluster sample. *Annals of Emergency Medicine.* 2008;51(4):426–432.
4. Centers for Disease Control and Prevention. Surveillance in hurricane evacuation centers—Louisiana, September–October 2005. *Morbidity and Mortality Weekly Report.* 2006;55(2):32–35.
5. Centers for Disease Control and Prevention. Early Aberration Reporting System. Available at: http://www.bt.cdc.gov/surveillance/ears/. Accessed March 7, 2010.
6. Rossi G, Lampugnani L, Marchi M. An approximate CUSUM procedure for surveillance of health events. *Statistics in Medicine.* 1999;18:2111–2122.
7. Cavey AMJ, Spector JM, Ehrhardt DT, et al. Mississippi's infectious disease hotline: A surveillance and education model for future disasters. *Prehospital Disaster Medicine.* 2009;24(1):11–17.
8. World Health Organization. Disease surveillance: WHO's role. *Weekly Epidemiologic Record.* 1998;73(43):333–334.
9. Marfin AA, Moore J, Collins C, et al. Infectious disease surveillance during emergency relief to Bhutanese refugees in Nepal. *Journal of the American Medical Association.* 1994;272(5):377–381.
10. Goma Epidemiology Group. Public health impact of Rwandan refugee crisis: What happened in Goma, Zaire in July, 1994? *Lancet.* 1995;345(8946):339–344.
11. Sphere Project. *Humanitarian charter and minimum standards in disaster response.* Geneva: Sphere Project, 2004.
12. Connolly MA (ed.). *Communicable disease control in emergencies: A field manual.* Geneva: World Health Organization; 2005.
13. McNabb SJN, Chungong S, Ryan M, et al. Conceptual framework of public health surveillance and action and its application in health sector reform. *BMC Public Health.* 2002;2. doi: 10.1186/1471-2458-2-2.
14. World Health Organization. *International health regulations (2005)* (2nd ed.). Geneva: World

Health Organization; 2008.

15. Aung M. Syndromic surveillance in major sporting event: Jamaican experience. *Advances in Disease Surveillance*. 2007;4:144.

16. Harvard Humanitarian Initiative, Oxfam America. *Diarrhea early warning system and cholera response assessment*. Cambridge, MA: Harvard Humanitarian Initiative, 2009. Available at: www.hhi.harvard.edu. Accessed April 7, 2010.

17. Centers for Disease Control and Prevention. Updated guidelines for evaluating public health surveillance systems: Recommendations from the Guidelines Working Group. *MMWR Recommendations and Reports*. 2001;50:RR-13.

18. Brahmbhatt D, Chan JL, Hsu EB, et al. Public health preparedness of post-Katrina and Rita shelter health staff. *Prehospital Disaster Medicine*. 2009;24(6):500–505.

CHAPTER 11

Rapid Needs Assessments

Hilarie H. Cranmer and Mary Pat McKay

INTRODUCTION

The first priority in a public health emergency is to assess needs, vulnerabilities, capacities, damages, and losses in the affected population. Essential information must be rapidly gathered and communicated to enable appropriate resource mobilization. Rapid needs assessments (RNA)—also known as rapid epidemiological assessments—are a means to reduce morbidity and mortality in a vulnerable population in the immediate aftermath of a disaster. RNA has developed into one of the most essential tools in managing public health emergencies.

The goal of RNA is to identify objectively health and humanitarian needs so that responders can take immediate action based on those needs. Ideally, the information gathered helps to direct resources to the affected population as soon as possible, thereby preventing, to the maximum extent possible, morbidity and mortality in the weeks and months after the crisis. Optimally, these assessments help prioritize, plan, coordinate, address gaps, avoid duplication, and target those persons who are most vulnerable and most severely affected by the public health emergency. When carried out recurrently over the initial time period following an event, RNA enables monitoring and evaluation of programs that have been implemented.

Due to the often difficult nature of accessing those persons who are affected by a disaster, public health professionals would find it nearly impossible to ask each and every person what they need most and when. Over the years, a population-based approach to assessment has been developed to handle this task in the aggregate. To accurately determine the most representative sample of the whole population's needs, the most simple and effective methodology of RNA is cluster sampling. Cluster sampling was first adapted by the World Health Organization (WHO) in its Expanded Programme on Immunization (EPI) to assess levels of immunization coverage during the era of smallpox eradication.[1]

To assess needs, rapid assessments are done using epidemiological methodology that has been developed over the last 30 years. Once on the ground, data are gathered from the site itself as well as from those persons affected from the disaster. This data collection is carried out by interviewing key informants, by walking around the sites, and by talking directly to the most vulnerable. One must ensure equality and non-discrimination when collecting data in this manner, with particular attention being paid to the most vulnerable populations (i.e., women, children, elderly, and ethnic minorities), who tend to be the most marginalized both before and after the disaster.

Maintaining preparedness and planning for RNA require a solid background in public health and epidemiology and familiarity with currently available needs assessment tools. Modifying the tool may be necessary for the disaster context, and training those who are to use it has to be taken into account. Most assessments are conducted in austere environments, and personal access and safety are of utmost concern. In addition, technological items that require recharging or access to cell towers may not function successfully. "Rapid" means a quick turnaround for the next phases of projects. Most public health emergencies will need rolling assessments, based on the type of emergency and the specific nature of the needs. Furthermore, the timing and frequency of assessments will depend on how rapidly the crisis is evolving.

The Hurricane Katrina disaster, which devastated much of the Gulf Coast in the United States in 2005, is illustrative of all the elements required in a rapid needs assessment. This case presented ongoing concerns about the safety of the assessment team due to flooding and lawlessness in the hurricane's wake. The response required a coordinated multidisciplinary effort and the inclusion of assistance from a number of actors so as to deliver the most efficient humanitarian aid. Turnaround of the data in a logical, informative, and transparent way, with coordination across sectors, is key for a successful response.

Case Study

Hurricane Katrina made landfall in the Gulf Coast of the southern United States on August 29, 2005, as a Category 3 hurricane.[2] Prior to its arrival, most of the area had undergone mandatory evacuation. While many residents with resources were successful in self-evacuating to distant locations to stay with friends or relatives or were able to afford temporary housing, more than 1 million people were evacuated to inter- and intra-state shelters. Thousands more were unable to evacuate and remained in New Orleans, with more than 9,000 taking shelter at the Louisiana Superdome. Overall, this group of New Orleans citizens was the most chronically ill, displaced population the world has ever seen. Although the immediate needs of a refugee population in the developing world typically include immediate health needs, diabetes care, dialysis, and hypertension are not usually among them.

If the levees had held, damage to the area would have been limited and the scope of the catastrophe similarly mitigated. Unfortunately, much of downtown New Orleans lies several feet or yards below sea level, where it is protected from routine flooding by levees—levees that failed in the early hours of the day following the hurricane.[3] The ensuing floodwaters from Lake Pontchartrain stranded thousands of citizens who had been unable or unwilling to evacuate and isolated thousands in shelters previously thought to be "safe harbors." As emergency rescue efforts began, airlifting families from roofs and rescuing thousands from the downtown arena, the scope of the public health crisis became more obvious, and more shelters were opened as more and more displaced people required assistance.[4]

As the most basic needs for escape from floodwaters, safety, food, water, and shelter began to be met, several additional health issues rose to the forefront of the disaster—primarily coping with the scope and severity of chronic illnesses in the displaced population. This is where the unique process of rapid needs assessment was best demonstrated. Two weeks after the hurricane, Greenough et al. performed a cluster survey of more than 500 evacuees living in Red Cross shelters in Louisiana.[5] The data confirmed the suspicion that the displaced populations living in shelters were likely to be economically disadvantaged. The researchers discovered that 53 percent of the refugees were under-employed or unemployed, and 38 percent were dependent on benefits or social assistance. Of those surveyed, 56 percent suffered from chronic disease, including hypertension, hypercholerolemia, diabetes, pulmonary disease, and psychiatric illness. Additionally, 48 percent of those patients did not have access to their medications. The consequences of chronic diseases on a displaced population were demonstrated by the fact that upon arriving at the shelters, more than one third of the surveyed population displayed acute symptoms requiring immediate medical intervention.

HISTORICAL PERSPECTIVES

Public health emergencies, both intentional and natural in origin, have been occurring for thousands of years. Each has unique characteristics, and the populations affected suffer specific problems related to geography, weather, preexisting conditions, the ability of help to reach them, and the effects of pre-event interventions such as notification and evacuation. The appropriate public health response to varied populations and situations—for example, the San Francisco earthquake in 1989; the terrorist attacks on New York City and Washington, D.C., in 2001; the Indian Ocean tsunami in 2004; and Hurricane Katrina in 2005—require public health professionals to be flexible, to identify existing health needs rapidly in real time, and, while responding to current needs, to predict and plan for health needs in the next phases of the emergency. To achieve these goals, public health practitioners must have the tools to perform a rapid needs assessment to identify and initially address local needs in a fashion that utilizes available information and technology. Moreover, these tools must be scalable, adaptable, and durable enough to withstand their use in resource-poor environments.

The origins of RNA lay in the frustrations of applying developed-world epidemiological methodology to developing world emergencies, as experienced by WHO investigators in the EPI initiative while investigating smallpox eradication in the

TABLE 11-1   World Health Organization's List of Protocols for Rapid Needs Assessment
Introduction to Rapid Health Assessment.
Rapid Health Assessment in Epidemics: First Steps
Rapid Health Assessment in Meningitis Outbreaks
Rapid Health Assessment in Outbreaks of Viral Hemorrhagic Fever, Including Yellow Fever
Rapid Health Assessment in Outbreaks of Acute Diarrheal Disease
Rapid Health Assessment in Sudden Impact Natural Disasters
Rapid Health Assessment in Sudden Populations Displacements
Rapid Health Assessment in Suspected Famine Situations
Rapid Health Assessment in Chemical Emergencies
Rapid Health Assessment in Complex Emergencies

Source: World Health Organization. *Rapid health assessment protocols for emergencies.* Geneva: World Health Organization; 1999.

1960s.[1] Barriers to effective assessment included inadequate census data, medical information on the baseline population, and logistics.[6,7] In the 1980s, RNA evolved by adopting techniques from health services research, operations research, and traditional epidemiology. Examples include lot quality assurance sampling, rapid ethnographic assessment, and the EPI cluster sample survey.[1,8] In 1990, WHO published nine protocols outlining best practices in rapid health assessment, specific to the threat. This work was updated in 1999 to include an additional chapter that discusses complex disasters where intense political issues occur in addition to a specific health concern.[9] (See Table 11-1.)

PREPAREDNESS

All disasters are local. The most effective means of mitigating the short- and long-term effects of disasters, no matter what their size, is local preparedness. In terms of preparations for performing RNA, several crucial connections need to be established long before a public health emergency occurs: coordination and communication, backup planning, and understanding existing health needs in the at-risk population.

The multidisciplinary team that is deployed needs to be experienced in public health and epidemiology, and the team members must be trained in standards of humanitarian aid delivery. They should be able to communicate the results of the assessment in an efficient and timely manner. In addition, the team should be able to adapt the survey tool to the public health emergency, whether intentional or natural; understand the baseline standards of the population in terms of morbidity and mortality; and be able to make recommendations related to affected sectors such as water, nutrition, health, and livelihoods.

Local officials can plan ahead by recognizing existing health needs in the at-risk population. In addition to information from the local health authority, useful information may be available from online resources. In the United States, the Census Bureau can provide information about the size of the population, the number of persons per vehicle available, and even the likely demographics (e.g., ethnicity, age) of the population. These demographic data may prove critical when putting assessment team members together because the most essential element of survey and interview work is the ability to communicate with the persons involved. Many high-income countries have similar information available online.

To better assess baseline health characteristics, the Behavioral Risk Factor Surveillance System (http://www.cdc.gov/brfss/index.htm), a telephone survey encoded to the county level, can be used to document local rates of diabetes, hypertension, and coronary disease in the United States.[10] In most metropolitan areas, the local transportation agency knows how many wheelchair-accessible rides are needed and from which locations. Possessing information about who needs to get out ahead of time (in case of an identifiable natural disaster, for example) and who will need special assistance in leaving can lead to better planning. If at all possible, local public health agencies should plan ahead and ensure that the people with complex medical needs, or those who will be unable to care for themselves, will be evacuated before the disaster begins. In the worst-case scenario, this information can be used to identify some needs even from a significant distance and even in the middle of the night.

A review article written by David Bradt evaluates the RNA protocols available in the literature and used most frequently by the largest humanitarian organizations. According to Bradt, there are 10 ideal components of RNA:[11]

1. Disaster application: should specify whether the disaster is natural versus human-made and describe the timing of the event.
2. Assessment focus: it is better to include both local site and system-wide data gathering, thereby capturing site-specific details such as immediate family needs as well as system-critical information such as water sources and road access.
3. Meta-data: capture of information that is available through census databases or through public health departments. These data must be characterized as to whether the source is reliable.
4. Information priorities are (1) appropriate and critical or (2) inappropriate or noncritical. For example, information priorities for health are typically morbidity and mortality. Directly related to this factor are the environmental determinants of health: water, sanitation, food, and shelters.
5. Performance indicators that are specific, measurable, accurate, realistic and time bounded (SMART).
6. Benchmarks or quantitative standards are present and able to be compared with performance indicators.
7. An explicit data structure: For example, a template or a checklist may be used.
8. Portability: maximized so there is minimal page length.
9. Time needed: should be minimized for data gathering and document completion.
10. Immediately deployable without further formatting or collation.

Bradt has developed a universally applicable, two-page tool based on these components, and many organizations have adapted this tool to meet their own needs during a time of crisis. In addition, WHO has published a comprehensive Initial Rapid Assessment (IRA) form that has six sections:[12]

1. Population description
2. Shelter and essential nonfood items

3. Water supply, sanitation, and hygiene
4. Food security and nutrition
5. Health risks and health status
6. Health facility/outreach site assessment

Rapid needs assessment is focused on exactly that—assessing needs quickly. Addressing these needs is a critical next step. Planning should begin early to assess which methods are available for addressing a given problem and efforts made to identify criteria for engaging a wider circle of assistance. When are local resources enough? When does the county or state need to be called for assistance? At what point (or based on which criteria) does the crisis warrant assistance from a federal resource (and which one)? Before a public health emergency occurs, public health officials must understand who has which kinds of support to offer.

RESPONSE

Each organization responding to a disaster has its mandates for response, including what to do with the data gathered. According to Bradt, relevant information for decision making focuses on four key areas:[11]

- The most severely affected geographic area ("where") and catchment population ("who")
- The unmet needs of that population ("what")
- The goods and services that are appropriate for the current phase of the post-disaster response ("what now")
- Whether the interventions are amenable to ongoing surveillance and monitoring ("what next")

Turnaround of the data in a logical, informative, and transparent way, with coordination across sectors, is key for response interventions. New technology using broadband communication strategies can make this task far easier to complete than previously, but a broadband network has to be available and electricity or solar power sources must also be available to recharge portable devices. Again, preplanning is a crucial step for coordination of data transfers in the event of a disaster.

Cluster Sampling

Cluster sampling is one of the tools used to assess a population in a rigorous and inclusive way. The EPI method for cluster sampling recommends a systematic evaluation of 30 clusters, or communities, for the question at hand. In the WHO EPI cluster sampling, the assessment question is "What is the vaccination rate for all the children in this community?"[13] To begin the sampling process, the public health provider selects 30 clusters from a known population estimate; this population estimate can be obtained from a recent census. When selecting the cluster, the public health provider will want to be able to choose each cluster in a way that allows for an equal likelihood that the population in that cluster is similar to the population in any other cluster chosen. The best example of this process involves using a map of the area with a known population and creating a grid over the assessment area, such that each square of the grid is symmetric with its neighbor. If sampling a town that has an area of 30 miles by 30 miles, the public health provider can make a grid that has 0.25-mile squares, for a total of 120 clusters. Each square will then be assigned a number.

The next step is determining the interval the study will need to end up with 30 clusters to sample. In this case, 120 total squares divided by 30 clusters is 4; thus the assessment team will randomly determine where to start by picking a number from 1 to 4. A random-number generator can be used to accomplish this task or, more simply, the numbers on the serial number of a U.S. dollar bill can be used as a place to start (U.S. currency serial numbers are 8 numbers long). The assessment team goes to the center of the first cluster that is randomly chosen. If the number 3 is selected, the team will go to cluster number 3 and begin there. In that cluster, the team starts at a central point, selects a random direction from that point (spin a bottle), then chooses a dwelling at random among those in the line from the center, where they are standing, to the edge of that cluster.

Researchers must also determine the sampling unit and number of units to be sampled in each cluster.[14] For the EPI sampling of vaccinations, all children in the household in the age range of 12 to 23 months are selected and the caregiver interviewed. The sampling unit is a child, and the number of units is 7. When the team has selected a multifamily dwelling, the members would visit the first occupied unit. Starting from this household, the next nearest household is visited until at least 7 children have been found. Then the team moves to the next cluster, located 4 clusters away from the first cluster, spins the bottle again, and starts asking questions of the next cluster. If no one is there, the members proceed to the next household. Because clusters are selected with a probability that is proportional to the estimated size of the population (from the census data), the households/dwellings are selected with equal probability, and all eligible children in households are selected, the overall likelihood of any child being selected is roughly equal and the design is roughly self-weighted. The numbers chosen in this example allow vaccine coverage to be estimated with a 95 percent confidence interval of ±10 percentage points.[14]

MITIGATION _____

Disaster planning and preparedness have been shown to be quite effective at mitigating disasters. An important component of preparedness for rapid assessment is familiarity with the tools of assessment. The critical first step in assessing the needs of a disaster-affected population is information gathering. Once public health professionals determine who is at highest risk of being affected by a disaster, they have a better chance of helping them avoid or recover from further injury.

Local Emergency Mitigation

Just as all disasters are local, so the initial response and subsequent mitigation efforts also begin with local public health professionals. In the state of Louisiana and the city of New Orleans, these local mitigation efforts were initiated prior to Hurricane Katrina. Local and federal emergency officials rated the possible filling of the bowl of New Orleans as the worst possible scenario for a natural disaster in the United States.[15] Therefore, this event was ranked near the top of the U.S. Federal Emergency Management Agency's (FEMA) list of most probable and worrisome disasters. Because of these concerns, FEMA sponsored the development of a comprehensive disaster response and mitigation plan to be instituted in case of a severe hurricane striking New Orleans. In July 2004, the "Hurricane Pam" exercise brought together more than 300 officials from southeast Louisiana parishes, Louisiana state agencies, and federal agencies for an 8-day planning workshop and scenario-based exercise.[16] The scenario presented included a slow-moving, Category 3 hurricane, levee breeches, and flooding of the New Orleans metropolitan region.

One stated goal was to bridge the gap between the new National Response Plan and the existing state and local emergency response plans. Out of the Hurricane Pam exercise came the first draft of the Southeast Louisiana Catastrophic Hurricane Functional Plan, which covered 14 aspects of disaster response. Additional workshops throughout 2004 provided more details and specifics to the document, but, according to one FEMA official, some areas were never fully completed due to budget issues.[17] A number of plans, including those pertaining to a possible levee breech, were never delineated. In these cases, it was assumed that local officials would turn to their emergency preparedness plans.

Under the Louisiana Emergency Assistance and Disaster Act of 1993, the Louisiana Office of Homeland Security and Emergency Preparedness (LOHSEP) was responsible for both the preparation and the implementation of Louisiana's state emergency operations plan. The act also mandated that each parish president establish an office of homeland security and emergency preparedness to develop local emergency plans. Two supplements of the state's emergency operations plan were devoted solely to hurricane preparedness. The Southeast Louisiana Hurricane Evacuation and Sheltering Plan specifically addressed the evacuation of the New Orleans region. Although the state plan was intended to provide an outline for an "orderly" response to a catastrophic hurricane, it specifically stated that this document did not "replace or supersede any local plans, nor usurp the authority of any local governing bodies."

Basic Principles for an Effective Assessment

For public health officials to be able to utilize RNA tools and methods effectively, certain underlying principles must be taken into account and certain resources must be made available prior to the event. If these assessment resources are available before the public health emergency occurs, they can serve as mitigation in reducing the overall impact of the emergency by providing useful assessment data that can guide life-saving interventions. The assessment must be conducted immediately after the event, in an organized and coordinated fashion. The information must cover three main areas:[18]

- *The quality of life of the victims:* Determine the geographic region affected; its population; access areas; modes of transportation; communications systems; availability of basic services (water, electricity, communications, sanitation facilities, housing, shelters); and availability of food.
- *The scope of the damage:* Determine the number of deaths; the number of persons injured, the number who have disappeared, the number displaced, and their location; the status and capacity of health facilities; urgent needs; and human and material resources in the area.
- *The secondary health hazards for the population:* Identify potential threats to the population's health.

In addition, public health officials must have the capabilities to fulfill the following responsibilities:

- Keep the entire population informed of changes in the situation as they occur
- Keep the international community and potential donors informed of different situations that arise
- Adequately organize the receipt of donations and the procurement of the necessary resources

Public health officials must ensure that their agencies and personnel embrace certain principles regarding RNA-collected data prior to an event occurring. In the first few days after the event onset, timely information must be collected while disaster relief is being provided. The assessment teams must provide correct, easy-to-access information that is summarized—preferably, in tables, figures, and maps—for ease in using the data. When seeking initial donations, public health agencies need to be very specific about the resources required for optimal management of the emergency. These agencies should attempt to maintain a flexible information system that can be accessed by the national and international community, and they should share the compiled data with relief agencies, in addition to other government agencies.[18] Furthermore, agencies and officials should avoid making requests for donations of materials not itemized as immediate needs by the assessment teams. They should also refrain from issuing exaggerated reports or reports beyond the scope of the assessed sectors in an attempt to obtain increased amounts of external supplies.

ANALYSIS OF CASE STUDY

The 2005 Hurricane Katrina disaster is illustrative of all the elements required in RNA. Its aftermath has raised major questions about the United States' ability to respond to large-scale natural disasters. The limitations in the government's response capacity were highlighted when Hurricane Rita placed additional demands on an already strained response effort just one month after Hurricane Katrina had struck. Numerous high-profile studies of the response and recovery efforts have identified the four areas in which domestic disaster response can be improved: communication, planning, preparation, and response—all of which have direct implications regarding RNA.

The RNA tool that was created for the Hurricane Katrina response was a demonstration of the ideals that Bradt has outlined and that were discussed earlier in this chapter. The tool that was applied to Hurricane Katrina (and subsequently adapted to Hurricane Rita) had the following characteristics:[5]

- Focused on the shelters that were accessible
- Compared data with known census information
- Gathered critical information about mental health and livelihoods before and after the disaster
- Included performance indicators such as the Sphere standards for water and hygiene
- Used only a two-page template

- Took 20 minutes to complete
- Allowed team members to enter data in a timely manner that enabled a rapid turnaround

The problematic issues in the response to Hurricane Katrina were multiple: failing to plan for flooding; failing to enable evacuation for those persons who could not self-evacuate prior to the flood; failing to call for appropriate levels of state, regional, or federal assistance soon enough; and failing to secure initial coordination among disparate sources of assistance. The location of a major shelter (the Louisiana Superdome) was chosen inappropriately (partly due to failure of planning for flooding) and thousands of people who should have been protected were instead placed at particular risk. Going back even further, the failure to ensure that those in the New Orleans floodplain (which was always known to be below sea level) were offered and required to maintain adequate flood insurance means that even now, many families are permanently displaced from the homes they occupied before the hurricane hit.

Many of the problems that arose during the response to Hurricane Katrina resulted from poor planning and communication. Within the realm of disaster preparedness, a greater emphasis has been placed on clearly defining leadership roles and the chain of command. Hurricane Katrina and its aftermath have also prompted a shift in the U.S. government's disaster response. In a radical departure from the previous bottom-up response plan, the government has modified its response to be more proactive in disasters. In the event of a future catastrophic incident, the federal government says it will be better able to anticipate the possible need to assume local and state responsibilities temporarily. In these situations, communication and collaboration will be vital. The federal government has also become increasingly involved in assessing local preparedness, which it has incentivized by offering grants for well-prepared locales. On a local level, the lessons learned from Hurricane Katrina have improved the understanding of the flow of communication—most importantly, when, how, and who to ask for assistance.

In addition to identifying the need to quickly provide routine medications and treatments for chronic medical problems, even in the absence of any medical records, rapid assessments of shelter populations shortly after the disaster revealed that one of the most important aspects facing the displaced population was urgent treatment of mental health issues. Even after arrival at distant locations, some evacuee groups needed further needs assessment. A small group of 106 family groups arrived in Denver, Colorado, and repeat RNA demonstrated specific needs within the group for assistance adjusting to altitude, medication, housing, dental care, and finding employment.[19]

CONCLUSION

Rapid needs assessments are a critical component of the preparedness, response, and mitigation for any public health emergency. Preparedness and planning of emergency responders include familiarization with these assessment tools as well as background work on the disaster itself and the affected population. Key methodological components include using cluster sampling methodology and applying tools that use SMART techniques. For public health professionals, understanding the "where, who, what, what now, and what next" aspects of the crisis is critical.

INTERNET RESOURCES

Centers for Disease Control and Prevention: Behavioral Risk Factor Surveillance System
http://www.cdc.gov/brfss/

Sphere Project: *The Sphere Handbook*
http://www.sphereproject.org/content/view/27/84/lang,english/

United Nations High Commissioner for Refugees: *UNHCR Handbook for Emergencies*
http://www.unhcr.org/472af2972.html

World Health Organization: *Health Cluster Guide*
http://www.who.int/hac/global_health_cluster/guide/en/index.html

World Health Organization: *Global Health Cluster Tools*
http://www.who.int/hac/global_health_cluster/guide/tools/en/index.html

World Health Organization: *Global Mid-level Management Modules*
http://www.who.int/immunization_delivery/systems_policy/training/en/index1.html

NOTES

1. Lemeshow S, Robinson D. Surveys to measure programme coverage and impact: A review of the methodology used by the Expanded Programme on Immunization. *World Health Statistics Quarterly*. 1985;38:65–75.
2. Hurricane Katrina makes landfall. *International Herald Tribune*. August 29, 2005. Available at: http://www.iht.com/articles/2005/08/29/america/web.0829katrina.php. Accessed December 10, 2009.
3. New Orleans inundated as levees break after Hurricane Katrina. *Bloomberg.com*. August 31, 2005. Available at: http://www.bloomberg.com/apps/news?pid=10000087&sid=at8E.YPX_.JA&refer=top_world_news. Accessed December 10, 2009.
4. Treaster JB, Kleinfield NR. Levee breaks devastate New Orleans: City virtually submerged as those remaining are told to leave. *International Herald Tribune*. Available at: http://www.iht.com/articles/2005/08/31/news/katrina.php. Accessed December 10, 2009.

5. Greenough G, Lappi MD, Hsu EB, et al. Burden of disease and health status among Hurricane Katrina–displaced persons in shelters: A population-based cluster sample. *Annals of Emergency Medicine*. 2008;51(4):426-432.

6. Tailhades M, Toole MJ. Disasters: What are the needs? How can they be assessed? *Tropical Doctor*. 1991;21(suppl 1):18–23.

7. Lemesow S, Tserkovnyi AG, Tulloch JL, et al. A computer simulation of the EPI survey strategy. *International Journal of Epidemiology*. 1985;14:473–481.

8. Henderson RH, Sundaresan T. Cluster sampling to assess immunization coverage: A review of experience with a simplified sampling method. *Bulletin of the World Health Organization*. 1982;60:253–260.

9. World Health Organization. *Rapid health assessment protocols for emergencies*. Geneva: World Health Organization; 1999.

10. Holt JB, Mokdad AH, Ford ES, Simoes EJ, Mensah GA, Bartoli WP. Use of BRFSS data and GIS technology for rapid public health response during natural disasters. *Prevention of Chronic Disease*. 2008;5(3):A97.

11. Bradt DA, Drummon CM. Rapid epidemiological assessment of health status in displaced populations: An evolution toward standardized minimum essential data sets. *Prehospital Disaster Medicine*. 2002;17(4):178–185.

12. World Health Organization. Initial Rapid Assessment (IRA): Field assessment form. Available at: http://www.who.int/hac/network/global_health_cluster/ira_form_v2_9_eng.pdf. Accessed March 22, 2010.

13. World Health Organization. Training for mid-level managers: The EPI coverage survey. Available at: http://www.who.int/immunization_delivery/systems_policy/MLM_module7.pdf. Accessed March 22, 2010.

14. Milligan P, Njie A, Bennett S. Comparison of two cluster sampling methods for health surveys in developing countries. *International Journal of Epidemiology*. 2004;33:469–476.

15. McQuaid J, Schleifstein M. In harm's way. *The Times-Picayune*. First in a five-part series, "Washing Away," June 23–27, 2002.

16. Beriwal M. Preparing for a catastrophe: The Hurricane Pam exercise. Statement before the Senate Homeland Security and Governmental Affairs Committee. January 24, 2006.

17. Shane S, Lipton E. Government saw flood risk but not flood levee failure. *The New York Times*. September 2, 2005. Available at: www.nytimes.com/2005/09/02/national/nationalspecial/02response.htm. Accessed June 1, 2010.

18. Pan American Health Organization. Rapid needs assessment. Available at: http://new.paho.org/disasters/index.php?option=com_content&task=view&id=744&Itemid=800. Accessed March 20, 2010.

19. Ghosh TS, Patnaik JL, Vogt RL. Rapid needs assessment among Hurricane Katrina evacuees in metro-Denver. *Journal of Health Care for the Poor and Underserved*. 2007;18(2):362–368.

SECTION 4

Infectious Diseases Emergencies

CHAPTER 12

Contagious Diseases Epidemics

Terry Mulligan and G. Bobby Kapur

INTRODUCTION

The community response to any contagious disease outbreak must be an integrated effort involving the entire public health and medical resources. Infectious diseases occur commonly, regardless of region, socioeconomic status, or stage of urban development. Wherever public health officials or healthcare providers practice, they will be confronted with patients who have been exposed to contagious diseases through a variety of means. Given the extraordinary changes in immigration patterns, interstate and international commerce and shipping, national and international travel, and the numbers of asylum seekers and refugees, public health professionals now frequently encounter patients with contagious diseases that historically were confined to foreign and isolated parts of the world. For this reason, it has become even more important for emergency healthcare providers to become experts in recognition, stabilization, and treatment of many different contagious diseases, both common and uncommon, and to serve both patients and the general public through surveillance and monitoring.

Most healthcare professionals involved in acute care are comfortable and well trained in the process of evaluating patients of all ages who have fever or other signs of infection. However, recognition of the cause of an illness can become complicated when evaluating the same symptoms in a patient with a history of immigration, international travel, or refugee status. Even under usual circumstances, patients are exposed to any number of infectious agents through travel, food, and normal interactions with the many hundreds of individuals with whom they come in contact every day. In addition to more common diseases, healthcare providers should consider the possibility of unusual and rare pathogens, especially in recent travelers. Travel exposes an individual to a different environment and leads to different behaviors, and some travelers may take fewer precautions while on vacation and, therefore, may be exposed to less common respiratory, gastrointestinal, or sexually transmitted diseases.[1] The hospital's emergency department (ED) possesses its own unique set of variables, owing to the diverse mixture of nonspecific signs and symptoms exhibited by patients and the high risk of exposure from invasive procedures. The ED faces additional challenges as a vital component in limiting disease transmission by maintaining a high index of suspicion, sequestering high-risk patients, and strictly adhering to clearly defined infection control measures.[2]

In examining the major public health concerns surrounding contagious disease epidemics, this chapter addresses the important historical characteristics affecting immigrants, travelers, and local populations. It also provides an overview of major contagious diseases to assist public health and emergency healthcare professionals in monitoring for and surveillance of these diseases. Finally, this chapter discusses the public health implications of these contagious diseases and the role of public health and emergency responders in the recognition, treatment, and reporting of contagious diseases.

Case Study

On February 12, 2008, an adult visitor from Switzerland was hospitalized in Arizona with a rash and pneumonia. The disease was eventually identified as measles and linked to an outbreak occurring in Switzerland at the same time.[3] The patient's hospital admission prompted the verification of approximately 1,800 healthcare personnel's immunization status, and those without immunity were vaccinated. Through March 31, 2008, nine measles cases were reported to the Arizona Department of Health, and all but one were infected in healthcare settings. All cases were not vaccinated for measles at the time of exposure.

From January to July in 2008, 131 cases of measles were reported to the Centers for Disease Control and Prevention (CDC) from the following states:[4]

- District of Columbia: 15 cases
- Illinois: 32 cases
- New York: 27 cases
- Washington: 19 cases
- Arizona: 14 cases
- California: 14 cases
- Wisconsin: 7 cases
- Hawaii: 5 cases

- Michigan: 4 cases
- Arkansas: 2 cases
- Georgia: 1 case
- Louisiana: 1 case
- Missouri: 1 case
- New Mexico: 1 case
- Pennsylvania: 1 case
- Virginia: 1 case

From 2000 to 2007, on average, 63 measles cases were reported each year in the United States. During 2008, seven outbreaks occurred where three or more cases were linked to the same time and place; these outbreaks accounted for 106 (81 percent) of the cases. Fortunately, no deaths occurred during this measles epidemic. The findings indicate that measles outbreaks can occur in communities with unvaccinated persons and that maintaining high overall measles vaccination rates in the United States is necessary to limit future outbreaks of measles.

HISTORICAL PERSPECTIVES

Travel-Related Illnesses

Every year increasing numbers of people travel outside the United States. According to the CDC, more than 65 million U.S. residents traveled abroad in 2008 alone. Larger numbers of people are also traveling to the United States from other countries.[5,6] A large number of these travelers are at risk for travel-related illness and for being carriers of contagious diseases back to their communities. Nearly 70 percent of people traveling from industrialized countries to low-income countries become ill as a result of diseases contracted during their journeys, and at least 8 percent will seek medical care.[7-9] A specific study of 784 U.S. travelers found that 64 percent experienced at least one travel-related illness.[10] Common symptoms of travel-related illness include vomiting, diarrhea, fever, rash, and respiratory illness, although symptoms can vary widely. These illnesses can arise from a number of different sources: contaminated food or water, insect bites from vectors (mosquitoes, ticks), infected humans, or infected animals. Most source exposures are unknown, however.

Efficient evaluation of the ill traveler requires a systematic approach. The healthcare provider must obtain an appropriate and pertinent history such as pre-travel immunizations, regions and specific locations visited, and time spent in each region or country (Table 12-1). Likewise, the public health professional must be aware of the

TABLE 12-1   Important Historical Facts to Obtain from Travelers with Contagious Diseases

- Illness after travel does not always mean illness is travel related.

- Obtain the patient's specific itinerary to determine which diseases are endemic to the area(s) visited.

- Check up-to-date information on any disease outbreaks in locations of travel.

- Determine the amount of time spent at each location to take advantage of known incubation times in identifying specific diseases.

- Review the type of travel (rural, urban) and ask about ingestion of untreated water, raw foods, or specific exposures.

- Identify any pre-travel vaccines or prophylaxis for specific diseases the patient has been given. Also ask about normal childhood vaccinations.

- Always consider malaria after travel to regions where this disease is endemic, especially Africa. Also remember that the incubation time for malaria can be months long.

- Remember to obtain sexual history for the traveler and consider acute HIV or other sexually transmitted diseases as a source.

- Ask about any illnesses in fellow travelers and about any medical treatment given during the trip.

- Ask about any insect bites (especially ticks).

- Notify local health departments for concerns of transmissible disease outbreaks.

Source: Hals G, Davis D. The traveler in the ED: Initial evaluation. *Emergency Medicine Reports.* 2008;29(14).

diseases that are endemic in different regions around the world and the specific etiologic and physiologic details of these conditions or diseases.[6]

Fever Patterns and Febrile Illnesses

Fever is a frequent presenting complaint in post-travel medical visits. In one British study of 1,084 admitted patients, 50 percent of travelers had a chief complaint of fever.[11] A larger study of almost 25,000 ill travelers found that 26 percent of patients with fever were admitted, compared to only 3 percent of those without fever.[12] The majority of patients presenting with fever after travel will ultimately have common, non-travel-related dis-

TABLE 12-2   Fever Patterns in Contagious Diseases

Episodic fever: classic for malaria

- Tertian fever (fever every other day) with *Plasmodium malariae*
- Quartan fever (fever every 3 days) with *P. falciparum, P. ovale,* and *P. vivax*
  - These patterns are uncommon in travelers with malarial infection, being seen in only 33% of cases.

Saddleback fever: common in dengue patients with early infection

- Brief (1 to 2 days) afebrile period between two longer periods of fever
- Also seen with leptospirosis, chikungunya fever, and brucellosis

Diurnal fever patterns: usually normal and do not usually represent exotic disease

- Temperatures higher in the afternoon/early evening and lower in the morning
- Morning fever spikes suggests typhoid fever

eases, such as upper respiratory infections or urinary tract infections.[13] As much as 25 percent of all travel-related febrile illnesses involves self-limited viruses that resolve spontaneously within 48 to 72 hours.[14,16] Although they are not diagnostic alone, fever patterns can provide helpful clues to suggest specific diseases (Table 12-2).[15–18]

Certain contagious diseases may be rapidly fatal and will require early identification to prevent morbidity or mortality (Table 12-3).

Immigration-Related Illnesses

The United States is a nation of immigrants. In the year 2000, it was estimated that 30 million immigrants resided in the United States[7, 8] and 93 percent of the U.S. population is descended from immigrants.[9,10] The U.S. immigrant population from 1900 to 1950 were 90 percent from Europe; in contrast, the latter half of the twentieth century brought increasing numbers of Asian and Latin American immigrants to the United States. Further, certain subgroups such as migrant workers also bring their particular set of travel, immigration, and exposure disease patterns.[10]

As the number of foreign-born individuals in the United States continues to grow, public health and healthcare providers must become ever more adept at handling the medical issues unique to this population. Many immigrants arrive in the United States with limited resources and little access to health care. Approximately 60 percent of low-income immigrants are uninsured, compared with 30 percent of

TABLE 12-3   Rapidly Fatal Contagious Diseases

Specific Treatment Available

- Malaria
- *Neisseria meningitis*/septicemia
- Rickettsial (spotted fevers, typhus)
- Leptospirosis
- Lassa fever
- Typhoid
- Amebiasis
- East African trypanosomiasis

Supportive Treatment Only

- Dengue hemorrhagic fever
- Yellow fever
- Japanese encephalitis
- Viral hemorrhagic fevers (Ebola, Marburg)

Reportable Due to Public Health Risk

- Active tuberculosis/multidrug-resistant tuberculosis
- Viral hemorrhagic fevers (Ebola, Lassa, Marburg)
- *Neisseria meningitis*/septicemia
- Severe acute respiratory syndrome (SARS)
- Plague (pneumonic)
- Cholera
- Potential agents of bioterrorism (e.g., anthrax)

Source: McLellan SLF. Evaluation of fever in the returned traveler. *Primary Care Clinical Office Practice.* 2002; 29:947–969.

individuals born in the United States with the same income.[19] In addition, over the past decades, the federal government and states have reduced access to health coverage and care for immigrants, leaving the ED as the safety net for this significant segment of the population. Often, a disease process in an immigrant patient may be predicted by country of origin; nevertheless, while certain illnesses may predominate in some geographic regions, they may occur sporadically around the globe.[20]

Under-immunization

Although children born in the United States may not receive appropriate vaccinations despite rigorous public health vaccination campaigns, under-immunization affects immigrant populations at higher levels. Data from the CDC indicate that more than 50 percent of new arrivals in 1998 had an incomplete vaccination series.[9,20] Vaccination for diphtheria, pertussis, tetanus, and polio is common in most countries; however, vaccination for measles, mumps, and rubella is much more sporadic.[21–23] One survey of Guatemalan and Salvadoran refugees in Belize indicated that only 50 percent of children had received measles immunization.[23] In addition, U.S. immigrant children have *H. influenza* B (Hib) and hepatitis B vaccinations less frequently than non-immigrants.[24] In one New York immunization clinic, Hib coverage was 12 percent for foreign-born Latino children as compared to 78 percent for U.S.-born Latino children.[24] Many immigrants do not know if they have received a full vaccination series. One study of internationally adopted children showed that 65 percent had no written records of immunizations.[25]

PREPAREDNESS

The response to any disease outbreak must be an integrated effort involving the entire public health community. In addition to institutional protocols, public health departments should develop policy guidelines for such events, tailored specifically for application in an emergency public health setting. These guidelines should cover all essential areas:

1. Basic information on the clinical and pathophysiological characteristics of contagious diseases and their initial management
2. Definitions of contagious disease alert levels and their respective responses
3. Criteria for isolation
4. Equipment and physical materials for healthcare providers to receive, manage, and treat potentially infected patients
5. A training model regarding education, exercises, surveillance, prophylaxis, treatment, and communications

Public health and healthcare professionals need to apply these principles for their departments, depending on local needs, regulations, resources, and professional principles.[2]

Global Preparedness

At the global level, the World Health Organization (WHO) coordinates epidemic intelligence for contagious diseases through its Global Alert and Response (GAR) operations; the GAR focuses on a specific set of contagious diseases (Table 12-4). The International Health Regulations (IHR) have been in effect since June 15, 2007, in

TABLE 12-4   Contagious Diseases Monitored by the World Health Organization for Outbreaks

Acute diarrheal syndrome	Lassa fever
Acute febrile syndrome	Legionellosis
Acute hemorrhagic fever syndrome	Leishmaniasis
Acute neurological syndrome	Leptospirosis
Acute respiratory syndrome	Listeriosis
Acute watery diarrheal syndrome	Louseborne typhus
Anthrax	
Avian influenza	Malaria
	Marburg hemorrhagic fever
Botulism	Measles
Buffalopox	Meningococcal disease
	Monkeypox
Chikungunya	Myocarditis
Cholera	
Coccidioidomycosis	Nipah virus
Creutzfeldt-Jakob disease	
Crimean-Congo hemorrhagic fever	O'Nyong-Nyong fever
Dengue fever	Pertussis
Dengue hemorrhagic fever	Plague
Diphtheria	Poliomyelitis
Ebola	Rabies
Ehec (*Escherischia coli* 0157)	Relapsing fever
Encephalitis, Saint-Louis	Rift Valley fever
Enterohaemorrhagic *E. coli* infection	
Enterovirus	Severe acute respiratory syndrome (SARS)
	Shigellosis
Foodborne disease	Smallpox vaccine—accidental exposure
	Staphylococcal food intoxication
Hantavirus pulmonary syndrome	
Hemorrhagic fever with renal syndrome	Tularemia
Hepatitis	Typhoid fever
Influenza	West Nile fever
Influenza A (H1N1)	
	Yellow fever
Japanese encephalitis	

Source: World Health Organization Global Alert and Response. Available at: http://www.who.int/csr/don/archive/disease/en/index.html. Accessed February 2010.

194 countries and serve as legally binding international legislation. The IHR requires countries to report specific disease outbreaks to the WHO, and the WHO then implements established procedures to protect against the further spread of diseases (Figure 12-1).[26] These operational interventions include the following provisions:[27]

- Procedures for outbreak notification, consultation, and reporting
- Permanent communication channels 24 hours per day between countries and the WHO
- The availability of the WHO to accept account reports from sources other than notifications or consultations
- Verification requests by the WHO to national health authorities if an outbreak report occurs within a country
- Establishment of an Emergency Committee that reports to the WHO Director General regarding outbreaks that may indicate an international epidemic
- Collaboration of the WHO with other intergovernmental organizations or international bodies

The Global Public Health Intelligence Network (GPHIN) is a secure, Internet-based, early-warning instrument that constantly searches global media sources such as news wires and Web sites to locate information about disease outbreaks. GPHIN is a critical source for informal information about outbreaks, and more than 60 percent of initial outbreak reports come from unofficial and informal sources that require verification.[28] Once an outbreak has been identified by the WHO, the Global Outbreak Alert and Response Network (GOARN), a technical collaboration of existing institutions and networks, is activated to rapidly identify, confirm, and respond to international outbreaks. The GOARN provides an operational framework to interconnect personnel and technical expertise and skills within the international community, and allows countries to be alert and responsive to the threat of outbreaks.[29]

U.S. Surveillance Systems

Public health surveillance systems serve as a critical component of the preparedness for contagious diseases at the national, state, and local levels. These systems utilize a diverse set of sources to identify and locate disease outbreaks. These networks of surveillance systems attempt to identify contagious diseases at the outset prior to their expanding to the broader population. The bulk of most of the United States' surveillance lies with the local public health departments, which receive complaints from local individuals or providers in the community or notifications regarding reportable diseases.

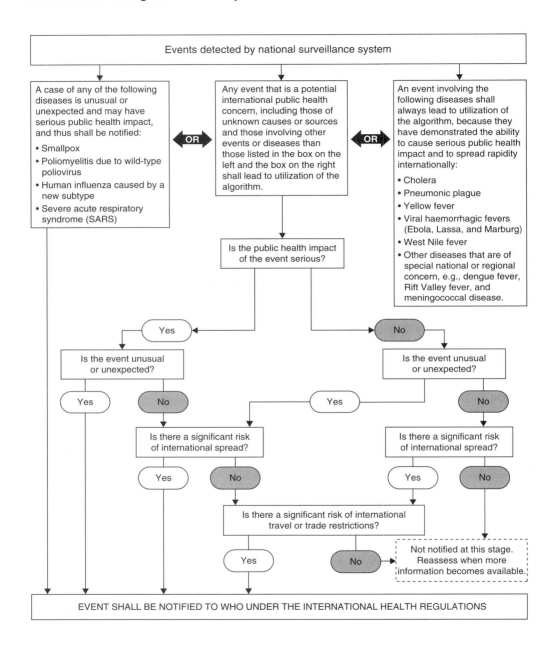

FIGURE 12-1   International Health Regulations Outbreak Notification Instrument
Source: WHO. Towards a Safer Future. In *World Health Report 2007: Global Public Health Security,* Chapter 5. Geneva:2007. Available at: http://www.who.int/whr/2007/en/index.html. Accessed February 2010.

At the national level, the CDC maintains a National Notifiable Disease Surveillance System that receives disease outbreak information from local and state public health agencies. Each individual state determines the specific conditions that are reportable, and reporting of diseases by the states to the CDC is done on a voluntary basis. The CDC annually updates the list of diseases it recommends for reporting (Table 12-5).

TABLE 12-5   CDC Nationally Notifiable Infectious Conditions, 2010

- Anthrax
- Arboviral neuroinvasive and non-neuroinvasive diseases
  - California serogroup virus disease
  - Eastern equine encephalitis virus disease
  - Powassan virus disease
  - St. Louis encephalitis virus disease
  - West Nile virus disease
  - Western equine encephalitis virus disease

- Botulism
- Brucellosis

- Chancroid
- *Chlamydia trachomatis* infection
- Cholera
- Cryptosporidiosis
- Cyclosporiasis

- Dengue
- Diphtheria

- Ehrlichiosis/anaplasmosis
  - *Ehrlichia chaffeensis*
  - *Ehrlichia ewingii*
  - *Anaplasma phagocytophilum*
  - Undetermined

- Giardiasis
- Gonorrhea

- *Haemophilus influenzae*, invasive disease
- Hansen disease (leprosy)
- Hantavirus pulmonary syndrome
- Hemolytic uremic syndrome, post-diarrheal

- Hepatitis
  - Hepatitis A, acute
  - Hepatitis B, acute
  - Hepatitis B, chronic
  - Hepatitis B, perinatal infection
  - Hepatitis C, acute
  - Hepatitis C, chronic
- HIV infection

- Influenza-associated pediatric mortality

- Legionellosis
- Listeriosis
- Lyme disease

- Malaria
- Measles
- Meningococcal disease
- Mumps

- Novel influenza A virus infections

- Pertussis
- Plague
- Poliomyelitis, paralytic
- Poliovirus infection, nonparalytic
- Psittacosis

- Q fever

- Rabies
- Rubella
- Rubella, congenital syndrome

- Salmonellosis
- Severe acute respiratory syndrome-associated coronavirus (SARS-CoV) disease

(continues)

TABLE 12-5 (*cont.*)   CDC Nationally Notifiable Infectious Conditions, 2010

- Shiga toxin-producing *Escherichia coli* (STEC)
- Shigellosis
- Smallpox
- Spotted fever rickettsiosis
- Streptococcal toxic-shock syndrome
- *Streptococcus pneumoniae*, invasive disease
- Syphilis

- Tetanus
- Toxic-shock syndrome (other than streptococcal)
- Trichinellosis (trichinosis)
- Tuberculosis
- Tularemia
- Typhoid fever

- Vancomycin-intermediate *Staphylococcus aureus* (VISA)
- Vancomycin-resistant *Staphylococcus aureus* (VRSA)
- Varicella (morbidity or deaths)
- Vibriosis
- Viral hemorrhagic fevers
  - Arenavirus
  - Crimean-Congo hemorrhagic fever virus
  - Ebola virus
  - Lassa virus
  - Marburg virus
- Yellow fever

Source: CDC National Notifiable Diseases Surveillance System. Available at: http://www.cdc.gov/ncphi/disss/nndss/phs/infdis2010.htm. Accessed February 2010.

Other components of the U.S. contagious diseases surveillance system focus on a broad spectrum of possible sources including food, water, or insect vectors. Food-based complaints and illnesses are tracked by local and state public health agencies, and each jurisdiction manages the reports and investigates the findings differently. Michigan has launched a Web-based reporting system that allows the public to file concerns any time of day.[30]

The CDC, in addition, manages the Foodborne Outbreak Reporting System, which is accessible through the Internet. In 2009, the CDC expanded the sources of reportable infections to contagious diseases due to water-borne, person-to-person contact, and animal contact, and the web-based reporting system was renamed the National Outbreak Reporting System (http://www.cdc.gov/healthywater/statistics/wbdoss/nors/).[30] In addition, the CDC funds the Foodborne Diseases Active Surveillance System (FoodNet), which serves as an enhanced sentinel surveillance system with 10 partner sites. FoodNet focuses on enteric diseases that are verified by laboratory testing and is an active surveillance process because investigators routinely contact area laboratories to enhance reporting of foodborne diseases. The CDC also coordinates the nationwide collaboration of local, state, and federal laboratories that can compare pathogens and their subtypes that are isolated from humans, animals, and foods throughout all jurisdictions. This collaboration is called the National Molecular Subtyping Network for Foodborne Disease Surveillance (PulseNet).

Agency Preparedness

Local public health agencies have numerous responsibilities preparing for a contagious disease outbreak that include implementing surveillance activities, registering and investigating complaints, communicating with local healthcare providers, regulating and inspecting food-service operations, implementing control measures to halt outbreaks, educating food workers on preventing outbreaks, and informing the public and media about outbreaks.[30] They also act as liaisons with local industry representatives and with the state and federal public health agencies. Many also provide advanced laboratory testing, including subtyping, such as the molecular fingerprinting available through PulseNet.

State public health agencies also conduct surveillance activities, but they often detect and coordinate the preparedness and response to outbreaks that occur across multiple jurisdictions such as cities or counties. Importantly, the state agencies establish policies and regulations for food safety and for disease reporting. In addition, they frequently have more advanced laboratory capabilities and personnel with expertise in epidemiologic and environmental outbreak investigation. State agencies serve as liaisons between local and federal agencies, and they can assist local agencies with communications and legal support.

At the federal level, the CDC serves as the lead agency for outbreak preparedness. The national surveillance systems have already been described in this chapter, and the CDC continuously develops and implements improved public health tools and methods to monitor for outbreaks. These advances are shared with state and local agencies. The CDC also standardizes the laboratory testing methods to maintain uniform tracking across jurisdictions. Additional resources include a large cadre of experts, training programs for public health professionals, educational materials for the public, and the capacity to address surges seen with epidemics.

RESPONSE

Once sentinel cases have been identified for a contagious disease, public health authorities will need to initiate control measures to limit the number of people affected by the disease, to communicate with the public about preventive measures, to discuss treatment options with healthcare providers, and to eradicate the source of the infection. In doing so, these officials will need to balance personal freedoms with population measures, especially if the disease has a high incidence of morbidity or fatality. Often, public health agencies will be required to act rapidly based on limited data, and response activities will be focused on population-wide measures and hospital-based measures, including surge capacity.

After an outbreak has been confirmed, usually with a cluster of cases of the same disease that can be traced to a single source, public health officials will initiate different responses based on the modes of transmission. For food- or water-based infections, officials will remove the affected consumable items from the food distribution network. If the disease is transmitted through a vector, such as the mosquito, then vector control measures will be implemented. If the transmission occurs in a person-to-person manner, then isolation measures may need to be enforced. Although a long list of contagious diseases are tracked by both the WHO and the CDC, this section focuses on the response measures to diseases that can spread rapidly through person-to-person contact (tuberculosis, measles, and bacterial meningitis) or through infected food or water (hepatitis A) and that have caused epidemics previously in the United States, leading to contagious disease public health emergencies.

Tuberculosis

Tuberculosis (TB) is the second most common infectious cause of death in adults globally, after HIV. Approximately one third of the world's population (nearly 2 billion people), is infected with *Mycobacterium tuberculosis* bacteria, and nearly 10 million people have symptoms of active disease.[31] The emergence of multidrug-resistant tuberculosis, the ongoing HIV epidemic, and social issues such as poverty and homelessness influence the increasing prevalence and global disease burden of TB. The WHO estimates that 95 percent of all cases of this disease occur in developing countries, mostly in sub-Saharan Africa and Asia. Therefore, the risk of an epidemic TB outbreak remains high either from a U.S. traveler returning from an area where TB is endemic or a visitor or immigrant from one of these countries serving as a carrier.

Tuberculosis is spread via airborne droplet transmission. Droplets are produced when patients with pulmonary tuberculosis speak, cough, or sneeze, or during medical interventions such as sputum induction, aerosol treatments, or bronchoscopy. Aerosolized particles are capable of remaining in the air for periods lasting from minutes to hours. Droplets deposited on intact skin are not infectious, as the organisms are unable to invade tissue. Of the patients with a primary infection, 90 percent will minimize (contain) the infection and develop a latent (non-active) tuberculosis infection that is not contagious to others.[32]

The classical systemic findings seen in TB are fever, weight loss, night sweats, loss of appetite, and weakness. In studies, fever has been observed in as many as 80 percent of patients with TB.[33] The clinical presentations of TB vary with the type of TB the patient has: pulmonary, miliary (disseminated), and extra-pulmonary. Pulmonary TB is the typical presentation of the disease; it may be either asymptomatic or manifested as pneumonia with productive cough and fevers. Pulmonary TB can eventually lead to cough with bloody sputum (hemoptysis) due to inflammation and tissue necrosis.

Pulmonary TB is frequently diagnosed on a chest x-ray, and the diagnostic finding is a Ghon complex: a calcified focus of infection in the lung. However, not all patients with TB have radiographic findings, and studies show that 10 percent of patients have normal chest x-rays. The definitive method of diagnosing TB is the finding of the infectious organism in sputum collected from the patient.

Treatment is usually started after a definitive diagnosis of TB. For pulmonary TB, the therapeutic regimen includes four drugs for the initial 2 months, followed by 18 weeks of continued therapy with a two-drug regimen of isoniazid and rifampin.[33] Isolation is recommended until at least 2 weeks of therapy have been completed, but, if a patient has multidrug-resistant (MDR) TB, isolation should end only when the sputum smears are negative.

At the global level, the WHO is working with partner countries through the Stop TB Strategy to limit the spread of TB. The primary components of this global plan include six actions:[34]

1. Pursue high-quality DOTS (directly observed treatment, short course) expansion and enhancement
2. Address TB-HIV, MDR TB, and the needs of poor and vulnerable populations
3. Contribute to health system strengthening based on primary health care
4. Engage all care providers
5. Empower people with TB and communities through partnership
6. Enable and promote research

For public health officials and healthcare providers, control measures at the local level begin by maintaining a high index of suspicion for TB in patients with a history and clinical presentation suggestive of the disease, especially for immunocompromised patients.[33] Patients suspected of having TB should be placed in respiratory isolation, with healthcare workers taking respiratory precautions as well. Patients should be admitted, and diagnosis of both pulmonary and extra-pulmonary TB should be aggressively pursued to prevent further transmission of these forms of the disease. In addition, public health officials should be notified, and individuals with possible exposures will need to be identified and tested.

Measles

Measles (rubeola) is a highly contagious viral illness transmitted via respiratory secretions. The CDC has instituted a policy that requires two doses of measles vaccine for every child.[35] The first dose is administered between 12 and 15 months of age, and the second between 4 and 5 years of age. If a suspected case is encountered by a public health professional or a healthcare provider, rapid interventions must be taken to prevent secondary cases because the virus is extremely contagious, with epidemics originating from only one or two index cases.

The incubation period for measles ranges from 7 to 18 days, and the diagnosis of measles should be considered in any person with a generalized maculo-papular rash lasting more than 3 days.[36] This rash typically begins at the hairline and behind the ears and gradually spreads down the entire body. In addition, patients may have a fever, cough, vomiting, diarrhea, or conjunctivitis. After the fourth day, the rash begins to disappear. In contrast to the pattern just described, immunocompromised patients may not present with a rash or may have the presence of an atypical rash. The appearance of Koplik spots—white spots located on the oral mucosa just adjacent to the molars—is indicative of the disease and can aid in clinical diagnosis. Secondary bacterial infections also are common, and prolonged fever may indicate ear infection, pneumonia, or encephalitis.

Measles is usually diagnosed based on clinical signs and symptoms, but the diagnosis may be confirmed with immunoglobulin M (IgM) antibody titer levels. Treatment of measles primarily includes supportive care. Some trials have shown that high doses of vitamin A may prevent morbidity and mortality in infants, and the American Academy of Pediatrics recommends vitamin A supplements for children aged 6 months to 2 years.[37]

Rapid and aggressive public health action is needed in response to measles cases. Case investigation and vaccination of household or other close contacts without evidence of immunity should not be delayed pending the return of laboratory results. Moreover, preparation for other control activities may need to be initiated before laboratory results are known. Control activities include isolation of known and suspected cases/patients plus administration of vaccine (at any interval following exposure) or immune globulin (within 6 days of exposure, particularly among contacts who are 6 months of age or younger, pregnant women, and immunocompromised people, for whom the risk of complications is highest) to susceptible contacts.[38] For contacts who remain unvaccinated, control activities include exclusion from day care, school, or work and voluntary home quarantine for 7 to 21 days following exposure. Persons who are known contacts of patients with measles and who develop fever and rash should be considered suspected measles patients and be appropriately evaluated by a healthcare provider.

To prevent transmission of measles in healthcare settings, infection control measures should be followed stringently. Patients who are suspected of having measles should be removed from ED and waiting areas as soon as they are identified and placed in an isolation room. If admitted as inpatients to the hospital, individuals with suspected measles should be placed immediately in a negative-pressure, isolation room and, if possible, should not be sent to other parts of the hospital for examination or testing purposes.

All healthcare personnel should have documented evidence of measles immunity on file at their work locations. Having high levels of measles immunity among healthcare personnel and such documentation on file minimizes the work needed in response to measles exposures. Recent measles exposures in hospital settings in three states necessitated verifying records of measles immunity for hundreds or thousands of hospital staff, drawing blood samples for serologic evidence of immunity when documentation was not on file at the work site, and vaccinating personnel who did not show evidence of immunity.

Bacterial Meningitis

Approximately 3,000 people in the United States are diagnosed with bacterial meningitis each year. The prevalence of the asymptomatic carrier state varies from less than 2 percent in children younger than two years of age to as high as 40 percent among certain groups of adolescents and young adults.[39] The highest carrier prevalence is found among people living in close proximity, such as college students and military recruits. Case fatality rates vary between 8 and 13 percent. Patients who recover from meningitis may sustain considerable long-term morbidity, and 12 to 19 percent experience sequelae such as hearing loss or brain injury.

The bacterium *Neisseria meningitidis* is the causative agent of meningococcal meningitis. In children and adults, clinical findings may include the following signs and symptoms:[40]

- Fever, pallor, rigors, and sweats
- Headache, neck stiffness, photophobia, or backache
- Nausea and vomiting, and sometimes diarrhea
- Lethargy, drowsiness, irritability, confusion, agitation, seizure, or altered mental status
- Painful or swollen joints, myalgias, and difficulty walking
- Hemorrhagic rash

In infants and young children, the following clinical findings may also occur:

- Irritability, dislike of being handled, or unwillingness to interact or make eye contact
- Loss of interest in the surroundings

- Tiredness, floppiness, drowsiness, and altered mental state
- Twitching or convulsions
- Grunting or moaning
- Turning from light
- Pallor despite a high temperature

The most specific and sensitive means of diagnosing bacterial meningitis is the evaluation of a patient's cerebrospinal fluid (CSF) for the causative bacterial agent through Gram stain and culture. In addition, the CSF may be evaluated for inflammatory markers such as white blood cells (WBCs), glucose, and protein levels to begin suspecting a bacterial cause for a patient's clinical presentation.[41] In the case of rapidly progressing meningococcal disease, laboratory tests are not available fast enough to be helpful, and they may remain within normal ranges early in the precipitous course of this disease. However, healthcare providers should not delay administration of antibiotics and resuscitative interventions to wait for the results of the lumbar puncture. Treatment consists of intravenous antibiotics of a third-generation cephalosporin with steroids to improve meningeal penetration of the antibiotics.[41]

Preventing spread of bacterial meningitis infections after a case has been confirmed will require personnel and logistical resources. The primary public health interventions will focus on targeted vaccinations and chemoprophylaxis. As recommended by the CDC, the decision to begin a population vaccination campaign should be based on the attack rate.[42] The attack rate per 100,000 = [(number of primary confirmed or probable cases during a three-month period) ÷ (number of population at risk)] × 100,000. At-risk populations should be vaccinated if the attack rate is greater than 10 cases per 100,000 population. Given that bacterial meningitis typically affects persons younger than 30 years of age and vaccines are not available for children younger than 2 years of age, targeted vaccinations emphasize people aged 2 to 30 years. However, public health authorities should consider the following variables before initiating such vaccinations:

- Thoroughness of case reporting and the number of possible cases of meningococcal disease that do not have bacteriologic or serotype confirmation
- The number of additional cases of meningococcal disease after the initial cluster of cases in the suspected outbreak
- Logistic and financial considerations

The primary method for prevention of meningococcal disease among close contacts of a patient with bacterial meningitis is antimicrobial chemoprophylaxis. Close contacts include the following persons:

- Household members
- Childcare center contacts
- Persons directly exposed to the patient's oral secretions (through kissing, mouth-to-mouth resuscitation, or endotracheal intubation)
- Travelers who had direct contact with respiratory secretions from an index patient
- Travelers seated directly next to an index patient on a prolonged flight (greater than 8 hours)

Because the probability of secondary infection for close contacts is greatest immediately after onset of disease in the index patient, chemoprophylaxis should be initiated in less than 24 hours after identification of the index case. Rifampin, ciprofloxacin, and ceftriaxone are approximately 95 percent effective in reducing nasopharyngeal carriage of *N. meningitidis* and are all acceptable antimicrobial agents for chemoprophylaxis.[42]

Viral Hepatitis A

Hepatitis A virus is a pathogenic RNA virus, and humans appear to be the only natural reservoir. Infection occurs through fecal–oral contamination, often through person-to-person contact, or as a result of poor hygiene and improper handling of food. Hepatitis A is the most common cause of acute hepatitis in the world, and subsequently a very common disease among travelers. Hepatitis A is also considered the most common travel-related infection that can be prevented by vaccination.[1]

Patients who are exposed to hepatitis A become symptomatic within 30 days. Interestingly, 90 percent of children with acute infection are asymptomatic, whereas 75 percent of adults who are infected develop a clinical syndrome.[43] Classic symptoms include sudden onset of fever, headache, anorexia, vomiting, abdominal pain, and dark urine. Jaundice is variable and is seen in 40 to 80 percent of cases. Most individuals recover after 2 to 3 weeks of illness, but in some cases relapses occur and symptoms may last as long as 6 months, usually in older patients.

Diagnosis of acute hepatitis A infection is by identification of IgM antibodies in the serum, and these IgM antibodies persist for 3 to 12 months after disease resolution. IgG antibodies appear after IgM antibodies and confer long-term immunity for the disease. Treatment for hepatitis A consists of supportive care. While symptoms persist, administration of other agents that may damage the liver—such as alcohol and acetaminophen—should be avoided.

Two vaccines are available in the United States against the hepatitis A virus, and they are recommended for travelers to high-risk areas. The first of the two doses of the vaccines should be given four weeks prior to travel. Hepatitis A immunoglobulin is also available for post-exposure prophylaxis and is usually given to close contacts of newly diagnosed patients. If given within two weeks of exposure, it is 85 percent effective in preventing illness.[43]

MITIGATION

Strategies to limit the impact of a contagious disease epidemic on a population will require interventions that reduce the exponential spread of the infectious agents through a series of multiple carriers. The critical means of mitigating the contagious disease include the following measures:

- Protecting uninfected individuals through vaccinations or chemoprophylaxis
- Vector control measures (eradicating mosquitoes)
- Removal of infected food and water products from the population
- Effective communications to the public about the disease, modes of transmission, and prevention
- Increases in healthcare workforce capacity for a limited duration

Vaccinations and chemoprophylaxis have already been discussed in this chapter. Thus this section focuses primarily on effective communications and healthcare surge capacity.

Effective Communications During an Outbreak

Contagious disease outbreaks possess unique characteristics that make communications critically important in mitigating the effects of the public health emergency within the population.[44] First, outbreaks require rapid interventions to prevent the spread of the disease among an unsuspecting population. Second, even familiar diseases, such as meningitis, may undergo mutations or present with varying subtypes that makes controlling their spread more challenging. Third, epidemics tend to illicit fear and anxiety in the public and lead to sudden changes in social patterns and behaviors. Finally, outbreaks can cause significant political and economic ramifications that can have a lasting impact on the population even after the outbreak has been contained or eradicated.

A crucial decision that frequently confronts public health professionals at the beginning of an outbreak is the timing of the announcement of the outbreak. Officials may want to delay the disclosure of a potential outbreak to limit panic and drastic activities by the public or government authorities. However, prompt disclosure has certain benefits:[44]

- When avoidable behaviors in the population are contributing to disease spread: Warn the public.
- When a defined risk group, such as healthcare workers or college students, is known to be especially vulnerable: Alert them to the risk and explain ways to reduce it.
- When neighboring countries may be at risk: Warn them to be alert for imported cases.
- When the affected country can benefit from international knowledge and expertise: Start the information flow.
- When local authorities know they will require international assistance: Reporting quickly produces a public expectation that interventions will follow.

The WHO outlines five best practices for communications during an epidemic: build trust, announce early, be transparent, respect public concerns, and plan in advance. From the public's perception, confidence in the motivations and actions of government agencies and officials will determine how well both the government and the population respond to an epidemic. Recommendations for both prevention and control measures that are provided by the public health authorities will be implemented only if the general public understands and accepts the validity of this information. If the public health agencies provide conflicting or delayed information during the outbreak, then the public will not trust any of the guidance that authorities communicate at the later stages of the outbreak. The initial announcement will have the largest impact on the public, and early disclosure has numerous benefits, as already described. Transparent communications are clear, accurate, and thorough, and they help build trust between the public and government agencies. Communications regarding an outbreak should address the public's concerns and attempt to counter any myths or false notions that may be spreading through the population. Finally, advance planning for effective communications strategies should occur in parallel with advance planning for other interventions such as vaccinations and treatments.

At the healthcare level, a contagious disease outbreak situation is an extremely stressful period for healthcare providers just as it is for the general public. To maximize morale and daily attendance, communication from departmental leadership on a daily basis, welfare activities, and identification of scope for frequent debriefings and feedback are all issues that need to be managed carefully and sensitively.[2] The heads of major departments within a hospital will also need to be closely involved with the hospital's outbreak planning process, including the determination of clinical protocols for management of suspected and probable cases. Such clinical protocols will also need to be disseminated to the staff on a regular basis.[2] Preparing training pamphlets, slides, and online documents for staff training have immense value in this realm because they can be used repeatedly, and learning materials for infection control procedures will be necessary for staff education to function in times of a disease outbreak.

Hospital Surge Capacity

The additional evaluation of patients required during a contagious disease outbreak, together with the slower pace of work that occurs when staff have to be completely gowned with full personal protective equipment (PPE), results in a longer time to manage each patient and an increased need for medical, nursing, and ancillary staff in the hospital, and particularly in the ED. There will be a need to determine the additional staffing required to manage not only the routine number of patients coming to the hospital, but also the extra numbers of patients who will be expected from the community. For planning purposes, the additional staffing during a contagious disease outbreak should be 50 percent higher than during non-outbreak periods based on experience during the SARS outbreak.[2]

The hospital will also be expected to maintain large observation areas separate from the ED owing to the surge of inpatient admissions and the difficulty in obtaining isolation beds for patients requiring inpatient care. Such areas, located close to the ED, will need to be pre-identified and the 24-hour staffing for these areas will need to be determined.

The sudden challenges faced by their workforce will cause hospitals to consider changing staffing patterns from the usual two or three shifts per day system to a modified per-day system to allow for hospital capacity and staff needs. Longer work hours can usually be tolerated if limited from a few weeks to a few months and if associated with other measures to improve staff welfare and communication.[2]

Consideration needs to be given to staff scheduling of fixed composite teams with little (if any) mixing between teams. This practice maximizes team integrity and minimizes losses to the department as a result of one member falling sick with an infection. It also simplifies contact tracing activities within the department. Of course, hospital administrators will need to be able to respond if staff members become ill. However, where infection control practices have been strictly complied with, the probability of infectious disease transmission and the likelihood of staff contracting the contagious disease or common diseases decrease significantly.

The additional staffing requirements would usually be met by preplanning and decreases in workload in the surgical areas of the hospital. Detailed pre-allocation would be important, and briefings for potential staff who may have to work in the ED during outbreaks allow for a smoother transition of these staff to the ED.[2] Planning for the additional staffing of the ED should be done commensurately with the increased need for outbreak-associated logistics such as PPE and positive-pressure respirators. Stockpiles of these items should be identified and secured by the hospital's Materials Management department. There will also be a need for additional patient stretchers, wheelchairs, and beds during the period of the outbreak. Sources of these items will need to be identified and arrangements made to have them delivered promptly in the event of the outbreak situation.

ANALYSIS OF CASE STUDY

Although measles is no longer an endemic disease in the United States, it remains endemic in most countries of the world, including some countries in Europe. In the United States, from January 1 to March 28, 2008, 24 confirmed cases of measles resulting from importations from endemic countries were reported to the CDC. The number of measles cases reported from January 1 to July 31, 2008, was the highest year-to-date total since 1996. This increase was not the result of a greater number of imported cases, but rather reflected greater viral transmission after the disease's importation into the United States, leading to a greater number of importation-associated cases. For the foreseeable future, measles importations into the United States will continue to occur because measles is still common in Europe and other regions of the world. Measles is one of the first diseases to reappear when vaccination coverage rates fall.

Within the United States, the current national measles, mumps, and rubella (MMR) vaccine coverage rate is adequate to prevent the sustained spread of measles. Unfortunately, importations of measles likely will continue to cause outbreaks in communities that have sizable clusters of unvaccinated persons; such clusters are often found in urban populations. These cases highlight the ongoing risk of measles spread in susceptible populations and the need for a prompt and appropriate public health response to measles cases. Because of the severity of the disease, people with measles commonly present in physicians' offices or emergency departments, and pose a risk of transmission to other patients and healthcare personnel both in these venues and in inpatient hospital settings. Healthcare providers should remain aware that measles cases may occur in their facility and that transmission risks can be minimized by ensuring that all healthcare personnel have evidence of measles immunity and that appropriate infection control practices are followed.

CONCLUSION

Infectious diseases occur on a routine basis in almost every community, and public health agencies need to be prepared for the possibility of a contagious disease epidemic. Changes in global trends for travel, commerce, and immigration will continue to affect modes of transmission of diseases that have historically been confined to certain regions. The WHO's International Health Regulations, the CDC, and state and local public health agencies all play critical roles in the surveillance and monitoring for disease outbreaks.

All health professionals involved in acute care should be aware of the larger public health risks that are posed by communicable diseases that present to the healthcare system, and should be familiar with the proper preparation, response, and mitigation procedures surrounding the recognition, stabilization, treatment, monitoring, reporting and surveillance of contagious diseases. Acting on the front line of the healthcare system and as the safety net for the majority of the public, acute care medical providers play an integral role in the arena of emergency public health.

INTERNET RESOURCES

CDC, National Center for Zoonotic, Vector-Borne, and Enteric Diseases: http://www.cdcgov/nczved/

CDC, recent outbreaks and incidents: http://emergency.cdc.gov/recentincidents.asp

U.S. Department of Health and Human Services, National Vaccine Program Office: http://www.hhs.gov/nvpo/publichealth.html

U.S. National Institutes for Health, National Institute of Allergy and Infectious Diseases: http://www3.niaid.nih.gov/

World Health Organization, Global Alert and Response: http://www.who.int/csr/en/

NOTES

1. Hals G, Davis D. A global perspective on infectious diseases. *Emergency Medicine Reports*. 2008;29(15).
2. International Federation for Emergency Medicine. Pandemic flu guidelines for emergency medicine. 2009. Available at: http://www.ifem.cc/Resources/PoliciesandGuidelines/Pandemic_Flu_Guidelines_for_Emergency_Medicine.aspx. Accessed February 2010.
3. CDC health advisory: Measles outbreaks in the United States: Public health preparedness, control and response in healthcare settings and the community. April 2, 2008. Available at: http://www2a.cdc.gov/han/archivesys/ViewMsgV.asp?AlertNum=00273. Accessed January 2010.
4. Update: Measles US January–July, 2008. *Morbidity and Mortality Weekly Report*. 2008;57(33): 893-896. Available at: http://www.cdc.gov/mmwr/preview/mmwrhtml/mm5733a1.htm. Accessed January 2010.

5. Bacaner N, Stauffer WM, Boulware DR, et al. Travel medical considerations for North American immigrants visiting friends and relatives. *Journal of the American Medical Association.* 2004;291: 2856–2864.

6. Hals G, Davis D. The traveler in the ED: Initial evaluation. *Emergency Medicine Reports.* 2008;29(14).

7. Lillie-Blanton M, Hudman, J. Untangling the web: Race/ethnicity, immigration, and the nation's health. *American Journal of Public Health.* 2001;91:1736–1738.

8. Walker P, Jaranson J. Refugee and immigrant health care. *Medical Clinics of North America.* 1999;4:1103–1120.

9. Meyer M, Barron D, Carter Clements R. Immigrant medicine: The emergency department perspective. Part I: Evaluation, diagnosis, and treatment of commonly encountered diseases. *Emergency Medicine Reports.* 2003;24(4).

10. Garcia H, Del Brutto O. *Taenia solium* cysticercosis: Emerging and re-emerging diseases in Latin America. *Infectious Diseases Clinics of North America.* 2000;14:97–116.

11. Harries AD. Fever. In: Cohen J, Powderly WG, et al. (Eds.), *Cohen & Powderly: Infectious diseases* (2nd ed.). New York: Mosby; 2004, pp. 1453–1458.

12. Wilson ME, Freedman DO. Etiology of travel-related fever. *Current Opinion in Infectious Diseases.* 2007;20:449–453.

13. O'Brien D, Tobin S, Brown GV, et al. Fever in returned travelers: Review of hospital admissions for a 3-year period. *Clinical Infectious Diseases.* 001;33:603–609.

14. Freedman DO, Weld LH, Kozanrsky PE, et al. Spectrum of disease and relation to place of exposure among ill returning travelers. *New England Journal of Medicine.* 2006;354:119–130.

15. Thompson MJ. Travel-related infections in primary care. *Clinical Family Practice.* 2004;6: 235–264.

16. Stanley J. Travel related emergencies: Malaria. *Emergency Medicine Clinics of North America.* 1997;15:113–155.

17. Sideridis K. Dengue fever: Diagnostic importance of a camelback fever pattern. *Heart and Lung.* 2003;32:414–418.

18. Cunha BA. Fever of unknown origin: Clinical overview of classic and current concepts. *Infectious Diseases Clinics of North America.* 2007;21:867–915.

19. Meyer M, Barron D, Carter Clements R. Immigrant medicine: The emergency department perspective. Part II: Commonly encountered diseases of Latin America, Asia, and Africa. *Emergency Medicine Reports.* 2003;24(5).

20. Walker P, Jaranson J. Refugee and immigrant health care. *Medical Clinics of North America.* 1999;4:1103–1120.

21. Gavagan T, Brodyaga L. Medical care for immigrants and refugees. *American Family Physician.* 1998;57:1061–1068.

22. Hurie, MB, Gennis MA, Hernandez LV, et al. Prevalence of hepatitis B markers, and measles, mumps, and rubella antibodies among Jewish refugees from the former Soviet Union. *Journal of the American Medical Association.* 1995;273:954–956.

23. Moss N, Stone M, Smith J. Child health outcomes among Central American refugees and immigrants in Belize. *Social Science and Medicine.* 1992;2:161–167.

24. Findley S, Irigoyen M, Schulman A. Children on the move and vaccination coverage in a low-income urban Latino population. *American Journal of Public Health.* 1999;89:1728–1731.

25. Schulte JM, Maloney S, Aronson J, et al. Evaluating acceptability and completeness of overseas immunization records of internationally adopted children. *Pediatrics.* 2002;109:E22.

26. World Health Organization (WHO). What are the International Health Regulations? Available at: http://www.who.int/features/qa/39/en/index.html. Accessed February 2010.

27. World Health Organization (WHO). International Health Regulations: Global alert and response. Available at: http://www.who.int/ihr/global_alert/en/. Accessed February 2010.

28. World Health Organization (WHO).Epidemic intelligence: Systematic event detection. Available at: http://www.who.int/csr/alertresponse/epidemicintelligence/en/index.html. Accessed February 2010.

29. World Health Organization (WHO). Global Outbreak Alert and Response Network. Available at: http://www.who.int/csr/outbreaknetwork/en/. Accessed February 2010.

30. Council to Improve Foodborne Outbreak Response (CIFOR). *Guidelines for foodborne disease outbreak response.* Atlanta, GA: Council of State and Territorial Epidemiologists; 2009.

31. World Health Organization (WHO). *Global tuberculosis control: A short update to the 2009 report.* Geneva: Author; 2009. Available at: http://whqlibdoc.who.int/publications/2009/9789241598866_eng.pdf. Accessed February 2010.

32. Centers for Disease Control and Prevention (CDC). Tuberculosis facts. Available at: http://www.cdc.gov/tb/topic/basics/default.htm. Accessed February 2010.

33. Wang E, Sohoni A. Tuberculosis: A primer for the emergency physician. *Emergency Medicine Reports.* 2007;21(1).

34. World Health Organization (WHO). *Global tuberculosis control: Epidemiology, strategy, financing.* Geneva: Author; 2009. Available at: http://www.who.int/tb/publications/global_report/2009/pdf/full_report.pdf. Accessed February 2010.

35. Centers for Disease Control and Prevention (CDC); Atkinson W, Wolfe S, Hamborsky J, McIntyre L (Eds.). *Epidemiology and prevention of vaccine-preventable diseases* (11th ed.). Washington, DC: Public Health Foundation; 2009.

36. Perry RT, Halsey NA. The clinical significance of measles: A review. *Journal of Infectious Diseases.* 2004;189(suppl 1):S4–S16.

37. Duke T, Mgone CS. Measles: Not just another viral exanthem. *Lancet.* 2003;361:763–773.

38. Centers for Disease Control and Prevention (CDC). *Manual for the surveillance of vaccine-preventable diseases.* Atlanta, GA: Author; 2008.

39. Humiston S, Brayer A. Meningococcal disease, Part I: Epidemiology, etiology, pathophysiology, and clinical features. *Emergency Medicine Reports.* 2005;26(6).

40. Yung AP, McDonald MI. Early clinical clues to meningococcaemia. *Medical Journal of America.* 2003;178:135.

41. Humiston S, Brayer A. Meningococcal disease. Part II: Diagnostic studies, differential diagnosis, and management. *Emergency Medicine Reports.* 2006;27(1).

42. Bilukha OO, Rosenstein N. Prevention and control of meningococcal disease: Recommendations of the Advisory Committee on Immunization Practices (ACIP). *Morbidity and Mortality Weekly Report.* 2005;54(RR07):1–21.

43. Brundage SC, Fitzpatrick AN. Hepatitis A. *American Family Physician.* 2006;73(12):2162–2169.

44. World Health Organization (WHO). *Outbreak communication: Best practices for communicating with the public during an outbreak.* Geneva: Author; 2005.

CHAPTER 13

Pandemic Influenza

Terry Mulligan and G. Bobby Kapur

INTRODUCTION

The large number of severely ill patients with influenza A H1N1 in 2009 who survived their illness serves as an important indicator that the public health response to an influenza pandemic today differs significantly from that noted during the 1918 influenza pandemic. In 2009, the surveillance, prevention measures, and antiviral treatments employed allowed countries to reduce mortality numbers from this potentially deadly infectious disease to the point that they were well below those observed in the devastating 1918 outbreak.[1] Given their more effective and widely available resources, nations have the obligation to develop collaborative strategies among hospitals and public health systems to ensure that, if the resurgence of a pandemic influenza occurs, the benefits of public health and healthcare infrastructures can be offered to the greatest number of people. Although it is difficult to predict the exact components of the next pandemic influenza virus, the current global experiences with influenza A H1N1 will serve as the framework and basis of discussions about pandemic influenza for this chapter.

Case Study

In April 2009, public health authorities in Mexico noted that the number of seasonal influenza cases was not decreasing as might be expected from March to May, and the healthcare divisions of the Mexican Institute for Social Security (Instituto Mexicano del Seguro Social [IMSS]) were informed of this aberration.

In addition, certain sentinel events occurred in Mexico from March to April that initiated increased surveillance epidemiological studies:[2]

- Outbreaks of influenza-like illness in the state of Veracruz
- Outbreaks of influenza-like illness in the state of Tlaxcala
- Outbreaks of influenza-like illness in the state of San Luis Potosí
- A suspected case of nontypical pneumonia in the state of Oaxaca

On April 23, 2009, public health officials in Mexico declared that a novel influenza A H1N1 virus (H1N1) had been isolated in samples from patients in Veracruz and Oaxaca.

Through the end of September 2009, more than 4,100 deaths were associated with the H1N1 pandemic globally, including 3,020 deaths in the Western Hemisphere. As of December 2, 2009, Mexico had 66,070 confirmed cases of pandemic H1N1 flu and reported 671 deaths from this cause.[3] The IMSS serves as Mexico's national public healthcare institution, providing health services to approximately 40 million people through nearly 1,100 primary healthcare centers and 259 hospitals. IMSS facilities treated the largest number of H1N1 cases and experienced the largest number of deaths from this influenza variant in Mexico during this episode.[2] Multiple factors played a role in the variation of both morbidity and mortality among patients in Mexico:

- Patient factors (comorbid diseases, nutritional status, immune levels)
- Population factors (density, number of people in community with H1N1)
- Health policy (access to care, quality of care)

In Mexico, many of the patients with flu symptoms would self-diagnose and select and purchase medications for their disease on their own; prescriptions are not required in this country. At the onset of the epidemic, prior to scaling up of the Mexican healthcare system, people with H1N1 infection might take as long as nine days to see a physician.[3] At the beginning of the H1N1 pandemic, Mexico was the only country to implement a large-scale strategy for school closures and bans on public gatherings. Mexico City, the world's third largest city, banned all nonessential activities. Estimates show that the pandemic cost Mexico approximately $4 billion.[3] On June 11, 2009, the World Health Organization (WHO) confirmed that this event qualified as the first influenza pandemic in 40 years.[4]

BACKGROUND

For the 2009–2010 flu season, more than 99 percent of circulating influenza viruses identified in the United States were influenza A H1N1 (2009 H1N1).[5] The clinical presentation of patients with uncomplicated 2009 H1N1 influenza virus infection is generally similar to that of patients with seasonal influenza and includes abrupt onset of fever, cough, sore throat, myalgias, arthralgias, chills, headache, and fatigue. Vomiting and diarrhea are reported more often with 2009 H1N1 than with seasonal influenza.[6] As is common with seasonal influenza, some patients with 2009 H1N1 may present without fever. Clinical judgment and local surveillance data for influenza and other respiratory pathogens are important in considering the differential diagnosis of patients presenting with an influenza-like illness. The 2009 H1N1 variant, although widespread globally, has not yet reached the mortality levels of prior pandemics in the past 100 years (Table 13-1).

Differential Diagnosis and Clinical Presentation of Influenza

The fever and respiratory manifestations of influenza are not specific, and similar findings can present with several other pathogens:

- Respiratory syncytial virus (RSV)
- Parainfluenza viruses
- Adenoviruses
- Rhinoviruses
- Coronaviruses
- *Mycoplasma pneumonia*

In contrast to influenza viruses, most of these pathogens do not usually cause severe disease, particularly in previously healthy adults. RSV and parainfluenza viruses can, however, lead to severe respiratory illnesses in young children and the elderly, and they should be considered in the differential diagnosis if these pathogens are known to be circulating in the community.[7] Because the clinical picture of seasonal influenza can often be indistinguishable from illnesses caused by other respiratory infections, management can be challenging even when the diagnosis of influenza is confirmed. Influenza virus infections can span the spectrum from subclinical infection to severe deterioration and can result in a wide variety of complications.

Even if an alternative etiology is determined, viral or bacterial co-infections can occur. The tendency for influenza to arise in community epidemics and to affect persons

TABLE 13-1   Characteristics of the Three Pandemics of the Twentieth Century

Pandemic (Date and Common Name)	Area of Emergence	Influenza A Virus Subtype	Estimated Reproductive Number	Estimated Case Fatality Rate	Estimated Attributable Excess Mortality Worldwide	Age Groups Most Affected (Simulated Attack Rates)	GDP Loss (Percentage Change)
1918–1919 "Spanish Flu"	Unclear	H1N1	1.5–1.8	2–3%	20–50 million	Young adults	−16.9 to 2.4
1957–1958 "Asian Flu"	Southern China	H2N2	1.5	<0.2%	1–4 million	Children	−3.5 to 0.4
1968–1969 "Hong Kong Flu"	Southern China	H3N2	1.3–1.6	<0.2%	1–4 million	All age groups	−0.4 to (−1.5)

Source: WHO Global Influenza Program. Pandemic influenza preparedness and response: A WHO guidance document. 2009. Available at: http://www .who.int/csr/disease/influenza/PIPGuidance09.pdf. Accessed January 2010.

of all ages may sometimes allow the clinician to diagnose influenza with reasonable certainty even in the absence of laboratory testing (Table 13-2). Nevertheless, definitive diagnosis requires laboratory testing. Rapid influenza diagnostic tests and immunofluorescence assay testing using a panel of respiratory pathogens have become increasingly available for aiding clinical management of patients with suspected influenza.[8]

TABLE 13-2   Key Clinical Features of Influenza

A typical case often begins abruptly with systemic symptoms such as fever, chills, myalgias, anorexia, headache, and extreme fatigue.

Fever typically lasts 2–3 days and usually reaches 38–40°C, but can be higher, particularly in children.

Nonproductive cough, sore throat, and upper respiratory congestion can occur at the same time, although these symptoms may be overshadowed by systemic complaints.

Physical examination reveals fever, weakness, mild inflammation of the upper respiratory tract, and rare crackles on lung examination, but none of these findings is specific for influenza.

In uncomplicated illness, major symptoms typically resolve after a limited number of days, but cough, weakness, and malaise may persist for as long as 2 weeks.

In the elderly and infants, presenting signs can include the following:

- Respiratory symptoms with or without fever
- Fever only
- Anorexia only
- Lassitude
- Altered mental status

In children:

- In children, fevers are often higher than in adults and can lead to febrile seizures.
- Gastrointestinal manifestations occur more frequently in children.
- Fever or apnea without other respiratory symptoms might be the only manifestations in young children, particularly in neonates.

Influenza is difficult to distinguish from illnesses caused by other respiratory pathogens on the basis of symptoms alone.

Source: Centers for Disease Control and Prevention (CDC). Interim recommendations for clinical use of influenza diagnostic tests during the 2009–10 influenza season. September 29, 2009. Available at: http://www.cdc.gov/h1n1flu/guidance/diagnostic_tests.htm. Accessed December 2009.

The WHO Pandemic Phases

The WHO has established a six-phase classification system for pandemics. This classification system allows countries to apply appropriate surveillance and monitoring resources based on global patterns of disease epidemiology. The phases provide a framework to aid countries in pandemic preparedness and response planning. The use of a six-phase approach has been utilized to facilitate incorporation of new recommendations into existing national plans.[9]

The six WHO pandemic phases are outlined here:[10]

- No animal influenza virus circulating among animals has been reported to cause infection in humans.
- An animal influenza virus circulating in domesticated or wild animals is known to have caused infection in humans and, therefore, is considered a specific potential pandemic threat.
- An animal or human-animal influenza reassortant virus has caused sporadic cases or small clusters of disease in people, but has not resulted in human-to-human transmission sufficient to sustain community-level outbreaks.
- Human-to-human transmission of an animal or human-animal influenza reassortant virus able to sustain community-level outbreaks has been verified.
- The same identified virus has caused sustained community-level outbreaks in two or more countries in one WHO region.

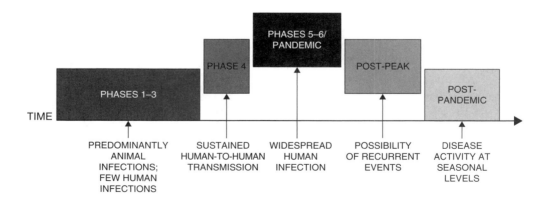

FIGURE 13-1   Pandemic Influenza Phases 2009
Source: WHO. Global Influenza Program. In Pandemic Influenza Preparedness and Response: A WHO Guidance Document, 2009. Available at: http://www.who.int/csr/disease/influenza/PIPGuidance09 .pdf. Accessed February 2010.

- In addition to the criteria defined in Phase 5, the same virus has caused sustained community-level outbreaks in at least one other country in another WHO region.

In addition, the WHO defines a "post-peak period" when levels of pandemic influenza have dropped below peak levels in most countries with adequate surveillance. It further defines a "post-pandemic period" when levels of influenza in most countries return to levels seen for seasonal influenza (Figure 13-1).

PREPAREDNESS

The WHO advocates a "whole society" approach to preparedness for pandemic influenza. In this concept, the national government serves as the lead entity for communications and coordination of efforts. To help nations with pandemic influenza preparations, the WHO has provided a checklist that divides government interventions into essential and desirable tasks for effective preparedness (Table 13-3). WHO officials will work with countries to coordinate the international public health response and will take responsibility for the following tasks:[10]

- Designate the current global pandemic phase
- Assist with the selection of the pandemic vaccine strain and recommend the timing to start pandemic vaccine production
- Assist with national pandemic rapid-containment efforts
- Assess pandemic severity
- Aggregate global key epidemiologic, virologic, and clinical information about the pandemic virus to help national authorities in deciding on the optimal response
- Provide guidance and technical assistance

Within the framework of the government policies and legislation, the WHO "whole society" model divides the main sectors into three subcategories:[10]

- Health sector
- Nonhealth sectors
- Individuals, families, and communities (civilian population)

The health sector includes public health and medical providers, including both public and private health sector components. This sector has the responsibility to communicate the risks of disease, to provide prevention measures, to develop the capacity to continue delivering medical care even during a pandemic, and to implement plans that halt the spread of the disease if surveillance systems indicate an approaching pandemic.

TABLE 13-3   Country Pandemic Influenza Preparedness Checklist

Section	Essential	Desirable
1. Preparing for an emergency		
1.1 Getting started	X	
1.2 Command and control	X	
1.3 Risk assessment	X	
1.4 Communication	X	
1.5 Legal and ethical issues		
1.5.1 Legal issues	X	
1.5.2 Ethical issues		X
1.6 Response plan by pandemic phase	X	
2. Surveillance		
2.1 Interpandemic surveillance		
2.1.1 General		X
2.1.2 Early warning	X	
2.2 Enhanced surveillance	X	
2.3 Pandemic surveillance		X
3. Case investigation and treatment		
3.1 Diagnostic capacity		
3.1.1 Local laboratory capacity		X
3.1.2 Reference laboratory availability	X	
3.2 Epidemiological investigation and contact management	X	
3.3 Clinical management	X	
4. Preventing spread of the disease in the community		
4.1 Public health measures	X	
4.2 Vaccine programs		X
4.3 Antiviral use as a prevention method		X
5. Maintaining essential services		
5.1 Health services	X	
5.2 Other essential services	X	
5.3 Recovery		X
6. Research and evaluation		X
7. Implementation, testing, and revision of the national plan	X	

Source: World Health Organization, Global Influenza Program. WHO checklist for influenza pandemic preparedness planning. Geneva: Author; 2005. Available at: http://www.who.int/csr/resources/publications/influenza/FluCheck6web.pdf. Accessed February 2010.

As part of the logistics and communications preparedness for influenza pandemics, the health sector must first identify those populations at highest risk for contracting influenza and for having severe complications from the disease, such as hospitalization or death (Table 13-4). At the community level, public health officials need to focus on preparing and planning for two primary interventions: vaccinations and antiviral stockpiles. Public health messages should advise the population to become vaccinated against the seasonal flu, and officials should recommend vaccines that are effective against novel or pandemic flu strains for high-risk groups. The second population-wide preparedness task will be having available stockpiles of antivirals to dispense to high-risk groups who have either been exposed to or have contracted the pandemic virus. The Centers for Disease Control and Prevention (CDC) maintains a Strategic National Stockpile that contains antivirals effective against H1N1, for example, and these resources are available to local public health officials within 12 hours of a large-scale pandemic flu emergency.[11]

TABLE 13-4   Groups at Risk for Complications of Influenza

The following groups are currently recognized by the Advisory Committee on Immunization Practices (ACIP) as being at higher-than-normal risk for complications of influenza compared to healthy older children and younger adults:

- Residents of nursing homes and other chronic-care facilities that house persons of any age who have chronic medical conditions

- Adults and children who have chronic disorders of the pulmonary or cardiovascular systems, including asthma

- Adults and children who required regular medical follow-up or hospitalization during the previous year because of chronic metabolic diseases

- Children and adolescents (aged 6 months to 18 years) who are receiving long-term aspirin therapy (and, therefore, are at risk for Reye syndrome)

- Pregnant women

- All children younger than 2 years of age

- All persons with conditions that can compromise respiratory function or the handling of respiratory secretions, or that can increase the risk of aspiration

Excluding the last group, in 2003 approximately 85 million persons in the United States belonged to one or more of these target groups.

Source: Centers for Disease Control and Prevention. Interim recommendations for clinical use of influenza diagnostic tests during the 2009–10 influenza season. September 29, 2009. Available at: http://www.cdc.gov/h1n1flu/guidance/diagnostic_tests.htm. Accessed January 2010.

The nonhealth sector will have the responsibility to prepare for contingency plans in the event of a pandemic and to protect employees so that business operations in all other sectors can continue, even if at a reduced capacity. Preparedness will be essential to prevent economic and financial disruption for the country. The U.S. Department of Homeland Security (DHS) provides recommendations for the business sector to assist with preparedness and planning for pandemic flu (Table 13-5).[12]

TABLE 13-5   Recommendations for Business-Sector Preparedness for Pandemic Influenza
Develop policies that encourage ill workers to stay at home without fear of any reprisal.
Develop flexible policies to allow workers to telecommute (if appropriate) and create other leave policies to allow workers to stay home to care for sick family members or care for children if schools close.
Provide resources and a work environment that promote personal hygiene: tissues, no-touch trashcans, hand soap, hand sanitizer, and disinfectants and disposable towels for workers to clean work surfaces.
Provide education and training materials in an easy-to-understand format, in the appropriate language, and at the appropriate literacy level for all employees.
Instruct employees who are well but who have an ill family member at home with the flu that they can go to work as usual.
Encourage workers to obtain a seasonal influenza vaccination.
Encourage employees to get the pandemic influenza vaccine when it becomes available if they are in a priority group according to government recommendations.
Provide workers with up-to-date information about influenza risk factors, protective behaviors, and instruction on proper hygiene.
Plan to implement practices to minimize face-to-face contact between workers if so advised by the local health department. Consider the use of such strategies as extended use of email, Web sites, and teleconferences. Encourage flexible work arrangements (e.g., telecommuting or flexible work hours) to reduce the number of workers who must be at the work site at the same time or in one specific location.
If an employee does become sick while at work, place the employee in a separate room or area away from other workers until they can go home.
Source: U.S. Department of Homeland Security. Planning for 2009 H1N1 influenza: A preparedness guide for small business. Washington, DC: Author; September 2009. Available at: http://www.flu.gov/professional/business/smallbiz.pdf. Accessed February 2010.

Individuals, civil society organizations, and nongovernmental organizations (NGOs) will be instrumental in stopping the spread of the disease by following strict hygiene guidelines and complying with immunization recommendations. Local organizations can assist with enhanced communications to members of local communities by providing information on disease prevention measures and on vaccination sites. Often these organizations have better outreach and penetration into communities, and they possess high credibility that will persuade individuals to take appropriate actions. The U.S. Department of Health and Human Services (DHHS), for example, collaborates with community and faith-based organizations to improve their effectiveness.[13] These organizations can provide facts and prevention measures in their own newsletters, and they can present the material in a format and language that are appropriate to the members of the organization. In addition, community and faith-based organizations might take steps such as sponsoring a lecture series on pandemic flu and related health topics, or they might provide a system whereby the organization corresponds intermittently with high-risk members, such as elderly individuals living alone, to evaluate how they are doing during a flu outbreak.

Even though an influenza pandemic may occur at any time, pandemic preparedness in many communities remains incomplete. The precise timing and impact of a future influenza pandemic remain unknown. Although developing and sustaining a

---

TABLE 13-6   Potential Consequences of Pandemic Influenza

Rapid spread of pandemic disease, leaving little time to implement ad hoc measures

Medical facilities struggling to cope with a possible large surge in demand

Serious shortages of personnel and products, resulting in disruption of key infrastructure and services, and problems in continuity affecting all sectors of business and government

Delayed and limited availability of pandemic influenza vaccines, antivirals, and antibiotics, as well as common medical supplies for treatment of other illnesses

Negative impact on social and economic activities of communities, which could persist long after the end of the pandemic period

Intense scrutiny from the public, government agencies, and the media on the state of national preparedness

A global emergency limiting the potential for international assistance

Source: World Health Organization, Global Influenza Program. WHO checklist for influenza pandemic preparedness planning. Geneva: Author; 2005. Available at: http://www.who.int/csr/resources/publications/influenza/FluCheck6web.pdf. Accessed February 2010.

community's preparedness is certainly challenging, communities should confront the risks posed by complacency so as to help their members avoid the emergency public health consequences of a full-scale pandemic flu (Table 13-6).

RESPONSE

The DHHS has outlined a three-part plan for responding to an influenza pandemic: a strategic plan, public health guidance for state and local partners, and DHHS agencies' operational plans.[14] The DHHS strategic plan focuses on protective public health measures, vaccines and antivirals, healthcare and emergency response, and communications and outreach (Table 13-7).

At the state and local levels, pandemic influenza response will require management of scarce resources and clarification of local laws, regulations, and statutes pertaining to closures, quarantine measures, and worker's compensation. The actual surveillance, diagnostic testing, infection control, and delivery of care will occur at the local and state

TABLE 13-7 DHHS Pandemic Influenza Strategic Plan Components	
Strategic Plan Component	**Pandemic Response Action**
Surveillance, investigation, and protective public health measures	1. Increase international surveillance and collaboration to track the emerging epidemiological patterns and effects of the novel influenza virus. 2. Determine the feasibility of containing the initial outbreak of a potential pandemic, working in consultation with international partners and implement containment activities. 3. Obtain samples of the potential pandemic virus from infected people and distribute them to laboratories for genetic, antigenic, and antiviral resistance analysis. Prepare reference strains for distribution to vaccine manufacturers. Assess the efficacy of stockpiled vaccine (if available) against the pandemic virus. 4. Implement surveillance and control measures at points of entry into the country to decrease introduction and spread of the pandemic virus in the United States. 5. Enhance domestic surveillance to detect pandemic outbreaks, track the spread of virus in near real time, and assess its effects on health and infrastructure. 6. Implement public health measures to limit the spread of infection as well as individual measures to decrease the risk of acquiring or spreading infection. 7. Monitor pandemic response actions and assess their effectiveness.

TABLE 13-7 *(cont.)*   DHHS Pandemic Influenza Strategic Plan Components

Strategic Plan Component	Pandemic Response Action
Vaccines and antiviral medications	1. Consider administration of pre-pandemic stockpiled vaccine (if available) to predefined groups critical to the pandemic response. This could provide partial immune protection. 2. In conjunction with other parties, manufacture, test, license, and produce a vaccine against the specific pandemic virus strain. 3. Allocate and administer the pandemic vaccine to predefined priority groups. Ensure security for protection of scarce vaccines. 4. Monitor vaccine coverage and track vaccine use so that persons who receive initial pandemic vaccine can return for a second dose, if required. Monitor for adverse events following vaccination, and conduct studies to assess vaccine safety and effectiveness. 5. Allocate stockpiled antiviral drugs for use in predefined high-risk and critical-infrastructure populations. 6. Monitor antiviral drug distribution and adverse events, and conduct studies to further assess safety and effectiveness.
Healthcare and emergency response	1. Distribute stockpiled ventilators and other medical materials needed to treat and care for infected individuals to health departments and federal agencies that provide direct patient care. 2. Deploy Federal Medical Stations, as available, to handle the healthcare surge capacity in the hardest-hit areas. 3. Test patient specimens using highly accurate, rapid diagnostic tests to identify pandemic outbreaks in communities and contribute to management decisions. 4. Assist communities with surge mortuary services to accommodate a large number of expected fatalities. 5. Provide psychosocial support to responders and affected communities.
Communications and outreach	1. Communicate measures the public can implement to minimize risk of contracting the disease and decrease the spread of infection. 2. Provide honest, accurate, understandable, and timely information. 3. Counter confusion and panic.

Source: Modified from U.S. Department of Health and Human Services. HHS pandemic influenza plan. Available at: http://www.hhs.gov/pandemicflu/plan/pdf/Overview.pdf. Accessed February 2010.

levels, and public health authorities in these jurisdictions will need to ensure they have adequate financial and personnel resources to respond effectively (Table 13-8). One of the critical response initiatives carried out at the local level will be vaccination campaigns. Specifically, local public health authorities will need to establish collaborations with healthcare partners and stakeholders to distribute, deliver, and administer vaccines to high-priority groups.[15] In addition, local authorities will be required to monitor vaccine supplies and watch for adverse events due to vaccinations. After high-priority groups have been vaccinated, public health officials will initiate vaccinations of the general population and provide updated information as the pandemic evolves.

Pandemic Influenza Control Measures

Control measures that need to be initiated in healthcare facilities and possibly in large gathering areas include early identification, early isolation, and early implementation.[16]

TABLE 13-8   Pandemic Influenza Response Summary Points at Local and State Levels
Public health officials should consider influenza diagnostic testing for the following groups: • Hospitalized patients with suspected influenza • Patients for whom a diagnosis of influenza will inform decisions regarding clinical care, infection control, or management of close contacts
Most individuals who have clinical signs and symptoms of uncomplicated influenza and who reside in a community where influenza viruses are circulating will not require diagnostic influenza testing.
When a decision is made to use antiviral treatment for influenza, treatment should be initiated as soon as possible without waiting for influenza test results because treatment is most effective when provided early in the course of illness.
Public health officials should be aware when using rapid influenza diagnostic tests that negative results do not necessarily indicate absence of influenza virus infection.
Laboratory tests to diagnose pandemic influenza with high specificity, such as real-time reverse transcriptase polymerase chain reaction (RRT-PCR), should be prioritized for hospitalized patients and immunocompromised persons with suspected influenza where rapid diagnostic tests are negative.
Source: Centers for Disease Control and Prevention (CDC). Interim recommendations for clinical use of influenza diagnostic tests during the 2009–10 influenza season. September 29, 2009. Available at: http://www.cdc.gov/h1n1flu/guidance/diagnostic_tests.htm. Accessed January 2010.

Early identification of persons infected or suspected to be infected with influenza can be accomplished through fever screening conducted at the entrance of healthcare facilities for all presenting patients. Fever screening consists of the following steps:

- Rapid temperature measurement of all patients by the use of tympanic membrane (TM) thermometers or thermal scans ("walk-through" sensors)
- Completion of fever-screening questionnaire:
  - Patient demographic information
  - Temperature measurement
  - History of fever documentation
  - Travel history documentation, especially in regard to travel to areas known to have patients with current flu infection
  - Contact history documentation
  - Documentation of related symptoms of flu
  - Particulars of accompanying persons, including contact particulars

All patients who fail the fever screening test are to be directed to the "fever zone" of the facility (discussed next) to help separate febrile and potentially infectious cases from other patients.

Early isolation of persons infected or suspected to be infected with influenza can occur in an area called a "fever zone," where all patients with fever, positive contact history, and history of travel to infected communities and those with associated symptoms will receive care. The fever zone should have facilities for full triage, patient registration, and management of both ambulatory and stretcher patients. A number of observation beds will also be useful in this zone. In addition, this zone will require its own radiology facility, patient toilets, and separate access to a discharge pharmacy. Ventilation systems in the fever zone need to be kept separate from those serving the rest of the facility. While air entering the fever zone may come from the same source as the remainder of the building, the effluent air from these fever zones should be channeled out of the facility and into the external air after being passed through suitable bacterial and viral filters. Such air should not be recirculated to air-conditioning systems.[16]

While all patients failing the fever screening test should be seen in a separate fever zone, it may not be feasible to have dedicated resuscitation areas in the fever zone. Patients requiring acute resuscitation may have to be directed to a designated portion of the hospital's resuscitation area that will need to be set aside for possibly infected patients.[16] If the patient were to require inpatient admission, then arrangements will need to be made to move the patient along distinct channels of the hospital, including pre-identified elevators, to the isolation wards.

Early implementation of preventive measures will limit the transmission of pandemic influenza, and they should be put into place in all areas of healthcare facilities and in large public venues. Hospitals and emergency departments (EDs) in particular will be the healthcare facilities that will serve the highest volume of influenza patients and will bear the greatest burden in responding to a surge in patients in the event of a pandemic. Healthcare centers, hospitals, and EDs should not wait for an outbreak to trigger the implementation of infection control measures. All EDs should routinely institute basic infection control measures that will need to be systematically enhanced if the local community moves closer to a pandemic flu situation.[16] These routine measures should include the following steps:[9,16]

1. Screening of all patients at the entrance of the ED to identify those who are at high risk of having a communicable infectious illness.
2. Isolation of all such patients screened as infectious in a separate area of the ED with its separate ventilation system.
3. Use of—at the least—basic personal protective equipment (PPE: surgical masks, hospital scrubs, gloves) when attending to patients who are potentially infectious.
4. Hand-washing or use of disinfectants before and after attending to any patient presenting to the ED.
5. Arrangement of special isolation facilities for those patients who require inpatient care and likely to be having active infection with a highly communicable illness.
6. Screening surveillance—a measure that may be implemented in normal times. Such surveillance measures achieve two objectives:
   • They provide early warning of an impending infectious disease outbreak.
   • They serve as a regular reminder to staff of the need to remain vigilant for such outbreaks. To maintain such vigilance, weekly reports recounting surveillance data need to be disseminated to all staff through various channels of communication in the hospital.

Many exposures to influenza occur in hospitals or other healthcare settings. Influenza-infected healthcare workers (HCW), patients, and visitors can spread infection both within and outside healthcare facilities. Transmission risks primarily come from unprotected exposure to unrecognized cases in inpatient and outpatient settings. Exposure to influenza pathogens can also occur through large respiratory droplets and close contact with infected patients. Also, exposure during aerosol-generating procedures may increase the risk of infection. Strict adherence to appropriate infection control practices, including the use of PPE, will help prevent transmission.[16]

MITIGATION

Any fatalities from a pandemic influenza episode will be tragic, but any deaths caused by insufficient planning or inadequate preparation will be difficult to defend.[1] Mitigation for reducing the negative consequences of a pandemic influenza outbreak will focus on the appropriate use of scarce resources and on the specific community-wide, nonpharmaceutical interventions that will lower the morbidity and mortality of an influenza public health emergency.

Although the Strategic National Stockpile of antivirals and the campaigns for population-wide immunizations will be available, communities will still face scarcities of both providers and equipment for treating respiratory diseases. One concept that may alleviate some of these problems is the regionalization of care for patients with advanced respiratory failure. Just as many regions have designated centers for trauma care, cardiac care, and stroke care, so large municipalities and regions within states may benefit from a similar designation of centers with the equipment, resources, and personnel to care for large surges in the number of patients with severe, contagious respiratory symptoms seen in influenza pandemics. Development of such respiratory centers would allow a few healthcare facilities to accumulate experience in managing the sickest patients, while preserving the resources available at outlying hospitals for other patients. Strengths of this approach include the potential for improved outcomes due to accumulated experience at the specialty care center and the potential for streamlined conduct of clinical trials of promising treatments.[8]

Other mitigation efforts may include the utilization of advanced telemedicine, now that the technology supporting this type of care has become more accessible and less expensive. Rural or remote hospitals may want to establish telemedicine initiatives that would allow their physicians to communicate with infectious diseases and pulmonary experts for clinical guidance with severely ill patients. Demonstration projects related to use of telemedicine during a public health emergency are currently ongoing in the United States.[17]

An analysis of national pandemic influenza plans in the Asia-Pacific region that included Australia, Cambodia, China, Hong Kong, Indonesia, Laos, New Zealand, Thailand, and Vietnam noted that the following mitigation efforts were particularly effective:[18]

- Give political support to preparedness planning.
- Link surveillance and response measures for animals and humans.
- Incorporate wide multisector cooperation, involving major stakeholders from the health, animal, and civil response sectors.
- Propose measures for early containment.

- Discuss the use of various social distancing measures, including travel restrictions (both domestic and international).
- Outline strategies for organization of the response from health services, relying mainly on specialized units. Several countries have made advanced preparations for cooperation with other countries in their geographic region.
- Address education and awareness for the population.
- Outline ethical principles that govern access to scarce resources.
- Include the private healthcare sector in preparation and implementation steps.

Similar strategies can be implemented at the local and state levels for many jurisdictions across the United States.

Non-pharmaceutical Interventions

As part of their overall strategy, public health officials can plan to mitigate a community-wide epidemic through the use of nonpharmaceutical interventions (NPIs). NPIs may decrease influenza transmissions by reducing contact between infected and uninfected persons, thereby decreasing the overall number of infected persons. Such a decline in incidence will, in turn, diminish the demand for healthcare services and minimize the impact of a pandemic on the economy and the population. Reshaping the demand for healthcare services by using NPIs is an important component of the overall mitigation strategy.[19] NPI strategies include the following measures:

- Voluntary isolation of persons
- Voluntary quarantine of household members of ill persons
- Child social distancing
- Adult social distancing

The goal of voluntary isolation of persons is to decrease influenza transmission by minimizing contact between those persons who are ill and those who are not. Individuals whose symptoms do not require hospitalization will be requested to remain at home for 7 to 10 days after the onset of symptoms. These efforts will be successful if the influenza infection is recognized early, the individual and household members use hygiene and infection control practices, and the employer supports the recommendation that ill employees stay home. Voluntary home isolation may be combined with antiviral medications if appropriate. Additionally, public health authorities need to provide concise information about when to seek additional care, and they need to make provisions for people living alone. Furthermore, public health officials may institute another NPI by requesting the voluntary quarantine of all household members in families where one member is ill with influenza. A large proportion of these household contacts may shed virus and present a risk of infecting others in the community despite having asymptomatic or only minimally symptomatic illness that is not recognized as pandemic influenza disease.[19]

Child social distancing attempts to prevent spread of pandemic influenza in the setting of dense classrooms and to protect vulnerable children. Social distancing interventions for children include dismissal from schools and closure of childcare programs; these measures, in combination with social distancing in the community, also seek to achieve reductions of out-of-school social contacts and community mixing.[19] Childcare facilities and schools represent an important point of epidemic amplification, and the children themselves are efficient transmitters of disease in any setting.

Similarly, adult social distancing measures include recommendations for both workplaces and the community, and these measures may have an important role in lowering community transmission pressure. The goals of workplace measures are to decrease infections within the occupational setting and the likelihood of their transfer into the larger community, to establish a healthy working environment and promote confidence in the workplace, and to maintain business continuity, especially for critical infrastructure. Workplace measures such as encouragement of telecommuting and other alternatives to in-person meetings may be important in reducing social contacts and the accompanying increased risk of transmission. Also, modifications of employee schedules, such as staggered shifts, may decrease infection transmission probabilities. Cancellation or postponement of large gatherings, such as indoor venue performances, may reduce transmission risk. Moreover, changes in mass-transit policies, such as reducing the numbers of passengers in a single vehicle, may reduce transmission risk, but these modifications may require running additional trains and buses, which may be an obstacle due to transit employees' absences, equipment availability, and the transit authority's financial ability to operate nearly empty vehicles.[19]

ANALYSIS OF CASE STUDY

By July 31, 2009, the Mexican Institute for Social Security had identified 63,479 reported cases of influenza-like illness, and 6,945 (11 percent) cases were confirmed to be the H1N1 strain.[2] Among these patients with influenza A H1N1, 6,407 (92 percent) were treated as outpatients, 475 (7 percent) were admitted and survived, and 63 (less than 1 percent) died. The findings also showed that individuals aged 10 to 39 years were most affected by the infection, and those aged 70 years and older were at greatest risk for mortality. Also, patients with delayed admission or with co-morbid chronic diseases were at an increased risk of dying. By comparison, people who had been vaccinated for seasonal influenza had a decreased risk of infection.

Fortunately, Mexico had a public health system in place that was capable of monitoring the H1N1 epidemic and was able to track epidemiological statistics from the event. These data have proved valuable in understanding the influenza epidemic and in guiding future interventions. Like many other countries, Mexico faced many obstacles attempting to acquire sufficient doses of vaccines effective against H1N1. Interestingly, for many decades, Mexico possessed the capacity to produce sufficient vaccines for internal distribution, but political and economic decisions led to a loss of this capacity. The government of Mexico has invested $250 million in a vaccine plant and has established an agreement with Sanofi-Aventis for the technology transfer to be able to produce 25 million vaccine doses by 2012.[3]

To respond to the surge in volume due to the H1N1 epidemic, Mexico attempted to expand its healthcare system's capacity to evaluate and treat patients. First, officials mandated that 12 percent of capacity at government hospitals be designated for H1N1 influenza patients. In addition, hospital capacity was increased by extending care areas into parking lots and by cancelling elective surgeries and procedures. In Mexico City, two hospitals were designated specifically for influenza patients, and the 220 outpatient clinics extended hours into evenings and weekends.[3] Two years earlier, in 2007, Mexico had launched a national mobile healthcare system, and these mobile units were expanded and tailored to provide outreach for the H1N1 epidemic.

At the outset of the epidemic, the Institute of Epidemiological Diagnosis and Reference (InDRE—Mexico's National Public Health Laboratory) in Mexico was the only laboratory that was able to conduct RRT-PCR studies to confirm the presence of the influenza A (H1N1) 2009 virus strain. Meeting the demands for rapid diagnosis of H1N1 around the country proved to be a significant public health issue. The Mexican government dedicated large amounts of investments to upgrade the country's diagnostic laboratory network. Now that these additional resources have become operational, 27 of Mexico's 31 state public health laboratories, 1 laboratory in the Mexican Institute for Social Security network, and 3 of the 12 National Institutes of Health in Mexico City are capable of using RRT-PCR to detect the H1N1 virus.[3]

CONCLUSION

The 2009 H1N1 influenza pandemic was challenging for several reasons. First, the H1N1 influenza virus infection can span the spectrum from subclinical infection to severe deterioration with a wide array of complications. Moreover, the ability of public health systems and emergency health professionals to prepare for and respond to the disease was tested on an unprecedented global scale. The lessons learned after a challenge of this type promise to inform potential improvements in surveillance, recognition, treatment, diagnostics, public health, and health policy. Public health officials and all emergency healthcare providers can learn from these experiences to improve their preparedness, response, and mitigation of pandemic influenza in the future to assure the highest quality of care for patients and the highest level of health for the public.

INTERNET RESOURCES

Planning and Coordination

Centers for Disease Control and Prevention, H1N1 flu provider planning:
http://www.cdc.gov/h1n1flu/clinicians/planning/

U.S. Department of Health and Human Services, pandemic influenza plan:
http://www.hhs.gov/pandemicflu/plan/

World Health Organization, International Health Regulations:
http://www.who.int/ihr/finalversion9Nov07.pdf

World Health Organization, pandemic influenza preparedness and response:
http://www.who.int/csr/disease/influenza/pipguidance2009/en/index.html

Situation Monitoring and Assessment

Centers for Disease Control and Prevention, situation update:
http://www.cdc.gov/h1n1flu/update.htm

Interim World Health Organization guidance for the surveillance of human infection with influenza A (H1N1) virus:
http://www.who.int/csr/resources/publications/swineflu/interim_guidance/en/index.html

World Health Organization, countries able to perform PCR to diagnose influenza A (H1N1) virus infection in humans:
http://www.who.int/csr/resources/publications/swineflu/country_pcr_capacity/en/index.html

World Health Organization, global surveillance during an influenza pandemic:
http://www.who.int/csr/resources/publications/swineflu/surveillance/en/index.html

World Health Organization, technical consultation on the severity of disease caused by the new influenza A (H1N1) virus infections:
http://www.who.int/csr/resources/publications/swineflu/technical_consultation_2009_05_06/en/index.html

Reducing the Spread of the Disease

Centers for Disease Control and Prevention, infection control:
http://www.cdc.gov/h1n1flu/infectioncontrol/

World Health Organization, case management of influenza A(H1N1) in air transport:
http://www.who.int/csr/resources/publications/swineflu/air_transport/en/index.html

World Health Organization, infection prevention and control in health care in providing care for confirmed or suspected cases of pandemic (H1N1) 2009 and influenza-like illnesses:
http://www.who.int/csr/resources/publications/swineflu/swineinfinfcont/en/index.html

World Health Organization, influenza A (H1N1) patient care checklist:
http://www.who.int/csr/resources/publications/swineflu/patient_care_checklist/en/index.html

World Health Organization, pandemic influenza prevention and mitigation in low-resource communities:
http://www.who.int/csr/resources/publications/swineflu/low_resource_measures/en/index.html

World Health Organization, reducing excess mortality from common illnesses during an influenza pandemic:
http://www.who.int/csr/resources/publications/swineflu/commonillnesses_pandemic/en/index.html

World Health Organization, reducing transmission of pandemic (H1N1) 2009 in school settings:
http://www.who.int/csr/resources/publications/swineflu/reducing_transmission_h1n1_2009/en/index.html

Communications

Centers for Disease Control and Prevention, patient education:
http://www.cdc.gov/h1n1flu/clinicians/patient_education/

World Health Organization, behavioral interventions for reducing the transmission and impact of influenza A(H1N1) virus: a framework for communication strategies:
http://www.who.int/csr/resources/publications/swineflu/framework/en/index.html

World Health Organization, *Outbreak Communication Planning Guide:* http://www.who.int/ihr/elibrary/WHOOutbreakCommsPlanngGuide.pdf

NOTES

1. White D, Angus D. Preparing for the sickest patients with 2009 influenza A (H1N1). *Journal of the American Medical Association.* 2009;302(17):1905–1906.
2. Echevarría-Zuno S, Mejía-Aranguré JM, et al. Infection and death from influenza A H1N1 virus in Mexico: A retrospective analysis. *Lancet.* 2009;374:2072–2079.
3. Vargas-Parada L. H1N1: A Mexican perspective. *Cell.* 2009;139:1203–1205.
4. Chan M. World now at start of 2009 influenza pandemic. World Health Organization; June 2009. Available at: www.who.int/mediacentre/news/statements/2009/h1n1_pandemic_phase6_20090611/en/index.html. Accessed February 2010.
5. Centers for Disease Control and Prevention (CDC). FluView. Available at: http://www.cdc.gov/flu/weekly/. Accessed February 2010.

6. Centers for Disease Control and Prevention (CDC), Novel Swine-Origin Influenza A (H1N1) Virus Investigation Team. Emergence of a novel swine-origin influenza A (H1N1) virus in humans. *New England Journal of Medicine.* 2009;360:2605–2615.

7. Centers for Disease Control and Prevention (CDC). Interim recommendations for clinical use of influenza diagnostic tests during the 2009–10 influenza season. September 29, 2009. Available at: http://www.cdc.gov/h1n1flu/guidance/diagnostic_tests.htm. Accessed January 2010.

8. Centers for Disease Control and Prevention (CDC). Clinical description and lab diagnosis of influenza. 2010. Available at: http://www.cdc.gov/flu/professionals/diagnosis/. Accessed February 2010.

9. U.S. Department of Health and Human Services. Pandemic influenza plan. Available at: http://www.hhs.gov/pandemicflu/plan/pdf/S05.pdf. Accessed January 2010.

10. World Health Organization, Global Influenza Program. Pandemic influenza preparedness and response: A WHO guidance document. 2009. Available at: http://www.who.int/csr/disease/influenza/PIPGuidance09.pdf. Accessed January 2010.

11. Centers for Disease Control and Prevention (CDC). Strategic national stockpile. Available at: http://www.bt.cdc.gov/stockpile/. Accessed February 2010.

12. U.S. Department of Homeland Security. *Planning for 2009 H1N1 influenza: A preparedness guide for small business.* Washington, DC: Author; September 2009. Available at: http://www.flu.gov/professional/business/smallbiz.pdf. Accessed February 2010.

13. U.S. Department of Health and Human Services. H1N1 flu: A guide for community and faith-based organizations. Available at: http://pandemicflu.gov/professional/community/cfboguidance.html. Accessed February 2010.

14. U.S. Department of Health and Human Services. HHS pandemic influenza plan. Available at: http://www.hhs.gov/pandemicflu/plan/pdf/Overview.pdf. Accessed February 2010.

15. U.S. Department of Health and Human Services. Pandemic influenza plan supplement 6: Vaccine distribution and use. Available at: http://www.hhs.gov/pandemicflu/plan/pdf/S06.pdf. Accessed February 2010.

16. International Federation for Emergency Medicine. Pandemic flu guidelines for emergency medicine. May 2009. Available at: http://www.ifem.cc/site/DefaultSite/filesystem/documents/IFEM%20Documents/IFEM%20Pandemic%20Flu%20Guidelines%20May%2009.pdf. Accessed January 2010.

17. Meade K, Lam DM. A deployable telemedicine capability in support of humanitarian operations. *Telemedicine and e-Health.* 2007;13(3):331–340.

18. Coker R, Mounier-Jack S. Pandemic influenza preparedness in the Asia-Pacific region. *Lancet.* 2006;368:886–889.

19. U.S. Department of Health and Human Services. Community strategy for pandemic influenza mitigation. February 2007. Available at: http://www.flu.gov/professional/community/commitigation.html. Accessed February 2010.

CHAPTER 14

Emerging and Re-emerging Infectious Diseases

Larissa May

INTRODUCTION

An emerging infectious disease is either a novel pathogen or one whose incidence has increased, expanded its geographic range, or will pose a threat to humans in the near future. Since 1967, approximately 40 new pathogens have been identified as diseases of clinical importance. This chapter discusses the factors leading to the emergence and re-emergence of infectious diseases, their detection, and recommendations for public health surveillance, using as examples some key emerging infections with important implications for public health. Approaches to public health preparedness, response to emerging infectious disease outbreaks and epidemics, and tools for mitigation, including surveillance systems and outbreak reporting tools, are covered from national and international perspectives. A case study of an emerging respiratory disease illustrates these important principles.

Case Study

In November 2002, the first cases of atypical pneumonia subsequently determined to be a novel coronavirus were reported in Guangdong Province in China; eventually, a total of 305 cases would be identified in the province.[1-3] This illness was characterized by fever greater than 38°C, myalgias, cough with subsequent respiratory failure, and occasionally diarrhea.[4-6] The worldwide outbreak of severe acute respiratory syndrome (SARS) began when a physician from the Guangdong Province traveled to Hong Kong for his daughter's wedding, ultimately infecting 16 persons from at least 6 different countries at the Metropole Hotel. This outbreak led to a global pandemic of more than 8,000 cases, including 1,700 cases in healthcare workers. Half of the cases occurred in Singapore and Toronto, with approximately 800 fatalities resulting in Hong Kong, Canada, Singapore, and Vietnam.[7,8] The high case fatality rate of 10 to 15 percent, coupled with the fact that as many as 30 percent of patients required critical care, led to worldwide panic and a rapid response to the pandemic, including travel restrictions, quarantine measures, and collaborative research leading to the discovery of a new virus.[4,9]

In February 2003, Canada received the first of 5 imported SARS case. Two cases arrived before the March 12 global alert issued by the World Health Organization (WHO). Although only 2 were imported to Toronto, they ultimately led to 245 cases in the city. One patient was incorrectly presumed to have tuberculosis and received nebulized aerosols.[10,11] Of the 251 total number of cases in Canada, 43 percent involved healthcare workers, among whom the mortality rate was 17 percent.[4,11] Although most of these cases could be attributed to inadequate infection control, at least two documented transmissions occurred despite the use of full barrier precautions. Overcrowded emergency departments with limited resources became sites for transmission of the virus. SARS was spread by respiratory droplets, although airborne transmission could not be ruled out. High-risk procedures, such as intubations, led to the infection of many healthcare workers. Despite the high rate of nosocomial transmission, few SARS cases turned out to be superspreaders, based on a high rate of secondary transmission. The typical number of patients infected per primary case was 2 to 4 cases.[11]

The SARS outbreak was eventually controlled, in large part due to strict infection control and quarantine programs—but not until significant public fear and economic repercussions had occurred. Even though difficult to estimate, the economic impact of SARS was approximately 2 percent of affected countries' gross domestic product (GDP), with the largest effects noted in Hong Kong and Singapore due to their high levels of consumer trade and retail.[12]

HISTORICAL PERSPECTIVES

Background

An emerging infectious disease is either a novel pathogen or one whose incidence in humans has increased over the past two decades, has expanded its geographic range, or will pose a threat in the near future. Three categories of emerging infectious diseases exist: known agents in a new geographic locale, known agents in an unsusceptible species, and previously unknown agents discovered for the first time.[13] Since the late 1960s, nearly 40 new human pathogens have been discovered.[14,15]

Emerging infections have quadrupled over the past two decades, with wildlife zoonoses accounting for approximately three fourths of these diseases.[13,16] A zoonosis is a pathogen that has its reservoir in the animal population and can spread from animal to human populations (or vice versa). A review of 1,415 known human pathogens revealed that 62 percent have an animal origin. Many of these zoonotic pathogens are able to infect multiple species. This kind of variable infectivity is possible for 77 percent of pathogens affecting domestic livestock and for 90 percent of those pathogens affecting carnivores.[17]

Newly discovered pathogens have included all types of organisms, including bacteria (*Legionella*, toxic shock syndrome, *Helicobacter pylori*, *E. coli* O157:H7, community-acquired methicillin-resistant *Staphylococcus aureus*) as well as viral diseases (Marburg, Ebola, HIV, hantavirus, Chikungunya, and SARS).[18] Re-emerging diseases are those that have increased in incidence or are occurring in new geographic regions. An example is the re-emergence of cholera in the Western Hemisphere with the El Nino climate phenomenon in the early 1990s and the resurgence of dengue fever in the Western Hemisphere.[19,20]

Inciting Factors

Public health concerns regarding emerging and re-emerging infectious diseases, antimicrobial resistance, and agents of bioterrorism have been increasing in recent years. The Institute of Medicine's 1992 report titled *Microbial Threats to Health: Emergence, Detection and Response* outlined five factors that have facilitated the emergence and spread of infectious diseases. Public health professionals and governments officials need to address these factors to decrease the risk of emerging and re-emerging infections causing widespread illness:

1. Changes in the physical environment: climate and weather changes affecting the ecology of vectors, animal reservoirs, and the transmissibility of microbes
2. Human behavioral activities: global travel, land use, contact with animal reservoirs, globalization of the food supply, increasing human crowding, reforestation, and irrigation practices

3. Social/political/economic factors: war and famine leading to population movements, and broken-down public health infrastructure
4. Bioterrorism
5. Increased use of antimicrobials and pesticides leading to increased resistance[21–23]

International business travelers and tourists, military personnel, and immigrants may all carry new diseases to areas where they were not previously endemic. Furthermore, with increasing airline travel, the potential for rapid international spread of new pathogens to vulnerable populations is very high.[24] Additional demographic factors involved in the rise of emerging infectious diseases include rapid population growth, overcrowding, an aging population with increasing susceptibility to infectious agents, and increasing numbers of individuals with immune suppression due to advances in cancer treatment and improved survival of persons infected with human immunodeficiency virus (HIV).[18]

Control of emerging infectious diseases is a challenging prospect considering the great number of pathogens and the opportunity for drug resistance.[25] The incidence of foodborne diseases and waterborne diseases is also increasing owing to trends favoring food importation and globalization of the food supply. Changes in land use and environmental transformations have led to increases in vector-borne diseases such as malaria and dengue fever. Parasites are continually emerging and have a great impact on endemic areas. Although they represent minimal threat to the United States, disasters and instability in resource-poor areas of the developing world affect control of parasites in those areas, which in turn increases the chance of transmission to travelers. For example, the number of cases of imported malaria due to inadequate compliance with prophylaxis is increasing, as is the incidence of leishmaniasis among U.S. military personnel.[26] In 1994, six cases of imported malaria occurred in Paris, all of which arose in airport workers or their neighbors. None of the workers had traveled to malaria-endemic regions.[27] These "runway" cases illustrate the potential for rapid spread of diseases to non-immune populations.

Incurable, highly contagious diseases that can spread from person to person may also spread across borders. For example, Lassa fever, a highly contagious and potentially lethal hemorrhagic fever virus, was imported into New Jersey in 1994.[28]

Identification of Outbreaks

Early detection and response to emerging infectious diseases is critical, but challenging, in an era characterized by decreased funding for public health infrastructure.

Early detection occurs via public health surveillance, defined as the ongoing, systematic collection, analysis, interpretation, and dissemination of health data.[29] Astute clinicians also play a role in reporting unusual presentations of disease or clusters of cases. New technologies are currently supplementing traditional surveillance—in particular, advances in information technology, improvements in laboratory testing and surveillance, and molecular techniques for bacterial typing. One such surveillance and response network for foodborne diseases based on molecular typing of organisms is PulseNet. PulseNet is a national network of local, state, and federal public health and food regulatory agency laboratories coordinated by the Centers for Disease Control and Prevention (CDC). DNA "fingerprints" of organisms such as salmonella or *E. coli* O157:H7 are electronically shared with participants in this network via a CDC database that allows for rapid comparison of strains and enhances epidemiologic investigations and response.[30,31]

Unfortunately, routine surveillance may not always detect emerging infectious diseases. Although laboratory testing has traditionally been the means to characterize and identify new pathogens, clinicians are often the first to recognize a novel or re-emerging pathogen. For example, an alert clinician recognized the outbreak of West Nile virus in New York City in 1999. In spite of significantly increased incidence above baseline for both meningitis (172 cases) and encephalitis (9 cases), traditional surveillance did not detect this outbreak. Because many of these emerging diseases are zoonoses, laboratory surveillance for animal outbreaks may, in fact, be the best way to detect outbreaks.[32] Testing of wildlife has been used in surveillance of many diseases, including West Nile virus and, more recently, avian influenza H5N1.[33]

Achievement of the optimal surveillance approach necessitates a multidisciplinary collaboration between infectious disease, emergency medicine, travel medicine, and public health authorities.[34] Although preventive measures for known diseases may include vaccines or other prophylactic measures, they also include the control of antimicrobial resistance and minimization of food practices that encourage the development of resistance. Public health professionals should pursue collaboration with their peers in other disciplines such as agriculture, health care, and the pharmaceutical industry to develop a strategy of prevention and control for emerging infectious diseases. Effective and timely public health surveillance should be a part of this cooperative strategy. Indeed, prior experience with smallpox in Africa demonstrates that a vaccine program without routine public health surveillance is not effective.[30,35] Multiple emerging infectious diseases are of critical importance for public health professionals (Table 14-1).

TABLE 14-1   Selected Emerging Infectious Diseases of Public Health Importance

Organism	Characteristics	Signs and Symptoms	Containment and Prevention
Ebola and Marburg viruses	• Filoviruses with single-stranded RNA that cause severe hemorrhagic illnesses • Endemic to Central Africa • No vaccine[36,37]	Initial symptoms are nonspecific, flu-like illness and can progress to severe hemorrhage, shock, central nervous system malfunction, and multisystem organ failure	• Isolation of infected cases (contact and air-borne precautions) • Supportive treatment; no vaccine or cure
Hantavirus	• Endemic to southwestern United States • Transmitted by a single rodent species, and infection occurs via inhalation of dried rodent feces or urine; not usually transmitted from person to person[38,39]	Febrile phase with nonspecific flu-like symptoms, a hemorrhagic phase characterized by hypotension and hypovolemic shock, and an oliguric phase followed by a diuretic phase, characterized by renal dysfunction, then convalescence[40]	• No vaccine or cure • Rodent control
Rift Valley fever	• Endemic to East Africa, spread to Arabian peninsula • More than 30 species of mosquito can transmit the disease • Possible spread from the parent mosquito to its offspring; eggs typically hatch during rainfall • Sheep are usual host[41]	Flu-like illness with hemorrhagic fever syndrome	• Increased incidence related to rainfall patterns[42] • Vector control
Human metapneumovirus	• Recently discovered paramyxovirus associated with respiratory illness during the winter months	Lower respiratory tract disease that is typically more severe in infants and young children[43,44]	• Droplet precautions
Monkeypox	• Relative of the smallpox virus • Was first isolated in 1958, with the first documented human infection in 1970 • Case fatality rate reported to be as high as 10%[45] • Imported into the United States via exotic pet trade[46]	Fever, headache, myalgias, and lymphadenopathy, as well as a characteristic vesicular rash, lasting two to four weeks	• Trade control • Smallpox vaccine • Cidofovir use is controversial[47]

West Nile virus	• First isolated Uganda in 1937 and then emerged in New York City in 1999 • Vector is the Culex mosquito[48–50]	• 20% of cases show signs of clinical disease including fever, rash, lymphadenopathy, headache, myalgias, and persistent fatigue • 1% of cases present with severe neurologic manifestations such as flaccid paralysis, seizures, aseptic meningitis, and encephalitis[51]	• Supportive therapy only • Vector control
Nipah virus	• Paramyxovirus with reservoir in fruit bat • Outbreak in Malaysia in pigs preceded human outbreak • Case fatality rate is estimated at 40% to 75%[52]	• Initially develop flu-like symptoms of fever, headaches, myalgias, vomiting and sore throat • May progress to acute encephalitis with dizziness, drowsiness, altered consciousness, and neurological signs	• Climatic change (ENSO drought) and slash-and-burn deforestation have contributed to its emergence[53]
Community-acquired methicillin-resistant *Staphylococcus aureus* (CA-MRSA)	• Virulent "superbug" that attacks healthy people • National Nosocomial Infections Surveillance Program data for 1998–2002 showed that of 18,397 S. aureus infections, 51% were MRSA[54]	• Serious skin abscesses to severe pneumonia[55] • Not acquired in hospitals or long-term care facilities, compared to nosocomial MRSA	• Infection control • Education • Decolonization strategies
Chikungunya virus	• Alphivirus that is transmitted to humans via the *Aedes aegypti* mosquito • Found in Africa, Indian subcontinent, and Southeast Asia[56]	• Abrupt fever accompanied by joint pain, muscle pain, headache, nausea, fatigue, and rash • Long-term complications may include severe arthritis, fatigue	No vaccine or treatment

PREPAREDNESS

Planning is imperative to prevent the spread of emerging infectious agents, particularly respiratory pathogens. In addition to transmission in the public setting, sites for transmission in the clinical setting include outside of the healthcare facility, triage areas, the waiting room, the emergency department (ED) treatment area, and the hospital. Policies to address emerging pathogens are necessary, including a critical need for readiness plans with preemptive planning and knowledge of healthcare and ED resources availability.[57] The absence of resource planning played a contributory role in the spread of SARS.[58]

Healthcare facilities are responsible for accepting and treating victims of public health emergencies, including those affected by an outbreak of an emerging infectious disease. Unfortunately, no agency or authority is solely responsible for coordinating resources and facilities, and very little surge capacity is available.[59] A hospital survey in 2001 reported that few hospitals had surge capacity and fewer than 20 percent had a plan for dealing with a biological disaster.[60]

The Joint Commission requires healthcare organizations to develop, implement, and conduct exercises for emergency operations plans. Unfortunately, a survey by the American Hospital Association reported that one third of community hospitals had negative financial margins in 2008.[61] Lack of funding poses a challenge to many hospitals in terms of completing their daily operations, much less handling an unexpected outbreak. Preparedness for an emerging infectious disease outbreak includes hazard and vulnerability assessment, the determination of facility capability and capacity, and identification of staff competencies.[60,61]

Surge Capacity

Public health surge capacity is defined as the facility of the public health infrastructure to accommodate the evaluation and treatment of unexpectedly large numbers of patients, whether from a contagious disease outbreak or from a mass casualty or natural disaster. Healthcare and facility-based surge capacity refers to the local ability to increase significantly the ability to care for patients.[59] This capacity is usually limited due to the financial constraints that prohibit healthcare institutions from stockpiling of equipment and pharmaceuticals and due to the existing shortage of healthcare providers and ancillary staff. Designated alternative sites of care for increased numbers of patients typically consist of "flat spaces" such as lobbies, waiting rooms, conference rooms, stadiums, or mobile units.[59] In previous epidemics, such as in pandemic flu and smallpox outbreaks, auxiliary hospitals were used. In today's market economy, however, few private hospitals would be willing to serve as auxiliary hospitals for an infectious disease outbreak without economic assurances (i.e., adequate compensation) and liability protections from the federal government. Furthermore, surge capacity should not be confused with surge capability, which refers to an institution's ability to care for patients requiring specific interventions not normally available at that site, such as care for an excess number of burn victims, who would normally be treated in specialized burn centers.[59]

Hospital Emergency Incident Command System

Based on the Incident Command System (ICS) developed by fire fighters to respond to mass casualties, the Hospital Emergency Incident Command System (HEICS) incorporates contagious outbreak plans into existing internal emergency operations preparedness in an "all hazards" approach. This system should be compliant with the National Incident Management System (NIMS), which establishes standard procedures for responding to incidents.[62,63] In the Incident Command System, one incident commander is designated as the leader and authority for an event. Sub-chiefs are designated responsible for logistics, operations, finance, and planning. HEICS provides a common organizational structure to coordinate response for a mass-casualty event or outbreak.[62] The ICS structure should be clearly identified in the planning stages with specific positions, rather than individuals, designated to perform tasks.

Hospital Response Plans

The CDC has developed guidelines for readiness for bioterrorism.[64] These same guidelines can be applied to preparing for emerging infectious disease outbreaks, as both bioterrorism events and contagious outbreaks involve biological agents, which are likely highly transmissible and have no definitive treatment. A contagious disease outbreak plan should be ready prior to any actual event's occurrence. It should be activated by key personnel, including the healthcare organization's administration and infectious disease specialist, when syndrome-based criteria are met, such as cases involving severe respiratory illnesses, severe gastrointestinal illnesses, or unexplained fevers and rashes. The plan should take into account infection control, isolation precautions, patient placement, patient transport, cleaning, disinfection, sterilization, discharge management, postmortem care, post-exposure management, triage of large-scale exposures and suspected exposures, and psychological aspects and counseling (Table 14-2).[61,64]

Laboratory Capabilities

Diagnosis of emerging or re-emerging infectious diseases is frequently difficult, as most emerging infectious diseases present with nonspecific, flu-like symptoms. Moreover, testing for these diseases may not be routinely available, or may not be

TABLE 14-2   Hospital Response Plan Components for an Emerging Infectious Disease Outbreak

Component	Characteristics
Activation/notification	• Notification of administration, security, laboratory and pathology, respiratory therapy, pharmacy, infection control, facilities management, and the emergency department should be included. • Media relations should be involved in reporting information to the public. • Local and state departments of health should be notified for assistance and epidemiological investigation.
Facility protection	• Security should be responsible for the lockdown of the hospital, including controlled entry and exit points and a controlled, unidirectional flow of patients. • Visitor access to the facility should be restricted. • Separate external triage sites should be established for staff and patients.
Decontamination	• In the event of a contagious disease outbreak, self-decontamination is usually sufficient as days often pass between the initial exposure and the onset of clinical symptoms. • Decontamination via shower is not necessary with a contagious disease outbreak, unlike with a biologic attack.
Supplies/logistics	• Review supplies of pharmaceuticals, personal protective equipment (PPE), and equipment. • Develop stockpiles of antibiotics, vaccines, biohazard bags, masks, gloves, ventilators, and routine supplies such as linens in advance.
Alternative care sites	• Identify sites that can accommodate increased surge capacity within the healthcare facility. • Prepare for expedient discharge of patients from the emergency department and inpatient wards and the cancellation of elective cases. • Institute a strict review by infection control to determine which patients may be taken off isolation or boarded together. • Identify alternative external sites for delivery of care, and develop memoranda of understanding with neighboring organizations and facilities.
Staff education/ training	• As part of emergency preparedness, healthcare organizations are responsible for including training and practice drills on contagious disease outbreak events as part of their routine mass-casualty protocols and drills. Education and training on the proper use of PPE needs to be undertaken in accordance with occupational health and safety guidelines.

TABLE 14-2 (*cont.*)	Hospital Response Plan Components for an Emerging Infectious Disease Outbreak
Command/Control	• Incident Command System structure. • Logistics, operations, finance, planning.
Coordination and communication	• Ensure timely communication and cooperation among emergency medical services (EMS), fire department, police, and government. • Provide for media updates.
Recovery	• Reimbursement by the Federal Emergency Management Agency (FEMA) may be warranted. • Plan for ongoing disease surveillance of staff. • Ensure psychological support for staff and patients is available through cooperation with mental health officials.

available at all in the case of a novel pathogen. Identification of many emerging pathogens requires the use of expensive and specialized molecular techniques such as amplification with reverse transcriptase polymerase chain reaction (RT-PCR), which must be conducted in specialized laboratories. Furthermore, laboratories working with these highly transmissible agents must follow specific isolation precautions and ensure that the chain of custody remains intact.[65]

Agents of bioterrorism are of national security importance and a leading public health issue. Biologic agents not only can cause high fatality rates, but also have the ability to surpass the capacity of healthcare institutions to provide care for patients who become ill through contact with these infectious agents as well as other patients. Accurate and timely identification of biologic agents is critical in the emergency public health response to an infectious disease outbreak or intentional attack.

Approximately 2,000 public health laboratories are currently in operation in the United States. These laboratories collectively form the Laboratory Response Network (LRN), which was created in 1999 by the CDC as a means to ensure laboratory biopreparedness.[65,66] Hospital laboratories are Level A laboratories that can refer problematic testing issues to the next level of safety and containment.[65] Level B laboratories are often public health laboratories that can provide confirmatory and susceptibility testing, and Level C laboratories provide advanced molecular techniques. Level D laboratories include CDC or Department of Defense (DOD) laboratories that utilize advanced techniques and can offer special surge capacity.[65,66]

The LRN recommends that hospital-based laboratories restrict their testing to human specimens under diagnostic protocols developed with the American Society for Microbiology, the CDC, and the Association of Public Health Laboratories. These laboratories' main focus is the detection, characterization, identification, and susceptibility testing of the biologic agent.[66] The main role of the microbiology laboratory in planning for a bioterrorism event or emerging infectious disease outbreak is to maintain a high level of suspicion and, working in coordination with infection control and hospital administration, to develop laboratory and institution response plans. These plans should include diagnostic testing protocols regarding utilization of the LRN and communication and notification protocols.[65] Electronic order entry, tracking, and notification for agents of bioterrorism, as well as other infectious disease agents such as avian influenza, are key components of biopreparedness plans and satisfy the requirements of the LRN. Processes that enable expedited collection, analysis, and reporting of microbial pathogen and susceptibility data can aid in timely detection of a bioterrorism agent.[67]

Disease Surveillance Systems

Based on public health experiences with SARS and other respiratory infections, it has become clear that strategic planning for emerging respiratory pathogens requires case containment via early diagnosis of sporadic cases. A detailed and well-thought-out strategy for patient triaging and testing should be in place, particularly during the winter season, when baseline rates of respiratory illnesses that mimic emerging infectious diseases are at their peak. Border control with an infrared temperature device may be effective, as 15 imported cases of dengue and malaria were found in 2003 (although no cases of SARS were detected).[68] Laboratory diagnoses can be strengthened through increased availability of PCR and creation of improved alert, reporting, and surveillance systems. Once an emerging infectious disease is known, it should be added to a preexisting Web-based reporting system to be accessed by regional hospitals and healthcare centers. Telephone reporting may facilitate early detection, as will ED-based syndromic surveillance for fever, cough, and respiratory diseases; such a system has been established in Taiwan, for example.[68]

Because few surplus resources exist, plans for surge capacity should be realistic, yet flexible. Examples of such resources include the auxiliary hospitals used in treating cases of smallpox and pandemic flu in the past.

Syndromic Surveillance

Epidemiologic surveillance with current systems is difficult due to the need to wait for confirmed diagnoses, reliance on passive reporting, and delays in both patients seeking care and authorities recognizing the existence of an outbreak. Syndromic surveillance, or the use of prediagnostic information, may mitigate these factors. Syndromic surveillance is a recently developed public health surveillance tool emphasizing the use of near "real-time" prediagnostic data and statistical tools to detect and characterize unusual activity for further public health investigation.[69] In the response to a bioterrorism or contagious disease outbreak, time is critical: A speedy response is essential to contain the outbreak and minimize the potential spread of the infection to other individuals. Most agents with outbreak or bioterrorism potential present as "flu-like illness;" thus it would be extremely difficult to detect a low-level outbreak by traditional surveillance methods.

Syndromic surveillance aims to decrease the time to detection of an outbreak compared to traditional surveillance methods.[69] During the syndrome grouping stage, data are collected and organized using complaint or diagnostic codes, such as the ICD-9 (*International Classification of Disease*, version 9). Based on data collected over a defined period of time, during which there is no contagious disease outbreak, a historical model can be built. In the detection stage, differences between predictions from the model and the actual visits recorded are evaluated.[70] Detection of a large outbreak is obvious, whereas a small outbreak is more difficult to discern. A basic syndromic surveillance model may look at the daily numbers of patients with flu-like symptoms and then add a hypothetical number of cases to simulate an attack or outbreak. An excess of cases is chosen at which point the alarm will be triggered.[71]

Syndromic surveillance systems have inherent trade-offs between sensitivity, timeliness, and false-positive rates.[69] The goal is to have a sensitive system but to minimize false alarms, as these will be costly from both economic and time perspectives.[69] Syndromic surveillance encompasses a broad range of activities, including monitoring illness syndromes or events. Alarms are triggered by "flags," signaling that a statistical threshold has been reached.[72] Such triggers are based on a certain number of markers, such as medication purchases or a diagnosis of "viral syndrome." In an outbreak involving severe disease, hospital admissions and patient deaths may be more useful than early indicators of care. During the clinician reporting stage, the individual clinician informs the local department of health of any cases of interest.[72] In turn, those data are fed into a larger reporting system. The CDC's BioSense program is a "national program intended to enhance national capabilities for conducting real-time bio-surveillance and enabling health situational awareness through access to existing data from healthcare organizations across the country."[73] This type of system may allow the early identification of emerging infectious disease outbreaks by integrating emergency department, hospital, and laboratory data from state surveillance systems, local healthcare organizations, national laboratories, the Department of Defense, and Veterans Affairs facilities.

Proposed syndromic surveillance systems vary in their methodology and complexity. Data can be collected in several fashions: hospital data from a 24-hour period, a moving daily average with increased weight given to recent data, cumulative deviations from a constant expected value, or an expected daily value adjusted for seasonal variation in flu-like symptoms. The more advanced statistical methods have been predicted to increase the detection of a slow attack.[69] Integration of syndromic surveillance into the public health system is crucial. Traditional surveillance sets off alarms but limits the clinician's role in outbreak reporting. In contrast, physicians and other healthcare providers are essential for active syndromic surveillance and reporting to public health officials, assisting with epidemiological investigations, and implementing information technology.[72] Information technology facilitates real-time detection, communication between various entities (i.e., labs and clinicians), and use of database systems for epidemiologic intelligence.[65] The clinician's role in outbreak detection, therefore, is determination of "credible risk" by both epidemiological and clinical criteria, arrangement for rapid and efficient pathogen identification, and immediate reporting to public health authorities.[74]

Summary of Preparedness Activities

Preparing for an emerging infectious disease outbreak is first a local responsibility. Currently, most communities in the United States have disaster response systems and plans. The West Nile virus outbreak of 1999 demonstrated that an emerging infectious disease is primarily a local emergency public health and medical crisis. Event detection by surveillance is important because timely detection is critical, and this capacity initially requires knowledge of the baseline incidence in the case of a re-emerging disease. Sharing of local and regional information helps facilitate these processes.[75]

Preparedness for emerging infectious diseases for local and regional institutions includes completion of the following steps by a pre-formed planning committee:[75]

- Review of existing preparedness documents
- Hazard and vulnerability analysis of the facility
- System capacity and capability
- Identification of all tasks and requirements
- Plans to match facility capability to requirements
- Enhancement of capability and capacity based on the assessments
- Development of plans and procedures
- Education of staff with detailed and realistic exercises (tabletop, functional, full scale) and testing of plans in a variety of scenarios

- Evaluation of education and planning activities on an ongoing basis
- Establishment of continuous preparedness improvement program

RESPONSE

The response to an emerging infectious disease outbreak is similar to the response to an attack with a bioterrorism agent, with the main difference being the absence of a criminal component. Response to the outbreak should follow protocols instituted during the emergency preparedness phase; therefore, a robust and efficient response depends on the strength of the emergency preparedness phase. Protocols and plans should be flexible in nature, and they will need to be evaluated and modified to reflect the characteristics and extent of the outbreak in the context of situational awareness.

Outbreak Detection

Most outbreaks present as "flu-like illness." The size of an outbreak is related to the virulence of the organism or agent, the modes of transmission (e.g., contact versus aerosol), and the potential extent and mode of dissemination. The following clinical features should alert clinicians to the possibility of a sentinel case for a contagious outbreak or bioterrorism-associated event, especially if seen in large numbers of patients or in an unexpected patient population, geographic location, or time of the year:

- Gastroenteritis with bacterial origin: *Salmonella*, *Shigella*, *E. coli* O157:H7 (new or virulent strains)
- Pneumonia with sudden death in a healthy patient: pneumonic plague, SARS, avian influenza
- Acute neurologic illness with fever: botulism, viral hemorrhagic fever[76]

Epidemiological criteria for suspicion of an emerging infectious disease are similar to those for a bioterrorism event:[76]

1. Severe disease in a healthy patient
2. Increased numbers of patients with fever, respiratory, or gastrointestinal symptoms
3. Multiple patients presenting from a similar location with the same symptoms
4. Endemic disease at an unusual time of the year
5. Large numbers of rapidly fatal respiratory cases
6. Increasing numbers of ill or dead animals

7. A rapid rise and fall of the epidemic curve
8. Increased numbers of patients with sepsis, sepsis with coagulopathy, or fever with rash

These epidemiologic criteria should be used in deciding whether to activate emergency outbreak plans.

Outbreak Containment: Hospital Infection Control Practices Advisory Committee Infection Control Guidelines

Once clinicians and public health practitioners determine there is an emerging infectious disease outbreak, infection control precautions should be followed based on suspicion or knowledge of the agent's transmissibility (Table 14-3). In the United States, standard infection control guidelines were established by the CDC in 1991 as part of occupational safety for healthcare workers and are updated and revised by the Hospital Infection Control Practices Advisory Committee (HICPAC) of the CDC.[77]

Hospital Response to an Emerging Infectious Disease

Contact tracing, laboratory identification, and active monitoring of exposed persons are key features of an emergency public health response to an outbreak.[78] The public health authorities are responsible for tracing of contacts. However, in the event of an outbreak, physicians need to work closely with public health officials to identify, provide prophylaxis to, and treat contacts of ill patients. The hospital infection control officer or hospital epidemiologist is responsible for coordinating prophylaxis of exposed staff.

Engineering controls include negative-pressure isolation rooms and high-efficiency particulate air (HEPA) filtration to apply negative pressure. HEPA filters can remove fungi and bacteria larger than 0.1 micrometer in diameter. Physical separation of infected patients is another type of engineering control.[78] During the response to an outbreak of an emerging infectious disease, engineering controls not only include negative-pressure wards for respiratory isolation, but may also involve the following measures: dedication of units to infected patients with single rooms, the use of portable HEPA filters to increase available isolation space, heated tents outside the hospital for screening, and anterooms.[78] Closing doors and patient cohorting were found to be effective in Hong Kong in the SARS outbreak that occurred in early 2003. Cohorting of SARS patients into three separate isolation wards was instituted, with no secondary transmission occurring after appropriate precautions were taken.[79,80] Administrative and work practice controls include PPE with CDC- and Occupational Safety and

TABLE 14-3 Types of Infection Control Precautions and Their Characteristics

Type of Precaution	Characteristics
Standard	• Should be used when the healthcare provider expects exposure to blood and body fluids • Personal protective equipment (PPE) is to be used: gown, gloves, and mask with eye protection if splash of blood or other body fluids anticipated
Contact	• PPE is required for all healthcare workers • Patients are to be in private rooms • Dedicated patient equipment is to be used • Patient transport should occur only if necessary • Required for such emerging diseases as methicillin-resistant *Staphylococcus aureus* and *Clostridium difficile*
Droplet	• Designated for microbes less than 5 micrometers in diameter that are transmissible at a distance of less than 3 feet • Healthcare providers are to use PPE, including surgical masks, at all times while providing patient care. • Required for respiratory pathogens such as meningococcemia and influenza
Airborne	• Provides protection for exposure to small infectious particles. • Healthcare workers are to use PPE including N95 masks • Patients should remain in a private negative-pressure isolation room with 6–12 air changes per hour • Used for tuberculosis and for highly infectious and lethal respiratory pathogens such as SARS and avian influenza H5N1

Health Administration (OSHA)–approved N95 masks. In addition, early notification of emergency medical services (EMS) and ED personnel is important, as these caregivers will be on the front lines of any outbreak. ED treatment should involve early isolation of potentially infected patients and use of caution during high-risk airway procedures and transport.[78]

Workplace and administrative controls should follow written procedures and protocols, limit or restrict visitors, and assign staff to designated areas, thereby ensuring geographical and healthcare worker cohorting. Medical surveillance, limited transport through dedicated routes during which patient and transport personnel wear PPE, and restriction of interfacility transfers may decrease the potential for nosocomial transmission.

The use of PPE should follow infection control guidelines, and isolation should be initiated at the first point of contact. Powered air-purifying respirators (PAPR) should be considered for high-hazard procedures (e.g., intubation). PAPR may provide a higher level of protection in aerosol-generating procedures; however, this additional protection must be balanced against the increased likelihood of a needle stick while wearing it. Hand-washing policies should be strictly enforced during the outbreak as well. Organizational measures may include closure of the ED to EMS personnel, suspension of outpatient procedures and elective surgical cases, and restriction of staff employment at other institutions.[78] The hospital infection control office should work with the pharmacy staff to develop procedures for evaluating inpatient antimicrobial use and to discontinue using medications effective against specific outbreak pathogens for other pathogens whenever possible.

Diagnostic Testing

As described in the previous section on emergency preparedness, laboratory chain of custody is vital, with laboratories within the CDC's LRN providing public health support for laboratory testing of agents. Four biosafety levels have been developed by NIH, WHO, CDC, and the U.S. Army Medical Research Institute of Infectious Diseases (USAMRIID) for work with biological agents:

- Level 1: Educational facilities and teaching labs, involves work with strains not known to cause disease in healthy adults. Can provide basic containment of infectious agents.
- Level 2: Clinical, reference, and teaching labs that provide the capacity to work with indigenous moderate risk agents and human fluids and tissues.
- Level 3: Designated for clinical, diagnostic, reference, teaching, research, and production of indigenous or exotic agents with the potential for respiratory transmission causing serious infection, or recombinant molecules with the potential for transmission. This level requires biosafety cabinets and specialized ventilation.
- Level 4: Allows work with dangerous and exotic agents causing high-risk lethal disease, or that exhibit transmission by aerosols, and for which no vaccine or therapy available. These facilities provide biosafety cabinets and full-body, air-supplied, positive-pressure suits. Level 4 requires a separate building or its own ventilation and waste management.[81]

Emerging infectious diseases will continue to pose challenges in diagnosis given laboratory issues with chain of custody.[81]

Outbreak Containment: State and Federal Response

Local and state authorities are responsible for the first response to an outbreak. The Department of Health and Human Services' role is to identify and apply containment for epidemics. The Federal Emergency Management Agency (FEMA) coordinates federal assistance when local and state resources are overwhelmed by a crisis.[82] Responsibility for the control of epidemics and infectious disease lies with DHHS and the U.S. Public Health Service. A new office of Public Health Preparedness was established in 2001. The CDC and the Office of Emergency Preparedness (OEP) determine the amount and distribution of stockpiled materials, which include antibiotics for prophylaxis and treatment, medical equipment, and logistical supplies. While the CDC provides specific recommendations, the Surgeon General has the authority to enforce the quarantine to restrict the spread of an infectious disease across state lines and into and out of the United States.[83] Under the National Disaster Medical System (NDMS), multiple Disaster Medical Assistance Teams (DMATs) can be deployed from various locations as needed, including some with expertise in specific areas (pediatrics, chemical weapons, urban search and rescue).

During an outbreak, the CDC will provide epidemiological and laboratory expertise and recommend appropriate control measures and prophylactic regimens. The CDC and DHS maintain eight Strategic National Stockpile "pushpacks" in several locations across the United States, the contents and location of which are classified. Such a pushpack may be deployed upon a state's request if pharmaceuticals or other supplies are needed in a biological disaster. The pushpacks are programmed to arrive within 12 hours in the event of a public health emergency, and they would then be divided and distributed depending on the need in point of distribution centers (PODs). Should further or more specific supplies (e.g., ventilators, specific antibiotics) be necessary, Vendor Managed Inventory (VMI) is available within 24 to 36 hours.[83,84] Prior to and upon arrival of the necessary stockpile materials, local and state departments of health will be responsible for their distribution.[84]

MITIGATION

Most emerging infectious disease pandemics emerge randomly, and preparedness for an emerging infectious disease outbreak requires both pharmacologic and nonpharmacologic methods. Stockpiling of pharmaceuticals and planning for the distribution of vaccines and drugs in a timely fashion will serve a mitigating role, as discussed in the preparedness and response sections of this chapter.[85] Not to be overlooked, nonpharmacologic interventions—including an adequate and timely surveillance system, social distancing methods such as closure of schools and cancellation of public gatherings, travel restrictions, and quarantine—may mitigate the impact of an epidemic.

Although social distancing has mainly been advocated as a method for mitigating the effects of a pandemic influenza outbreak, it may also be useful for other emerging infectious diseases that are highly transmissible by contact, droplet, or aerosol. Within the United States, the CDC provides specific recommendations on quarantine practices, but the Surgeon General has the authority to recommend and provide enforcement for quarantine (or the restriction of exposed persons).[83] The use of PPE, such as surgical and N95 masks and gowns, will help decrease the rate of transmission among healthcare providers. In the event of a respiratory outbreak, portable ventilators will be needed. Communications networks and international teamwork to decrease transmission from infected regions will remain a challenge. Moreover, public education will be important to minimize panic.

SARS provided a real-life drill in terms of how these interventions might work; however, other agents with greater infectivity and a faster reproduction rate may prove less easy to control. Weaknesses in surveillance, poor population awareness, inadequate healthcare facilities, and practices that discourage reporting may all worsen the impact of an emerging infectious disease outbreak. As an example, consider the outbreaks of SARS in southern coastal areas of China in fall of 2002: They were initially not reported to health authorities, leading to a delay in diagnosis of this novel agent and potentially exacerbating the spread of the disease across borders.[86]

Both traditional and syndromic surveillance methods may be useful in early detection of the outbreak and prevention of its spread, provided adequate communication methods and cooperation of local and cross-national public health authorities exist. Establishing a sentinel surveillance system may counteract existing weaknesses by monitoring the situation in specific geographic regions more closely. Currently, sentinel surveillance exists for diseases such as cholera, plague, and dengue fever.[86] The revised International Health Regulations of 2005 call for the reporting of defined clinical syndromes of international importance, with the goal of mitigating global outbreaks such as occurred with SARS.[87] Despite this requirement, it appears that few existing systems now comply with this regulation.

Communication strategies, infection control guidelines to limit the transfer and management of more complex patients, resources such as critical care beds, and coordinated leadership and communication infrastructure may all be mitigating factors in the event of an infectious disease outbreak.[88] Epidemiologic surveillance has already highlighted difficulties with current systems (i.e., the need to await confirmed diagnoses, passive reporting, and delays). Event discovery is an important first step in addressing any outbreak, and should be based on syndromic and epidemiologic criteria. Diagnosis is often difficult in the early stages, as symptoms and signs are typically nonspecific, and identification of many emerging pathogens requires specialized laboratory testing methods, such as enzyme-linked immunosorbent assay (ELISA) or PCR, which are not widely available.[65]

Mitigation of the spread of an emerging infectious disease relies on early detection and response as well as established communication systems. Mitigating measures include the following:

- Expedient epidemiologic investigation
- Response with hospital activation and notification, containment procedures, mass prophylaxis and care, and the request for outside assistance
- Containment involving exposure avoidance, isolation, and quarantine for highly contagious diseases
- Governor's declaration of emergency
- Environmental controls (i.e., vector control, water supplies)
- Mass prophylaxis (points of distribution)
- Mass patient care/fixed site health care
- Expedient discharge, shared hospital rooms, use of flat spaces (cafeteria, auditorium), use of volunteers (credentialed), and mass-fatality management (local morgue capacity, temporary morgues)[89]

When surge capacity is required, usual standards of care may need to be modified to maximize the number of patients treated. Although some critics suggest that this strategy might increase healthcare worker infection, most public health professionals support it. Preparations for such an event include stockpiling supplies, adding ventilators, adapting inpatient beds to critical care capacity, conducting staff training and drills, and enhancing infection control procedures.[90]

Outbreak Reporting

Various national and international networks have been developed to facilitate recognition of infectious outbreaks and to mitigate the spread of emerging diseases. The following list outlines some of the U.S. and global surveillance networks currently in place:

- *EMERGency IDNET*: emergency department sentinel network for emerging infections.[91]

- *IDSA EIN* (Infectious Diseases Society of America Epidemic Intelligence Network: network of infectious disease consultants who monitor emerging and re-emerging infectious diseases.[92]
- *Geosentinel*: sentinel network of travelers' clinics that analyzes trends and develops travel advisories. Geosentinel provides a worldwide communication and data collection network for the surveillance of travel related morbidity.[93]
- *PROMED*: International Society of Infectious Diseases program for monitoring infectious diseases. An email list of registrants is maintained at the following Web site: www.promedmail.org. Front-line clinicians or public health staff may report puzzling or unusual infections on this site. A team of experts reviews these reports as well as news reports and posts notices to registrants.[94]
- *GOARN* (WHO Global Outbreak Alert and Response Network; 110 interlinked networks): A technical collaboration that collects new outbreak reports and provides resources for rapid identification, confirmation, and response to those outbreaks of international importance.[22,95]
- *GPHIN* (Global Public Health Intelligence Network): A secure, Internet-based "early warning" system for Health Canada and WHO that searches news reports and Web sites in seven languages on a continuous basis and is analyzed by the Public Health Agency of Canada. It collects information on a wide range of topics, such as infectious disease outbreaks, contaminated food or water, and bioterrorism. The output is made accessible to users, and notifications about health events with potential serious public health consequences are immediately forwarded to users.[96]
- *GEIS* (U.S. Department of Defense Global Emerging Infections Surveillance): An infectious disease surveillance network that links together U.S. and foreign public and private agencies and provides support for global surveillance, training, research, and response to emerging infectious disease threats.[97]
- *Intrepid:* A multidisciplinary team of government and academic scientists who use data from NASA's Earth Observing System (EOS) with the goal of building an early warning system based on climatic changes that may indicate early effects on ecological systems that could increase the transmission of existing pathogenic organisms or the development of emerging zoonotic infections. This system has been used to help track and predict outbreaks of infection with West Nile virus.[22,98]
- *International Emerging Infections Program of the CDC:* A program that seeks to prevent and control emerging infectious diseases, train public health professionals and clinicians in outbreak detection and control, and facilitate the

application of research and public health tools to the detection and response to emerging infections.[21,22]

CASE STUDY ANALYSIS

The worldwide pandemic of SARS in 2002–2003 provided many important lessons regarding the preparation, response, and mitigation to an emerging infectious disease. The response to SARS was a challenge given the lack of adequate infection control capacity, nonspecific clinical presentation, lack of rapid diagnostic testing, and necessity of a presumptive diagnosis based on clinical features and epidemiological criteria such as travel or a sick contact. Furthermore, the mechanism for transmission was unclear (although the pathogen was likely transmitted by large droplets), and no cure or vaccine was available.[78]

In Toronto, Ontario, restrictions on non-urgent use of hospital services were imposed in March 2003 to control the outbreak of SARS. A provincial health emergency was declared, and ambulatory and inpatient activity was restricted to urgent cases. Respiratory isolation rooms were expanded, visitor access was restricted, and the use of PPE in high-risk areas was enforced. A centralized system for screening for transfers was established, although this system lacked measures to mitigate the impact on vulnerable populations.[99]

A retrospective population-based study comparing the Greater Toronto Area and unaffected areas before, during, and after the SARS outbreak looked at data during the early and late SARS period. The study found that the rate of medical admissions decreased 10 to 12 percent in Toronto, with no change being observed in the comparison regions. Rates of elective surgery in Toronto fell by 22 percent and 15 percent during early and late restriction periods, respectively, versus 8 percent in comparative regions. High-acuity visits to EDs actually fell 37 percent in Toronto, and interhospital transfers declined by 44 percent. In summary, the restrictions achieved modest reductions in overall admissions, and they led to a brief reduction in admissions for serious conditions, high-acuity visits to EDs, and transfers, suggesting access to care for some potentially seriously ill patients was affected.[100]

One of the challenges in the early diagnosis of SARS was that the WHO case definition for SARS was found to be useful for epidemiological purposes but not very sensitive for the assessment of ED patients in triage areas. A Hong Kong study looking at cases in 2003 reported reliable results when the diagnostic criteria were combined with variables such as exposure history, symptoms, and laboratory data.[101] Thus clinical decision tools may prove to be more reliable for hospital use in the early stages of an emerging infectious disease outbreak than broad case definitions. Unfortunately, there was a lack of reliability of decision tools in non-endemic areas. In future scenarios, each new outbreak will require validation. EDs will be at the front line of access for patients presenting with emerging infectious diseases and should receive recognition as key sites for early detection surveillance systems.[102] Furthermore, the development and testing of novel molecular techniques is a public health approach that is recommended to facilitate ED evaluation of aerosolized infectious diseases.[103] Fortunately, few SARS cases turned out to be "superspreaders"—that is, individuals whose infection was characterized by a high rate of secondary transmission. The typical number of patients infected per primary case was only 2 to 4 cases.[11]

On February 23, 2003, Canada imported the first of 5 imported SARS cases, 2 of which were in Toronto, and 3 of which led to 245 cases. Two of these patients arrived in Canada before the March 12 global alert was issued. One patient was mistakenly presumed to have tuberculosis, was inadequately isolated, and received nebulized aerosols.[10] Of the 251 total number of cases in Canada, 43 percent involved healthcare workers, with a 17 percent mortality rate being noted.[104] In Hong Kong, 62 percent of cases occurred in healthcare workers; in Toronto, the corresponding proportion was 51 percent.[88] Most cases occurred because of inadequate infection control precautions, in part due to misdiagnosis of the nonspecific presentation of SARS. At least two documented transmissions occurred despite the use of full barrier precautions.[11]

In February 2003, when SARS arrived, Canada was unprepared for this emerging infectious disease. There was no curative treatment, and only supportive treatment was available. The country lacked trained infection control practitioners and limited ability to provide isolation. Lessons learned in Toronto focused on the use of the following measures to control the spread of the disease: effective isolation in a 15-person SARS acute treatment unit (SATU) with use of negative-pressure and HEPA filters, 24-hour patient care by dedicated providers, a heated tent for outdoor screening, and strict adherence to PPE.[105]

The Singapore experience led to ED implementation of facility, staff, and patient protection. The Ministry of Health centralized SARS cases, and it created a national ED screening center that screened 11,461 cases, with 12.9 percent of patients eventually being admitted. Of the admitted cases, 235 out of 1,386 were positive for SARS. No ED transmission was documented.[106] Strategies in Singapore included changing the length of caregivers' shifts from 8 hours to 12 hours and implementing strict protocols regarding use of PPE. Administrators retrofitted and redesigned the ED to create and partition separate areas for infectious and non-infectious patients. The hospital enforced staff temperature checks, set up a clinic for sick staff, established temperature-taking stations at triage entry points, and administered a risk factor questionnaire to all patients.[107] The workload increased significantly at first, with daily numbers of patients in the ED increasing from 330 to 500 during the early part of the outbreak. As more cases were diagnosed among healthcare providers, the number of visits decreased to 200 per day for a short period due to the public's perception of risk. Supplies and logistics were important considerations, with increased use of stretchers, biohazard containers and bags, and cleaning solution being noted. There was also an increased need for PPE as part of healthcare providers' infection control precautions against SARS.[107]

With the next emerging respiratory pathogen, healthcare facilities will once again quickly search for effective treatment. These containment methods should be devised in advance. N95 masks should be tested for efficacy against each emerging pathogen to determine the best form of isolation, and regulatory agencies are needed to implement and enforce these standards.[10]

In summary, infection control precautions are critical to prevent hospital-based transmission of any emerging disease with respiratory transmission. This hierarchy of control includes several types of engineering controls: isolation, negative pressure, ventilation with exhaust system removal, local ventilation to catch contaminants at the source, and filtration by HEPA filters. The CDC recommends devices that filter 99.97 percent of particles greater than or equal to 0.3 micrometer in diameter. This strategy has proved effective in protecting healthcare workers against acquiring tuberculosis, for example.[108] Administrative and work practice controls include standard operation procedures (SOPs) that minimize intensity and duration of exposure—a consideration that is particularly important for contagious respiratory outbreaks. Written policies and procedures and infection control precautions (hand washing, glove use) are important, and mechanisms should be in place to encourage compliance with recommended precautions.[78] Public health authorities, government leaders, and clinicians can all learn important lessons from past experiences with infectious diseases outbreaks that will enable them to respond more effectively to the next outbreak, whether it involves SARS or some novel pathogen.

CONCLUSION

Infectious diseases are emerging and re-emerging at unprecedented rates, fueled by human behavioral practices such as deforestation, population movements, use of antimicrobial agents, and modern farm practices. The global experience with SARS illustrates the impact of an emerging infectious disease on the public health infrastructure and emphasizes the importance of global cooperation in addressing any outbreak. Local and international surveillance systems must be in place to ensure early detection of emerging diseases, which often present with nonspecific febrile illness and are difficult to diagnose in a timely fashion. Strengthening global preparedness, response mechanisms, and laboratory capabilities will mitigate the effects of a future emerging disease outbreak. Given that each new pathogen may have different transmission patterns, geographic predisposition, and severity of illness, plans must be flexible and public health authorities and healthcare providers must be able to adapt to each outbreak. The basic public health tools of disease surveillance, prudent antimicrobial use and farming practices, public health resources, and infection control with isolation and quarantine will likely be our best defense and response to emerging infectious diseases.

ONLINE RESOURCES

Centers for Disease Control and Prevention, recent outbreaks and incidents: http://www.cdc.gov/ncidod/EID/index.htm

Centers for Disease Control and Prevention, recent outbreaks and incidents: http://www.bt.cdc.gov/recentincidents.asp

International Society for Infectious Diseases, Program for Monitoring Emerging Diseases: http://www.promedmail.org/pls/otn/f?p=2400:1000

U.S. Department of Health and Human Services, Pandemic Flu Plan: http://www.hhs.gov/pandemicflu/plan/

U.S. National Institutes of Health, emerging and re-emerging infectious diseases: http://www3.niaid.nih.gov/topics/emerging/

World Health Organization, Weekly Epidemiologic Record: http://www.who.int/wer/en/

NOTES

1. Xu R, He J, Evans M, et al. Epidemiologic clues to SARS origin in China. *Emerging Infectious Diseases*. 2004;10(6):1030–1037.
2. Rosling L, Rosling M. Pneumonia causes panic in Guangdong Province. *British Medical Journal*. 2003; 326(7386):416.
3. World Health Organization (WHO). Acute respiratory syndrome, China. *Weekly Epidemiologic Record*. 2003;78:44.
4. Peiris J, Yuen K, Osterhaus A, et al. The severe acute respiratory syndrome. *New England Journal of Medicine*. 2003;349(25):2431–2441.
5. Centers for Disease Control and Prevention (CDC). Fact sheet: Basic information about SARS. Available at: http://www.cdc.gov/ncidod/sars/factsheet.htm. Accessed June 17, 2008.
6. Ksiazek T, Erdman D, Goldsmith C, et al. A novel coronavirus associated with severe acute respiratory syndrome. *New England Journal of Medicine*. 2003;348(20):1953–1966.

7. Poon L, Guan Y, Nicholls J, et al. The aetiology, origins, and diagnosis of severe acute respiratory syndrome. *Lancet: Infectious Diseases*. 2004;4(11):663–671.

8. Phua GC, Govert J. Mechanical ventilation in an airborne epidemic. *Clinical Chest Medicine*. 2008;29(2):323–328.

9. Levy MM, Baylor MS, Bernard GR, et al. Clinical issues and research in respiratory failure from severe acute respiratory syndrome. *American Journal of Respiratory and Critical Care Medicine*. 2005;171:518–526.

10. Thiessen RJ. The impact of severe acute respiratory syndrome on the use of and requirements for filters in Canada. *Respiratory Care Clinics*. 2006;12:287–306.

11. World Health Organization (WHO). *Consensus document on the epidemiology of severe acute respiratory syndrome (SARS)*. Report WHO/CDS/CSR/GAR/2003. Geneva, Switzerland; Author; 2003.

12. U.S. General Accounting Office. Report to the Chairman, Subcommittee on Asia and the Pacific, Committee on International Relations, House of Representatives: Emerging infectious diseases: Asian SARS outbreak challenged: Available at: http://www.gao.gov/new.items/d04564.pdf. Accessed June 17, 2008.

13. Torres-Velez FT, Brown CB. Emerging infections in animals: Potential new zoonoses? *Clinical Laboratory Medicine*. 2004;24:825–828.

14. Hargreaves S. Better global cooperation needed to tackle emerging infectious diseases. *Lancet: Infectious Diseases*. 2007;7(10).

15. World Health Organization (WHO). International spread of disease threatens public health security. Available at: http://www.who.int/mediacentre/news/releases/2007/pr44/en.index.html. Accessed September 11, 2009.

16. Senior K. Global hot spots for emerging infectious diseases. *Lancet: Infectious Diseases*. 2008;8(4).

17. Cleaveland L, Laurenson MK, Taylor LH. Diseases of humans and their domestic mammals: pathogen characteristics, host range, and risk of emergence. *Philosophical Transactions of the Royal Society (London) B: Biological Sciences*. 2001;356(1411):991–999.

18. Church DL. Major factors affecting the emergence and re-emergence of infectious diseases. *Clinical Laboratory Medicine*. 2004;24:559–586.

19. Tauxe RV, Blake PA. Epidemic cholera in Latin America. *Journal of the American Medical Association*. 1992;267(10):1388–1390.

20. Mourino-Perez RR. Oceanography and the seventh cholera pandemic. *Epidemiology*. 1998;9(3):355–357.

21. Centers for Disease Control and Prevention (CDC). Preventing emerging infectious diseases: A strategy for the 21st century: Overview of the updated CDC plan. *Morbidity and Mortality Weekly Report*. September 1998;47(RR-15).

22. Global emerging crisis in infectious diseases: Challenges for the 21st century. *Pfizer Journal*. 2004;V(2).

23. Lederberg J, Shope RE, Oaks SC; Institute of Medicine Committee on Emerging Microbial Effects to Health. *Emerging infections: Microbial threats to health in the United States*. Washington, DC: National Academy Press; 1992.

24. Greenberg MI, Marty AM. Emerging natural threats and the deliberate use of biological agents. *Clinical Laboratory Medicine*. 2006;26:287–298.

25. McFee RB. Global infections: Avian influenza and other significant emerging pathogens: An overview. *Disease Monitoring*. 2007;53: 343–347.

26. Christie JD, Garcia LS. Emerging parasitic infections. *Clinical Laboratory Medicine*. 2004;24: 737–772.

27. Giacomini T, Mouchet J, Mathieu P, Perithory JC. Study of 6 cases of malaria acquired near Roissy-Charles-de-Gaulle in 1994. *Bulletin of the Academy of National Medicine*. 1995;179: 335–351.

28. Ufberg JW, Karras DJ, Talan DA, Moran GJ, Pinner R. Update on emerging infections: News from the Centers for Disease Control and Prevention. Imported Lassa fever—New Jersey, 2004. *Annals of Emergency Medicine*. 2005;45:3:323–326.

29. Centers for Disease Control and Prevention (CDC). HIV/AIDS statistics and surveillance. Available at: http://www.cdc.gov/hiv/topics/surveillance/. Accessed July 30, 2008.

30. Binder S, Levitt AM, Sacks JJ, Hughes JM. Emerging infectious diseases: Public health issues for the 21st century. *Science*. 1999;284:1311–1313.

31. Centers for Disease Control and Prevention (CDC). PulseNet. Available at: http://www.cdc .gov/pulsenet/. Accessed June 17, 2008.

32. Fine A, Layton M. Lessons from the West Nile viral encephalitis outbreak in New York City, 1999: implications for bioterrorism preparedness. *Clinical Infectious Diseases*. 2001;32:277.

33. U.S. Department of the Interior, U.S. Geological Survey. Surveillance for Asian H5N1 avian influenza in the United States. Fact sheet 2006–3025, February 2006. Available at: http://www .nwhc.usgs.gov/publications/fact_sheets/pdfs/ai/AIFEB06.pdf. Accessed July 30, 2008.

34. Talan DA, Moran GJ, Mower W, et al. EMERGEncy ID NET: An emergency department–based emerging infections sentinel network. *Annals of Emergency Medicine*. 1998;32:703–711.

35. *Report of the interim meeting of the Technical Consultative Group (TCG) on Global Eradication of Poliomyelitis*. WHO/V&B/30.04. Geneva: World Health Organization; November 13–14, 2002.

36. Centers for Disease Control (CDC), Special Pathogens Branch. What are viral hemorrhagic fevers? Available at: www.cdc.gov/ncidod/dvrd/spb/mnpages/dispages/vhf.htm. Accessed June 17, 2008.

37. Borio L, Inglesby T, Peters CJ, et al. Hemorrhagic fever viruses as biological weapons: Medical and public health management. *Journal of the American Medical Association*. May 8, 2002;287(18).

38. Chapman LE, Khabbaz RF. Etiology and epidemiology of the Four Corners hantavirus outbreak. *Infectious Agents and Disease*. 1994;3(5):234–244.

39. Su JR. Emerging viral infections. *Clinical Laboratory Medicine*. 2004;24:773–795.

40. Centers for Disease Control (CDC), National Center for Infectious Diseases, Special Pathogens Branch. All about hantaviruses. 2004. Available at: http://www.cdc.gov/ncidod/ diseases/hanta/hps/noframes/treating.htm. Accessed June 17, 2008.

41. Madani TA, Al Mazrou YY, Al-Jeffri MH, et al. Rift Valley fever epidemic in Saudi Arabia: Epidemiological, clinical, and laboratory characteristics. *Clinical Infectious Diseases*. 2003;37: 1084–1092.

42. Linthicum KJ, Anyamba A, Tucker CJ, et al. Climate and satellite indicators to forecast RVF epidemics in Kenya. *Science*. 1999;285:347–348.

43. Stockton J, Stephenson I, Fleming D, Zambon M. Human metapneumovirus as a cause of community-acquired respiratory illness. *Emerging Infectious Diseases*. 2002;8(9):897–901.

44. Su JR. Emerging viral infections. *Clinical Laboratory Medicine*. 2004;24:773–795.

45. Centers for Disease Control and Prevention (CDC). What you should know about monkeypox. Available at: http://www.cdc.gov/ncidod/monkeypox/factsheet2.htm.

46. Update: Multistate outbreak of monkeypox—Illinois, Indiana, Kansas, Missouri, Ohio and Wisconsin, 2003. *Morbidity and Mortality Weekly Report.* 2003;52(27):642–646.

47. Centers for Disease Control and Prevention (CDC). Updated interim CDC guidance for use of smallpox vaccine, cidofovir, and vaccinia immune globulin (VIG) for prevention and treatment in the setting of an outbreak of monkeypox. 2003. Available at: http://www.cdc.gov/ncidod/monkeypox/treatmentguidelines.htm. Accessed June 17, 2008.

48. Smithburn KC. Hughes TP, Burke AW, Paul JH. Neutropenic virus isolated from blood of native of Uganda. *American Journal of Tropical Medicine.* 1940;20(4):71–92.

49. Sampathkumar P. West Nile virus: Epidemiology, clinical presentation, diagnosis, and prevention. *Mayo Clinic Proceedings.* 2003;78(9):1137–1143.

50. Campbell GL, Marfin AA, Lanciotti RS, Gubler DJ. West Nile virus. Lancet: *Infectious Diseases.* 2002;2(9):519–529.

51. Weiss D, Carr D, Kellachan J, et al. Clinical findings of WNV infection in hospitalized patients, New York and New Jersey, 2000. *Emerging Infectious Diseases.* 2001;7(4):654–658.

52. Chua KB. Nipah outbreak in Malaysia. *Journal of Clinical Virology.* 2003;26:265–275.

53. Page SE, Seigert F, Rieley JO, Boehm HD, Jaya A, Limin S. The amount of carbon released from peat and forest fires in Indonesia during 1997. *Nature.* 2002;420(6911):61–65.

54. National Nosocomial Infections Surveillance (NNIS) system report: Data summary from January 1992 to June 2002, issued August 2002. *American Journal of Infection Control.* 2002; 30(8):458–475.

55. Zetola N, Francis JS, Nuermberger EL, Bishai WR. Community acquired methicillin resistant *Staphylococcus aureus*: An emerging threat. *Lancet: Infectious Diseases.* 2005;5:275–286.

56. Centers for Disease Control and Prevention (CDC). Chikunguya. 2008. Available at: http://www.cdc.gov/ncidod/dvbid/Chikungunya/. Accessed June 17, 2008.

57. Rothman RE, Irvin CB, Moran GJ, et al. Respiratory hygiene in the emergency department. *Annals of Emergency Medicine.* 2006;48(5):570–582.

58. Hawryluck L, Lapinsky SE, Stewart TE. Clinical review: SARS: Lessons in disaster management. *Critical Care.* 2005;9:384–389.

59. Hick J, Hanfling D, Burstein JL, et al. Health care facility and community strategies for patient surge capacity. *Annals of Emergency Medicine.* 2005;44(3):253–261.

60. Wetter DC, Daniell WE, Tresser CD. Hospital preparedness for victims of chemical or biological terrorism. *American Journal of Public Health.* 2001;91(5):724–726.

61. American Hospital Association. Trendwatch Chartbook 2010. Available at http://www.aha .org/aha/trendwatch/chartbook/2010/chapter4.pdf. Accessed June 16, 2010.

62. Pons PT, Catrill SV. Mass casualty management: A coordinated response. *Critical Decisions in Emergency Medicine.* Monthly CME publication by the American College of Emergency Physicians. November 2003.

63. National Incident Management System FEMA/501, draft August 2007. Available at: http://www.fema.gov/pdf/emergency/nrf/nrf-nims.pdf. Accessed July 30, 2008.

64. Centers for Disease Control and Prevention (CDC); English J, Cundiff M, Malone J, et al. APIC Bioterrorism Task Force, CDC Hospital Infections Program Bioterrorism Working

Group. Bioterrorism readiness plan: A template for healthcare facilities. 1999. Available at: http://www.cdc.gov/ncidod/dhqp/pdf/bt/13apr99APIC-CDCBioterrorism.PDF. Accessed June 17, 2008.

65. Snyder JW. Role of the hospital-based microbiology laboratory in preparation for and response to a bioterrorism agent. *Journal of Clinical Microbiology.* 2003;41(1):1–4.

66. Centers for Disease Control and Prevention (CDC). The Laboratory Response Network: Partners in preparedness. 2005. Available at: http://www.bt.cdc.gov/lrn/. Accessed July 31, 2010.

67. Agency for Healthcare Research and Quality. Bioterrorism preparedness and response: Use of information technologies and decision support systems. Evidence Report/Technology Assessment No. 59. Available at: http://www.ahrq.gov/clinic/epcsums/bioitsum.htm. Accessed June 17, 2008.

68. Ho MS, Su IJ. Preparing to prevent severe acute respiratory syndrome and other respiratory infections. *Lancet: Infectious Diseases.* 2004;4:684–689.

69. Stoto M, Schonlau M, & Mariano L. RAND Center for Domestic and International Health Security. Syndromic surveillance: Is it worth the effort? *Chance.* 2004;17(1):19–24.

70. Reise BY, Mandl KD. Syndromic surveillance: The effects of syndrome grouping on model accuracy and outbreak detection. *Annals of Emergency Medicine.* 2004;44(3):235–241.

71. RAND. Syndromic surveillance: An effective tool for detecting bioterrorism? Available at: http://www.rand.org/pubs/research-briefs/2005/RB9042.pdf. Accessed September 11, 2009.

72. Buehler JW, Berkelman RL, Hartley DM, et al. Syndromic surveillance and bioterrorism-related epidemics. *Emerging Infectious Diseases.* October 2003; 9:10.

73. Centers for Disease Control and Prevention (CDC). BioSense: Real-time biosurveillance. Available at: http://www.cdc.gov/BioSense/files/fact_sheet.pdf. Accessed June 17, 2008.

74. Katona P. Bioterrorism preparedness: A generic blueprint for health departments, hospitals and physicians. *Infectious Diseases in Clinical Practice.* 2002;11(3):2004.

75. Flowers LK, Mothershead JL, Blackwell TH. Bioterrorism preparedness II: The community and emergency medical services systems. *Emergency Medicine Clinics of North America.* 2002;20:457–476.

76. Rega P. *Bioterrorism: A statistical manual to identify and treat diseases of bioterrorism.* Maumee, Ohio: Mascap; 2000.

77. Centers for Disease Control and Prevention (CDC). Guideline for isolation precautions: Preventing transmission of infectious agents in healthcare settings. 2007. Available at: http://www.cdc.gov/ncidod/dhqp/pdf/guidelines/Isolation2007.pdf. Accessed July 31, 2010.

78. Thorne CD, Khozin, S, McDiarmid MA, et al. Using the hierarchy of control technologies to improve healthcare facility infection: Lessons from severe acute respiratory distress syndrome. *Journal of Occupational and Environmental Medicine.* July 2004;46(7):613–622.

79. Borgundvaag B, Ovens H, Goldman B, et al. SARS outbreak in the Greater Toronto area: The emergency department experience. *Canadian Medical Association Journal.* 2004;171:23.

80. Tan YM, Chow PK, Tan BH, et al. Management of inpatients exposed to an outbreak of severe acute respiratory syndrome (SARS). *Journal of Hospital Infection.* 2004;58:210–215.

81. Greenberg MI, Marty AM. Emerging natural threats and the deliberate use of biological agents. *Clinical Laboratory Medicine.* 2006;26:287–298.

82. Michael GE. National Disaster Medical System, Federal Emergency Management Agency, Department of Homeland Security. U.S. Medical Disaster Assistance Teams. Available at: http://www.dmat.org/teamlinks.html. Accessed July 10, 2008.

83. Mothershead JL, Tonat K, Koenig KL. Bioterrorism preparedness III: State and federal and response. *Emergency Medicine Clinics of North America.* May 2002;20(2):477–500.

84. May L, Cote T, Hardeman B, et al. A model "go-kit" for use at Strategic National Stockpile points of dispensing. *Journal of Public Health Management and Practice.* 2007;13(1):23–30.

85. Juckett G. Avian influenza: Preparing for a pandemic. *American Family Physician.* 2006;74(5): 783–790.

86. Arita I, Nakane M, Kojima K, Yoshihara N, Nakano T, El-Gohary A. Role of a sentinel surveillance system in the context of global surveillance of infectious diseases. *Lancet: Infectious Diseases.* 2004;4:171–177.

87. World Health Organization (WHO). The Fifty-Seventh Session of the Regional Committee for South-East Asia. Information documents. SEA/RC57/Inf.4. July 2004. Available at: http://www.searo.who.int/en/Section1430/Section1439/Section1638/Section1646/Section1648_6946.htm. Accessed June 17, 2008.

88. Booth CM, Stewart TE. Severe acute respiratory syndrome and critical care medicine: The Toronto experience. *Critical Care Medicine.* 2005;22(1 suppl):S53–S60.

89. Meltzer MI, Damon I, LeDuc JW, et al. Modeling potential responses to smallpox as a bioterrorist weapon. *Emerging Infectious Diseases.* 2001;7(6):959–969.

90. Rubinson L, Nuzzo JB, Talmor DS, et al. Augmentation of hospital critical care capacity after bioterrorist attack or epidemics: Recommendations of the Working Group on Emergency Mass Critical Care. *Critical Care Medicine.* 2005;33:2393–2403.

91. Talan DA, Moran GJ, Mower WR, et al. EMERGEncy ID NET: An emergency department–based emerging infections sentinel network. *Clinical Infectious Diseases.* 1999;28(2):401–402.

92. Busch DF, Gilbert DN, Liedtke LA, et al. Executive Committee of the Infectious Diseases Society of America Emerging Infections Network. The Emerging Infections Network: A new venture for the Infectious Diseases Society of America. *Clinical Infectious Diseases.* 1997;25: 34–36.

93. Geosentinel: The global surveillance network of the ISTM and CDC. Revised April 2008. Available at: http://www.istm.org/geosentinel/main.html. Accessed July 31, 2010.

94. International Society for Infectious Diseases. Promedmail. Available at: http://www.promedmail.org/pls/otn/f?p=2400:1000. Accessed July 31, 2010.

95. World Health Organization (WHO). Global Outbreak Alert and Response Network. Available at: http://www.who.int/csr/outbreaknetwork/en/. Accessed July 31, 2010.

96. Public Health Agency of Canada. Global Public Health Information Network. Available at: http://www.phac-aspc.gc.ca/media/nr-rp/2004/2004_gphin-rmispbk-eng.php. Accessed July 31, 2010.

97. U.S. Department of Defense. Global Emerging Infections Surveillance Program. Available at: http://www.geis.fhp.osd.mil/.

98. National Air and Space Administration. NASA researchers developing tools to help track and predict West Nile virus. *Earth Observatory.* October 2002. Available at: http://earthobservatory.nasa.gov/Newsroom/NasaNews/2002/2002100810843.html. Accessed July 31, 2010.

99. Public Health Agency of Canada. *Canadian SARS numbers: September 3, 2003.* Ottawa: Author; 2003. Available at: www.phac-aspc.gc.ca/sars-sras/cn-cc/20030903_e.html. Accessed June 17, 2008.

100. Schull MJ, Stukel TA, Vermeulen MJ, et al. Effect of widespread restrictions on the use of hospital services during an outbreak of severe acute respiratory syndrome. *Canadian Medical Association Journal*. 2007;176(13).

101. Leung L, Rainer T, Lau F, et al. A clinical prediction rule for diagnosing severe acute respiratory syndrome in the emergency department. *Annals of Internal Medicine*. 2004;141(5):333–342.

102. Rothman RE, Hsieh Y, Yang S. Communicable respiratory threats in the ED: Tuberculosis, influenza, SARS, and other aerosolized infections. *Emergency Medicine Clinics of North America*. 2006;24:989–1017.

103. Yang S, Rothman R. PCR-based diagnostics for infectious diseases: Uses, limitations, and future applications in acute-care settings. *Lancet: Infectious Diseases*. 2004;4(6):337–348.

104. World Health Organization (WHO). *Summary table of SARS cases by country, 1 November 2002–7 August 2003*. Geneva, Switzerland: Author; 2003. Available at: http://www.who.int/csr/sars/country/en/country2003_08_15.pdf. Accessed July 31, 2010.

105. Dwosh HA, Hong HH, Austfarden D, Herman S, Schabas R. Identification and containment of an outbreak of SARS in a community hospital. *Canadian Medical Association Journal*. 2003; 168:1415–1420.

106. Tham KY. An emergency department response to severe acute respiratory syndrome: A prototype response to bioterrorism. *Annals of Emergency Medicine*. 2004;43(1):6–14.

107. Lateef F. SARS changes the ED paradigm. *American Journal of Emergency Medicine*. 2004; 22:483–487.

108. Centers for Disease Control and Prevention (CDC). Guidelines for preventing the transmission of *Mycobacterium tuberculosis* in health-care facilities. *MMWR Recommendations and Reports*. 1994;43:1–132.

SECTION 5

Terrorism

CHAPTER 15

Bombing Events

G. Bobby Kapur

INTRODUCTION

Even in the twenty-first century, terrorist bombing events using rudimentary substances such as fertilizers or gunpowder remain the most prominent and likely threat of a public health emergency due to intentional violence against a population. Because of the ease of acquiring bomb-making materials and the ready access to detonation technology, terrorists can devise and implement a blast event more easily than a chemical, biological, or nuclear incident. Therefore, preparedness, response, and mitigation for bombing events will continue to be critical components of the public health infrastructure. In addition to public health authorities, a variety of other entities—such as local and state government agencies, healthcare providers, the private sector, and nongovernmental organizations (NGOs)—will play important roles in supporting a community's resilience and response to a potential bombing event.

Case Study

On April 19, 1995, at 9:02 A.M., at the North entrance of the Alfred P. Murrah Federal Building in Oklahoma City, Oklahoma, Timothy McVeigh detonated a truck bomb that contained more than 4,100 pounds (1816 kg) of ammonium nitrate fertilizer saturated with diesel fuel and nitromethane. The blast caused a partial collapse of the 9-story Murrah Building and produced an 8-foot by 30-foot crater on N.W. 5th Street. At the time of the bombing, approximately 600 employees and 250 visitors were present in the building. The damage extended to a 48-square-block area, and caused extensive damage to surrounding buildings including the 24-story Regency apartment complex, the 2-story Oklahoma Water Resources Board office building, the 6-story Journal Record Building, and the 3-story Athenian Building. At 9:45 A.M., the governor of Oklahoma, Frank Keating, declared a state of emergency and ordered all non-essential employees in Oklahoma City to evacuate government facilities.[1]

Immediately after the detonation of the truck bomb, the Oklahoma City Fire Department initiated the Incident Command System (ICS), and the Oklahoma City Police Department began coordinating security and traffic. The blast from the detonation destroyed both primary and secondary communications for the local ambulance system (Emergency Medical Services Authority); however, ambulance units responded without notification after hearing the blast.

Emergency personnel established two medical triage areas: a primary triage site at N.W. 5th Street and Robinson and a secondary triage site at the Murrah Building. The incident command post (ICP) was established at N.W. 6th Street and Harvey Avenue, and the Oklahoma City Fire Department staged a forward command post at the Murrah Building loading dock. The forward command post also became the operations site for the Federal Emergency Management Agency's (FEMA) incident support team (IST). Two additional "bomb scares" occurred after the initial detonation that required evacuation of emergency personnel, and these subsequent threats forced the relocation of the ICP two blocks north of the original location. At the new site, federal officials from the Federal Bureau of Investigation (FBI), Bureau of Alcohol, Tobacco, and Firearms (ATF), and Drug Enforcement Administration (DEA) joined local and state agencies. The state emergency operations center (SEOC) was located approximately 3 miles from the Murrah Building, and state agencies coordinating activities from the SEOC included the Oklahoma Department of Public Safety, Department of Human Services, Military Department, Department of Health, and Department of Education.

The State Medical Examiner's Office set up a family assistance center at the First Christian Church (N.W. 36th Street and N. Walker Avenue). The Medical Examiner's Office provided briefings twice a day, and additional support and counseling were provided by the American Red Cross, the Salvation Army, the Oklahoma Funeral Directors Association, and private volunteer professionals. Critical incident stress debriefings and mental health services were offered by experts from the Oklahoma City Fire Department and Police Department, Oklahoma Department of Mental Health, and FBI. Other support services for survivors and families included shelter, clothing, and meals. The American Red

Cross provided logistics support from its warehouses, and additional resources were supplied by the Oklahoma City–based Feed the Children organization and the Oklahoma Restaurant Association. By 4 P.M., President Bill Clinton had signed FEMA-3115-EM-OK, which designated the site of the bombing as a federally declared national disaster.

The terrorist bombing caused the deaths of 167 individuals and injured another 592 people. Of the people with injuries, 351 were evaluated in an emergency department (ED), 158 were treated by a private physician, and 83 were hospitalized.[2] The most common sites of injuries included the extremities, head and neck, and face. A study of building occupants revealed that 88 percent sustained injuries from the bombing, and location within the building had a significant impact on morbidity and mortality. Individuals in the collapsed portion of the building had a greater likelihood of death, and this risk increased on the upper floors (2 to 9): 72 of 74 people in these collapsed upper floors died.[3]

An analysis of hospital ED records revealed interesting findings regarding prehospital management of patients and patient care-seeking decisions. Of the people requiring medical care, nearly two-thirds went to hospitals within a 1.5-mile radius of the Murrah Building. More than 55 percent of patients arrived by privately owned vehicles, and only 33 percent arrived by ambulance. The median time from detonation of the bomb to arrival to a hospital was 91 minutes.[3] More critically ill patients typically arrived by ambulance at a longer time than the median; they were classified as a "second wave" of patients. Prehospital interventions mostly included spinal immobilization, field dressings, and intravenous fluids.

HISTORICAL PERSPECTIVES

Terrorist bombing events have been a public health threat for many decades; however, the sophistication and coordination of attacks in recent years have led to increasing concerns about the vulnerability of civilian populations. In addition, with the rise in the number of suicide bombings, traditional protections against bombing events are now serving as less of a deterrent against terrorists who are willing to lose their lives during a bombing event. Historically, bombing events have targeted government installations in an attempt either to force a change in policies or to overthrow the leadership. Current trends in terrorism incidents show that terrorists are targeting civilian populations—more so than government installations—in an attempt to induce psychological fear and private-sector instability as a means of undermining a country's authority and credibility on security issues.

According to the U.S. Department of State's Country Reports on Terrorism 2008, approximately 11,800 terrorist attacks occurred worldwide in 2008, and perpetrators injured or killed nearly 50,000 individuals in these incidents. The report also states:

> Most attacks in 2008 were perpetrated by terrorists applying conventional fighting methods such as armed attacks, bombings, and kidnappings. Terrorists continued their practice of coordinated attacks that included secondary attacks on first responders at attack sites, and they continued to reconfigure weapons and other materials to create improvised explosive devices.[4]

Although enormous attention and media coverage are directed toward weapons of mass destruction (WMD) such as nuclear, biological, and chemical threats, the risk is actually much higher that a conventional bombing event will occur, given the ease of access to bomb-making instructions and materials. For this reason, public health officials and emergency personnel need to emphasize preparedness, response, and mitigation for bombing incidents.

Internationally, the past decade has witnessed a series of horrific bombing events. Conflict regions such as Iraq, Afghanistan, Pakistan, and India have had to prepare and respond to multiple bombing events.[5] Even countries in Europe that are experiencing relative peace and have liberal policies toward diverse ethnic and religious groups have been struck by bombings. The Madrid subway bombings on March 11, 2004, on four commuter trains resulted in 177 deaths and more than 2,000 injuries, and the detonation of explosives on three trains of the London Underground on July 7, 2005, resulted in 56 deaths and nearly 700 injuries.[6,7] Similarly, Russia and Turkey have experienced multiple bombings carried out by militant groups working within their borders, and resort areas, such as Bali, Indonesia, have also been targets of bombings.[8,9]

Domestically, the United States has experienced only a small number of large-scale bombing events in the past few decades, including the attacks on the World Trade Center towers in New York City in 1993 and the Alfred P. Murrah Federal Building in Oklahoma City in 1995. Nevertheless, the terrorist attacks on the World Trade Center towers and the Pentagon and the downing of another United Airlines flight on September 11, 2001, changed the U.S. government's and civilian population's engagement with terrorism. The nearly 7,500 injuries and 2,500 deaths resulting from these attacks spurred increased surveillance and preparedness for potential future bombing threats, and public health professionals are involved at each step of the planning and coordination of these activities.

In addition to these large-scale, mass-casualty events, studies show that a persistent, underlying threat of bombing events exists in the United States on a daily basis. A 20-year study of bombing events in this country revealed that from 1983 to 2002, 36,110 bombing incidents occurred. These incidents included 21,237 explosive bombings, 6,185 incendiary bombings (flammable materials), 1,107 premature bombings, and 7,581 attempted bombings.[10] These data indicate that both small-scale and large-scale bombing activities occur on a regular basis in the United States—which explains why local, state, and federal public health officials should have the knowledge and capabilities to respond to a bombing event.

PREPAREDNESS

Ensuring that the public health infrastructure has the ability to manage a potential bombing event effectively will require extensive preparations. In a mass-casualty bombing event, multiple services and personnel require coordination and communication; however, an effective response cannot be expected without pre-event planning. Preparedness and planning activities have been proven to influence the risk for events before they occur, and they accomplish horizontal coordination and vertical integration of separate plans from various levels and sectors. A shared preparedness and planning program results in greater collaboration of all parties involved before, during, and after a bombing event. The primary purpose of preparedness and planning is to confront complex risks and uncertainties through a logical and analytical process with an ongoing evaluation cycle (Figure 15-1).[11]

The Federal Emergency Management Agency (FEMA) has outlined several fundamental principles in planning for public health emergencies. According to its guidelines, such planning must involve all partners to achieve coordination and trust, and these stakeholders should also include senior officials and experts who can bring knowledge from prior experiences to the preparations. These preparedness activities need not begin with a blank slate, however: Public health planners should utilize existing plans as a framework for future initiatives. Most importantly, the plans should contain concrete details that identify tasks to be achieved, allocate resources to accomplish those tasks, and establish accountability to specific individuals for completing those tasks.[12]

FEMA also outlines two specific types of plans: concept plans (CONPLANs) and operations plans (OPLANs). CONPLANs integrate and synchronize the activities across multiple agencies, whereas OPLANs provide specific directives within individual agencies for personnel and assets. Effective preparedness will require completion of six steps:

- Form a collaborative planning team (public health, emergency medical services, fire, law enforcement, healthcare providers).

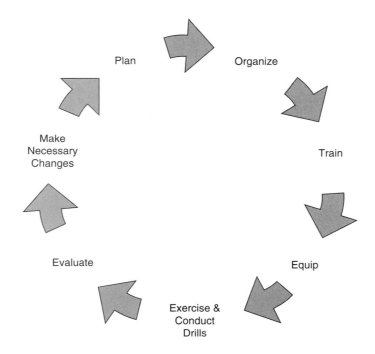

FIGURE 15-1   FEMA Disaster Preparedness Cycle
Source: Adapted from FEMA. Available at: www.fema.gov/emergency/nims/Preparedness. Accessed June 2010.

- Understand the situation (background research and hazard analysis).
- Determine goals and objectives.
- Develop response plan.
- Prepare and disseminate the plan.
- Refine and execute the plan.

Emergency planners and public health professionals must ensure that their emergency plans are not too detailed or lengthy; otherwise, they will be difficult to follow during an actual bombing event.

Government Agencies

Following FEMA recommendations, state and local governments will need to develop preparedness plans for potential bombing events, and individual agencies will also require specific plans. State and local executive administrations (e.g., governors, mayors) can follow the template of the National Response Framework (NRF) to implement preparedness plans and establish defined emergency support functions (ESFs; see Table 15-1).[13] The primary objectives will be the horizontal coordination of lead agencies (law enforcement, fire, EMS) and the vertical integration among other levels of government: local with state; state with national. In addition, government agencies should plan for how they will disseminate vital information to the public. If a bombing event occurs, the local government will need to use multiple forms of media such as television, radio, and the Internet to inform the general public about the event, ongoing hazards, locations to seek services, and sources of ongoing information.

For high-value targets (e.g., large commercial buildings, monuments, tourist attractions) at risk for a bombing incident, the fire department will need to develop site-specific plans for access and control, evacuation, incident command posts, and

TABLE 15-1　**Emergency Support Functions**
ESF 1: Transportation
ESF 2: Communications
ESF 3: Public Works and Engineering
ESF 4: Firefighting
ESF 5: Emergency Management
ESF 6: Mass Care, Emergency Assistance, Housing, and Human Resources
ESF 7: Logistics Management and Resource Support
ESF 8: Public Health and Medical Services
ESF 9: Search and Rescue
ESF 10: Oil and Hazardous Materials Response
ESF 11: Agriculture and Natural Resources
ESF 12: Energy
ESF 13: Public Safety and Security
ESF 14: Long-Term Community Recovery
ESF 15: External Affairs

Source: Modified from U.S. Department of Homeland Security. Overview: ESF and support annexes coordinating federal assistance in support of the National Response Framework. January 2008.

triage operations. Fire department personnel will also need to ensure they have the necessary supplies and equipment to manage a large-scale explosive event. Similarly, EMS systems will need to educate and train emergency medical technicians (EMTs) and paramedics to provide prehospital medical care for victims with bomb-related injuries.[14] Law enforcement agencies will need to prepare for handling scene security, personal security, and traffic control responsibilities in connection with a bombing event. A major threat after a terrorist bombing is the possibility of a secondary device detonating that will directly target emergency personnel and survivors: Law enforcement must be vigilant for this hazardous threat.

One important component of government preparedness is live simulations and drills. Through these pre-event engagements, lead agencies can evaluate the effectiveness of horizontal coordination among multiple agencies and focus on difficult areas of synchronization such as communications, resource sharing, and lines of command.

Health Care

In the event of a bombing, hospitals and emergency healthcare providers will be at the front lines for providing life-saving interventions for patients with injuries sustained during the blast event. Similar to prehospital care providers, hospital-based healthcare professionals should be trained to identify and treat specific injuries due to bombings. In addition, healthcare facilities will have to plan for the surge of patients that will occur if a mass-casualty bombing occurs. These contingency plans to manage the increased number of patients should account for the following possibilities:[15]

- Activating on-call or additional physicians and nurses
- Canceling elective surgeries and procedures
- Discharging non-urgent patients from the ED
- Discharging less-sick patients from inpatient beds
- Transferring patients from the intensive care unit (ICU) to regular hospital beds
- Bringing additional beds into the ED
- Having a dedicated blood supply for transfusions
- Establishing separate treatment areas within the ED for minor injuries because the large "first wave" of patients will mostly have minor trauma injuries
- Controlling patient and visitor flow through the ED

Hospitals will also face the challenge of trying to triage large numbers of patients simultaneously and differentiate acutely ill patients from those with minor injuries. Historical data from prior bombing events indicate that only one third of patients are likely to arrive by ambulance, and a majority of patients will not have any prehospital interventions when they arrive to the ED. In addition, previous bombings have shown that multiple individuals will present to private physicians' offices for treatment.[3]

Civilian Population, Nongovernmental Organizations, and Private-Sector Organizations

For the general public and private sector, the Centers for Disease Control and Prevention (CDC) and the American Red Cross have developed personal preparedness guidelines that focus on the need for home disaster kits, food and water supplies, evacuation routes and local maps, and prescription medications. In addition, individuals can receive further training and engage in preparedness activities by becoming members of a Community Emergency Response Team (CERT).[16,17] CERTs are community-based teams that function alongside government agencies during times of public health emergencies to provide resources for local neighborhoods.

The American Red Cross is probably the most recognizable example of a nongovernmental organization (NGO) that serves a critical role during public health emergencies. Of course, many other local and national NGOs may also play important roles during a large-scale crisis. These organizations may provide both material supplies and emotional support. Because nonprofit organizations have a long-standing history and presence in a community, they can utilize their informal networks for communications and relief efforts. Nonprofit organizations should have plans in place that allow for rapid scaling up of daily activities to provide resources to a larger population quickly in the event of a bombing.

Private-sector institutions (businesses, nonprofit organizations, faith-based institutions) should follow similar emergency planning principles as public agencies, such as those related to resource allocation, assigned tasks, and accountability. These private-sector plans should emphasize communications, evacuation, and first-aid training. One of the key objectives of any terrorist bombing is the disruption of business activity, with the goal being to inflict damage on the country's economy. Business continuity planning is an important component of private-sector preparedness and allows companies to rebound quickly after a public health emergency. To assist in these private-sector efforts, the US government instituted the Voluntary Private Sector Preparedness Accreditation and Certification Program as a mandate of the Implementing Recommendations of the 9/11 Commission Act of 2007.[18] The Department of Homeland Security (DHS) is in the process of establishing standards for the voluntary accreditation process, and DHS has signed an agreement with the ANSI-ASQ National Accreditation Board (ANAB) to manage the certification and accreditation process.[19]

RESPONSE

Government Agencies

The response system deployed by most municipal governments during a bombing event is the Incident Command System (ICS). Typically, the fire department oversees the ICS and will assume responsibility for managing the overall logistics of a municipal response to a bombing event.[20] The ICS is lead by an incident commander; in most municipal governments, this role is filled by the fire department chief. The ICS commander typically has command officers who directly report to him or her and fill the roles of public information officer, safety officer, and liaison officer (Figure 15-2).

The ICS has four main sections: Operations, Planning, Logistics, and Finance/Administration. Each section is led by a chief of the section. The Operations section conducts the actual response operations, such as firefighting, security, and medical care. The subunits of the Operations section that carry out these specific objectives are called branches. The Planning section prepares and documents the action plans to accomplish the designated objectives, gathers and evaluates information, maintains information about the status of resources, and keeps documents for incident records. The Logistics section provides the supplies and resources required to accomplish the goals of each branch of the Operations section. The Finance/Administration section monitors expenses incurred in

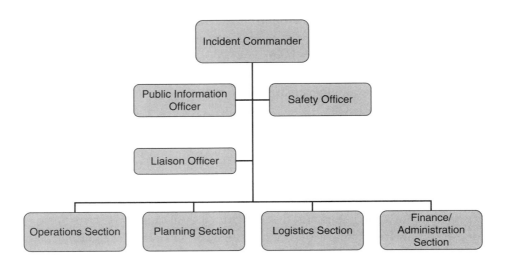

FIGURE 15-2   Incident Command System
Source: Modified from Incident Command System Training. Washington, D.C.: Federal Emergency Management Administration; 2008.

preparation and response to an incident and also assists with accounting, procurement, and personnel issues.[14]

Once a bombing event has occurred and the ICS has been activated, the Operations branches will need to begin a coordinated response to the incident. For a bombing event, the main Operations branches will include firefighting, law enforcement, and EMS. The Logistics section will include parallel branches that provide the supplies and resources required for each Operations branch to achieve its objectives. Activities directed toward these Operations objectives will be carried out simultaneously; therefore, logistics and communications will be essential. During this phase of the incident, the fire department will focus on controlling and extinguishing the subsequent fires from the initial blast, law enforcement will begin conducting criminal investigations and securing the incident site, and EMS personnel will be treating injured people and transporting them to local healthcare facilities.

Many large cities have established permanent emergency operations centers to coordinate planning and response to public health emergencies such as bombings. However, once the event occurs, an on-site command center will also need to be established to provide direct "scene management."[21,22] In addition, the EMS system will need to establish a triage site to evaluate people from the scene, provide urgent treatment measures, and determine who requires transport to a hospital to receive a higher level of medical care. Bombing events are immediately classified as crime scenes, and the criminal investigations will often include all possible levels of law enforcement, from federal to local agencies. If the blast event leads to a large area of destruction or if the local firefighting agency does not have the capacity to respond to the event, mutual aid from surrounding fire departments may be incorporated into the response.

Health Care

Studies have shown that the type of bombing event can affect the patterns of injuries and numbers of mortalities from the blast. This epidemiology of the type of bombing can help guide healthcare response to an event. Bombings can be classified as either confined-space bombings, open-air bombings, or structural-collapse bombings.[23] Confined-space bombings produce blasts that shatter windows and cause injuries, but the dynamics and magnitude of the blast do not lead to ceilings or walls collapsing. Open-air bombings occur when explosives are placed outside a building or on a person ("suicide bombing"). These events typically produce a biphasic mortality pattern, with deaths occurring either immediately after the event or at later stages, such as days or weeks from the incident. Structural-collapse bombings tend to produce higher numbers of deaths in the immediate stage, whereas confined-space and open-air bombings tend to be associated with more deaths in the later stages. Structural-collapse victims have higher rates of orthopedic injuries and inhalation injuries, confined-space victims have higher rates of blast lung injuries, and open-air victims have high rates of wound injuries (lacerations and penetrating shrapnel injuries).[23] These findings can direct public health professionals and emergency department providers in scaling up their specific response efforts appropriately based on the type of bombing that has occurred.

Similar to the ICS, a Hospital Emergency Incident Command System (HEICS) can be deployed once the healthcare facility receives notification of a bombing event.[24] In the hospital setting, the emphasis will be on patient care areas and ancillary services such as laboratory, radiology, and materials supply. The key components of the healthcare response to a mass-casualty bombing event are resource mobilization, additional healthcare providers and personnel, triage, identification and management of specific blast injuries, patient flow, and disposition.[25] Hospitals usually have a small delay in time from the actual bombing event to the arrival of patients, and this brief interval allows these facilities to begin rapid resource mobilization. For example, they may discharge less-acute patients from the ED and the inpatient hospital beds, and they may transfer less-ill patients out of the ICU. They may also bring extra supplies from central supply areas to the ED and the operating rooms. In addition, they can cease conducting non-emergent radiology studies, laboratory tests, and surgeries. Finally, hospitals anticipating a large number of patients may need to call in additional providers and support staff.

Once the surge of patients arrives, the hospital will need to designate low-acuity and high-acuity areas in the ED. A large proportion of patients will be "walking wounded" and will have arrived by personal transportation for treatment of minor injuries or just an assessment of potential injury. Some patients may be suffering panic symptoms or acute mental health issues. All of these patients will need to be rapidly triaged and assigned to the appropriate care area. Healthcare providers will then need to judiciously use the limited resources and beds at their disposal to treat the soft-tissue wounds, orthopedic injuries, and lung injuries usually seen in bombing victims. The healthcare leadership will need to manage the flow of patients through the various elements of the hospital system, such as the drawing of blood samples, starting of intravenous lines, transporting to radiology, and admitting to inpatient beds. One key factor will be the pace of disposition of patients. If the providers can quickly either discharge or admit patients, then they will be able to increase the number of patients seen each hour in the facility and reduce the overall morbidity and mortality from the bombing event.

Bombing events produce specific types of injuries, and healthcare providers will need to know the mechanisms of injury and the types of injuries associated with these incidents to provide the most effective care. Primary blast injuries (PBI) are caused by the direct effects of the atmospheric pressure differentials that result from a blast wave.[26] Secondary blast injuries arise when projectiles from the explosion strike a patient and cause blunt or penetrating injuries. Tertiary blast injuries occur when the patient's body is displaced by the blast wave. Other indirect injuries or morbidities include burns from secondary fires started by the bombing event or exacerbation of chronic illnesses, such as asthma or diabetes, by the incident. To improve the response to bombing events, healthcare providers can reduce the number of injuries and deaths by recognizing and treating these blast injuries in a timely manner.

Civilian Population, Nongovernmental Organizations, and Private-Sector Organizations

The initial response from the civilian population and the private sector will be to focus on personal safety. Individuals should seek medical assistance only if they believe they have suffered an injury; otherwise, they should refrain from unnecessary utilization of scarce resources. Businesses at or near the site of the bombing event should implement their internal emergency plans. The NGO community will have a limited role in the immediate aftermath of the bombing event. Nevertheless, in the hours and days after the mass-casualty event, NGOs may provide key psychological and social support services to the victims of the event. For example, individuals may need assistance locating family members if large numbers of injuries and deaths have occurred. People may be separated from one another, especially if they were transported to a hospital in an acute medical condition that requires surgery or hospitalization.

In addition to providing reunification services, NGOs may help with long-term mental health effects of the bombing event. These issues may be especially pronounced in children. If a residential structure is involved in the event, such as high-rise apartment complex, then NGOs may assist in supplying personal needs such as food, shelter, and temporary housing. These organizations will have the responsibility to provide indirect services and fill any voids in this area, because government agencies will not be able to meet the specific needs and supply necessary resources to all individuals affected by the bombing event. Finally, the civilian population, NGOs, and private-sector organizations will provide an enormous resilience and support framework for the victims of the bombing. By simply returning to normal activities and daily routines quickly, they will have a high impact on the long-term response to the event.

MITIGATION

Government Agencies

Government's primary means of mitigating bombing events is to find and capture potential terrorists who have the intention to carry out a bombing event before they are able to initiate the incident. Since September 11, 2001, the U.S. government has attempted to maintain a delicate balance between ensuring security and respecting civil liberties while trying to increase surveillance measures and to identify potential perpetrators through means such as psychological profiling. The federal government has also invested large amounts of funds into mitigation technology in two domains: hazards identification and infrastructure resilience. Hazards identification is simply the use of advanced technology to locate bomb-related materials before they are detonated. Infrastructure resilience involves instituting engineering standards to prevent structural collapse and developing materials that can withstand potential bomb blasts, such as glazing on windows to prevent shatter. Often this technology originates in the military sector and is then transferred to the private sector.[27] In addition, building design measures can help secure the structure to prevent criminal entry.[28]

After the August 7, 1998, terrorist bombings of U.S. embassies in Tanzania and Kenya, the U.S. Congress passed the Secure Embassy Construction and Counterterrorism Act of 1999 to mitigate against the impacts of a potential bomb detonation at or near a U.S. embassy.[29] This legislation charges the Secretary of State with ensuring that all new embassy and consulate compounds meet strict security standards that include perimeter defenses, building distances from entrances, and blast resistance (Figure 15-3). Using its past experiences as a guide, the U.S. government has taken its hard-learned lessons to heart and mandated changes that will help protect against future losses through proactive measures. Similar design and construction features can be translated into the private sector.

Health Care

The health sector assists with mitigation of bombing events by increasing coordination among healthcare facilities prior to any such event, so that multiple hospitals can share the surge of patients effectively and reduce morbidity and mortality. In addition, through increased training of prehospital care and hospital-based providers in the management of specific bomb-related injuries, such as blast lung injuries, the medical community can mitigate the long-term disabilities from these specific pathologies.

Improved triage methodologies for mass-casualty incidents in general, and for bomb events specifically, can also improve patient flow through the healthcare system

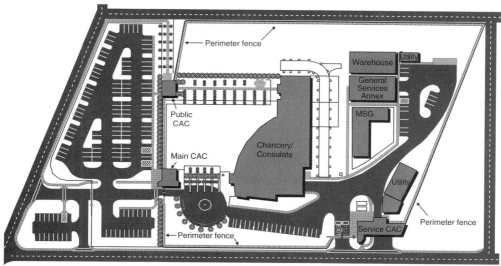

CAC Compound Access Control
MSG Marine Security Guard Quarters

FIGURE 15-3 Example of New Embassy Compound Security Features
Source: US GAO. Embassy Construction, June 2006. Available at: http://www.gao.gov/new.items/ d06641.pdf. Accessed June 2010.

after the bombing incident and improve the quality of patient care. If patients are "over-triaged" (assessed as being likely to have a critical injury when in reality only a low-acuity injury exists), then they may receive unnecessary tests and studies rather than an individual who truly needs those scarce resources. If they are "under-triaged" (assessed as having a low-acuity injury when in reality a critical injury exists), then they may wait for treatment, and this delay may lead to increased morbidity or death. In the Madrid 2004 subway bombings, many of the patients seen at the closest hospital to the event were over-triaged.[6] Preventing triage errors can mitigate against poor clinical outcomes after a bombing event.

Civilian Population, Nongovernmental Organizations, and Private-Sector Organizations

Just as the military is developing mitigation strategies to reduce the number of bombings and to diminish the physical impact of blast events, so the private sector is also actively engaged in these pursuits. The government is seeking to foster public–private partnerships that will enhance technology transfer related to this issue and reduce the time from research and development to real-world application of new technologies. Private-sector organizations are also trying to reduce risks and hazards by improving security measures and investing in resilient engineering and design strategies.

CASE STUDY ANALYSIS

The 1995 Oklahoma City bombing exemplifies some of the traditional vulnerabilities to bombing events and the multiple actors involved in the critical response to the public health emergency caused by bombing events. Evaluating the planning and response of the different sectors can help guide future preparedness and mitigation efforts.

Government Agencies

Because the target of the Oklahoma City bombing was a federal building, the primary government responsibility was security of the infrastructure. Had Timothy McVeigh not been able to approach the building, he might have been deterred from targeting this structure—for example, if a large barrier wall had protected the facility or if the building had been offset from the exterior entrance. These design elements are being modeled into newly built federal buildings. In addition, if tracking and surveillance measures had been implemented, government authorities might have been able to intervene when McVeigh began purchasing large quantities of ammonium nitrate fertilizer. His ability to purchase the bomb materials supports the contention that improved intelligence is a fundamental component of terrorist bombing prevention and mitigation.

The Oklahoma City Fire Department ICS and the Oklahoma City Police Department security operations provided an effective initial response to the event. However, the incident command post was relocated after further bomb threats, and this scenario reveals the balance authorities face between providing leadership on site and maintaining security for first responders. Furthermore, local authorities had to share responsibilities and coordinate responses with state and federal officials. Finally, the blast event affected critical communications infrastructure, and the local EMS system could not communicate with participants in the field operations. Coordination of multiple jurisdictions and communications within and among agencies remain two key areas that are the focus of ongoing emergency public health improvements for many municipalities.

Health Care

Only one third of the Oklahoma City bombing victims were able to utilize the pre-hospital care system. Moreover, this case study highlights the findings from other blast events that bombing victims tend to suffer either very severe injuries or only minor complaints. Most of the people who arrive by personal transportation (foot or vehicle) at hospitals will have non-acute injuries, and they will overwhelm the facilities closest to the event site. In the 1995 incident, the large majority of the victims arrived at hospitals within a 1.5-mile radius of the Murrah Federal Building. These hospitals had to quickly triage large numbers of patients, and the providers had to make critical decisions on which patients needed to be treated immediately and which patients could receive deferred care. In addition, knowing the location within the building and specifics about blast injuries would have helped guide clinical management of patients.

Civilian Population, Nongovernmental Organizations, and Private-Sector Organizations

Multiple nonprofit NGOs helped with the immediate response to the bombing incident in Oklahoma City. The American Red Cross provided both resources from its warehouses and counseling through its staff. In addition, other NGOs were able to offer support to victims and family members. The Oklahoma City event shows the ancillary services that NGOs and the private sector provide to fill in gaps that government agencies cannot address during the immediate aftermath of an incident. Often these NGOs have longstanding relations with members of local communities, and these informal relations and communications can prove valuable resources in the response to a public health emergency.

CONCLUSIONS

Bombing events continue to be the high-probability terrorist threat for most communities, and public health authorities will be integral in the preparedness and response to these potential events. Effective planning and response capabilities will require the coordination and communications of multiple key actors, and public health professionals will play valuable roles in guiding these interactions. Knowing which resources each entity is able to provide will help guide how these resources are best utilized during a bombing event. A community's resilience to a terrorist bombing incident will be a function of both planning and mitigation strategies.

INTERNET RESOURCES

American Red Cross, civilian preparedness resources:
http://www.redcross.org/preparedness

Centers for Disease Control and Preparedness, emergency preparedness and response for terrorist bombings: http://www.bt.cdc.gov/masscasualties/preparingterroristbombing.asp

Citizen Corps: www.citizencorps.gov

Emergency Management Assistance Compact (a Congressionally ratified site that serves as a resource for interstate mutual aid): www.emacweb.org

U.S. Department of Health and Human Services, Agency for Healthcare Research and Quality (AHRQ)—public health emergency preparedness: http://www.ahrq.gov/prep/

U.S. Department of Health and Human Services, Center for Domestic Preparedness:
http://cdp.dhs.gov/

U.S. Department of Homeland Security, protecting infrastructure:
http://www.dhs.gov/files/programs/critical-infrastructure.shtm

U.S. Federal Emergency Management Agency (FEMA), Emergency Management Institute:
http://training.fema.gov/EMICourses/

U.S. Federal Emergency Management Agency (FEMA), National Incident Management System (NIMS) resource center: http://www.fema.gov/emergency/nims/

U.S. Federal Emergency Management Agency (FEMA), National Response Framework:
www.fema.gov/emergency/nrf/

NOTES

1. The Oklahoma Department of Civil Emergency Management. After action report: Alfred P. Murrah Federal Building bombing 19 April 1995 in Oklahoma City, Oklahoma. Oklahoma City: Department of Central Services Central Printing Division; 1995. Available at: http://www.ok.gov/OEM/documents/Bombing%20After%20Action%20Report.pdf. Accessed September 2, 2009.
2. Mallonee S, Shariat S, Stennies G, Waxweiler R, Higan D, Jordan F. Physical injuries and fatalities resulting from the Oklahoma City bombing. *Journal of the American Medical Association*. 1996;276:382–387.
3. Hogan D, Waeckerle JF, Dire DJ, Lillibridge SR. Emergency department impact of the Oklahoma City terrorist bombing. *Annals of Emergency Medicine*. 1999;34:160–167.
4. Office of the Coordinator for Counterterrorism. *Country reports on terrorism 2008*. Washington, DC: U.S. Department of State; 2009.
5. Gause FG. Can democracy stop terrorism. *Foreign Affairs*. 2005:84;62–76.
6. Gutierrez de Ceballos JP, Turégano Fuentes F, Diaz DP, Sanchez MS, Llorente CM, Sanz JEG. Casualties treated at the closest hospital in the Madrid, March 11, terrorist bombings. *Critical Care Medicine*. 2005;33:S107–S112.

7. Arnold JL. The 2005 London bombings and the Haddon matrix. *Prehospital and Disaster Medicine*. 2005;20:278–281.

8. Arnold J, Tsai MC, Halpern P, Smithline H, Stok E, Ersoy G. Mass-casualty, terrorist bombings: Epidemiological outcomes, resource utilization, and time-course of emergency needs (Part I). *Prehospital and Disaster Medicine*. 2003;18(3):220–234.

9. Lerner EB, O'Connor RE, Schwartz R, et al. Blast-related injuries from terrorism: An international perspective. *Prehospital Emergency Care*. 2007;11:137–153.

10. Kapur GB, Hutson HR, Davis MA, Rice PL. The United States twenty-year experience with bombing incidents: Implications for terrorism preparedness and medical response. *Journal of Trauma*. 2005;59:1436–1444.

11. Federal Emergency Management Agency. *Preparedness*. Available at: http://www.fema.gov/emergency/nims/Preparedness.shtm#item1. Accessed September 1, 2009.

12. Federal Emergency Management Agency. *Comprehensive Preparedness guide 101*. Washington, DC: Author; March 2009.

13. Overview: ESF and Support Annexes Coordinating Federal Assistance in Support of the National Response Framework. Department of Homeland Security; January 2008. Available at: www.fema.gov/pdf/emergency/nrf/nrf-overview.pdf. Accessed January 23, 2010.

14. Sasser SM, Sattin RW, Hunt RC, Krohmer J. Blast lung injury. *Prehospital Emergency Care*. 2006;10(2):165–172.

15. Halpern P, Tsai M, Arnold JL, Stok E, Ersoy G. Mass-casualty, terrorist bombings: Implications for emergency department and hospital emergency response (Part II). *Prehospital and Disaster Medicine*. 2003;18(3):235–241.

16. American Red Cross, CDC. *Preparedness today*. Available at: http://www.redcross.org/preparedness/cdc_english/home.asp. Accessed September 1, 2009.

17. Community Emergency Response Team (CERT). Available at: https://www.citizencorps.gov/cert/index.shtm. Accessed on September 1, 2009.

18. Public Law 110-53, Implementing the Recommendations of the 9/11 Commission Act of 2007, Title IX, August 3, 2007.

19. Federal Emergency Management Agency. *Voluntary private sector preparedness accreditation and certification program*. Available at: http://www.fema.gov/media/fact_sheets/vpsp.shtm. Accessed on September 15, 2009.

20. Emergency Management Institute. *Incident Command System training*. Washington, DC: Federal Emergency Management Agency; 2008. Available at: http://training.fema.gov/EMIWeb/IS/ICSResource/assets/reviewMaterials.pdf. Accessed September 1, 2009.

21. Frykeberg ER. Principles of mass casualty management following terrorist disasters. *Annals of Surgery*. 2004;239(3):319–321.

22. Simon R, Teperman S. The World Trade Center attack: Lessons for disaster management. *Critical Care*. 2001;5:318–320.

23. Arnold JL, Halpern P, Tsai MC, Smithline H. Mass casualty terrorist bombings: A comparison of outcomes by bombing type. *Annals of Emergency Medicine*. 2004;43:263–273.

24. Hospital Incident Command System. Available at: www.heics.com. Accessed January 23, 2010.

25. Halpern P, Tsai MC, Arnold J, Stok E, Ersoy G. Mass-casualty, terrorist bombings: Implications for emergency department and hospital emergency response (Part II). *Prehospital and Disaster Medicine*. 2003;18(3):235–241.

26. Wightman JM, Gladish SL. Explosions and blast injuries. *Annals of Emergency Medicine.* 2001;37:664–678.

27. National Academy of Sciences. *Protecting buildings from bomb damage: Transfer of blast-effects mitigation technologies from military to civilian applications.* Washington, DC: National Academies Press; 1995.

28. Sevin E, Little RG. Mitigating terrorist hazards. *The Bridge.* 1998;28(3):3–8.

29. U.S. Government Accountability Office. Embassy construction: State has made progress constructing new embassies, but better planning is needed for operations and maintenance requirements. June 2006. Available at: http://www.gao.gov/new.items/d06641.pdf. Accessed January 27, 2010.

CHAPTER 16

Biological Agents

L. Kristian Arnold

INTRODUCTION

Preparation of biological agents for mass dispersal often requires sophisticated laboratory and production facilities, which historically made it less likely that such agents would be procured by nongovernment groups or individuals. More recently, the scope of potential users of these agents as weapons has increased. At the same time, considering the continued reliance on conventional explosive devices by terrorist groups during the first decade of the twenty-first century, the minimal history of use of biological agents by groups, and little suspicion in the international defense community of state-level biological programs, discussions have developed regarding the optimal balance between cost-effectiveness and vigilance in preparing for potential biological weapon assaults.

Case Study

Dr. Johansson was fortunate that he had recently attended a public health review course covering toxic exposures—because without it, he was not sure he would have been able to determine the etiology of the problem with the man presenting with choking symptoms and difficulty speaking. Although the patient could not make a lot of sense, Dr. Johansson had noted that he seemed to be "cross-eyed" and not used to this condition: He kept twisting his head around as if he was trying to get a better look at his surroundings. Other healthcare providers thought the patient might have been using drugs alone in a hotel while attending a convention. The concerns for an unusual pathology increased when the patient started gesturing with his arms as if something was wrong with his fingertips. In addition, he was too alert and oriented to be under the influence of a drug of abuse. Dr. Johansson realized that he had to go through the rest of the evaluation to rule out other diagnoses with progressive neurologic deficits. All of the other options, however, were either ascending paralyses or indications with bulbar signs that come later in the disease, such as Guillain-Barré syndrome. As for the suggestion by the medical student that the patient might have suffered a stroke, a brain stem stroke might give some bulbar findings but not in this pattern and with the bilateral upper extremity weakness.

At midnight, one hour after the end of his emergency department (ED) shift, Dr. Johansson was still at the hospital—and trying valiantly to convince the skeptical critical care specialist that he had a bona fide case of botulism. The public health official's reaction, when Dr. Johansson told him he needed to get botulinum antitoxin from the state public health department immediately, was to insist on laboratory confirmation because the patient's dietary history was not suggestive of ingestion.

A news flash brought Dr. Johansson out of his musings. Two men had been found dead in separate rooms at the hotel next to the convention center when room service came to deliver their food orders. There were no signs of foul play or trauma. As almost an afterthought, the newscaster mentioned that both victims had been attending the National Conference on Strategic Internet Security, which had just finished after four days of meetings. Police had begun questioning other conference attendees, although most had already left to return home. Even though Dr. Johansson's patient could not talk and was unable to write, paramedics had reported transporting him from the same hotel. When Dr. Johansson walked into the waiting room, he noticed that a rush of people had arrived from the hotel with a variety of complaints. Other healthcare professionals asked if Dr. Johansson would return to work and help out with the surge. He quickly told the triage nurse of his concern that there might be a botulism outbreak at the hotel. His next call was to the public health official who had given him a hard time about getting botulinum antitoxin.

HISTORICAL PERSPECTIVES

Biological agents have been the basis for some of the most terrifying threats to human well-being in recorded history—leprosy, the black plague, smallpox, anthrax, Ebola, severe acute respiratory syndrome (SARS), locust swarms, mad cow disease, poison darts, botulism, and tetrodotoxin (puffer fish), to name but a few. They also represent some of the oldest agents of warfare, with recorded uses dating from the Peloponnesian War.[1] Biologically derived toxins have been used since before recorded history for hunting and warfare. In the 1990s, a North Atlantic Treaty Organization (NATO) handbook dealing with biowarfare listed 39 agents of concern.[2] Biological agents have been used for mass aggression as well as for strategic individual aggressions, including assassinations. The U.S. defense analysis community believes that biological agents are the most likely class of weapon of mass destruction to be employed, given the technologies involved and the potential impact of such an attack.[3]

Several characteristics of biological agents allow them to be weaponized, historically based on military use, which explains why these agents are a critical concern for public health officials. These characteristics include ease of dispersion to a large number of people (aerosolization being the most rapid delivery method); ease of preparation in a stable form; endemic presence (creating confusion between attack and natural disease); frightening conditions produced in humans, which are associated with high morbidity and mortality; and often a lack of preventive measures or treatments for infection with the agents. Militia or terrorist groups having social disruption (as opposed to incapacitation of military forces) as a primary goal may be drawn to these agents.

A more insidious manner in which biological agents have been used as agents of aggression for societal destabilization involves deploying agents that harm the food supply without causing direct human disease. For example, members of the Mau Mau tribe were suspected of using oils from *Synadenium grantii*—a plant known to be used as a hunting poison in Africa—to poison cattle belonging to neighboring tribes during a 1952 revolt in Kenya.[4,5] The discovery of animal diseases such as hoof and mouth disease at critical junctures in the food processing chain can lead to financially devastating slaughter of herds, disruption of international trade, and lack of food resources for the public.[6]

Although military forces have used biological agents as weapons for centuries, modern research and production programs date from the mid-twentieth century, coincident with availability of improved laboratory technologies. The U.S. military biological warfare program was established in 1943 based on concerns about similar programs in Japan and Germany. President Richard Nixon formally terminated the offensive biological warfare program in 1969, leaving a defensive program, which operates under the aegis of the U.S. Army Medical Research Institute for Infectious Diseases (AMRIID).[7] Internationally, the United Nations Biological Weapons Convention, which became effective in 1975, was intended to end the Cold War buildup of biological and chemical

TABLE 16-1   CDC Classification of Bioterrorism Agents and Diseases

Category	Definition	Basis	Agents/Diseases
A	High-priority agents, including organisms that pose a risk to national security	• Can be easily disseminated or transmitted from person to person • Result in high mortality rates and have the potential for major public health impact • Might cause public panic and social disruption • Require special action for public health preparedness	• Anthrax • Botulism • Plague • Smallpox • Tularemia • Viral hemorrhagic fevers
B	Second-highest-priority agents	• Are moderately easy to disseminate • Result in moderate morbidity rates and low mortality rates • Require specific enhancements of CDC's diagnostic capacity and enhanced disease surveillance	• Brucellosis • Epsilon toxin of Clostridium perfringens • Food safety threats • Glanders • Melioidosis • Psittacosis • Q fever • Ricin toxin • Staphylococcal enterotoxin B • Typhus fever • Viral encephalitis • Water safety threats
C	Third-highest-priority agents, including emerging pathogens that could be engineered for mass dissemination	• Availability • Ease of production and dissemination • Potential for high morbidity and mortality rates and major health impact	• Emerging infectious diseases such as Nipah virus and hantavirus

Source: Adapted from Centers for Disease Control and Prevention. Available at: http://emergency.cdc.gov/agent/agentlist-category.asp. Accessed July 31, 2010.

weapons as well as to discourage other nations from undertaking such programs. As of 2010, almost all countries, with a few exceptions, had ratified it.[8]

In the latter part of the 1990s, the U.S. Congress undertook to bolster the United States' bio-defensive capabilities through funding initiatives in response to several events:[9–16]

- Revelation of a 1979 outbreak of anthrax in the Soviet Union
- Discovery of the clandestine Soviet Biopreparat program for bioweapons development
- Claims by Iraq of pursuing bioweapon development
- Attempted anthrax attacks by the same group that had executed a chemical attack in the Tokyo subway
- Deliberate contamination of a salad bar in Oregon by a group intent on influencing local elections
- Multiple hoax allegations of anthrax terrorist attacks

In 1997, the Johns Hopkins School of Public Health presented a conference on biological warfare; as part of this effort, it developed a Working Group on Civilian Biodefense by calling together a number of scientific experts and stakeholders, who ultimately published a series of papers on five potential bioweapon agents.[17–22] In 1999, the Centers for Disease Control and Prevention (CDC), in cooperation with the Working Group on Civilian Biodefense, developed a list of 16 biological agents of concern in regard to possible terrorist acts and prioritized them according to their perceived ability to affect public health and medical infrastructure on a large scale (Table 16-1).[23] They also specified two general categories of food and water contamination, under which they refer to microorganism dissemination via these media for direct infection of human targets. Other agencies and organizations including the North Atlantic Treaty Organization (NATO) and National Institute for Occupational Safety and Health (NIOSH) have also developed lists of potential bioweapons that include agents not in the CDC listing.[24,25]

This chapter primarily addresses Category A, B, and C biological agents on the CDC bioterrorism list. In addition, it provides specific recommendations for preparedness (identification and diagnosis of agents) and response (treatment) for these biological agents.

PREPAREDNESS AND RESPONSE: CATEGORY A AGENTS

Anthrax

The term "anthrax" comes from Greek word for "coal," referring to the black eschars that form in cutaneous anthrax. Anthrax has been recognized as a medical condition through the ages, owing to the potential for animal skin exposure among shepherds and people in the tannery and leather working trades. Anthrax is endemic in many parts of the world as a zoonotic infection with occasional, primarily cutaneous human infection.

Bacillus anthracis grows as large (1–1.5 µm × 4.5–10 µm), Gram-positive, non-motile, encapsulated, rectangular chain-forming cells (with a box-car train appearance) on most laboratory media. The virulent strains form ragged, mildly hemolytic colonies, whereas the nonvirulent strains form smooth colonies.[11] Under the proper environmental conditions, *B. anthracis* creates a dormant and resilient spore that can last years, giving it the potential to be used as a weapon.[26–28] Effective infection via air dispersion requires adequate respiratory tract penetration, and usually particles with sizes in the range of 5 micrometers (microns, µm) or smaller can cause respiratory infections. Anthrax spores are between 0.4 and 0.6 µm in diameter, making them ideal for air dispersion delivery into the respiratory tree. Anthrax produces two toxins that become activated when bacterial factors bind to the host antigens to form an edema toxin and a "lethal" toxin.

Three relatively distinct clinical syndromes of anthrax infection exist: cutaneous, gastrointestinal, and pulmonary (Table 16-2). The incubation period for all syndromes is between 4 and 6 days. The pulmonary form is generally considered the most lethal. Inhalation-based pulmonary infection usually begins with a nonspecific, flu-like syndrome with cough and can rapidly progress to respiratory failure without treatment. The radiologic hallmarks for early detection of pulmonary anthrax on chest x-ray include irregular mediastinal widening and pleural effusion.

TABLE 16-2 Clinical Syndromes Produced by *Bacillus anthracis*	
Pulmonary	• 2–4 days incubation (up to 60 days) • Prodrome of flu-like symptoms • None/minimally productive cough • May have nausea/vomiting • Rapidly progressing respiratory failure • Specific hallmark of widened mediastinum on chest x-ray • Lymphadenopathy • Septicemia • Multiple-organ failure
Cutaneous	• 1–7 days incubation • Localized itching followed by a papular lesion that turns vesicular, and within 2–6 days develops into a depressed black eschar • Commonly observed on hands, forearms, or head
Gastrointestinal	• 1–7 days incubation • Abdominal pain, nausea, vomiting and fever • Bloody diarrhea, hematemesis • Commonly fatal

When any clinical suspicion of anthrax arises, antibiotic treatment must be initiated without delay; healthcare providers should not wait for further confirmatory testing to start treatment. Recommendations for treatment and prophylaxis are subject to change and are not based on any large randomized trials. Treatment and post-exposure prophy- laxis recommendations from the CDC were updated following the experience with anthrax exposures and infections in 2001.[29,30] Currently, the combination of ciprofloxacin with another drug to which anthrax is normally sensitive is recommended as initial treat- ment for ill patients with suspected inhalation or gastrointestinal anthrax.[31] Prophylaxis should be initiated upon confirmation of an anthrax exposure. Some evidence suggests that combined post-exposure treatment with vaccine and antibiotics may allow for a shorter length of antibiotic prophylaxis.[32] If available, post-exposure vaccination consists of three doses of vaccine at 0, 2, and 4 weeks after exposure.

Anthrax jumped to the forefront of issues related to biological weapons in the fall of 2001, when a series of envelopes containing highly refined anthrax spores were sent through the U.S. Postal Service to commercial and government locations. This expo- sure led to 11 cases of inhalation anthrax with 5 deaths ,and 11 cases of cutaneous anthrax with no deaths. One of the earliest cases was identified by an emergency physician who had recently been to a seminar on bioterrorism, demonstrating the importance of educational activities and highlighting the potential for emergency departments and public health authorities to serve as a front line of defense for the community. The ultimate response involved multiple agencies and raised a number of systems-related issues, particularly regarding the interface between public health and public safety agencies in performing investigations. The origin of the letters had still not been determined at the time of this writing.[33] Experience gained from these cases brought up questions regarding some of the clinical descriptions presented by the Working Group on Civilian Biodefense, whose members had obtained most of their information from reports of unintentional infection.[34]

Botulism

Clostridium botulinum toxin was first recognized as causing a clinical syndrome and named *botulism* (Latin for "sausage") following ingestion of undercooked sausage- stuffed pig stomach by German villagers in the early 1800s.[35] The toxin has been iden- tified as a family of seven antigenically distinct dual-chain, heat-labile proteins, designated as types A through G; human toxicity is mostly attributed to types A, B, E, and F.[36] In addition to four genetically distinct strains of *C. botulinum*, members of two other species—*C. baratii* and *C. butyricum*—produce botulinum toxin. *Clostridae* are spore-forming natural residents of soil throughout the world. Human illness normally occurs through ingestion of toxin or spores or through contamination of wounds by dirt. Inhalation is not recognized to occur in the wild.

Toxicity is based on selective penetration of nerve cells and permanent blocking of acetylcholine (ACh)-containing vacuoles from binding with the cell wall to release the ACh to the neuromuscular junction. Recovery occurs by regrowth of the motor endplates. Botulinum toxin is one of the most lethal biological toxins, with findings from primate studies suggesting that a lethal dose of type A toxin for adult humans would be on the order of 70 μg through ingestion and between 0.7 and 0.9 μg through inhalation.[12]

Clinically, intoxication most often begins with bulbar paralysis (diplopia, dysphagia, dysarthria, dysphonia), classically with diplopia resulting from weakness of the lateral rectus eye muscle. Affected individuals are afebrile with a normal mental status, but develop a descending symmetrical motor paralysis.[37] Clinical symptoms from ingestions generally occur within 6 to 72 hours after exposure, but symptom onset may sometimes be delayed up to several days. Abdominal cramps, nausea, vomiting, and diarrhea may be associated with ingestion. Animal toxin inhalation studies have also demonstrated a variable time to symptom onset, ranging from 12 to 80 hours in one simian study.[12] Confirmatory laboratory diagnosis depends on identifying toxin in serum, feces, or wound tissue, or by identifying bacteria in samples of gastrointestinal (GI) contents, suspected food, or wound tissue. The process is not rapid, which suggests that initial treatment decisions be based on clinical findings.

Intentional deployment of *C. botulinum* would likely be difficult to differentiate from a naturally occurring contamination of food sources. Historically, most botulism was associated with insufficiently sterilized home-preserved (home-canned) foods; however, in recent years, incidents have increasingly involved commercially prepared foods. Even with inhalation, differentiation of intentional and accidental intoxication may be difficult considering the variability in timing of symptom onset.

Botulinum antitoxin may lessen the full impact of an exposure if administered early. Otherwise, treatment is based on respiratory support. As of the time of this writing, antitoxins were equine derived and, therefore, carried a risk of allergic reaction. Some countries do not stock antitoxin due to questions regarding this treatment's efficacy and safety as well as the exit of commercial producers from the antitoxin market.[38] In the United States, antitoxin is stocked in regional "quarantine stations" under the auspices of the CDC and the control of state health officials. The local health department or the CDC should be contacted in all suspected cases and will assist with locating antitoxin. Initial care in suspected botulinum intoxication should include frequent objective measuring of respiratory function using vital capacity and maximal inspiratory force.

Plague

Plague—that is, infection with *Yersinia pestis*—manifests in three forms: bubonic, septicemic, and pneumonic. *Y. pestis* is probably the earliest recorded bioweapon: Mongol troops reportedly catapulted their plague dead into the besieged Crimean city of Caffa in 1346 with resultant infection of the Genoese, leading to their departure.[39] The United States and the Union of Soviet Socialist Republics (USSR) both weaponized plague during the Cold War. Of the three forms of plague, pneumonic plague is the only form that can lead to person-to-person transmission. Because it can be aerosolized and is contagious, pneumonic plague has the potential to be a serious public health threat.

Pneumonic plague usually follows inhalation of aerosolized germs, although it may also develop as an advancement of bubonic plague. Patients with pneumonic plague rapidly progress to pneumonia symptoms. Clinical features of pneumonic plague include cough with purulent sputum, fever, chest pain, and bloody sputum. A chest x-ray will show evidence of bronchopneumonia. Treatment consists of antibiotics such as doxycycline or ciprofloxacin. Persons symptomatic with pneumonic plague are contagious through droplet transmission. Thus, in terms of risk assessment for co-workers or healthcare workers, anyone who has maintained a distance of less than approximately 3 feet from a contagious individual should be considered at high risk (Table 16-3). Because the initial symptoms are nonspecific, infected persons may

TABLE 16-3 Airborne Infectious Disease Transmission Protection		
Level of Transmission	**Particle size/Character**	**Protection**
Droplet	> 5 μm	> 3 feet separation
	Droplets produced by cough, sneeze, talking	Standard surgical mask with face shield to prevent conjunctival exposure.
Airborne	< 5 μm	N95 mask
	Droplet nuclei (evaporated droplets) containing microorganisms that remain suspended in the air for long periods of time; dust particles containing the infectious agent	High-efficiency particulate air (HEPA) filter

not always be recognized as posing a contagious threat. Given this fact, pneumonic plague can escalate to a serious public health crisis once a large number of infected people become carriers.

Bubonic and septicemic plague result from transmission by infected fleas. Symptoms include swollen and tender lymph glands (called buboes), fever, headache, chills, and weakness. Bubonic plague is easily treated when identified early in the disease process. Treatment options include streptomycin or gentamicin; alternative antibiotics include doxycycline, ciprofloxacin, or cloramphenicol. If treatment is delayed, the mortality increases significantly.

Post-exposure prophylaxis should be initiated following confirmed or suspected unprotected *Y. pestis* exposure and for healthcare workers and others who have unprotected close (less than 3 feet) contact with symptomatic patients with pneumonic plague. Doxycycline is the recommended antibiotic for post-exposure prophylaxis, and ciprofloxacin is approved as a second-line agent. Prophylaxis should continue for 7 days after the last known or suspected *Y. pestis* exposure. No effective vaccine currently exists for *Y. pestis*.

Smallpox

Smallpox is known for having been a major global health burden as well as one of the greatest success stories in public health history with eradication of its natural state in 1977.[40] In the 30 years since this disease's eradication through a massive international vaccination program, most countries in the world have eliminated their surveillance and immunization programs. Therefore, following anthrax, many authorities consider smallpox the next most likely bioterrorism agent to be used on larger population groups. The majority of practicing physicians in the world at this time are unlikely to have seen smallpox or to have administered a smallpox vaccination—a task that requires that the technique be followed closely to achieve effective and safe vaccination. This loss of the global healthcare system's capacity to react to a resurgence of smallpox, coupled with the decreasing numbers of persons alive with active immunity, increases the relative concern regarding any release of smallpox into the general population.

The variola virus causes smallpox. It is a member of the same poxvirus family that includes monkeypox and vaccinia—the biggest and most complex viruses to infect humans.[41] The virulence of smallpox is, in part, linked to production of immune-modulating proteins. Infection for all forms of smallpox occurs via the respiratory tree, with the incubation period lasting 10 to 14 days. Clinical disease begins with a

2- to 4-day prodrome of fever and myalgia. A papular rash then appears; it becomes vesicular, then pustular, then ulcerated, and finally covered with eschar. Each stage of progression takes 1 to 3 days. Individuals are infectious for several days before the development of the rash and remain infectious until all lesions have scabs. Transmission occurs via both droplet and airborne mechanisms. Death is usually due to multiple-organ failure[42] and respiratory compromise.[42,43]

The smallpox rash might be confused with different rashes at different stages in its evolution. The overall disease picture is most likely to be confused with varicella (chickenpox). Smallpox advances in waves over the body, starting on the face and moving to the trunk, then affecting the limbs, with all lesions being in the same stage of maturation. With chickenpox, the lesions are in various stages of maturation throughout the body, and they tend to develop initially at the trunk of the body and spread to the face and limbs.[4]

Smallpox is relatively easily weaponized because it does not lose virulence on drying and it stands up well to lyophilization. Given that the organism will remain infectious after drying, potentially contaminated clothing, equipment, and environments must be sterilized carefully and thoroughly. Currently there are no therapeutic agents for smallpox. Research is limited due to the eradication of the wild disease and limited access to official stocks of virus. Most experimentation since the 1960s, for which public records are available, has been done using monkeypox as a surrogate. Following the 2001 anthrax incident, the CDC, in conjunction with the Department of Defense, set up a smallpox vaccination program involving a cadre of 500,000 vaccinated professionals likely to be involved in responding to a smallpox outbreak and undertook vaccination of some members of the community in an attempt to execute a response plan of "ring immunization" around every identified case.[44] More than 500,000 individuals—mostly members of the military—were vaccinated.[43,45] Among the civilians vaccinated, 21 developed inflammation around the heart as a side effect, a complication not seen with prior vaccination programs.[46] The initiative was downgraded following the initial surge of vaccination in association with poor response from many healthcare workers.

Tularemia

Tularemia was named after Tulare County, California, following its identification in 1911 as the cause of the deaths of squirrels in that geographic area. Subsequently, it was identified in humans and noted to have as much as a 50 percent mortality rate prior to development of effective antibiotics.[47] In the 1930s and 1940s, tularemia was found to be the cause of large waterborne epidemics in two countries that would become the leaders in bioweapons development: the United States and the USSR.[22]

Tularemia is caused by *Francisella tularensis*, a small (0.2–0.5 μm × 0.7–1.0 μm), pleiomorphic, aerobic, facultative, intracellular, Gram-negative coccobacillus with particular affinity for macrophages and neutrophils.[48] Of the four biochemically and genetically distinct subspecies, *tularensis* is the primary and most virulent human pathogen. The leading modes of transmission involve handling infected animals (primarily rabbits) and being bitten by infected ticks. *F. tularensis* has also been associated with ingestion of infected meat, inhalation, laboratory exposure, and aquatic transmission.[49]

Clinical presentation of *F. tularensis* infection varies with the route of infection, dose, and host factors.[22,49,50] Tularemia can infect the lungs, skin, GI tract, or mucous membranes, and it has an incubation period of 3 to 5 days. Each of these clinical scenarios is similar to those associated with some naturally occurring infectious diseases, as well as with other potential bioweapon-based infectious agents.[30] The most likely scenario for intentional bioweapon use of tularemia focuses on aerosol delivery, presumably leading to a preponderance of cases of pneumonic tularemia, with lesser numbers of persons manifesting one of the other types of clinical presentations. The relatively nonspecific nature of the initial phases of infection, coupled with a significant decrease in the efficacy of antibiotics with treatment delay, makes tularemia a potential bioweapon threat.

Rapid diagnosis can be accomplished with polymerase chain reaction (PCR) testing, thereby allowing for early differentiation and antibiotic delivery. At this time, however, PCR testing is available only for rapid diagnosis of infected wounds and in a limited number of clinical locations. The first-line choice of antibiotic treatment is streptomycin or gentamicin, although these agents are usually reserved for isolated cases. In mass-casualty situations, doxycycline or ciprofloxacin has been recommended.[22,51] Doxycycline is also the recommended medication for post-exposure prophylaxis.[22] A live attenuated virus vaccine has been used on a limited basis in the United States (military and laboratory workers) since the USSR gifted its vaccine strain to the United States in the 1960s.

Viral Hemorrhagic Fevers

Little known to the general public in much of the Northern Hemisphere, this group of primarily zoonotic, single-strand RNA viruses cause hemorrhagic febrile illnesses that have been developed as bioweapons by both the United States and Russia. They are also poorly studied in the largely rural and resource-poor countries where they occur most frequently (and naturally). The viral hemorrhagic fevers meet several criteria for use as biological weapons.[52] Most of them can be spread by aerosol and grow relatively easily on simple cell cultures. They are endemic in several geographic regions, although some are not easily isolated for research purposes because their natural reservoir is unknown or outbreaks tend to be sporadic. Finally, they are severe, frightening diseases with high morbidity and mortality, no preventive vaccine, and, for most of these viruses, no known treatment (Table 16-4).

Although some of the viruses have known linkage with an animal vector or reservoir, the natural origins of Ebola and Marburg are not known. For all these viruses, person-to-person transmission can occur via body fluids, and weak evidence exists that aerosols from bed clothing may be infectious as well. The finding of Marburg and Ebola in skin and sweat orifices suggests possible simple physical contact may transfer the virus, even without a portal in the form of broken skin. Although all of these viruses produce a coagulopathy effect, they are taxonomically diverse. The clinical courses for the individual viruses share some characteristics, based on aspects of their individual biology. The hemorrhagic reactions also appear to be driven by different mechanisms among the different viruses. The more virulent of the viruses have rapid and severe courses, particularly if the route of infection is transcutaneous.

Based on World Health Organization (WHO) screening guidance, viral hemorrhagic fever should be strongly considered in someone with fever (temperature

TABLE 16-4 Hemorrhagic Fever Viruses	
Virus	**Clinical Features**
Ebola	Severely ill, high fever, rapid onset, diffuse maculopapular rash around day 5, coagulopathy with disseminated intravascular coagulation (DIC) common.
Marburg	Severely ill, high fever, rapid onset, diffuse maculopapular rash around day 5, coagulopathy with DIC common.
Lassa fever	Nausea, abdominal pain, pharyngitis, cough, mucosal ulcerations—all accompany slower elevation of temperature. Characteristic late head/neck swelling. Fewer hemorrhagic complications than observed with Ebola or Marburg.
New World arenaviruses (Machupo, Junin, Guanarito, Sabia)	Similar to Lassa fever, but more involvement of central nervous system findings.

Source: Adapted from Borio L, Inglesby T, Peters CJ, et al.; Working Group on Civilian Biodefense. Hemorrhagic fever viruses as biological weapons: Medical and public health management. Journal of the American Medical Association. 2002;287:2391–2405.

greater than 38°C) for less than 3 weeks and at least two of the following hemorrhagic symptoms: ecchymotic or purpuric rash, epistaxis, hematemesis, hemoptysis, and blood in stools. Supportive care is the foundation of treatment for infection with this group of viruses as a whole. For infections with Lassa fever and New World arenaviruses, early diagnosis is important because they respond to the antiviral ribavirin.[53] Immunologic tests—either enzyme-linked immunosorbent assay (ELISA) or PCR—can be used to make the diagnosis. Due to the high infectivity, the use of bedside testing is recommended if at all possible. A number of lab technicians have been infected while performing routine clinical lab work on infected blood. Currently, no treatment exists for infection with the Ebola and Marburg viruses.

Clinical personnel should wear appropriate personal protective equipment when viral hemorrhagic fever is suspected. For some situations, an N95 mask with face shield is adequate; however, a powered air-purifying respirator (PAPR) will provide increased protection.

PREPAREDNESS AND RESPONSE: CATEGORY B AGENTS

Brucellosis

Brucellosis has been recognized for centuries and is one of the most common zoonotic diseases around the world, with several hundred thousand new cases occurring each year.[54] Although it has a low mortality, this disease is often chronically debilitating. In addition, the bacteria are highly virulent, only 10 to 100 organisms being required to create an active infection. Of the eight known species of *Brucellae*, only four cause human disease: *B. melitensis*, *B. suis*, *B. abortus*, and, rarely, *B. canis*. *B. melitensis* accounts for the majority of human pathologies.[55] *B. suis* holds the distinction of having been the first U.S. bioweapon developed, with research into this agent beginning in 1942 and bomb tests being pursued in 1944 and 1945.[56] This U.S. experience also identified potential hazards related to the management of bioweapons programs: Several unexploded and unaccounted-for brucellosis bombs were found in 1995 at a U.S. military base.[56]

The different *Brucellae* species have reservoirs in specific domestic mammals, particularly in sheep, goats, and cows. The bacteria are able to survive outside a host for some time. Also, although the organisms are sensitive to daylight, they can be deployed in an aerosol. The majority of human disease occurs from ingestion of inadequately pasteurized milk products made from infected sheep and goats. The routes of infection include inhalation, via breaks in the skin, or direct penetration of mucosa (e.g., conjunctiva); the clinical manifestations do not vary depending on this route.

Early diagnosis can be challenging because clinical manifestations of brucellosis vary. They include fever, malaise, and a variety of GI, respiratory, neurologic and rheumatologic symptoms, with no distinguishing single feature or constellation of findings. A high degree of clinical suspicion is necessary unless the individual is located in an area where infection with *Brucellae* pathogens is endemic.[57] Given that the incubation period is variable and potentially protracted (60 to 90 days), in the event of an attack with aerosolized material, it may be difficult to recognize the presence of a cluster of cases immediately. Brucellosis is rarely fatal but frequently causes chronic and disabling symptoms, and it may result in significant economic burden if an attack affects a large sector of a population.

Definitive diagnosis is made by culturing the organism from body fluids, especially bone marrow. Because culture growth can take 3 to 6 weeks, immune (ELISA and agglutination) testing is used most commonly for initial screening, although its utility is hampered by the tendency of these tests to produce both false negatives and false positives.

Single and short-term drug therapy courses for brucellosis are associated with failure and relapses. Treatment has historically involved dual or triple antibiotic treatment for at least 6 weeks with doxycyline and rifampin, supplemented with streptomycin in either more chronic or severe acute cases.[58,59] In the event of a verified aerosol attack, recommendations for prophylaxis are a 3- to 6-week course of dual antibiotics used for treatment of confirmed disease. No vaccination exists at this time.

Despite the initial interest in this pathogen as a potential biologic weapon, *Brucellae* is rarely lethal and is characterized mostly as being of historical interest as a weapon. Current importance for public health awareness is that *Brucellae* is the world's most common zoonosis, and outbreaks may be identified with foreign travel, consumption of exotic foods, and border region populations.

Clostridium perfringens Epsilon Toxin

Epsilon toxin is a theoretical bioweapon because no documented human disease or evidence of weapons use exists. Among the five types (A–E) of *Clostridium perfringens*, each produces one or more of four major toxins: alpha (α), beta (β), epsilon (ε), and iota (ι). Types B and D are the only ones that produce the epsilon toxin. These two types of *C. perfringens* cause illness in cattle, goats and sheep, but have not been found in humans. Epsilon toxin is a "pore-forming" toxin, referring to the "pores" it creates in cell walls; these pores destroy the chemical integrity of the cell wall, thus leading to ion leakage. In animal experiments, infection with *C. perfringens* proves rapidly fatal when the virus is administered by either inhalation or an intravenous route.[60] Currently an animals-only vaccine exists, but development of a human vaccine is under way.[61]

Food Safety Threats

"I, for the life of me, cannot understand why the terrorists have not, you know, attacked our food supply because it is so easy to do," Health and Human Services Secretary Tommy G. Thompson commented on his primary concerns at his resignation.[62] Food security involves a discussion of two components: the food chain and potential contaminants. The 1990s and beginning years of the twenty-first century have seen a number of instances of adulteration of the food supply on both small and large scales. Most notorious in recent years, perhaps, was the intentional contamination of a salad bar with *Salmonella* by a religious cult with the intent of influencing a local election—one of only two recorded episodes of intentional addition of a pathogen to food in the United States. By contrast, there have been several significant contaminations that appear to have been unintentional and where current surveillance procedures in the food safety system proved inadequate, such as contamination of fresh salad with *Escherichia coli* traced back to the use of manure to fertilize the fields in which the lettuce grew.

The modern global "food chain" does not actually match up well with the "chain" metaphor. It is much more like a matrix than a chain, particularly when considering processed foods with multiple ingredients. Fifteen or more U.S. federal agencies share the responsibility of implementing the numerous statutes (more than 30) directing food inspection. Over the years there have been many calls to reorganize and simplify the federal food safety system, but no action has been taken to date.[63] To at least partially address the problem of complexity, in the late 1990s the FDA instituted the Hazard Analysis and Critical Control Point (HACCP) program, which involves identifying strategic safety "nodes" in the food system and developing monitoring systems, feedback loops, and training to execute the monitoring.[64]

The other component of food biosecurity concerns agents of adulteration. The CDC has listed agents that might potentially be harmful to the food supply on its Web site: botulinum toxin, *E. coli* O157:H7, *Salmonella*, *Shigella dysenteriae* type 1, *Typhi* (typhoid fever), and *Vibrio cholerae* (cholera). This list includes some of the more debilitating agents currently known to have contaminated commercially processed foods. Modeling exercises have predicted hundreds of thousands of hospitalizations and even deaths from strategically placed food adulteration.[65] The models attribute a significant number of the deaths to the overburdening of the hospital systems, including inability to meet the demand for resources such as respirators.

Glanders

Glanders is a disease primarily of equines, with rare passage to humans being noted. It is of historical interest in the bioweapon domain because Germany began a multiple-continent campaign in World War I to infect horses, mules, and donkeys intended for service with the Allies. The animals targeted were in Norway, Spain, Argentina, and the United States. With robust testing and culling programs now being in place in most developed countries, glanders is presumed to exist mostly in some of the poorer countries of Central America, the Middle East, and some Eastern European and Central Asian areas.[66–68]

Human infection with the *Burkholderia mallei* via skin and mucous membranes produces a local suppurative reaction, followed by fever and dispersed additional suppurative lesions. Historically, many patients with this disease have reported fevers, malaise, headache, and diarrhea with abdominal pain.[69] *B. mallei* infection manifests as either a lethal sepsis or a chronic mucous membrane infection in animals and humans. Several human infections have occurred in laboratory personnel since World War II, with most presumably involving inhalation, the most likely route for a biological attack. In a recent transcutaneous infection at a military research facility, it took several weeks before optimal treatment was instituted.[70] *B. mallei* is sensitive in culture to aminoglycocides, erythromycins, and tetracyclines and shows resistance to penicillins and first-generation cephalosporins.

Melioidosis

The causative agent of melioidosis, *Burkholderia pseudomallei* is a close relative to *Burkholderia mallei*, the causative agent for glanders. Despite the genetic relationship, the two diseases have some marked differences, starting with the pathogens' distribution among animal hosts. Unlike *B. mallei*, *B. pseudomallei* is widely distributed in mammals, reptiles (crocodiles), and birds, leading to a difference in global presence of the diseases and in human infection. Like *B. mallei*, *B. pseudomallei* is easily manipulated to form an infectious aerosol, leading to its consideration as a potential weapon.[71] However, *B. pseudomallei* is not known to have ever been used as a weapon.

Melioidosis is endemic to Thailand and northern Australia, producing enough cases to permit more investigation of this disease. In endemic areas, the bacteria are present in the general environment, including in standing water such as found in rice paddies, with the major route of infection being through skin breaks. Localized melioidosis manifests as suppurative lesions in all tissues, but shows a particular affinity for the lungs. Focal pulmonary disease is of particular interest in bioterrorism preparedness. Reportedly, the most common presentation can be confused with tuberculosis or lung abscess (e.g., cavitating pneumonia with marked weight loss). Overall mortality reported for clinical melioidosis ranges from 20 to 70 percent. Antibiotic treatment regimens for melioidosis have been studied in small clinical trials in Thailand and Australia, leading to a two-phase approach to therapy: an initial disease-arresting phase based on intravenous medications and lasting 2 to 4 weeks, followed by an eradicative phase to prevent relapse.

Psittacosis (*Chlamydia psittaci*)

Psittacosis, also known as parrot fever and ornithosis, is caused by infection with *Chlamydia psittaci* and is named after the parrot species that was originally identified as the source of this occasional human pathogen. As the name implies, the primary host is birds. *C. psittaci* is passed to humans from aerosolization of bacteria in dried feces or nasal discharge and through direct contact with the beaks or feathers of infected birds.

The incubation period for psittacosis lasts from 5 to 14 days. Clinical disease may vary from subclinical to severe multisystem involvement. Human infection commonly manifests as an initial nonspecific febrile illness, which is followed by pneumonia with possible multiple-organ involvement. The presence of liver or spleen enlargement in a patient with what appears to be community-acquired pneumonia is suggestive of *C. psittaci* infection.[72] The pneumonia may progress because the disease is uncommon and difficult to diagnose and because the first-line antibiotics commonly used to treat community-acquired pneumonia will be ineffective against psittacosis.[73] Doxycycline is the antibiotic of choice.

Q Fever

Q fever (originally called query fever, as its cause was unknown) is caused by infection with *Coxiella burnetii*. Following genetic typing, this organism has been reclassified as a *Legionella* species. The bacterium is very resistant to heat, pressure, and chemicals, particularly antiseptic materials. It normally persists as a chronic infection in a variety of animals around the world that shed it in urine and feces. Although it is passed among the animals by a tick vector, humans are infected by inspiration of aerosolized dried animal droppings. Q fever is highly infectious, with only a single bacterium needed to kick off the full-fledged disease.

The incubation period is from 1 to 3 weeks, with the initial disease manifesting as a flu-like illness that may involve atypical appearing pneumonia. There may also be liver involvement. If not treated, most patients recover, but they may have relapses or develop chronic infection. As many as 50 percent of persons in a cluster infection may not have any clinical findings. Immunocompromised patients are more susceptible to developing chronic Q fever that will prove fatal if left untreated. Early diagnosis is difficult due to the nonspecific symptoms, but immunologic and PCR testing can be used to confirm the presence of this pathogen.[74]

Treatment is effective and consists of tetracyclines, macrolides, and fluoro-quinolones;[75] these agents should be administered for 14 to 21 days. In chronic Q fever, 18 months of treatment with dual antibiotics (doxycycline with chloroquine) is necessary to prevent relapses. Although *C. burnetii* is highly infectious, survives outside the body, and is easily aerosolized, the fact that the acute clinical syndrome is relatively benign and resolves easily with treatment consisting of simple antibiotics decreases its strategic value as a biologic weapon.

Ricin Toxin

Ricin toxin, which is derived from the fibrous portion of seeds from castor bean plants (*Ricinus communis*), is a ribosome-inactivating toxin. While toxicity related to ingesting castor bean seeds has long been recognized, the use of purified toxin as a weapon largely developed following World War II. It gained international attention after having been determined to be the agent responsible for the murder of a Soviet Bloc defector in 1978.[76] Ricin toxin exerts its effect by blocking protein synthesis through damage to the endothelial reticulum. This agent is considered a potential bioweapon owing to the relative ease with which it can be produced. The toxin is stable in liquid and crystalline forms. It can be detoxified by heating to 80°C for 10 minutes or to 50°C for an hour at a slightly elevated pH of 7.8. Chlorine bleach can also inactivate it.[77]

Ricin's clinical toxicity depends on the route of entry. Inhalation of the toxin leads to pulmonary epithelial necrosis with resultant inflammation of all levels of the pulmonary tree. Victims develop interstitial pneumonia with perivascular and alveolar edema, along with acute respiratory distress syndrome (ARDS). Ingestion of ricin toxin leads to gastrointestinal mucosal necrosis with secondary abdominal pain, GI bleeding, and liver, spleen, and kidney necrosis. There is no antidote or vaccine available, and treatment is symptomatic and supportive. Some sources recommend GI decontamination based largely on literature reports related to ingestion of the whole seed.

Staphylococcal Enterotoxin B

Staphylococcal enterotoxin B (SEB) is a member of the bacterial superantigen (SAg) protein family. Although the biochemical mechanisms underlying its toxicity have not been determined, animal studies show that this agent leads to mucosal cellular disruption. In the intestines, this damage repairs itself over the course of 24 to 48 hours. The typical clinical scenario involves acute vomiting with cramps, diarrhea, and fever following a meal, often at a buffet or an eatery where food is kept warmed. Occasionally, victims may suffer shock. When experimental animals are exposed to an aerosol of SEB, however, mortality is generally 100 percent—hence this pathogen's potential as a bioweapon. Molecular studies to date have demonstrated that when SEB comes in contact with T cells, they release massive amounts of cytokines and are depleted. At present, there is no specific treatment or pre-exposure treatment, although several groups are working on a vaccine for SEB.[61]

Water Safety Threats

Public water processing plants in the United States are designed around the principle of removing certain designated microorganisms through a process of filtration and treatment with chemicals, largely chlorine. The Environmental Protection Agency (EPA) sets minimum drinking water standards based on size of population served (fewer or more than 10,000) and whether the water source is ground water or deep well water.[78] The CDC lists two agents, *Vibrio cholerae* and *Cryptosporidium parvum*, as example contaminants that might pose a threat to the water supply. Other sources have suggested that other bioweapon agents might target water safety, in part because of the likelihood of delayed diagnosis by clinicians given that the clinical effects of the agents may be quite different when they are ingested than when they are inhaled.[79]

PREPAREDNESS AND RESPONSE: CATEGORY C AGENTS

The CDC's Web site describes Category C pathogens as emerging agents. Several viral agents are classed in this category. Other listings have characterized this category as including not only emerging agents, but also agents potentially amenable to laboratory manipulation.[2] In addition, other publications have addressed the future possibility of genome attacks using benign viruses as vectors. Two primary modes of attack have been proposed: short- and long-latency ("stealth") attacks. The former leads to essentially an immediate change in cell function or death; the latter scenario would produce a dormant genetic insertion from the initial attack that would be activated at a later time.[80] Because these agents are potentially a future threat and do not pose an immediate risk related to bioweapons use, specific preparedness and response measures will not be discussed in detail here. The two agents frequently cited in this category are the emerging infectious diseases Nipah virus and hantavirus.

MITIGATION

The U.S. Biodefense Structure

The back-to-back terrorism-related events that occurred in the fall of 2001—multiple simultaneous aircraft hijackings and dispersion of anthrax spores via the postal service—led to intense interaction between law enforcement and public health agencies.[81,82] These interactions highlighted some of the differences in methodology and operating procedures between the two domains, while also providing an opportunity for evaluation to develop more integrated procedures. Following analysis of the two events, including assessment of preceding events by the National Commission on Terrorist Attacks Upon the United States (9-11 Commission), the U.S. Congress developed a multipronged approach to mitigate the risks of a biological weapons attack.[83] Currently, U.S. government policy for responding to biological weapon aggression is based on the National Strategy to Combat Weapons of Mass Destruction and the National Strategy for Homeland Security, published in 2002 and updated in 2007.[84–86] This policy is complemented by the National Military Strategy to Combat WMD (weapons of mass destruction).[87] Collectively, these policies outline a multiple-front approach for dealing with various threats to the United States.

The response to the "anthrax episode" of 2001, for example, revealed difficulties in investigating a disease outbreak with potential intentional implications. Due to realized conflicts between public health and law enforcement philosophies and investigational operating procedures, the U.S. bioresponse capacity was reevaluated, with a resultant division of responsibilities being instituted. The Department of Health and Human Services' Office of the Assistant Secretary for Preparedness and Response is charged with coordinating and overseeing the federal government programs for biosecurity, ranging from research and development programs to deployment of Strategic National Stockpile medications.[88] The Department of Homeland Security (DHS) has overall jurisdiction over federal responses to an acute biological attack. Most federal law enforcement agencies, as well as the Federal Emergency Management Agency (FEMA), have been placed under the jurisdiction of DHS.

One of the primary projects undertaken by DHS for improving U.S. biosecurity is the Project Bio-Surveillance system. It consists of a set of biological environmental monitors placed in population centers, along with mobile units that can be deployed to major gatherings. Currently, sensors have been deployed in 30 population centers. These sensors require daily removal of filters, transportation to laboratories, and testing for specific agents to determine either their presence or increases in their presence over baseline levels. Project Bio-Surveillance has come under criticism on a number of grounds regarding its effectiveness.[89] Additionally, the program has been criticized for diverting resources from state public health laboratories, which are

---

TABLE 16-5   NIOSH Recommendations for the Selection and Use of Protective Clothing and Respirators Against Biological Agents Resulting from a Suspected or Known Terrorism Event

1. Responders should use a NIOSH-approved, chemical/biological/radiological/nuclear (CBRN) self-contained breathing apparatus (SCBA) in conjunction with a Level A, protective ensemble (use equipment certified to NFPA 1991 when available as a first choice) in responding to a suspected biological incident where any of the following information is unknown or the event is uncontrolled:
   - The type(s) of airborne agent(s)
   - The dissemination method(s)
   - If dissemination via an aerosol-generating device is still occurring, or if it has stopped but there is no information on the duration of dissemination or what the exposure concentration might be
   - Other conditions may present a vapor or splash hazard

2. Responders may use a Level B protective ensemble (use equipment certified as NFPA 1994 Class 2, NFPA 1992, or NFPA 1971 CBRN protective ensembles when available as a first choice) with an exposed or enclosed NIOSH-certified CBRN SCBA if the situation can be defined in which:
   - The suspected biological aerosol is no longer being generated
   - Other conditions may present additional hazards, such as a splash hazard (Note: NFPA 1994 Class 4 does not have a requirement to provide limited protection against liquid or chemical hazards)

3. Responders may use a Level C protective ensemble (use equipment certified to NFPA 1994 class 3 or 4 or certified as NFPA 1999 protective ensemble when available as a first choice) with a CBRN full face piece air-purifying respirator (APR) or CBRN full face piece powered air-purifying respirator (PAPR) when it can be determined that:
   - The suspected biological aerosol is no longer being generated
   - The biological agent and hazard level have been defined
   - Dissemination was by a letter or package that can be easily bagged

Source: Recommendations for the selection and use of respirators and protective clothing for protection against biological agents. NIOSH Publication No. 2009-132. April 2009. Available at: http://www.cdc .gov/niosh/docs/2009-132/. Accessed July 31, 2010.

charged with housing the surveillance testing laboratories and lending support to the program.

Project Bio-Shield—a complementary strategy to accelerate research, development, purchase, and availability of effective medical countermeasures against biological, chemical, radiological, and nuclear agents—is overseen by the Assistant Secretary for Preparedness of HHS. This program has funded research and development in a number of areas. Nevertheless, the primary responsibility for identifying and providing treatment for victims of a biological attack remains with local healthcare providers and public health officials, supported, when suspicion of malicious intent arises, by local police.

Taking Care of Healthcare Providers

Many of the biological attack scenarios involve agents or clinical states that involve a pulmonary component with a differential diagnosis that includes highly virulent organisms. For this reason, protection of the medical workforce in the wake of a bioterrorism attack is a critical issue. NIOSH has developed guidelines for personal protective equipment and airway protection (Table 16-5). Combining the information available through NIOSH with that available through the CDC for control of hospital infections will be useful for individuals involved in bioterrorism planning, response, and mitigation activities.

CASE STUDY ANALYSIS _____

Although a hypothetical case, the chapter-opening narrative describes many of the challenges associated with identifying and treating a potential bioterrorism event. Bioweapons may cause either unique or nonspecific symptoms, and many initial findings may not be categorized into classic patterns of disease. Healthcare providers will need to consider potential bioterrorism agents if one or more patients present with unusual clinical findings. In addition, if the biological agent has a delayed time of onset, such as 2 to 3 days, then patients may begin arriving at healthcare facilities at different stages of the disease process. Furthermore, once a bioterrorism attack is suspected, personal protective gear should be utilized immediately by everyone caring for patients.

This case study also highlights the criminal nature of a bioterrorism attack and the potential for an attacker to target either a high-profile gathering or a large public venue. Communications between healthcare providers, public health officials, and law enforcement should begin immediately, and all three should have low thresholds for suspecting a bioterrorism event. Consequently, local authorities should be prepared to initiate large-scale treatment and prophylaxis regimens without necessarily receiving laboratory testing and confirmation if a significant number of cases occur within a short period of time.

CONCLUSION

Public health and medicine are on a steep learning curve in regard to known bioterrorism agents and those that may be developed through redirection of current research in genomics and biotechnology. For the public health professional on the front lines with a mild to moderately ill patient, the question is whether the case represents a "routine viral syndrome" or a case of bio-aggression. Differentiation of these two circumstances may simply not be possible without some additional information. Several core concepts have been proposed as representing situations in which an "unusual" infectious disease should raise the suspicion that a bioweapon may be involved. Indicators suggestive of a biologic attack would include a sudden or unusual cluster of cases, especially involving an exotic disease, which is out of the normal temporal, geographic, or demographic distribution. Various analyses have repeatedly emphasized that recognition of a biological attack may not occur until a pattern is seen with multiple victims, similar to many natural epidemic outbreaks.

Given the levels of funding that have been directed toward homeland security in the United States in the past decade, greater basic sciences knowledge, including genetic and immunologic advances, is likely to be gained with regard to potential biologic weapons in the coming years. Through this new information, public health professionals and healthcare providers will become armed with more refined tools to assist with rapid diagnosis of illness due to intentionally distributed biological agents. As has happened in the past, medical advances made possible through crisis funding for wars ultimately may lead to many additional nonconflict advances.

INTERNET RESOURCES

Centers for Disease Control and Prevention, bioterrorism emergency preparedness and response: http://www.bt.cdc.gov/bioterrorism

Federal Emergency Management Agency, biological threats: http://www.fema.gov/hazard/terrorism/bio/index.shtm

U.S. Army Medical Department Borden Institute, *Medical Aspects of Biological Warfare:* http://www.bordeninstitute.army.mil/published.html

U.S. Department of Homeland Security, Weapons of Mass Destruction and Biodefense Office: http://www.dhs.gov/xabout/structure/gc_1205180907841.shtm

U.S. Food and Drug Administration, bioterrorism and drug preparedness: http://www.fda.gov/EmergencyPreparedness/Counterterrorism/default.htm

World Health Organization, bioterrorism: http://www.who.int/topics/bioterrorism/en/

NOTES

1. Martin JW, Christopher GW, Eitzen EM Jr. History of biological weapons: From poisoned darts to intentional epidemics. In: Dembek ZF (Ed.), *Medical aspects of biological warfare.* Washington, DC: Borden Institute, Walter Reed Army Medical Center; 2007, pp. 1–20.
2. Kortepeter MG, Parker GW. Potential biological weapons threats. *Emerging Infectious Diseases.* 1999;5:523–527.
3. Center for the Study of Weapons of Mass Destruction. *Are we prepared? Four WMD crises that could transform U.S. security.* Washington, DC: National Defense University, Center for the Study of Weapons of Mass Destruction; 2009. Available at: http://www.ndu.edu/WMD Center/docUploaded/Are%20We%20Prepared.pdf. Accessed October 3, 2009.
4. Carus WS. *Bioterrorism and biocrimes: The illicit use of biological agents since 1900.* Washington, DC: Center for Counter-Proliferation Research (renamed to Center for the Study of Weapons of Mass Destruction), National Defense University; 1999 (revised February 2001). Available at: http://www.ndu.edu/WMDCenter/Full_Doc.pdf. Accessed October 3, 2009.
5. Neuwinger HD. *African ethnobotany: Poisons and drugs: Chemistry, pharmacology, toxicology.* London: Chapman & Hall; 1996.
6. Ekboir JM. *Potential impact of foot-and-mouth disease in California: The role and contribution of animal health surveillance and monitoring systems.* Davis, CA: Agricultural Issues Center, Division of Agriculture and Natural Resources, University of California; 1999. Available at: http://aic.ucdavis.edu/pub/EkboirFMD-part1.pdf. Accessed October 3, 2009.
7. Henry L. Stimson Center. History of the US offensive biological warfare program (1941–1973). 2007. Available at: http://www.stimson.org/cbw/?sn=CB2001121275. Accessed October 3, 2009.
8. United Nations Office for Disarmament Affairs. *Status of multilateral arms regulation and disarmament agreements.* United Nations; 2009. Available at: http://disarmament.un.org/Treaty Status.nsf. Accessed October 3, 2008.
9. Meselson M, Guillemin J, Hugh-Jones M, Langmuir A, Popova I, Shelokov A, et al. The Sverdlovsk anthrax outbreak of 1979. *Science.* 1994;266(5188):1202–1208.
10. Alibek K. *Biohazard.* New York: Random House; 1999.
11. Davis CJ. Nuclear blindness: An overview of the biological weapons programs of the former Soviet Union and Iraq. *Emerging Infectious Diseases.* 1999;5:509–512.
12. WuDunn S, Miller J, Broad WJ. How Japan germ terror alerted world. *New York Times.* May 26, 1998. Available at: http://query.nytimes.com/gst/fullpage.html?res=9D00EFDE1438F935 A15756C0A96E958260. Accessed October 3, 2009.
13. Torok TJ, Tauxe RV, Wise RP, Livengood JR, Sokolow R, Mauvais S, et al. A large community outbreak of salmonellosis caused by intentional contamination of restaurant salad bars. *Journal of the American Medical Association.* 1997;278(5):389–395.
14. Stephenson J. Experts focus on infective agents of bioterrorism. *Journal of the American Medical Association.* 2002;287(5):575–576.

15. Stephenson J. Confronting a biological Armageddon: Experts tackle prospect of bioterrorism. *Journal of the American Medical Association.* 1996;276(5):349–351.

16. Bellamy RJ, Freedman AR. Bioterrorism. *Quarterly Journal of Medicine.* 2001;94(4):227–234.

17. Marwick C. Scary scenarios spark action at bioterrorism symposium. *Journal of the American Medical Association.* 1999;281:1071–1073.

18. Inglesby TV, Henderson DA, Bartlett JG, Ascher MS, Eitzen E, Friedlander AM, et al.; Working Group on Civilian Biodefense. Anthrax as a biological weapon: Medical and public health management. *Journal of the American Medical Association.* 1999;281:1735–1745.

19. Henderson DA, Inglesby TV, Bartlett JG, Ascher MS, Eitzen E, Jahrling PB, et al.; Working Group on Civilian Biodefense. Smallpox as a biological weapon: Medical and public health management. *Journal of the American Medical Association.* 1999;281:2127–2137.

20. Inglesby TV, Dennis DT, Henderson DA, Bartlett JG, Ascher MS, Eitzen E, et al.; Working Group on Civilian Biodefense. Plague as a biological weapon: Medical and public health management. *Journal of the American Medical Association.* 2000;283:2281–2290.

21. Arnon SS, Schechter R, Inglesby TV, Henderson DA, Bartlett JG, Ascher MS, et al.; Working Group on Civilian Biodefense. Botulinum toxin as a biological weapon: Medical and public health management. *Journal of the American Medical Association.* 2001;285:1059–1070.

22. Dennis DT, Inglesby TV, Henderson DA, Bartlett JG, Ascher MS, Eitzen E, et al.; Working Group on Civilian Biodefense. Tularemia as a biological weapon: Medical and public health management. *Journal of the American Medical Association.* 2001;285:2763–2773.

23. Rotz LD, Khan AS, Lillibridge SR, Ostroff SM, Hughes JM. Public health assessment of potential biological terrorism agents. *Emerging Infectious Diseases.* 2002;8:225–230.

24. NATO. Annex A: Medical classification of potential biological warfare agents. In: *NATO handbook on medical aspects of NBC defensive operations AMedP-6(B).* North Atlantic Treaty Organization; 1996. Available at: http://library.enlisted.info/field-manuals/series-1/FM8_9/APPA2 .PDF. Accessed: October 3, 2008. (To navigate the pdf sections, users must enter through the portal of http://library.enlisted.info/field-manuals/series-1/FM8_9/TOC2.PDF.)

25. National Institute of Occupational Health and Safety Education and Information Division. The emergency response safety and health database. Last updated August 22, 2008. Available at: http://www.cdc.gov/NIOSH/ershdb/AgentListCategory.html. Accessed October 3, 2009.

26. Center for Non-proliferation Studies. Russia announces plans to participate in research on Vozrozhdeniye Island. March 18, 2002. Available at: http://cns.miis.edu/stories/020318.htm. Accessed October 3, 2009.

27. Treverton GF, Jones SG. *Measuring national power.* Santa Monica, CA: Rand Corporation; 2005. Available at: http://www.rand.org/pubs/conf_proceedings/2005/RAND_CF215.pdf. Accessed May 23, 2008.

28. Redmond C, Pearce MJ, Manchee RJ, Berdal BP. Deadly relic of the great war. *Nature.* 1998; 393:747–748.

29. CDC. Update: Investigation of bioterrorism-related anthrax and interim guidelines for exposure management and antimicrobial therapy, October 2001. *Morbidity and Mortality Weekly Report.* 2001;50:909–919.

30. CDC. Update: Investigation of anthrax associated with intentional exposure and interim public health guidelines, October 2001. *Morbidity and Mortality Weekly Report.* 2001;50:889–893.

31. Bell DM, Kozarsky PE, Stephens DS. Conference summary: Clinical issues in the prophylaxis, diagnosis, and treatment of anthrax. *Emerging Infectious Diseases.* 2002;8(2):222–225.

32. CDC Advisory Committee on Immunization Practices. From the Centers for Disease Control and Prevention: Use of anthrax vaccine in response to terrorism: Supplemental recommendations of the advisory committee on immunization practices. *Journal of the American Medical Association.* 2002;288:2681–2682.

33. Shane S, Lichtblau E. Scientist's suicide linked to anthrax inquiry. *New York Times.* August 2, 2008. Available at: http://www.nytimes.com/2008/08/02/washington/02anthrax.html?pagewanted=1&_r=1. Accessed October 3, 2009.

34. Mayer TA, Bersoff-Matcha S, Murphy C, Earls J, Harper S, Pauze D, et al. Clinical presentation of inhalational anthrax following bioterrorism exposure: Report of 2 surviving patients. *Journal of the American Medical Association.* 2001;286:2549–2553.

35. Erbguth FJ. Historical notes on botulism, *Clostridium botulinum*, botulinum toxin, and the idea of the therapeutic use of the toxin. *Movement Disorders.* 2004;19(suppl 8):S2–S6.

36. Dembek ZF, Smith LA, Rusna JM. Botulinum toxin. In: Dembek ZF (Ed.), *Medical aspects of biological warfare.* Washington, DC: Borden Institute, Walter Reed Army Medical Center; 2007, pp. 337–353.

37. Arnon SS, Schechter R, Inglesby TV, Henderson DA, Bartlett JG, Ascher MS, et al.; Working Group on Civilian Biodefense. Botulinum toxin as a biological weapon: Medical and public health management. *Journal of the American Medical Association.* 2001;285(8):1059–1070.

38. Annex 5: Botulism reference service for Canada. Canadian Ministry of Health; May 2, 2006. Available at: http://www.hc-sc.gc.ca/ed-ud/respond/food-aliment/fiorp-priti_11-eng.php. Accessed October 3, 2009.

39. Wheelis M. Biological warfare at the 1346 siege of Caffa. *Emerging Infectious Diseases.* 2002;8:971–975.

40. Fenner F, Henderson DA, Arita I, Jezek Z, Ladnyi ID. Ch 5 The history of smallpox and its spread around the world. In: *Smallpox and its eradication.* Geneva: World Health Organization; 1988, pp. 209–s44.

41. Moore ZS, Seward JF, Lane JM. Smallpox. *Lancet* 2006;367:425–435.

42. Leitenberg M. *Assessing the biological weapons and bioterrorism threat.* Carlisle, PA: Strategic Studies Institute of the U.S. Army War College; 2005. Available at: http://www.strategicstudiesinstitute.army.mil/pubs/display.cfm?pubID=639. Accessed October 3, 2008.

43. Jahrling PB, Huggins JW, Ibrahim S, Lawler JV, Martin JW. Smallpox and related orthopoxviruses. In: Dembek ZF (Ed.), *Medical aspects of biological warfare.* Washington, DC: Borden Institute, Walter Reed Army Medical Center; 2007, pp. 215– s40.

44. Strikas R, Neff L, Rotz L, Cono J, Knutson D, Henderson J, et al. US civilian smallpox preparedness and response program, 2003. *Clinical Infectious Diseases.* 2008;46:S157–S167.

45. Centers for Disease Control and Prevention (CDC). Smallpox vaccination program status by state. October 31, 2005. Available at: http://www.cdc.gov/media/pressrel/smallpox/spvaccin.htm. Accessed October 3, 2009.

46. Centers for Disease Control and Prevention (CDC). Adverse events associated with smallpox vaccination among civilians. October 31, 2005. Available at: http://www.cdc.gov/media/pressrel/smallpox/spcivil.htm. Accessed October 3, 2009.

47. Sjostedt A. Tularemia: History, epidemiology, pathogen physiology, and clinical manifestations. *Annals of the New York Academy of Science.* 2007;1105:1–29.

48. Conlan WJ, Oyston PCF. Vaccines against *Francisella tularensis. Annals of the New York Academy of Science.* 2007;1105:325–350.

49. Hepburn MJ, Friedlander AM, Dembek ZF. Tularemia. In: Dembek ZF (Ed.), *Medical aspects of biological warfare*. Washington, DC: Borden Institute, Walter Reed Army Medical Center; 2007, pp. 167–184.

50. Centers for Disease Control and Prevention (CDC). Recognition of illness associated with the intentional release of a biologic agent. *Journal of the American Medical Association*. 2001;286: 2088–2090.

51. Perez-Castrillon JL, Bachiller-Luque P, Martin-Luquero M, Mena-Martin FJ, Herreros V. Tularemia epidemic in northwestern Spain: Clinical description and therapeutic response. *Clinical Infectious Diseases*. 2001;33:573–576.

52. Borio L, Inglesby T, Peters CJ, Schmaljohn AL, Hughes JM, Jahrling PB, et al.; Working Group on Civilian Biodefense. Hemorrhagic fever viruses as biological weapons: Medical and public health management. *Journal of the American Medical Association*. 2002;287:2391–2405.

53. Khan AS, Morse S, Lillibridge S. Public-health preparedness for biological terrorism in the USA. *Lancet*. 2000;356:1179–1182.

54. Pappas G, Papadimitriou P, Akritidis N, Christou L, Tsianos EV. The new global map of human brucellosis. *Lancet: Infectious Diseases*. 2006;6:91–99.

55. Pappas G, Panagopoulou P, Christou L, Akritidis N. *Brucella* as a biological weapon. *Cellular and Molecular Life Sciences*. 2006;63:2229–2236.

56. Purcell BK, Hoover DL, Friedlander AM. Brucellosis. In: Dembek ZF (Ed.), *Medical aspects of biological warfare*. Washington, DC: Borden Institute, Walter Reed Army Medical Center; 2007, pp. 185–198.

57. Troy SB, Rickman LS, Davis CE. Brucellosis in San Diego: Epidemiology and species-related differences in acute clinical presentations. *Medicine (Baltimore)*. 2005;84:174–187.

58. Demirturk N, Demirdal T, Erben N, Demir S, Asci Z, Kilit TP, et al. Brucellosis: A retrospective evaluation of 99 cases and review of brucellosis treatment. *Tropical Doctor*. 2008;38: 59–62.

59. Skalsky K, Yahav D, Bishara J, Pitlik S, Leibovici L, Paul M. Treatment of human brucellosis: Systematic review and meta-analysis of randomised controlled trials. *British Medical Journal*. 2008;336:701–704.

60. Huebner KD, Wannemacher RW, Stiles BG, Popoff MR, Poli MA. Additional toxins of concern. In: Dembek ZF (Ed.), *Medical aspects of biological warfare*. Washington, DC: Borden Institute, Walter Reed Army Medical Center; 2007, pp. 355–389.

61. Mantis NJ. Vaccines against the category B toxins: Staphylococcal enterotoxin B, epsilon toxin and ricin. *Advanced Drug Delivery Reviews*. 2005;57:1424–1439.

62. Branigin W, Allen M, Mintz J. Tommy Thompson resigns from HHS: Bush asks Defense Secretary Rumsfeld to stay. *The Washington Post*. December 3, 2004. Available at: http://www.washingtonpost.com/wp-dyn/articles/A31377-2004Dec3.html. Accessed October 3, 2009.

63. Forum on Microbial Threats. *Addressing foodborne threats to health: Policies, practices, and global coordination: Workshop summary*. Washington, DC: Institute of Medicine of the National Academies; 2006.

64. Hazard analysis and critical control point (HACCP). 2001. Available at: http://www.fda.gov/Food/FoodSafety/HazardAnalysisCriticalControlPointsHACCP/default.htm. Accessed October 3, 2008.

65. Wein LM, Liu Y. Analyzing a bioterror attack on the food supply: The case of botulinum toxin in milk. *Proceedings of the National Academy of Science USA.* 2005;102(28):9984–9989.

66. Waag DM, DeShazer D. Glanders: New insights into an old disease. In: Lindler LE, Lebeda FJ, Korch GW (Eds.), *Biological weapons of defense: Infectious diseases and counterbioterrorism.* Totowa, NJ: Humana Press; 2005, pp. 209–237.

67. Dance DAB. Melioidosis and glanders as possible biological weapons. In: Fong IW, Alibek K (Eds.), *Bioterrorism and infectious agents: A new dilemma for the 21st century.* New York: Springer; 2005, pp. 99–145.

68. Cheng AC, Dance DAB, Currie BJ. Bioterrorism, glanders and melioidosis [comment]. *European Surveillance.* 2005;10:E1–E2.

69. Gregory BC, Waag DM. Glanders. In: Dembek ZF (Ed.), *Medical aspects of biological warfare.* Washington, DC: Borden Institute, Walter Reed Army Medical Center; 2007, pp. 121–a46.

70. Srinivasan A, Kraus CN, DeShazer D, Becker PM, Dick JD, Spacek L, et al. Glanders in a military research microbiologist. *New England Journal of Medicine.* 2001;345:256–258.

71. Bossi P, Tegnell A, Baka A, Van Loock F, Hendriks J, Werner A, et al. BICHAT guidelines for the clinical management of glanders and melioidosis and bioterrorism-related glanders and melioidosis. *European Surveillance.* 2004;9:E17–E8.

72. Centers for Disease Control and Prevention (CDC). Compendium of measures to control *Chlamydia psittaci* infection among humans (psittacosis) and pet birds (avian chlamydiosis). *MMWR Recommendations and Reports.* 2000;49:3–17.

73. Case records of the Massachusetts General Hospital: Weekly clinicopathological exercises. Case 16-1998: Pneumonia and the acute respiratory distress syndrome in a 24-year-old man. *New England Journal of Medicine.* 1998;338:1527–1535.

74. Kazar J. *Coxiella burnetii* infection. *Annals of the New York Academy of Science.* 2005;1063: 105–114.

75. Morovic M. Q fever pneumonia: Are clarithromycin and moxifloxacin alternative treatments only? *American Journal of Tropical Medicine and Hygiene.* 2005;73:947–948.

76. Franz DR, Jaax NK. Ricin toxin. In: Sidell FR, Takafuji ET, Franz DR (Eds.), *Medical aspects of chemical and biological warfare.* Washington, DC: Borden Institute, Walter Reed Army Medical Center; 1997, pp. 631–642.

77. Maman M, Yehezkelli Y. Ricin: A possible, noninfectious biological weapon. In: Fong IW, Alibek K (Eds.), *Bioterrorism and infectious agents: A new dilemma for the 21st century.* New York: Springer; 2005, pp. 205–s16.

78. U.S. Environmental Protection Agency. Drinking water contaminants. June 5, 2008. Available at: http://www.epa.gov/safewater/contaminants/index.html. Accessed October 3, 2009.

79. Burrows WD, Renner SE. Biological warfare agents as threats to potable water. *Environmental Health Perspectives.* 1999;107. Available at: http://www.ehponline.org/members/1999/107p975-984burrows/burrows-full.html. Accessed October 3, 2009.

80. Black JL 3rd. Genome projects and gene therapy: Gateways to next generation biological weapons. *Military Medicine.* 2003;168(11):864–871.

81. Butler JC, Cohen ML, Friedman CR, Scripp RM, Watz CG. Collaboration between public health and law enforcement: New paradigms and partnerships for bioterrorism planning and response. *Emerging Infectious Diseases.* 2002;8(10):1152–1156.

82. Richards EP. Collaboration between public health and law enforcement: the constitutional challenge. *Emerging Infectious Diseases.* 2002;8(10):1157–1159.

83. Kean TH, Hamilton LH, Ben-Veniste R, Fielding FF, Gorelick JS, Gorton S, et al. *Report of the National Commission on Terrorist Attacks Upon the United States.* Washington, DC: National Commission on Terrorist Attacks Upon the United States; 2004. Available at: http://www.9-11commission.gov/. Accessed October 3, 2009.

84. U.S. Department of State. *National strategy to combat weapons of mass destruction.* Washington, DC: Author; 2002. Available at: http://www.state.gov/documents/organization/16092.pdf. Accessed October 3, 2009.

85. Office of Homeland Security. *National strategy for homeland security.* Washington, DC: White House; 2002. Available at: http://www.dhs.gov/xlibrary/assets/nat_strat_hls.pdf. Accessed October 3, 2009.

86. Homeland Security Council. *National strategy for homeland security.* Washington, DC: White House; 2007. Available at: http://www.dhs.gov/xlibrary/assets/nat_strat_homelandsecurity_2007.pdf. Accessed October 3, 2009.

87. Chairman of the Joint Chiefs of Staff. *National military strategy to combat weapons of mass destruction.* Washington, DC: Joint Chiefs of Staff; 2006. Available at: http://www.defenselink.mil/pdf/NMS-CWMD2006.pdf. Accessed October 3, 2008.

88. Office of the Assistant Secretary for Preparedness and Response. Available at: http://www.hhs.gov/aspr/index.html. Accessed July 31, 2010.

89. Nuzzo JB. Biosecurity and bioterrorism: Special feature: Biosecurity memos to the Obama administration. *Biosecurity and Bioterrorism: Biodefense Strategy, Practice, and Science.* 7(1). Pittsburgh, PA: Center for Biosecurity UPMC; 2009. Available at: http://www.upmc-biosecurity.org/website/resources/publications/2009/biomemo/PDF/2009-03-27-develop_natl_biosurveillance.pdf. Accessed October 3, 2009.

CHAPTER 17

Chemical Agents

Katherine Douglass and Rodney Omron

INTRODUCTION

Chemical agents remain a persistent emergency public health threat, and recent events have shown that even a small amount of certain chemicals on civilian populations can have an enormous impact. Although many countries have banned the use of chemical agents for wartime use, certain countries continue to stockpile chemical weapons. One major concern is the acquisition of weapons-grade chemical agents by terrorist groups either from a country's stockpile or from a private laboratory. In addition to the direct injuries and deaths due to these agents, chemical terrorist attacks may induce widespread fear and panic that will disrupt a population and perpetuate the large-scale crisis even after the chemical agents have been neutralized.

Case Study

On March 20, 1995, at 7:55 A.M., an unprecedented chemical terrorist attack was carried out on a civilian population in Tokyo, Japan. The calculated release of the chemical warfare agent sarin took place on the subway system during the morning rush hour at a convergence point underneath the offices of the Japanese Government Ministry. This calculated timing and location was intentionally planned to maximize the impact of the event and to impart as much potential death, injury, and fear as possible. Twelve people died in the attack, and more than 5,000 people sought emergency medical evaluation.[1]

The Tokyo attack was orchestrated by a religiously motivated cult with the intention of inflicting both physical and emotional harm. Sarin was first developed in the late 1930s as a potent compound for use during conventional warfare. Exposure of a population to this agent within a confined space is the ideal method to increase both the number of persons affected and the severity of their injuries. In the case of the Tokyo subway attack, the release of sarin gas took place at multiple subway locations at one time, on three separate lines in five subway cars.

The first victims began arriving at local emergency departments by foot within one hour of the attack, and the majority of victims presented for emergency evaluation and care on the day of the attack. The first responders to the scene encountered significant chaos and did not have a preconceived plan to manage such an event. Triage was not performed properly, there was no established decontamination site, and the first responders did not protect themselves by donning chemical-resistant clothing or using chemical-resistant equipment.[2] Although most exposed patients complained of eye irritation and visual disturbance, the more severely affected persons suffered various degrees of respiratory compromise. A significant number of patients did not suffer physical injury, but rather sought medical attention because of the psychological stress and concern for potential injury due to proximity to the chemical agent.[3] This event set a new precedent for chemical attacks on civilians, and it confirmed the potential for chemical warfare agents to wreak tremendous physical and psychological havoc on large populations, in both the short and long terms.

HISTORICAL PERSPECTIVES

The use of chemical weapons in warfare dates as far back as 423 B.C. when allies of Sparta in the Peloponnesian War overtook an Athenian-held fort by introducing the smoke from lighted coals and sulfur into the occupied rooms.[4] Various tactics using chemical agents have been employed throughout history, including the notable Greek fire of the Byzantine empire, which likely was fed by a combination of rosin, sulfur, pitch, naphtha, lime, and saltpeter.[4–6] This chemical-based fireball can travel on top of water, rendering it a tactical and decisive weapon that allowed multiple victories while imparting tremendous fear in its users' enemies and according its developers great military respect.

The development of more modern-day chemical agents continued throughout the late eighteenth and early nineteenth centuries, alongside an ongoing debate regarding the ethics of chemical warfare.[3] No international consensus on the use of chemical agents had been achieved by the beginning of World War I, which witnessed a historical and deadly usage of chemical agents in warfare. The first wartime usage of mustard gas occurred in 1915, when the German army released 160 tons of chlorine gas against British forces at Ypres, Belgium.[7,8] This event killed approximately 1,000 soldiers and injured 4,000 more, causing a chaotic, terrorized response among those exposed persons. The usage of chemical agents including chlorine, phosgene, and mustard gas during World War I was both pervasive and deadly, ultimately being responsible for more than 90,000 deaths and 1.3 million wounded by the time peace was achieved.[8]

Scattered usage of chemical agents in warfare has been persistent over time, up to and including reported cases in recent conflicts in the Middle East. The nerve gas sarin was first developed by a German scientist in 1937 as an insecticide, but its potential as an agent of warfare was recognized quickly. German forces developed and stored large quantities of nerve gas at the time of World War II, but it was not used as a warfare agent during this conflict.[9] Hitler himself was a mustard gas casualty during World War I, which is one potential explanation for the German decision not to utilize this stockpile.[5] The first wartime use of nerve gas occurred in the Iran–Iraq conflict in the 1980s, and it resulted in significant death and disability. To this day, a consistent and ongoing threat of potential usage of chemical agents in wartime exists, as well as the proven threat of chemical agents in terrorist actions in times of peace.

PREPAREDNESS AND PLANNING

The first step in preparation and planning for a chemical terrorist event is recognition of the existence of a potential threat. Only then can the preparedness step begin. Nonetheless, despite the clear threat posed by chemical agents, a significant number of healthcare workers and public health professionals remain under-educated in the recognition and management of chemical agent events. Various researchers have confirmed that prehospital care providers are inadequately trained in public health emergency and disaster response.[10] Since the September 11, 2001, terrorist attacks in the United States, national standards for training and preparedness have increased, as has government funding. For example, the 2003 Homeland Security Bill and the Nunn–Lugar–Domenici Amendment of 1997 both called for increased preparedness and training for first responders to help them deal with terrorist events.[11] Even with these governmental initiatives, however, training and education on this front remain inadequate.

Improved training and education remain a major focus of preparing for potential chemical events. Training should occur at all levels, from community laypersons, to first responders, to sophisticated response teams, to hospital employees and clinical staff, and to public health professionals. Evidence and knowledge gathered from previous experiences in public health emergencies can be used to guide training objectives and priorities.[12,13] Curricula must be focused to the particular responsibilities of the trainee. For example, past experience with disaster events has demonstrated that a significant portion of the initial response to large-scale crisis is provided by uninjured laypersons on the scene. Training initiatives such as the Citizen Corps Program can effectively bring relevant information to the community level.[14] For prehospital professionals, training should focus on scene safety, decontamination, extrication, chain of command, communication, basic and advanced life support, and transport priorities. In the hospital setting, training focuses on decontamination, chain of command, communication with subspecialists and field personnel, antidotes, definitive treatment, psychiatric care, personnel safety, family member communication, and public relations.

Timely antidote therapy can be the life-saving intervention in a chemical terrorist event, depending on which chemical agent is involved. In particular, exposure to nerve agents and cyanide requires immediate recognition and treatment to increase the chance of survival for exposed victims. Antidote stockpiling is an important strategy of preparation, so as to make the life-saving intervention rapidly available to the affected population. These antidotes will be useful only if they can be administered easily, have not expired, and can be accessed in a timely manner.[2,15] Thus regional and national public health planners must consider an accessible location for their storage, steps for mobilization, contingency planning, and communication. The initiation of antidote therapy may often precede final confirmation of the offending agent; therefore, it is essential that the mechanism of antidote mobilization accommodate these potential confounding circumstances.[16]

An antidote stockpile will serve the community effectively only if it is readily available—which clearly poses a challenge in planning and preparedness for public health professionals. The Centers for Disease Control and Prevention (CDC) and the U.S. Department of Homeland Security (DHS) have developed stockpiles of medicines and antidotes located throughout the United States. These "push packages" ("pushpacks") are made to be delivered within 12 hours of getting the request from the governor of the state in need. If a local organization requires such a push package, the governor's office must be contacted first. Along with this package comes a technical advisory response unit whose members will help the local government officials use the resources in the most efficient way. Furthermore, each state maintains a Web site with links to its emergency operations plan.

RESPONSE

Rapid recognition of a chemical agent is essential for both effective treatment of exposed victims and implementation of proper protective measures on the part of those responding to the incident. As is always the case when responding to a disaster or terrorist situation, providing adequate safety for those persons responding to the event is essential, both at the scene and in the hospital setting. Past experiences have demonstrated that while it may be immediately obvious that some event has taken place, the nature of the event in terms of severity of injury and number of persons affected will rarely be clear immediately. The particular agent may not be identified for hours or even days, long after the critical time period for initiation of life-saving interventions such as decontamination and antidote administration has passed. To provide the best safety for responders and the best care for patients, initial response steps must begin based on presumptive information.[16]

Personal protective equipment (PPE) must be used by rescuers caring for persons who have potentially been exposed to a chemical agent (Table 17-1). Level A PPE is recommended until initial decontamination efforts are achieved, at which time Level B equipment is sufficiently effective. Decontamination must begin at the scene of the incident, and must be initiated by the first responders to the event. No strict consensus exists regarding the level of PPE necessary at hospitals and similar healthcare facilities. A large proportion of persons involved in mass-casualty events usually arrive at the hospital by foot, bypassing the prehospital care system and, therefore, bypassing the prehospital decontamination system. At least Level C PPE is necessary, and some advocate even stricter precautions.[17,18]

Exposed persons must remove clothing and then wash with copious, sequential warm-water rinses and a mild soap. Staff members must similarly decontaminate critically ill patients, being sure to decontaminate both the back and the front of a supine patient, along with removing the clothes and blankets that have come into contact

TABLE 17-1	Levels of Personal Protective Equipment
Level A	Completely encapsulated suit and self-contained breathing apparatus (SCBA)
Level B	Encapsulated suit or junction seams sealed, supplied-air respirator or SCBA
Level C	Splash suit and air-purifying respirator
Level D	Work clothes, including standard precautions for healthcare workers (e.g., gloves, eye protection)

with the patient.[19] The joint tenets of personal protection of non-exposed persons and decontamination of exposed patients are fundamental strategies to ensure maximum survival for first responders, healthcare providers, and patients.

The Agency for Toxic Substances and Disease Registry provides medical management guidelines for unidentified chemical exposures. Notably, the triage and decontamination procedures in the prehospital and emergency department (ED) settings operate differently. In the prehospital setting, the potential for secondary contamination must be assessed. The scene must be secured by law enforcement officials. A "hot zone" (area of high probability of contamination) needs to be established, and rescuers should be appropriately trained and attired before entering this area. Worst-case possibilities must be assumed, and first responders ideally should wear Level A PPE. Initial stabilization measures include a quick assessment of airway, breathing, and circulation (the "ABCs") and utilization of adjunct interventions such as oxygen, a cervical collar, and a backboard. Basic decontamination includes removal of clothing and flushing exposed areas with plain water for 3 to 5 minutes. Contact lenses should be removed if they are easily and safely removable. After basic decontamination, patients should be moved to a support zone. Further treatment can be provided in the support zone prior to transport, including advanced airway interventions (e.g., intubation of the trachea, cricothyroidotomy, aerosolized bronchodilators) and advanced cardiac, trauma, and pediatric life support protocols.

In the ED, basic decontamination should occur outside the treatment area, when possible. Realistically, many patients arrive by personal vehicle, making it difficult to secure the ED. Triage personnel must be informed and able to recognize toxidromes. Decontamination strategies in the ED setting are similar to those employed in the prehospital setting. Although more resources to provide definitive care are available, caution must be used to prevent the ED from becoming contaminated. Entrances should be secured, and entry and exit points should be monitored and controlled. Management of unidentified chemical exposures is outlined in the Agency for Toxic Substances and Disease Registry's guidelines.

Medical care should be initiated in accordance with standard protocols, starting with a triage procedure at the scene of the incident to identify and prioritize the most critically ill, yet salvageable patients. For this reason, a standardized triage protocol should be included in basic disaster training and education for first responders. Medical providers should approach patients using the standard approach to a critically ill patient, while maintaining proper personal protective measures. Rapid recognition of classic signs and symptoms of exposure to a chemical toxin should prompt antidote administration as well as notification of public health and public service officials. Some authorities recommend incorporation of antidote administration in the triage protocol because of the extremely time-dependent nature of treatment in the case of severe toxicity. Particularly in the case of a nerve agent exposure, early administration of an antidote kit (MARK I) may prove life-saving, and such care does not require use of other advanced measures such as establishment of intravenous access.[20] These advanced protocols are not yet the standard of care, but they should be carefully considered when planning so as to provide the best care for the affected individuals.

Hospitals and other healthcare facilities should have established disaster plans to accommodate the surge in patient volume associated with a large-scale incident. Interhospital communication is essential in distributing patients among those facilities equipped with the resources needed to care for them. Risk communication is of vital importance as well, so as to provide effective information to the public regarding the nature of the event and the need to seek emergency care. Moreover, effective recognition and treatment of the psychologically injured and the "worried-well" is an important component of medical care; oftentimes, these non-physically injured patients will account for a large proportion of those seeking medical care.[21]

Chemical exposures may be inflicted on patients either intentionally, industrially, or accidentally. A list of more than 80 chemicals that commonly cause harm in humans can be found on the CDC's Web site.[22] Toxic presentations can be delayed after exposure, and identification and treatment often must be initiated before definitive diagnostic testing is complete. For all these reasons, clinicians and public health officials must have a high index of suspicion if they are to identify the appropriate toxidromes and initiate care and public safety measures, even prior to an absolute diagnosis.

Irritant Gas Syndromes

Respiratory tract irritants include chloroacetophenone ("tear gas"), oleoresin capsicum (OC) ("pepper spray"), and choking agents such as chlorine or phosgene (Table 17-2). The clinical effects of these substances are directly correlated to their water solubility, dose, reflex stimulation, and tissue reactivity. Highly water-soluble substances, such as ammonia, are absorbed in the upper airway quickly, causing reflex stimulation and quick tissue reactivity and allowing for early detection of symptoms. By comparison, less water-soluble irritants, such as phosgene, penetrate deeply, causing mild reflex stimulation and slow tissue reactivity; they may produce acute lung injury as late as 15 to 48 hours after exposure.[23,24] Tear gas and other lacrimators cause immediate, severe, and usually self-limited burning to the mucous membranes.

Regardless of the agent or its solubility, a massive exposure can cause laryngeal edema and acute lung injury. Chlorine has minor irritant effects at low doses and can cause severe lung injury at higher concentrations. Phosgene has low water solubility,

TABLE 17-2 Characteristics of Irritant Gas/Respiratory Tract Agents	
Unintentional-event agents	Chloroacetophenone ("tear gas") Oleoresin capiscum (OC; "pepper spray") Ammonia
Terrorist-event agents	Phosgene Chlorine
Mild-exposure clinical presentation	Self-limited burning of mucous membranes
Severe-exposure clinical presentation	Laryngeal edema Acute lung injury
Time course of clinical syndrome	Highly water soluble (ammonia): quick onset Poorly water soluble (phosgene): late onset (15–48 hours)
Treatment options	Supportive therapy with or without nebulized sodium bicarbonate

Source: Kales S, Christiani D. Acute chemical emergencies. *New England Journal of Medicine.* 2004;350: 800–808.

so it maintains prolonged contact with the mucous membranes until it causes irritation. Although it is known to smell like "new-mown hay," neither its odor nor its irritability produces early warning symptoms. Pulmonary edema on chest x-ray or shortness of breath within 4 hours is suggestive of a poor prognosis, however, and requires ICU admission. When no findings are present at 8 hours after exposure, then acute lung injury is unlikely.[25]

Treatment of respiratory irritants is largely supportive. Copious irrigation of mucous membranes, bronchodilator medications, and endotracheal intubation may be required. Although controlled studies of nebulized sodium bicarbonate for this indication are lacking, this agent is often used to neutralize chlorine-based irritants.[26] Some researchers recommend corticosteroid use in phosgene exposure, but this therapy remains controversial.[24]

Chemical Burns/Vesicant Syndrome

Vesicants are blistering agents that are very destructive to the mucous membranes (Table 17-3). Nitrogen mustard is an example of this type of agent. Mustard is an alkylating agent that affects DNA chains and acts as an inflammatory activator.[19]

Although mustard is a liquid at room temperature, as the ambient temperature rises it becomes a gas. This agent has a latent period of 4 to 17 hours before symptoms and signs of exposure appear; consequently, exposure to mustard gas can be difficult to detect initially. Furthermore, it takes only a few minutes of contact with the mucous membranes for mustard to be systemically absorbed.[25]

Cutaneous and ophthalmic effects of mustard are the first to appear. Injuries to the eye may range from conjunctivitis to corneal damage and permanent blindness. Cutaneous bulla often form in the intertriginous areas as a result of mustard exposure, but pulmonary complications are the most common cause of death. Respiratory tract findings may include pharyngitis laryngitis, pulmonary edema, and pseudo-membrane formation with airway obstruction.[25] Hematopoietic suppression leads to leukopenia. A fatal prognosis is likely when any of the following are observed: respiratory symptoms in 6 hours, burns covering more than 25 percent of the patient's body, or an absolute white blood cell (WBC) count of less than 200 WBCs per cubic millimeter of blood.[25]

Treatment requires immediate decontamination with copious fluids. In some cases, a dry method of decontamination may give a better result in counteracting

TABLE 17-3 Characteristics of Chemical Burn and Vesicant Agents

Unintentional-event agents	Hydrofluoric acid Hydrochloric acid
Terrorist-event agents	Nitrogen mustard
Mild-exposure clinical presentation	Hydrofluoric and hydrochloric acid cause burning to skin
Severe-exposure clinical presentation (nitrogen mustard)	Initial cutaneous bullae and corneal conjunctivitis Pulmonary edema Pseudo-membrane formation Leukopenia
Time course of clinical syndrome	Nitrogen mustard has a period of latency of 4–17 hours, but is almost instantaneously absorbed
Treatment options	Supportive burn care Fuller's Earth (nitrogen mustard) Thiosulfate (nitrogen mustard) Granulocyte-stimulating hormone (nitrogen mustard) Intravenous and local calcium (hydrofluoric acid)

Source: Kales S, Christiani D. Acute chemical emergencies. *New England Journal of Medicine.* 2004;350: 800–808.

deeply penetrated agents. For example, a dry powder such as Bentonite or "Fuller's Earth" is useful for decontamination of thickened agents because it adheres to the semi-liquid substance, making it easier to remove. Fuller's Earth is a fine-grained, naturally occurring, earthy substance that has a substantial ability to absorb impurities or coloring bodies from fats, grease, or oils. This material consists chiefly of hydrated aluminum silicates that contain metal ions such as magnesium, sodium, and calcium within their structure.[27,28]

Supportive care is necessary for pulmonary findings and burn care following mustard exposure, in addition to antibiotic ointment for eye involvement. Large blisters should be unroofed. Large volumes of intravenous fluid resuscitation should be avoided because mustard burns have less fluid loss than thermal burns. Nonsteriodal anti-inflammatory drugs (NSAIDs) have proved successful in pain relief.[29] Thiosulfate has been shown to decrease mortality in animal models.[19] Granulocyte-stimulating hormone should be considered for severe leukopenia, in consultation with an inpatient medical team.[25]

Most other chemical burns do not involve vesicants and, therefore, are not associated with the systemic toxicity of mustard. Initial treatment of such burns consists of copious irrigation with water. Burns from hydrofluoric acid (a component of household rust removers) can result in life-threatening hypocalcemia and hypomagnesemia. Treatment for severe exposure requires intake of large amounts of local and intravenous (IV) calcium and admission to an intensive care unit.[25]

Asphyxiants/Metabolic Poisoning Syndromes

Asphyxiants are defined as substances that decrease oxygen delivery to vital organs; they include carbon monoxide, hydrogen sulfide, and cyanide (Table 17-4). The cardiovascular and neurologic systems are most affected by these agents, because they are the body's most oxygen-sensitive systems. Affected persons may complain of a variety of symptoms, including shortness of breath, chest pain, generalized weakness, seizures, or complete unresponsiveness. A "cherry red" skin color is classically seen secondary to increased venous oxygen saturation. Asphyxiants are grouped into simple and chemical types. Simple-type asphyxiants displace oxygen and include methane and nitrogen. Chemical types interfere with metabolic oxygen transport at the cellular level and include carbon monoxide, hydrogen sulfide, and cyanide. The chemical types pose the greatest risk for public health exposures.[25,30,31]

Carbon monoxide is the most common etiology for fatal inhalation injuries in the United States.[32] Incidence is higher in the winter, when poisonings are often attributable to malfunction of the exhaust mechanisms on heating systems and combustion

TABLE 17-4 Asphyxiants and Metabolic Poisoning Agents	
Unintentional-event agents	Carbon monoxide Cyanide Hydrogen sulfide
Terrorist-event agents	Cyanide Hydrogen sulfide
Mild-exposure clinical presentation	Shortness of breath
Severe-exposure clinical presentation	Shortness of breath Weakness Seizure Coma Narrowed arterial–venous saturation gap Metabolic lactic acidosis
Time course of clinical syndrome	Immediate onset of symptoms
Treatment options	Sodium nitrite and sodium thiosulfate (cyanide) Hydroxocobalamin (cyanide) Sodium nitrite without thiocyanate (hydrogen sulfide) Hyperbaric oxygen (carbon monoxide)

Source: Kales S, Christiani D. Acute chemical emergencies. *New England Journal of Medicine.* 2004;350: 800–808.

engines. Carbon monoxide poisoning can be defined as an elevated carboxyhemoglobin level greater than 3 percent in nonsmokers and greater than 10 percent in smokers. These percentages should be used cautiously, as measurement may not occur until significantly later than the actual exposure. The typical presentation is hypoxia in a patient who has adequate arterial oxygenation and an elevated lactate level.[25]

Hydrogen sulfide exposure has a similar presentation. This gas is released from decaying organic matter and is known to affect exposed victims and those who come to rescue them. Hydrogen sulfide is very irritating and can cause very severe lung and eye irritation.[33,34]

Cyanide can cause acute toxicity from multiple routes of exposure, including dermal contact, parenteral intake, inhalation, and ingestion. Toxicity may occur secondary to industrial accidents, smoke inhalation, or intentional criminal poisoning. As little as 50 mg of cyanide can be lethal. This agent's primary toxicity derives from its inhibition of cytochrome oxidase, an enzyme necessary for aerobic respiration. Cyanide toxicity should be considered in anyone who suffers sudden collapse and seizure without a definitive cause. Cyanide smells like bitter almonds. No rapid diagnostic test is available to confirm cyanide toxicity; therefore, a clinician must rely on surrogate markers and clinical presentation when deciding on treatment.[16] Surrogate markers of cyanide poisoning include elevated serum lactate levels, profound metabolic acidosis, and arterial and venous oxygen saturation rates that are close in number, especially in the setting of a closed-space fire and sudden loss of consciousness.

The cyanide antidote kit contains sodium nitrite and amyl nitrite pearls and sodium thiosulfate. The nitrites induce methemoglobinemia; cyanide has a higher affinity for methemoglobin, which allows the mitochondria to perform oxidative phosphorylation. Thiosulfate converts cyanide to the less toxic thiocyanate, which is excreted renally. Amyl nitrite is intended to be inhaled while intravenous access is being established. Once IV access is established, sodium nitrite can be administered—this agent induces methemoglobinemia more reliably than amyl nitrite. Sodium thiosulfate can then be administered. It has a very slow onset of action, however, and this property limits its utility as a single agent. Oral administration of charcoal is indicated for oral exposures only. Early supportive treatment is vital in case of cyanide exposure, including correction of the profound metabolic acidosis.[16]

The nitrites have been shown to cause vasodilation and hypotension, which can be harmful in a hemodynamically unstable patient. The methemoglobinemia induced by these agents may also worsen hypoxia in patients with concomitant carbon monoxide poisoning, such as occurs in closed-space fires with smoke inhalation. Therefore, if the patient has severe anemia or high carbon monoxide exposure, consideration should be given to lowering the dose or foregoing treatment. In pregnant women, all treatments can be used except the absolutely contraindicated amyl nitrite.

Hydroxocobalamin has been licensed in France as a cyanide antidote since 1996 and has been recently approved by the FDA as a cyanide antidote. It combines with cyanide to form cyanocobalamine (vitamin B_{12}), a nontoxic metabolite that is excreted renally. This medication should be given to anyone suspected of having cyanide exposure or anyone with serious smoke inhalation. Hydroxocobalamin is extremely safe, so it can be administered if there is any suspected cyanide exposure. It acts synergistically when co-administered with sodium thiosulfate. Hydroxocobalamin should not be infused through the same site as the thiosulfate, however, because it can be inactivated by this interaction. Instead, the recommended treatment is to give hydroxocobalamin first, followed by thiocyanate. When they receive hydroxocobalamin, patients may have discoloration of mucous membranes, skin, and urine; the drug may also interfere with serum iron, bilirubin, creatinine and magnesium testing. A pustular rash may develop, which typically resolves in 6 to 38 days.[16,30,35]

In hydrogen sulfide poisoning, the chemical bonds preferentially to methemoglobin. Thus the recommendation is to use sodium nitrite and oxygen as treatment, without using thiosulfate, to induce the formation of methemoglobinemia.[34,36] Hyperbaric oxygen has been shown to work in carbon monoxide, cyanide, and hydrogen sulfide toxicity.[37–41]

Organophosphate Syndrome

Examples of cholinesterase inhibitors include carbamate and organophosphorous pesticides, soman, sarin, and VX (Table 17-5). These agents irreversibly inhibit the release of acetylcholinesterase, which leads to excessive buildup of acetylcholine in the body.[42] Two types of receptors are affected by acetylcholine: muscarinic and nicotinic. Muscarinic receptors are located in the parasympathetic and central nervous system. Nicotinic receptors are in found neurosynaptic junctions, the autonomic ganglia, and the central nervous system (CNS).[42]

Muscarinic stimulation leads to stimulation of excessive secretions, as evidenced by tearing, rhinorrhea, bronchorrhea, and salivation. It also affects the eyes, leading

TABLE 17-5 Characteristics of Organophosphate Agents	
Unintentional-event agents	Insecticides
Terrorist-event agents	Soman Sarin VX
Mild-exposure clinical presentation	Mild shortness of breath Rhinorrhea Lacrimation
Severe-exposure clinical presentation	Severe shortness of breath Muscle fasciculations Nausea and vomiting Generalized weakness
Time course of clinical syndrome	Immediate onset of symptoms
Treatment options	Atropine Pralidoxime Benzodiazepines

Source: Kales S, Christiani D. Acute chemical emergencies. *New England Journal of Medicine.* 2004;350: 800–808.

to miosis (pinpoint pupils), dim vision, and headache. A mnemonic device for remembering muscarinic effects is "DUMBBELS":

Muscarinic Effects

D: Diarrhea

U: Urination

M: Miosis (contraction of the iris), lack of accommodation

B: Bradycardia

B: Bronchoconstriction, bronchorrhea

E: Emesis

L: Lacrimation

S: Salivations

Nicotinic effects include muscle fasciculation, weakness, and paralysis. Cardiac symptoms initially consist of tachycardia and hypertension, as nicotinic stimulation predominates immediately after exposure, rather than muscarinic effects. Exposure to these chemicals causes diarrhea, abdominal cramping, nausea, vomiting, and fecal and urinary incontinence. Central nervous system findings range from altered mental status to convulsions to coma. Although depression of erythrocyte levels and serum cholinesterase is diagnostic for exposure to cholinesterase inhibitors, these tests are usually not available during the initial assessment and treatment period.[16]

Dermal exposure can delay the effects of cholinesterase inhibitors for as long as 18 hours as compared to inhalational exposure. The concentration of the agent in conjunction with the route of exposure will determine the time of its onset of action. For example, a droplet of VX the size of one-fifth the Lincoln Memorial on a penny when placed on unbroken skin can kill a human in 30 minutes; in contrast, significantly larger-volume exposures of a less concentrated agent may cause only mild symptoms.[43] The most common cause of death from exposures to these chemicals is respiratory failure due to bronchospasm, paralysis in muscles of respiration, and central apnea.[44,45] Notably, emergency personnel who lack proper personal protection may become contaminated by direct skin contact or inhaling nerve agents.[16]

Treatment involves the use of atropine, pralidoxime, and diazepam. The antidote most available and effective for organophosphate exposure is atropine. Atropine works most significantly on the muscarinic receptors. The atropine dose is 6 mg or three auto-injectors, with retreatment then occurring every 10 minutes to minimize shortness of breath, airway resistance, and respiratory secretions. The IV dose is 2 mg for adults and 0.02 mg/kg body weight for children. According to case reports, the typical dose of atropine for nerve exposure is in the range of 5 to 20 mg, but some cases have required doses as large as 200 mg.[16]

Pralidoxime (2PAM) reactivates acetylcholinesterase and works on the muscarinic, nicotinic, and CNS receptors. In a process called "aging," nerve agents will form an irreversible covalent bond with acetylcholinesterase over time. Soman ages quickly and its bonds become irreversible in 2 to 6 minutes. Sarin and VX age more slowly, with only 50 percent of acetylcholinesterase being affected by these agents over 5 hours and 48 hours, respectively. Aged receptors cannot be restored to their previous state; the patient will not regain use of acetylcholinesterase receptors until new receptors are synthesized. Pralidoxime can reactivate acetylcholinesterase if administered before aging.[46] This medication should be given to anyone showing signs of systemic nerve agent toxicity, especially if weakness or muscle fasciculations are evident. Ideally, this drug will be given by the IV route, but use of auto-injectors—which deliver intramuscular doses—is considered acceptable in the prehospital setting. Eighty to 90 percent of the pralidoxime dose will be excreted into the kidneys in 3 hours; thus a continuous infusion is recommended.[16]

Benzodiazapines, such as diazepam, are GABA-receptor agonists. Such medications should be administered to patients who have a large exposure resulting in coma, seizures, or two or more organ systems affected. After 5 minutes of exposure, atropine alone will not reverse seizures. Seizures can be reversed with benzodiazepines, however.[16]

Insecticides are less volatile and have slower onset of toxicity, but have longer duration of symptoms and require more atropine than nerve agents. Carbamate insecticides are milder and have fewer CNS side effects than organophosphorous types. They also inhibit acetylcholinesterase reversibly, which results in less severe symptoms.[25]

If a large number of victims are affected in a chemical attack, caring for them might quickly overwhelm a treatment facility. Limited supplies of antidotes are available, because it is costly to keep these medications on the shelf and replace them when unused drugs expire. To meet these needs, the CDC has provided a CHEMPACK push package as part of the Strategic National Stockpile. It contains a large number of MARK I kits and needles to augment local supplies. A MARK I kit is an individual antidote kit that includes two auto-injectors: one containing atropine and one containing pralidoxime. These kits are often carried by first responders or military personnel for self-administration after potential exposure. The availability of supplies from the Strategic National Stockpile should be integrated by local planners into their chemical casualty plans.[16] If a hospital is running low on atropine, alternatives can be used. For example, glycopyrrolate, scopolamine, diphenhydramine, and jimson weed extract have all been used are potential alternative antidotes.[16]

MITIGATION

Various steps have been taken at the governmental and international levels to introduce and uphold treaties to ban the development and use of chemical warfare agents. After the tremendous human toll exacted by the use of chemical agents during World War I, a series of conferences were held to try to limit or outlaw chemical weapons: the Washington Conference (1921–1922), the Geneva Conference (1923–1925), and the World Disarmament Conference (1933).[7] The Geneva Protocol, which was established in 1925, states: "The use in war of asphyxiating, poisonous or other gases, and of all analogous liquids materials or devices, has been justly condemned by the general opinion of the civilized world."[47] Nevertheless, chemical agents are still used today (albeit rarely), and they continue to pose a significant threat in both military usage and potential terrorist events.

On April 29, 1997, the Chemical Weapons Convention of the United Nations entered into force; it has been signed by at least 130 states. This convention prohibits states from undertaking any of the following actions:

> (a) To develop, produce, otherwise acquire, stockpile or retain chemical weapons, or transfer, directly or indirectly, chemical weapons to anyone; (b) To use chemical weapons; (c) To engage in any military preparations to use chemical weapons; (d) To assist, encourage or induce, in any way, anyone to engage in any activity prohibited to a State Party under this Convention.[48]

The destruction of international chemical weapons stockpiles has proven complicated, however. Indeed, as of April 2004, the United States lagged behind deadlines for destruction.[49] The need to maintain safety during the destruction process and efforts to avoid harmful events such as the accidental release of a chemical agent in part explain the delays in meeting the timeline. Progress continues, but the reality is that chemical agents still exist both in the United States and in some other countries. Therefore, the threat of a chemical agent event remains, particularly in the realm of potential terrorist activities. Mitigation efforts regarding overall elimination of terrorist activities and potential threats are important to obviate the risk of chemical events.

ANALYSIS OF CASE STUDY

A number of truly critical lessons were learned from the sarin attack in Tokyo. First and foremost, the attack proved to the international community that the potential for a chemical terrorist attack on a civilian population is real. Before this incident, the use of chemical agents had always occurred in wartime or, in an earlier 1994 event in Japan, was thought to be directed at a specific population. The 1995 attack was unique in being a calculated, undifferentiated attack on a civilian population. This type of incident reiterates the need for preparedness and the concept of universal vulnerability.

Second, the lack of proper usage of personal protective equipment and decontamination protocols in the response efforts to the event led to increased morbidity. Ten percent of first responders experienced secondary exposure while transporting victims; 23 percent of all hospital staff at St. Luke's International Hospital experienced secondary exposure symptoms. Strikingly, nearly 40 percent of all personnel in the hospital ICU experienced symptoms of secondary exposure.[50] Decontamination protocols are necessary in both the prehospital arena and the hospital setting in the event of a chemical agent attack, especially given that many patients will arrive at the hospital from the scene of the incident without interacting with prehospital care providers or first responders. It is of utmost importance for healthcare workers to remain safe in their efforts to provide care for exposed and injured persons. The Tokyo sarin experience clearly showed what can happen when proper precautions are forgotten—and is an experience that should not be repeated.

Third, many of those persons arriving for acute medical care did not suffer symptoms from the nerve gas release but rather were simply concerned about potential exposure. Reportedly, as many as 4,000 of the individuals seeking medical care had no symptoms of nerve gas exposure. The main receiving hospital had three separate entrances, and persons and patients descended upon all three entrances without order or separation, mixing the exposed and non-exposed patients with family members and media crews.[9] The importance of effective triage, prioritization of care for more severely injured victims, and separation of exposed persons from non-exposed individuals is very important in providing effective care. It should be expected that many asymptomatic, but potentially exposed persons will seek medical guidance after such a terrorist event because of the great fear of possible exposure. Preexisting plans must be in place at both prehospital and hospital levels to ensure appropriate triage and treatment, as well as communication of plans for potentially exposed persons, their family members, the public, and the media. Proper implementation of these plans can effectively protect those persons who are not exposed, while ensuring better care for those persons with true symptoms. These are the ultimate goals of providing care in any chemical exposure: protect those providing care, give the best care possible, protect those who are not exposed, and minimize overall death and disability, both psychologically and physically. As a result of the lessons learned in the Tokyo sarin terrorist event, it is hoped that future responses to potential chemical terrorist events will provide the best public health outcomes.

INTERNET RESOURCES

Centers for Disease Control and Prevention, chemical agents emergency preparedness and response: http://emergency.cdc.gov/chemical/

Centers for Disease Control and Prevention, chemical weapons eliminations: http://www.cdc.gov/nceh/demil/

Centers for Disease Control and Prevention, guide to local and state health departments: www.cdc.gov/mmwr/international/relres.html

Centers for Disease Control and Prevention, Strategic National Stockpile: http://www.bt.cdc.gov/stockpile

U.S. Department of Health and Human Services, Agency for Toxic Substances and Disease Registry—*Guide to Medical Management of Unidentified Chemical Substances:* www.atsdr.cdc.gov/mHmI/mmg170.html

Chemical Antidote and Decontamination Guide Books

Chemical Warfare Agents, National Library of Medicine: http://sis.nlm.nih.gov/enviro/chemicalwarfare.html

Medical Aspects of Chemical and Biological Warfare, U.S. Army Medical Department: http://www.bordeninstitute.army.mil/published_volumes/ChemBio/chembio.html

Medical Management of Chemical Casualties Handbook, third edition, August 1999: http://www.brooksidepress.org/Products/OperationalMedicine/DATA/operationalmed/manuals/RedHandbook/001TitlePage.htm

NATO Handbook on the Medical Aspects of NBC Defensive Operation, AMED P-6(B): http://www.fas.org/nuke/guide/usa/doctrine/dod/fm8-9/3toc.htm

NOTES

1. Okumura T, et al. Report on 640 victims of the Tokyo subway sarin attack. *Annals of Emergency Medicine.* 1996;28(2):129–135.
2. Tokuda Y, et al. Prehospital management of sarin nerve gas terrorism in urban settings: 10 years of progress since the Tokyo subway sarin attack. *Resuscitation.* 2006;68:193–202.
3. Brennan R, et al. Chemical warfare agents: Emergency medical and public health issues. *Annals of Emergency Medicine.* 1999;34(2):191–204.
4. U.S. Army Medical Research Institute of Chemical Defense. *Medical management of chemical casualties handbook* (3rd ed.). July 2000. Aberdeen Proving Ground, MD: Author.
5. Schecter W, et al. The surgeon and acts of civilian terrorism. *Journal of the American College of Surgeons.* 2000;200(1):128–135.
6. A brief history of chemical, biological, and radiological weapons. Available at: http://cbwinfo.com/History/ancto19th/shtml. Accessed July 21, 2008.

7. Reutter S. Hazards of chemical weapons release during war: New perspectives. *Environmental Health Perspectives.* 1999;107(12):985–990.

8. Fitzgerald GP. Public health then and now: Chemical warfare and medical response during World War I. *American Journal of Public Health.* 2008;98(4):611–625.

9. Lee EC. Clinical manifestations of sarin nerve gas exposure. *Journal of the American Medical Association.* 2003;290(5):659–662.

10. Markenson D, et al. Public health department training of emergency medical technicians for bioterrorism and public health emergencies: Results of a national assessment. *Journal of Public Health Management Practice.* November 2005; S68–S74.

11. Nunn–Lugar–Domenici: Amendment to the FY 97 Defense Authorization Act, Pub L No. 104–201, Title XIV: Defense Against Weapons of Mass Destruction, Subtitle A; Domestic Preparedness. U.S. Congress, June 27, 1996.

12. Auf der Helde E. The importance of evidence-based disaster planning. *Annals of Emergency Medicine.* 2006;47(1):34–49.

13. Kirk M, Deaton M. Bringing order out of chaos: Effective strategies for medical response to mass chemical exposure. *Emergency Medical Clinics of North America.* 2007;25:527–548.

14. Citizen Corps. Uniting communities, preparing the nation. Available at: http://www.citizencorps .gov/. Accessed December 21, 2009.

15. Barelli A, et al. The comprehensive medical preparedness in chemical emergencies: "The chain of chemical survival." *European Journal of Emergency Medicine.* 2008;15(2):110–118.

16. Lawrence D, Kirk M. Chemical terrorism attacks: Update on antidotes. *Emergency Medicine Clinics of North America.* 2007;25:567–595.

17. Hick JL, et al. Protective equipment for health care facility decontamination personnel: Regulations, risks, and recommendations. *Annals of Emergency Medicine.* 2003;42 (3):370–380.

18. Koenig K. Strip and shower: The duck and cover for the 21st century. *Annals of Emergency Medicine.* 2003;42(3):391–394.

19. Borak J, Sidell FR. Agents of chemical warfare: Sulfur mustard. *Annals of Emergency Medicine.* 1992;21:303–308.

20. Cone D, Koenig K. Mass casualty triage in the chemical, biological, radiological, or nuclear environment. *European Journal of Emergency Medicine.* 2005;12(6):287–302.

21. Alexander DA, Klein S. Biochemical terrorism: Too awful to contemplate, too serious to ignore. *British Journal of Psychiatry.* 2003;183:491–497.

22. Chemical agents: Emergency preparedness and response. Available at: http://www.bt.cdc .gov/Agent/agentlistchem.asp. Accessed August 7, 2008.

23. Nelson LS. Simple asphyxiants and pulmonary irritants. In: Goldfrank LR, Flomenbaum NE, Lewin NA, Howland MA, Hoffman RS, Nelson LS (Eds.), *Goldfrank's toxicologic emergencies* (7th ed.). New York: McGraw-Hill, 2002, pp. 1453–1468.

24. Borak J, Diller WF. Phosgene exposure: Mechanisms of injury and treatment strategies. *Journal of Occupational and Environmental Medicine.* 2001; 43(2):110–119.

25. Kales S, Christiani D. Acute chemical emergencies. *New England Journal of Medicine.* 2004; 350:800–808.

26. Sexton JD, Pronchik DJ. Chlorine inhalation: The big picture. *Journal of Toxicology: Clinical Toxicology.* 1998;36:87–93.

27. Koening K, et al. Health care facility based decontamination of victims exposed to chemical, biological, and radiological materials. *American Journal of Emergency Medicine.* 2008;26:71–80.

28. Hurst CG. Decontamination. In: Zajtchuk R, Bellamy RF, Sidell FR, Takafuji ET, Franz DR (Eds.), *Medical aspects of chemical and biological warfare.* Washington, DC: Office of the Surgeon General, Department of the Army; 1997, pp. 351–360.

29. Dachir S, Fishbeine E, Meshulam Y, Sahar R, Amir A, Kadar T. Potential anti-inflammatory treatments against cutaneous sulfur mustard injury using the mouse ear vesicant model. *Human and Experimental Toxicology.* 2002;21:197–203.

30. Salkowski AA, Penney DG. Cyanide poisoning in animals and humans: A review. *Veterinary and Human Toxicology.* 1994;36:455–466.

31. Snyder JW, Safir EF, Summerville GP, Middleberg RA. Occupational fatality and persistent neurological sequelae after mass exposure to hydrogen sulfide. *American Journal of Emergency Medicine.* 1995;13:199–203.

32. Valent F, McGwin G Jr, Bovenzi M, Barbone F. Fatal work-related inhalation of harmful substances in the United States. *Chest.* 2002;121:969–975.

33. Gregorakos L, Dimopoulos G, Liberi S, Antipas G. Hydrogen sulfide poisoning: Management and complications. *Angiology.* 1995;46:1123–1131.

34. Gabbay DS, De Roos F, Perrone J. Twenty-foot fall averts fatality from massive hydrogen sulfide exposure. *Journal of Emergency Medicine.* 2001;20:141–144.

35. Kulig K. Cyanide antidotes and fire toxicology. *New England Journal of Medicine.* 1991;325:1801–1802.

36. Hall AH, Rumack BH. Hydrogen sulfide poisoning: An antidotal role for sodium nitrite? *Veterinary and Human Toxicology.* 1997;39:152–154.

37. Thom SR. Hyperbaric-oxygen therapy for acute carbon monoxide poisoning. *New England Journal of Medicine.* 2002;347:1105–1106.

38. Weaver LK, Hopkins RO, Chan RJ, et al. Hyperbaric oxygen for acute carbon monoxide poisoning. *New England Journal of Medicine.* 2002;347:1057–1067.

39. Tomaszewski CA, Thom SR. Use of hyperbaric oxygen in toxicology. *Emergency Medicine Clinics of North America.* 1994;12:437–459.

40. Scolnick B, Hamel D, Woolf AD. Successful treatment of life-threatening propionitrile exposure with sodium nitrite/sodium thiosulfate followed by hyperbaric oxygen. *Journal of Occupational Medicine.* 1993;35:577–580.

41. Gunn B, Wong R. Noxious gas exposure in the outback: Two cases of hydrogen sulfide toxicity. *Emergency Medicine.* 2001;13:240–246.

42. Cannard K. The acute treatment of nerve agent exposure. *Journal of the Neurological Sciences.* 2006;249(1):86–94.

43. Newmark J. Nerve agents. *Neurologic Clinics.* 2005;23(2):623–641.

44. Newmark J. Therapy for nerve agent poisoning. *Archives of Neurology.* 2004;61(5):649–652.

45. Bird SB, Gaspari RJ, Dickson EW. Early death due to severe organophosphate poisoning is a centrally mediated process. *Academy of Emergency Medicine.* 2003;10(4):295–298.

46. Eyer P. The role of oximes in the management of organophosphorus pesticide poisoning. *Toxicology Reviews.* 2003;22(3):165–190.

47. *Protocol for the prohibition of the use of asphyxiating, poisonous, or other gases, and of bacteriological methods of warfare.* Geneva, Switzerland; June 17, 1925. Available at: http://www.icrc.org. Accessed July 25, 2008.

48. Organization for the Prohibition of Chemical Weapons. Convention on the prohibition of the development, production, stockpiling, and use of chemical weapons and on their destruction. Available at: http://www.opcw.org/. Accessed July 25, 2008.

49. McCarthy C, Fischer J. *Inching away from Armageddon: Destroying the U.S. chemical weapons stockpile.* Henry L. Stimson Center; April 2004.

50. Okumura S, et al. Clinical review: Tokyo—Protecting the health care worker during a chemical mass casualty event: an important issue of continuing relevance. *Critical Care.* 2005;9: 397–400.

CHAPTER 18

Radiological Agents

Hamid Shokoohi, Mohammad Reza Soroush, and G. Bobby Kapur

INTRODUCTION

Considering recent increases in sophisticated terrorist activities, the concerns over the potential use of radiological or nuclear materials in terrorism activities are significant and growing. Indeed, there have already been terrorist threats to use radioactive materials to launch attacks, although no successful radiological attack has occurred to date. Intelligence data reveal that Al-Qaeda has expressed an interest in acquiring radioactive materials, and radiological dispersal devices (RDDs) planted by Chechen rebels were disarmed in 1995 and 1998.[1-3]

Radiological terrorism represents a major threat to the public's health and safety. Emergency preparedness and response to radiological activities, however, have unique characteristics that pose a particular challenge to public health and homeland security personnel.[4,5] As efforts are made to improve preparedness for this developing threat, it will be important for public health professionals and first responders to learn as much as possible about the characteristics of radiological crises and to study industrial experiences with radioactive materials emergencies. This chapter examines the potential impact of deliberate radiological emergencies on the public health infrastructure and the response to these growing threats.

Case Study

On an autumnal day in October, the Board of Governors of the International Monetary Fund (IMF) and the Boards of Governors of the World Bank Group are having their annual meetings in Washington, D.C. These meetings are usually targeted by protesters from around the world, and large crowds that require law enforcement to control their movements assemble each year near the site of the current meeting. At approximately 9:45 A.M., the nearest emergency department (ED) receives a call from emergency medical services (EMS) dispatch stating that a "suitcase-sized" explosive has been detonated near the World Bank headquarters on H Street. Four ambulances will be arriving at the ED with patients with critical injuries. Within 5 minutes, a second call arrives from EMS stating that detectors are recording the presence of radiological particles in the vicinity, and law enforcement and city officials are concerned about the detonation of a "dirty bomb." The ED staff begins preparing for decontamination of the victims outside the hospital so as to not contaminate other patients.

Within minutes, the Washington, D.C., Department of Health begins mobilizing a response team. The city's Fire Department establishes an incident command post approximately two blocks from the event and cordons off a two-block circumferential area where the highest levels of radioactive signals are being detected. Law enforcement personnel begin fulfilling the dual roles of public safety and evidence collection at the scene while wearing appropriate personal protective equipment. Fortunately, the weather is mild, with minimal winds and no rain. Municipal officials begin sending out communications via TV, radio, and Internet, warning tourists, residents, and workers to avoid the area. The officials inform individuals who were in the area to take the following steps:

- Change clothing
- Place contaminated clothes in plastic garbage bags
- Wash thoroughly with a warm shower
- Seek immediate medical care if individuals have injuries or signs of radiation illness such as burns or vomiting

The local authorities begin communications and coordination with the federal government and the surrounding states of Maryland and Virginia. They are given access to the Strategic National Stockpile to obtain radiation countermeasure medications. The city cancels all local sporting events, and spokespersons tell the public that a Radiation Response Center has been established at the Verizon Center for population monitoring.

The American Red Cross and local nonprofit assistance agencies begin assisting families with reunification with family members who have been in the vicinity of the radiological terrorist attack. In addition, these nongovernmental organizations (NGOs) begin providing a change of clothes and portable decontamination showers to the large numbers of people who had arrived from out of town to protest or attend the World Bank meetings. The NGOs also begin psychosocial counseling and attempt to reduce the hysteria in the crowds by dispelling false information and myths about the radiation.

BACKGROUND

Basics of Radiation Physiology

Radioactive materials are used every day in laboratories, medical centers, food-preparation industries, and other industrial operations. Radioactive materials are non-stable elements, and they contain excess energy in their nuclei. These materials release energy by emitting ionizing radiation. The radiating energy includes alpha particles, beta particles, gamma rays, neutrons, and x-rays.[3,4,6]

Alpha particles are heavy particles with high amounts of energy, a very short range (a few microns), and low penetration. Due to their minimal penetration, alpha particles can be blocked by the skin and even by a sheet of paper. These particles can cause a health hazard, however, if they are internalized by ingesting radioactive materials. Alpha particles promote double-stranded DNA breaks and multiply damaged sites, and this type of damage is more difficult to repair than the single-stranded DNA breaks typically caused by beta or gamma radiation. Exposure to alpha radiation is more likely to cause cellular changes that can lead to cancer than exposure to the same dose of beta or gamma radiation. For example, cesium-131 (Cs-131) is a radioactive isotope of cesium that emits alpha radiation and is used to treat prostate cancer,[7] but Cs-131 can induce severe cellular damage if ingested.[2–4,6]

Beta particles can travel a few meters in ambient air, but can be blocked by a thin sheet of aluminum. These particles can penetrate a few centimeters of tissue, but usually go no deeper than the outer layers of skin. Because of this limited external penetration, beta particles can cause a slow, evolving thermal burn called "beta burn" if particles remain on the body surface for a prolonged period of time. In addition, ingesting beta-emitting materials causes significant internal damage. Iodine-131 (I-131), for example, is a radioactive isotope of iodine that emits both beta and gamma radiation; it is used in many medical procedures such as the monitoring and tracing of thyroxin from the thyroid gland.

Gamma-rays and x-rays differ from alpha and beta particles in that they travel farther and penetrate tissue to great depths. The actual clinical damage from exposure to this type of radiation depends on the level of energy of the gamma rays. Because of its high penetrability, however, gamma radiation can result in total body exposure and illness. If the radiation ions contain sufficient energy, they can create ion pairs within living cells. These ion pairs, in turn, may damage the DNA. This damage can cause fatal mutations in the organism genome and result in cellular death. Persistent nonfatal damage will be passed on to the next generations of cells. Mutations in noncoding parts of the genome may cause no damage, whereas other mutations may cause cancers.[3,4,6,8]

The radioactive intensity of materials is indicated by their half-life. The half-life of a radioactive isotope is the time needed for the material to lose half of its radioactivity. The intensity of radioactivity from a point source is inversely proportional to the distance from the radioactive source. The amount of energy absorbed in an object depends on the intensity of the source, the proximity of the object to the source, the type of energy, the duration of exposure, the medium in between (shielding, for example), and the material from which the object is made. The units of radioactivity, the curie (Ci) and the becquerel (Bq), measure the rate at which radiation is emitted from a mass of radioactive materials. Long-lived isotopes decay slowly, so a relatively large amount is needed to give the same radiation dose found in smaller amounts of shorter-lived isotopes. For example, 1 gram of radium-226 (Ra-226; half-life = 1,600 years) contains the same amount of radioactivity (and the same curie content) as approximately 3 tons of depleted uranium-238 (U-238; half-life = 4.38 billion years).[4, 6]

Radiation dose is a measurement of the amount of energy deposited by ionizing radiation in an absorber such as water, air, and tissue. This energy produces ionization that damages the cell or DNA. It is more precisely referred to as the radiation absorbed dose, which accounts for only the amount of energy absorbed by the absorber—that absorber need not be a living organism. The radiation dose is measured in either of two units: the gray (Gy; the SI unit) or the rad (the U.S. unit).[2,4,6]

Radiological Terrorist Devices

Radiological materials have the potential to be used as weapons. The three agents most likely to be deployed in a terrorist attack are a radiological dispersal device (RDD), a radiation emission device (RED), or an improvised nuclear device (IND).[9]

A "dirty bomb" is a relatively unsophisticated RDD that combines radioactive materials with conventional explosives.[1,2,5,6,8] When exploded, these weapons spread radioactive materials into the environment, thereby exposing both the targeted population and the environment to the radiation. Although the terms "dirty bomb" and "RDD" are often used interchangeably in the literature, RDDs can also include other means of dispersal such as contamination of food and water supplies with radioactive material or use of an airplane to disperse powdered or aerosolized forms of radioactive material.[2,3,5,8,10] The actual medical risks may be low from a dirty bomb, but the psychological fear engendered by the combination of the explosion and the presence of radioactive material will cause mass panic, and large numbers of individuals will need to be monitored for radiation exposure.

An RED is simply a high-energy radiation source deployed in a concealed location that exposes individuals who come in close range of the device. The device does not disperse radiological particles over a widespread area, however. The intention in using an RED is to induce acute radiation syndrome or cutaneous radiation syndrome in unsuspecting civilians.

Unlike an RDD or an RED, an IND contains actual fissile or fissionable material (uranium-233, uranium-235, or plutonium-239) that will produce a nuclear detonation.[9] Such devices will not produce effects on the same scale as a tactical nuclear weapon used for military purposes. Even so, they may release large amounts of energy and heat and produce a cloud of radioactive material.

In contrast to a nuclear event, a dirty bomb explosion would affect only local areas, ranging from a city block to a few square miles. After obtaining radioactive materials, terrorist organizations could detonate a simplistic dirty bomb that would cause limited radiological exposure. In contrast, designing an RDD that can deliver high doses of radiation and produce large numbers of fatalities is actually very difficult. These devices need special preparation techniques and transportation that, in the majority of cases, could cause severe health consequences or even kill the terrorists themselves. For this reason, most experts believe that an RDD will most likely be used only to contaminate facilities or places where people live and work, with the goals being to disrupt daily life, to prevent the use of these places, and to arouse fear and a sense of chaos in the target population.

The range of the affected area depends not only on the size of the bomb and the type of radioactive materials employed, but also on the means of dispersal (spray, explosion, liquid) and the physical and chemical form of the radioactive material. Weather conditions, local topography, and landscape characteristics will also determine the level of dispersion and shielding. The direction of the wind is a major factor that affects the size and area covered by the radioactive plume. If the radioactive material is released as a shower of fine particles, the plume will spread roughly at the same speed and direction of the wind. [1,2,6,8,10]

PREPAREDNESS

Preparedness for radiological terrorism is an essential component of the U.S. public health surveillance and response system. Hospitals and public health agencies should prepare for radiological terrorism's unique features, such as mass casualties with blast injuries combined with burns, radioactive contamination, and acute radiation syndrome.

Radiological agents present distinct challenges to public health professionals and medical providers, and specific principles distinguish the planning for these events from planning for other terrorist attacks (Table 18-1).

The emergency preparedness for a radiological terrorist incident should be consistent with the planning that already exists for other public health emergencies, such as bombings, chemical agents, and bioterrorism. The preparedness for all terrorist events comprises an "all hazards" approach because the first responders and local officials initially may not be aware that a radiation incident has occurred. Once it is determined that radiation or radioactive material is involved in the public health emergency, specific countermeasures for a radiologic or nuclear incident—taking into account factors related to time, distance, and shielding—should be addressed.[1,2,5,8,10]

Local, State, and Federal Responsibilities

Rapid public health and medical response to a nuclear or radiological incident requires special preparation at the local, state, and federal levels. Emergency response authorities at the local level should determine the available resources, and then these local officials should identify whether assistance from the state or federal public health authorities might be needed. The primary responsibilities for local authorities are as follows:[9]

TABLE 18-1   Key Principles in Public Health Preparedness for Radiological Terrorism
The initial priority is to save lives by responding to and treating injured persons first.
First responders and law enforcement may not know that a radiation event has occurred.
Scalability and flexibility are critical components of a community's response plan.
The population generally has a greater fear of radiation than of other terrorist weapons.
Radiation exposure is not immediately life threatening.
Decontamination recommendations for radiological agents differ from those for chemical agents.
Initial population monitoring should emphasize prevention of acute radiation health effects.
The lead agency for the state's radiation control will be a key resource for population monitoring.

Source: Adapted from Centers for Disease Control and Prevention (CDC). *Population monitoring in radiation emergencies: A guide for state and local public health planners.* Washington, DC: Author; 2007.

- Establishing criteria for incident site entry and operations
- Producing radiation injury prevention and control measures
- Recommending treatment and management protocols for affected individuals

First responders, EMS systems, and local hospitals will be responsible for ensuring that contaminated persons, injured individuals, and those concerned about potential exposure are treated in an efficient manner. However, the widespread fear of exposure to radioactive materials, the disruption of everyday life, and the possible contamination of medical facilities will almost certainly affect the capacity to provide these services.[1,2,5,8,11] At the state level, the state agency that monitors industrial nuclear activities and radiation control measures can provide critical technical expertise in the planning and response to terrorist radiological emergencies.

The Department of Homeland Security (DHS) coordinates the federal response to incidents of national significance, such as a terrorist incident involving radioactive materials, and the Department of Health and Human Services (DHHS) coordinates public health aspects of the federal response to such incidents. The Centers for Disease Control and Prevention (CDC) coordinates its activities with state health agencies on issues related to health surveillance, public health information, disease control, and worker health and safety; this agency also provides public health and medical consultation, technical assistance, and support as necessary.

In the event of a nuclear or radiological incident, an overwhelmingly large number of patients, including both individuals who are injured and those who are concerned about potential exposure, will seek medical attention. The CDC, in conjunction with the local jurisdiction's incident command, is responsible for coordinating the availability of supplies, diagnostic tests, and hospital beds. The public health agencies should be prepared to implement the following objectives in the initial hours after the incident:[9]

- Provide radiation dose predictions based on the device and plume size involved
- Identify the geographic areas where victims may be present
- Distribute radiation survey equipment to first responders
- Perform blood tests (complete blood count with white cell differential) to assess the effects of whole-body exposure to the radiation

Prior preparedness and training among local, state, and federal agencies can improve the response to a radiological public health emergency. When predetermined plans that designate each agency's responsibilities and resources exist, the actual response will be better coordinated and more effective at reducing morbidity and mortality.

RESPONSE

Phases of Response

The emergency response to a radiological terrorist incident involves the coordinated contributions of multiple disciplines including emergency medical systems, fire, law enforcement, radiation experts, hazardous materials (HazMat) teams, public health officials, and healthcare providers. The DHHS has outlined a time frame for response to radiological terrorism that is divided into three phases: early, intermediate, and late (Figure 18-1).[12]

The early phase occurs during the first hours to few days after the incident, when decisions will be made with only preliminary radiation data or pre-event models. Protective response actions can be either primary or secondary. Primary actions involve sheltering-in-place, evacuation, or relocation. Secondary actions involve administration of medical countermeasures, decontamination, restrictions of food and water, soil guidance, access control, and victim extraction.

The intermediate phase occurs after the radiation device has been controlled and radiation is no longer being emitted into the environment. The goals of response activities during this phase include return of critical infrastructure to normal operations and the population's rapid return to normal activities. During this phase, primary and secondary protective actions are based on actual measurements of exposure and identification of radioactive materials.

The late phase begins during the latter stages of the intermediate phase and extends until all post-incident recovery operations have been completed. Response activities of the late phase focus on reducing environmental radiation levels to acceptable levels.

Scene Management

In the event that a dirty bomb is detonated, scene management will begin with controlling entry and exit from the scene site and identifying the presence and estimated dose of the radioactive materials. If first responders equipped with radiation dosimeters detect higher than expected levels of radiation, a team of radiation experts and HazMat personnel will be brought to the scene to determine the type and estimated amounts of radioactive materials. Experts from the state environmental protection department and public health department will estimate the geographic distribution of the radioactive plume. In addition, public health officials and first responders will establish a radiation control zone in which the emergency operations will take place (Figure 18-2). This zone will consist of a "central perimeter" that contains radiation levels greater than 10 R/h; only life-saving and critical emergency operations will be

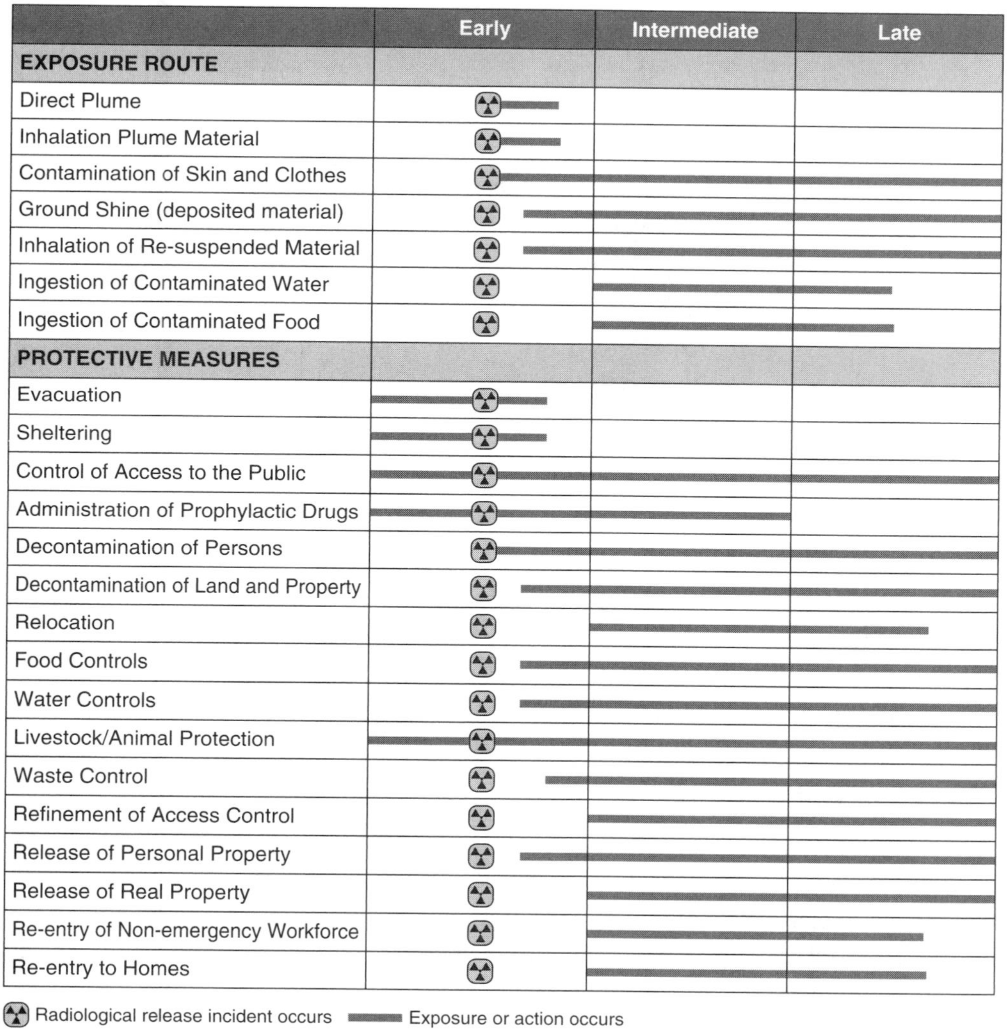

	Early	Intermediate	Late
EXPOSURE ROUTE			
Direct Plume	☢▬		
Inhalation Plume Material	☢▬		
Contamination of Skin and Clothes	☢▬▬▬▬▬▬▬▬▬▬▬▬		
Ground Shine (deposited material)	☢ ▬▬▬▬▬▬▬▬▬▬▬▬▬▬		
Inhalation of Re-suspended Material	☢ ▬▬▬▬		
Ingestion of Contaminated Water	☢	▬▬▬▬▬▬▬▬▬	
Ingestion of Contaminated Food	☢	▬▬▬▬▬▬▬▬▬▬▬▬▬▬	
PROTECTIVE MEASURES			
Evacuation	▬▬☢▬▬		
Sheltering	▬▬☢▬		
Control of Access to the Public	▬▬☢▬▬▬▬▬▬▬▬▬▬▬▬		
Administration of Prophylactic Drugs	▬▬☢▬▬▬▬▬▬▬		
Decontamination of Persons	☢▬▬▬▬▬▬▬▬▬▬▬▬▬		
Decontamination of Land and Property	☢ ▬▬▬▬▬▬▬▬▬▬		
Relocation	☢	▬▬▬▬▬▬▬▬	
Food Controls	☢ ▬▬▬▬▬▬▬▬▬▬▬		
Water Controls	☢ ▬▬▬▬▬▬▬▬▬▬▬		
Livestock/Animal Protection	▬☢▬▬▬▬▬▬▬▬▬▬▬		
Waste Control	☢ ▬▬▬▬▬▬▬▬▬▬▬▬		
Refinement of Access Control	☢	▬▬▬▬▬▬▬▬▬▬	
Release of Personal Property	☢	▬▬▬▬▬▬▬▬▬▬	
Release of Real Property	☢	▬▬▬▬▬▬▬▬▬▬	
Re-entry of Non-emergency Workforce	☢	▬▬▬▬▬▬▬▬	
Re-entry to Homes	☢	▬▬▬▬▬▬▬▬	

☢ Radiological release incident occurs ▬▬▬ Exposure or action occurs

FIGURE 18-1 Exposure and Protective Measures During Phases of Radiological Emergency
Source: From U.S. DHHS Radiation Event Medical Management. Available at: http://www.remm.nlm .gov/response_phases.htm. Accessed June 2010.

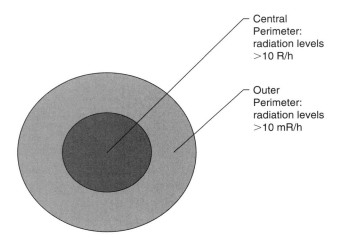

Central
Perimeter:
radiation levels
>10 R/h

Outer
Perimeter:
radiation levels
>10 mR/h

FIGURE 18-2   Radiation Control Zone

allowed within this area. Officials will also designate a second "outer perimeter" that contains radiation levels greater than 10 mR/h and should be isolated from all persons except for first responders and officials with appropriate protective equipment.

Evacuation and Decontamination

Medical management of a radiologic explosive event begins at the site with triage of casualties. Trained providers equipped with personal protective equipment (PPE) should start external decontamination of both injured and non-injured people.[1–3,5,6,13] Considering time, distance, and shielding principles, public health and public safety officials will then guide the affected population on whether to shelter in place or evacuate the scene.

The first step in external decontamination is to remove and double-bag clothing for future exposure analysis, followed by washing the exposed areas or full showering, depending on the nature of the exposure. Internal decontamination uses dilution, purging, diuretics, and laxatives to facilitate excretion and reduce absorption of radioactive materials. Use of medication countermeasures is part of internal decontamination. If the types of radioactive materials have been identified but the need for internal contamination has not yet been determined, medical providers may empirically treat contaminated victims with medication countermeasures. Healthcare providers should not withhold treatment until confirmation of exposure before beginning internal decontamination.

One of the most important roles fulfilled by public health officials is to ascertain the type of radiation exposure and determine the indications for medication countermeasures. Medication countermeasures for such exposures may include potassium iodide (KI), diethylene triamine pentaacetic acid (DTPA), or Prussian blue. These medication countermeasures are specific to contamination with particular radioisotopes:[14–16]

- Potassium iodide is a radioisotope-blocking agent for victims who are internally contaminated with radioisotopes of iodine.
- DTPA is a chelating agent available in calcium and zinc forms. Calcium and zinc DTPA are used for internal decontamination of victims exposed to plutonium, americium, and curium.
- Prussian blue, while taken orally, will stay within the digestive tract (it is not absorbed); there, it binds with cesium and thallium and accelerates their passage out of the body.[14–16]

These medications are part of the Strategic National Stockpile, and local and state authorities will coordinate with the federal government for distribution of these agents during a radiation-related incident.

Screening and Population Monitoring

One of the top priorities following a radiation incident is the screening of people for exposure and contamination. The safety of emergency healthcare providers is a major concern during the response phase. All workers should be screened for contamination at the end of their duty shift, after decontamination, or after time spent in the radiation control zone. Responders younger than age 18 or with known pregnancy must be allowed to work within the cold zone only. Health and safety officers for each agency will be responsible for maintaining records and recording radiation doses received by their agency workers.

In the first few hours after the incident occurs, the local and state public health officials will need to begin identifying individuals who either require immediate medical treatment for acute radiation syndrome (ARS) or need countermeasure treatment for exposure to radiological particles. This process is termed "population monitoring."[9] The three components essential to population monitoring are a location in which to conduct monitoring activities, a registry of affected individuals, and the collection of biological samples (urine and blood) for bioassays. In particular, local authorities will need to establish a radiation response center where population monitoring activities can take place. This site should be a large, covered area such as a sports arena or a convention center that can accommodate large populations. These venues usually also have adequate restroom and shower facilities and are compliant with the Americans with Disabilities Act (ADA). In addition, entry and exit control can be easily accomplished, and contamination detection can occur through portal (walk-through) or handheld radiation monitors.

Once individuals who may have been exposed to radiological materials begin arriving at the radiation response center, public health personnel should establish a registry of all potential patients and collect vital information and contact details for each person. All individuals should be given information and instructions about radiation contamination and physical signs to observe. In addition, people with a history of close proximity to the detonated device may be asked to provide blood or urine samples to run bioassay tests, and they may be provided with decontamination countermeasures if deemed appropriate.

Health Effects of Radiation

After a dirty bomb incident, patients may experience both acute and delayed effects. During the acute phase, in addition to the usual physical trauma, shrapnel, blast, and burn injuries, victims can suffer from ARS and internal contamination. The health effects of radiation tend to be directly proportional to the radiation dose. If a reasonable estimate can be made of the dose received, a tremendous amount of clinical information is available about the health effects at specific doses. In addition to the amount of radiation absorbed by the body, the radiation type, the means of exposure (absorbed through the skin, inhaled, or ingested), and the length of exposure are key factors determining the onset, duration, and severity of radiation sickness.[1,5,10,11]

Symptoms of ARS and radiation sickness evolve over time in three distinct phases: prodrome, latency, and clinical manifestations. The duration of each phase and the time of its onset are inversely proportional to the dose and duration of exposure. The prodromal phase is characterized by general symptoms such as nausea, vomiting, weakness, and fatigue that typically develop in hours to days after exposure. During the latency period, the patient may look and feel normal. This period can last for a few weeks, even with severe clinical manifestations such as bone marrow suppression or failure (Table 18-2).[13]

A unique association between the dose and the specific organ injuries is noted at different phases of ARS. White blood cells (WBCs) are among the most radiosensitive cells and are affected at the earlier stages following radiation exposure; thus the WBC count represents a useful laboratory test for determining the severity of ARS.[1,2,5,10,11,13] Following a radiation exposure that exceeds 0.5 Gy, a rapid fall in the number of WBC begins within hours. The trend of WBC depletion is proportional to the dose, and ranges between 1 Gy (mild) and 10 Gy (lethal).

In the latent phase, despite significant exposure, patients may remain asymptomatic. This period will follow with a period of symptomatic illness characterized by infection, bleeding, and gastrointestinal and cardiovascular symptoms (Table 18-2).[13]

Neupogen, one of the medication countermeasures available in the Strategic National Stockpile, can be used to improve a victim's chances for survival; it stimulates certain types of cells that remain in the bone marrow to produce mature WBCs.[14–16] In the management of hospitalized patients with severe ARS, consideration should be given to instituting neutropenic isolation precautions, antibiotic prophylaxis, aggressive hydration and electrolyte replacement, and, if needed, transfusion with irradiated blood products and platelets.

Communications and Psychosocial Assistance

Communication plays a key role in the successful management of a radiological event. By communicating in a manner that is clear, empathic, consistent, and meaningful to the public, important information can be provided that should help citizens make appropriate decisions to protect themselves from harm and to work collaboratively with public health and emergency officials during the response and recovery efforts. In addition, informative and effective communications can reduce fear and anxiety, and these efforts will help address psychosocial issues. The civilian population will most likely want to know the following information regarding the release of radiation particles into the population:[9]

- Was I exposed to radiation?
- Am I radioactive?
- Am I still carrying around radioactive materials on my body and clothing?
- Did I ingest radioactive materials and should I receive medical treatment?

The task of effectively communicating information about radiation exposure and related emergency issues is extremely challenging and requires considerable skill and preparation. Communication must be integrated into the agency's response plans to ensure that the general public remains well informed at all phases during a disaster. Communication must occur throughout the planning stages before an event occurs,

TABLE 18-2   Acute Radiation Syndromes

Syndrome	Dose*	Prodromal Stage	Latent Stage	Manifest Illness Stage	Recovery
Hematopoietic (bone marrow)	> 0.7 Gy (> 70 rad) (Mild symptoms may occur with exposures as low as 0.3 Gy or 30 rad)	• Symptoms include anorexia, nausea, and vomiting. • Onset occurs 1 hour to 2 days after exposure. • Stage lasts for minutes to days.	• Stem cells in bone marrow are dying, although the patient may appear and feel well. • Stage lasts 1 to 6 weeks.	• Symptoms include anorexia, fever, and malaise. • Drop in all blood cell counts occurs for several weeks. • Primary cause of death is infection and hemorrhage. • Survival decreases with increasing dose. • Most deaths occur within a few months after exposure.	• In most cases, bone marrow cells will begin to repopulate the marrow. • There should be full recovery for a large percentage of individuals from a few weeks up to 2 years after exposure. • Death may occur in some individuals at exposures of 1.2 Gy (120 rad). • The LD50/60† is in the range of 2.5 to 5 Gy (250 to 500 rad).

Gastrointestinal (GI)	>10 Gy (> 1,000 rad) (Some symptoms may occur with exposures as low as 6 Gy or 600 rad)	• Symptoms include anorexia, severe nausea, vomiting, cramps, and diarrhea. • Onset occurs within a few hours after exposure. • Stage lasts about 2 days.	• Stem cells in bone marrow and cells lining the GI tract are dying, although the patient may appear and feel well. • Stage lasts less than 1 week.	• Symptoms include malaise, anorexia, severe diarrhea, fever, dehydration, and electrolyte imbalance. • Death is due to infection, dehydration, and electrolyte imbalance. • Death occurs within 2 weeks of exposure.	• The LD100‡ is approximately 10 Gy (1,000 rad).
Cardiovascular (CV)/ central nervous system (CNS)	> 50 Gy (5,000 rad) (Some symptoms may occur with exposures as low as 20 Gy or 2,000 rad)	• Symptoms include extreme nervousness and confusion; severe nausea, vomiting, and watery diarrhea; loss of consciousness; and burning sensations of the skin. • Onset occurs within minutes of exposure. • Stage lasts for minutes to hours.	• The patient may return to partial functionality. • Stage may last for hours but often is shorter.	• Symptoms include return of watery diarrhea, convulsions, and coma. • Onset occurs 5 to 6 hours after exposure. • Death occurs within 3 days of exposure.	• No recovery is expected.

* The absorbed doses quoted here are "gamma equivalent" values. Neutrons or protons generally produce the same effects as gamma, beta, or x-rays but at lower doses. If the patient has been exposed to neutrons or protons, consult radiation experts on how to interpret the dose.

† The LD50/60 is the (lethal) dose necessary to kill 50 percent of the exposed population in 60 days.

‡ The LD100 is the (lethal) dose necessary to kill 100 percent of the exposed population.

Source: Acute radiation syndrome: A fact sheet for physicians. Available at: http://emergency.cdc.gov/radiation/arsphysicianfactsheet.asp#table1.

during an event to provide reliable and timely information about the situation, and after the event to foster as rapid a recovery to normal routines as possible.[2,5,8,11]

MITIGATION

As with all terrorist public health emergencies, mitigation of radiological terrorism begins with measures that prevent individuals from acquiring and deploying destructive materials against civilian populations. Although oversight and control of nuclear technology and materials have been historically tightly controlled by individual countries, the fall of the former Soviet Union and the development of nuclear technology by low-income countries where security measures may be lax, such as Pakistan and North Korea, have led to concerns that weapons-grade radiological materials may enter the possession of terrorists. The U.S. National Nuclear Security Administration recovers nuclear materials from primarily industrial sources and attempts to keep them from entering general circulation. In the 12 years that this agency has been operational, it has collected more than 20,000 sources of radiological materials within the United States.[17] In addition, the U.S. Nuclear Regulatory Commission (NRC) and state regulations require companies licensed to use or store radioactive materials to secure them from theft and unauthorized access. Since the terrorist attacks of September 11, 2001, these regulations have been strengthened, and lost or stolen high-risk radioactive material must now be reported immediately. Local authorities may also assist in finding and retrieving such sources. Fortunately, most reports of lost or stolen material involve small or short-lived radioactive sources that would not be useful for an RDD.[18,19]

At the international level, the United Nations' International Atomic Energy Agency (IAEA) provides oversight for member nations' nuclear programs. The IAEA has a critical objective—namely, to promote nuclear security. It works with countries to upgrade the security of their radiological materials through identification and protection against theft of radiological materials. The agency's terror mitigation efforts include the following measures:[20]

- Upgrades to physical security where radiological materials are located
- Increased accountability and control of radiological materials
- Strengthened legislation and regulation within countries
- Detection and interdiction of radiological materials trafficking

In the aftermath of a radiological attack, the affected community and public health system will face multiple medical, psychological, social, political, and economic challenges. During the earliest recovery phase, public service authorities and emergency response teams must manage both the scene and the municipality, so that the scene is stabilized, victims are cared for, and essential city services are maintained or resumed.[1,8,14,15] The psychological impact of spreading radioactivity, regardless of the actual damage inflicted by the radiation, is difficult to estimate. Most individuals in the affected community will prove resilient, but some will experience post-traumatic stress disorders. A majority will most likely possess some level of concern about delayed radiation health effects. Providing accurate information in a timely manner will improve public confidence. For this reason, restoration of public communication networks is one of the most crucial steps to mitigate the public impact of such an incident. If severe damage to the communications network disrupts communication from authorities, public anxiety and fear may be heightened.[2,3,5,10]

Following a radiological incident, the public infrastructure may be burdened by the high economic costs to decontaminate people and places, and possibly destroy and rebuild contaminated structures. The buildings and ground affected by the explosion will need to be decontaminated to mitigate against ongoing contamination and exposure. The extent to which decontamination will occur depends on the initial estimation of the scope of the plume and the evidence of contamination found in different areas. Methods for successful decontamination have been developed from previous experiences in mitigating industrial radiation accidents. Nevertheless, the cleanup will inevitably be both time-consuming and costly.[3,5,10,15,16]

CASE STUDY ANALYSIS

The hypothetical case study described at the beginning of this chapter highlights many of the challenges that will face local authorities in the immediate aftermath of a radiological terrorist event. As with any potential terrorist attack, the civilian population will be a high-risk target, and events with large crowds may be even more vulnerable if terrorists want to incite greater fear or panic. In this case, the event may occur at a very visible location, with many of the affected people residing outside the local region. The large numbers of visitors will make both immediate and long-term communications and follow-up difficult. The local authorities will use their resources to attempt control of entry and access and to alert local hospitals. In addition, they will begin coordination with federal authorities to obtain additional resources such as medications from the Strategic National Stockpile. Finally, they will begin providing high-impact messages to individuals who may have self-evacuated, and they will initiate population monitoring at a large venue with shower facilities that permits easy control of entry and exit patterns.

This case study is similar in certain ways to an accidental release of radiation materials that occurred in Goiania, Brazil. On September 13, 1987, sanitation workers pried open a metal canister from a cancer clinic that contained radioactive cesium-137 particles.[20] In the first two days after this event, hundreds of individuals were exposed. Among them, only 10 were seriously exposed and were hospitalized, with 4 deaths occurring. However, 112,800 people had to be medically screened. Almost 47,000 people had to be taken to decontamination showers and required follow-up over the next few years.

Recently, the Washington, D.C.-based Center for Strategic and International Studies simulated what would happen if terrorists detonated a 4,000-pound dirty bomb in a school bus parked outside the National Air and Space Museum.[21] In the simulation, the museum ended up mostly destroyed and many nearby buildings damaged. An estimated 10,000 people were in the immediate vicinity. How many would have died is not known, but the acute threat was confined to a few city blocks. In the simulation, the officials expected that contaminated citizens would absorb radiation at a rate of approximately 5 rem per hour. This exposure is the amount that the Environmental Protection Agency has determined is the maximum safe dose to absorb in one year—a standard that is considered very conservative. Even if individuals are exposed and radiation is absorbed in hours, the amount is not likely to make a person ill. Depending on the radioactive material used, the size of the explosive, wind conditions, and the effectiveness of the evacuation response, and not accounting for the damage inflicted by the blast itself, the numbers of deaths and injuries are likely to be minimal, according to the Center for Strategic and International Studies.

CONCLUSION

In the days following a radiological incident, authorities will be expected to establish a plan to conduct careful monitoring and assessment of affected areas, impose quarantines of contaminated areas, maintain decontamination procedures, and keep citizens informed about the progress during recovery. In addition, public health officials should investigate the possible contamination of water and food resources and act accordingly. The public health system will be responsible for establishing a surveillance system to monitor long-term health effects on contaminated individuals, many of whom could develop cancer within several years to decades after the radiological weapon attack. For example, the CDC's program on population monitoring following a mass-casualty radiological incident involves the process of identifying, screening, and monitoring people with exposure to or contamination from radioactive materials.[2,6,8,9,15,16] Only through a coordinated, multiagency response will a municipality be able to navigate the complex challenges of a radiological terrorist incident.

INTERNET RESOURCES

Centers for Disease Control and Prevention, radiation emergencies:
http://emergency.cdc.gov/radiation/

International Atomic Energy Agency, nuclear security:
http://www-ns.iaea.org/security/default.htm

U.S. Department of Health and Human Services, radiation event medical management:
http://www.remm.nlm.gov/

U.S. Department of Energy, Radiation Emergency Assistance Center:
http://orise.orau.gov/reacts/

U.S. Environmental Protection Agency, *Responding to Radiation Emergencies*:
http://www.epa.gov/radtown/emergencies.html

U.S. Nuclear Regulatory Commission, *Fact Sheet of Dirty Bombs*:
http://www.nrc.gov/reading-rm/doc-collections/fact-sheets/dirty-bombs.html

World Health Organization, nuclear terrorism and dirty bombs:
http://www.who.int/ionizing_radiation/a_e/terrorism/en/index.html

NOTES

1. Coleman CN, Hrdina C, Bader JL, Norwood A, Hayhurst R, Forsha J, Yeskey K, Knebel A. Medical response to a radiologic/nuclear event: Integrated plan from the Office of the Assistant Secretary for Preparedness and Response, Department of Health and Human Services. *Annals of Emergency Medicine*. 2009;53(2):213–222.
2. Barnett DJ, Parker CL, Blodgett DW, Wierzba RK, Links JM. Understanding radiologic and nuclear terrorism as public health threats: Preparedness and response perspectives. *Journal of Nuclear Medicine*. 2006;47(10):1653–1661.
3. U.S. Government Accountability Office. Combating nuclear terrorism (GAO-06-1015). Available at: http://www.gao.gov/. Accessed October 2009.
4. Federal Interagency Committee. Planning guidance for response to a nuclear detonation. First edit January 2009. Available at: www.ostp.org. Accessed October 2009.
5. Turai I, Veress K, Günalp B, Souchkevitch G. Medical response to radiation incidents and radionuclear threats. *British Medical Journal*. 2004;328:568–572.
6. Karam PA. Radiological terrorism. *Human and Ecological Risk Assessment*. 2005;11:501–523.
7. Kehwar TS. Use of cesium-131 radioactive seeds in prostate permanent implants. *Journal of Medical Physics*. 2009;34(4):191–193.
8. Bushberg JT, Kroger LA, Hartman MB, Leidholdt EM Jr, Miller KL, Derlet R, Wraa C. Nuclear/radiological terrorism: Emergency department management of radiation casualties. *Journal of Emergency Medicine*. 2007;32 (1):71–85.
9. Centers for Disease Control and Prevention (CDC). *Population monitoring in radiation emergencies: A guide for state and local public health planners*. Washington, DC: Author; 2007.

10. Hale JF. Managing a disaster scene and multiple casualties before help arrives. *Critical Care Nursing Clinics of North America*. 2008;20(1):91–102.

11. Moulder JE. Post-irradiation approaches to treatment of radiation injuries in the context of radiological terrorism and radiation accidents: A review. *International Journal of Radiation Biology*. 2004;80(1):3–10.

12. Radiation Event Medical Management. Three phases of the response to an RDD or IND. Washington, DC: U.S. Department of Health and Human Services; November 27, 2009. Available at: http://www.remm.nlm.gov/response_phases.htm. Accessed February 2010.

13. CDC. Acute radiation syndrome: A fact sheet for physicians. Available at: http:// emergency.cdc .gov/radiation/arsphysicianfactsheet.asp#table1. Accessed December 2009.

14. Bell WC, Dallas CE. Vulnerability of populations and the urban health care systems to nuclear weapon attack: Examples from four American cities. *International Journal of Health Geographics*. 2007;6:5.

15. Public health planning for radiological and nuclear terrorism. Available at: www.bt.cdc.gov/ radiation. Accessed January 2010.

16. How bad would a dirty blast be? Here's what the experts say. Available at: http://www .washingtonpost.com. Accessed December 2009.

17. Paddock RC. Little-known U.S. agency hunts down radioactive castoffs. *Los Angeles Times*. March 3, 2009. Available at: http://articles.latimes.com/2009/mar/03/local/me-plutonium3. Accessed February 2010.

18. U.S. Nuclear Regulatory Commission (NRC). Fact sheet on dirty bombs. February 20, 2007. Available at: http://www.nrc.gov/reading-rm/doc-collections/fact-sheets/dirty-bombs.html. Accessed February 2010.

19. International Atomic Energy Agency (IAEA). Promoting nuclear security: IAEA action against terrorism. June 1, 2004. Available at: http://www.iaea.org/NewsCenter/Features/Nuclear Security/terrorism.html. Accessed February 2010.

20. International Atomic Energy Agency (IAEA). *The radiological accident in Goiania*. Vienna: Author; 1988. Available at: http://www-pub.iaea.org/MTCD/publications/PDF/Pub815_web.pdf. Accessed February 2010.

21. How bad would a dirty bomb be? Here's what the experts say. Available at: http://www .memphistn.gov/pdf_forms/dirtyBlast.pdf. Accessed February 2010.

SECTION 6

Natural Emergencies

CHAPTER 19

Earthquakes

Christopher N. Mills

INTRODUCTION

Preparing for and responding to earthquakes is a challenge to emergency public health systems because of both their unpredictability and their great potential for widespread devastation. This chapter focuses on the challenges that earthquakes pose to the health and safety of affected populations. The 2005 earthquake in Pakistan-administered Kashmir serves as a case study because it exemplifies these challenges to an extreme degree—from preexisting poverty and instability in the region, to poor building design, to inadequate governmental preparedness, to extensive destruction of access, supply, and communications networks, to the urgency of responding to the humanitarian crisis before the encroaching Himalayan winter set in.

One key element of adequate preparation before an earthquake is the delivery of appropriate public health messages to the general population, such as the importance of maintaining supplies consisting of a few days' worth of food and water, knowing how to turn off gas and electric lines at home, and learning basic first aid. Preparedness at departmental and governmental levels includes developing an "all hazards" disaster response plan that incorporates coordination of all foreseeable facets of a disaster. Earthquake-prone areas should develop specific plans for how each public health entity is to respond after an earthquake. Plans should assume that telecommunications and transportation systems are likely to be crippled in the acute phase, in the immediate aftermath of the event.

The response to a major earthquake occurs in two phases. The first phase, when survivors are being pulled from the wreckage and in need of emergent medical care to save their lives, lasts for the first few days after an earthquake. The second phase consists of procuring goods and services to cover the basic humanitarian needs of the affected population. Often, these needs include shelter, nutrition, water, sanitation, and safety. This phase can last from months to years and blends into the recovery phase, which is aimed at restoring a state of normalcy to the population.

Successful mitigation of earthquake damage depends on both strength of leadership and the economic resources available in a given region. The construction of structures that are in compliance with earthquake-resistant building codes is critical to minimize morbidity and mortality after a major earthquake. In practice, such codes may not exist or may not be enforced, especially in economically disadvantaged areas. Economic development of a region also acts to mitigate the economic devastation (e.g., impact on livelihoods) after an earthquake: A more affluent population has greater capacity to rebuild after a crisis.

Maximizing survival after a deadly earthquake hinges on the existence of a functioning emergency public health system that plans for such an event beforehand and responds immediately after it strikes. This chapter explains characteristics of public health as it relates to earthquakes and methods employed to minimize the devastation they cause.

Case Study

Kashmir lies atop the junction of the Indian and Eurasian tectonic plates, which have been in the process of colliding for 50 million years. The ongoing crash between these plates has created the Himalayas, the highest landmass in the world, and continues to thrust the mountain range ever higher. Tectonic plates do not slide into each other smoothly. Instead, static friction maintains the plates' position as immense levels of tectonic potential energy mount along a geologic fault. When the force of collision surpasses the static friction, the plates slip suddenly past each other; this "slip" is felt as an earthquake.

The Earthquake in Kashmir

At 8:50 A.M. on Saturday morning, October 8, 2005, an earthquake measuring 7.6 on the Richter scale struck along the Indian–Eurasian fault in the mountainous Pakistan-administered Kashmir (PAK). Its epicenter lay 19 km northeast of the provincial capital, Muzaffarabad. Saturday is a normal business day in Pakistan, so children were in school and many people were at work when the earthquake struck. One minute later, 80 percent of the buildings of the 13,000 km² province had been damaged or destroyed, 2.8 million individuals had become homeless, and tens of thousands were dead or terminally trapped under collapsed structures. In total, an area encompassing more than 30,000 km^2 was affected by the earthquake. Because of the mountainous terrain, many areas of PAK are difficult to access even in the best of conditions. Most of the roads linking the villages of the province were destroyed either by the earthquake or by the landslides that it set off.[1]

The earthquake killed more than 80,000 people, with nearly the same number injured. Half of those killed or injured were children.[2] Although the majority of these people died immediately, many fell victim to the humanitarian disaster that followed the earthquake. More than a thousand people died in the surrounding territories as well, mostly in India-administered Kashmir. The quake hit just before the onset of the harsh Himalayan winter, increasing even further the urgency of securing shelter for the homeless. One month after the earthquake, 41 villages still remained cut off from all land-based aid because of the destroyed mountain roads.[2] Camps providing shelter to the persons displaced by the disaster were stricken by outbreaks of infectious diseases. Many thousands were still homeless as of 2009, lacking the livelihood to rebuild.

Pakistan's Minister of the Interior estimated that the infrastructure damage was approximately $5 billion. Although this figure is far lower than the infrastructure value that would be lost if a similar earthquake were to strike a developed city such as Tokyo or Los Angeles, it represents an enormous number of family homes destroyed, especially when considering the low face value of a dwelling in rural Pakistan in international monetary terms. Pakistan's ongoing conflict with India over control of Kashmir contributed to the economic depression that further worsened the impact on the region.

Challenges to Immediate Medical Response

At the time of the Kashmir earthquake, Pakistan effectively had no earthquake response plan.[1] Thus the primary responsibility for responding to an earthquake in this region fell to the surviving local inhabitants of each village and town, who sought to extricate those victims whom they could reach, individual by individual, and initiate whatever first-aid measures were available or known to them. Most hospitals were destroyed as well as most public buildings. Most of the people in these buildings were killed, leaving few local public officials alive to begin local-scale coordinated responses.[1] In the Muzaffarabad hospital, the patients had to be evacuated outside due to severe structural damage to the facility.[3] Numerous significant aftershocks continued to strike the region as the tectonic plates settled into a new configuration. Some of these aftershocks were quite significant in severity, registering more than 6.0 on the Richter scale.[1]

Approximately 90 percent of the victims of an earthquake who can be saved are extricated from the wreckage within 24 hours.[4] Unfortunately, the lack of heavy equipment in the PAK region decreased the number who could be extracted. Because the local healthcare system was disabled by the earthquake, very little immediate emergency management was available to the population of PAK in the first few days after the initial earthquake.

Challenges to Humanitarian Response

The obstacles facing relief organizations were immense. The United Nations Office for Coordination of Humanitarian Assistance identified the most pressing challenges of the aftermath of the earthquake to be providing shelter in the face of bitter winter conditions, providing food across broken transportation lines, airlifting supplies to needed locations, fomenting appropriate decentralization of aid, combating donor fatigue, and operating within an underfunded United Nations budget.[5] These challenges were undertaken in a high-terrain, remote region with very few roads left between villages, where freezing temperatures were only a few weeks away, with a decimated healthcare system, in an already war-torn and impoverished area, under a government ill prepared to meet a disaster on such a massive scale.

HISTORICAL PERSPECTIVES

Earthquakes are the most sudden of all natural disasters, occurring generally without warning and lasting only seconds. The amount of physical damage caused by an earthquake is determined by the energy released, the intensity and particular type of resultant motion, the distance from the epicenter, the duration of the earthquake, and the nature and quality of the buildings affected. Timing also matters because it affects whether people are more likely to be at home or at work. The second most deadly earthquake in history was in the city of Tangshan, China, in 1976, which killed at least 250,000 people.[6] It struck at 4 A.M., when most people were asleep inside their homes. More recently, the earthquake in May 2008 in Sichuan, China, struck at 2:28 P.M. on a Monday afternoon, when children were still in school. More than 7,000 classrooms collapsed, killing more than 10,000 schoolchildren.[7] In total, this earthquake killed at least 70,000 people and injured more than 350,000.[8]

Earthquake Characteristics

Earthquakes are commonly measured using the Richter scale, which is an estimate of the energy released. Each whole number represents a 10-fold increase in energy; thus a magnitude 7.0 quake is 10 times stronger than a magnitude 6.0 quake. Because the Richter scale becomes unable to differentiate earthquake strength above the 7.0 level, the moment magnitude scale was developed in the 1970s, which roughly approximates a continuation of the Richter scale into higher magnitudes.[9] On average, 17 earthquakes with magnitude greater than 7.0 occur each year worldwide, and one occurs each year with magnitude greater than 8.0.[6] A gestalt estimate of the human impact of earthquakes is provided by the Mercalli scale, which ranges from I (felt only by instruments) to XII (catastrophic with total destruction).[6]

Approximately 90 percent of all earthquakes in the world occur along the borders of the Pacific tectonic plate, called the "Pacific Ring of Fire" for its related association with active volcanoes.[6] The southern edge of the Eurasian tectonic plate, which passes through the Himalayas, Central Asia, and southern Europe, is a secondary focus of earthquakes. More than 500 million people live in urban zones near these geologic faults. Of the approximately 30 urban metropolitan areas in the world with populations exceeding 10 million, half are located in regions prone to severe earthquakes.[10] Urban locations are more lethal than rural ones not only because of higher population density, but also because most earthquake victims are killed by the collapse of buildings. An earthquake centered under a large city in the future could kill 3 million people or more and leave many millions injured.[11] Cities in developing countries are at greatest risk because of generally poor compliance with rigorous building codes.[4]

The fact that most deaths in earthquakes tend to result from collapsing buildings was manifested in horrific proportion in the deadliest earthquake in history: the 1556 earthquake in China's Shaanxi Province, which killed more than 800,000 people. The death toll was massive because a large proportion of the population at the time lived in dugout dwellings built into fragile loess cliffs that collapsed in huge numbers. In some counties in this area, more than half of the population was killed.[12]

Secondary Disasters

The immediate aftermath of earthquakes can kill and injure large numbers of people by multiple means besides building collapse. Fires, tsunamis, and violence are common; landslides and dam breaks are also possible. Later, in the weeks following an earthquake, humanitarian emergencies are prone to emerge, such as malnutrition from decreased food availability, exposure from lost housing, and disease from unsanitary conditions in temporary camps. Emergency public health response is required at all levels after a severe earthquake to minimize morbidity and mortality.

In the San Francisco earthquake in 1906, the largest proportion of the 3,000 victims were killed by fires that erupted throughout the city as a result of ruptured gas and electricity lines. A preponderance of wooden structures and burst water mains left the city without water pressure to combat fires, which in turn amplified the conflagration. Additionally, buildings were dynamited by untrained firefighters in a vain attempt to create a firebreak; this activity caused many additional fires.[13] In total, 80 percent of the city was destroyed by the earthquake and ensuing fire.

In 1755, Lisbon, Portugal, was destroyed by fires that erupted after an earthquake struck. More than 70,000 people were killed, representing one fourth of the population.[6] Half an hour after the Lisbon earthquake, a tsunami crashed against the coastline and killed many thousands more who had fled to the waterfront in an effort to escape the collapsing buildings and fires. In 2004, an extremely powerful earthquake shifted the ocean floor near Indonesia, giving rise to a tsunami that killed more than 225,000 people.

Disruption of civil society also factors into earthquake mortality, as with any large-scale disaster. After the 1906 San Francisco earthquake, numerous individuals purposely set fire to their own homes because insurance policies generally covered losses due to fire but not earthquakes.[14] Looting was rampant throughout the city as well. The mayor declared martial law, with police being given orders to shoot looters on sight. Approximately 500 people were shot and killed as a result, some of whom were found to be homeowners simply retrieving their own possessions from the ruins.[15] The annihilation of the health and social systems in Kashmir described earlier also serves as an example of the humanitarian emergency that can develop after an earthquake strikes remote or developing regions.

PREPAREDNESS AND PLANNING

Earthquake Warning and Prediction

Earthquakes cannot be prevented. The best way to limit morbidity and mortality from an earthquake is to accurately predict it so that the population has enough time to respond before it occurs. Unfortunately, the unpredictability of earthquakes makes establishment of an early warning system very difficult even with today's technology. Several strategies are currently used for early warning systems. In Mexico City, Taiwan, and Japan, authorities have installed a series of seismometers along nearby fault lines. The seismometers have the potential to electronically relay information about the onset of an earthquake to warning sirens within cities, which can give up to a minute of advance notice of an earthquake propagating through the ground. That period may be long enough to evacuate from structures, find locations of relative safety before the earthquake strikes, and trigger automated shutdowns of gas and electricity lines that might otherwise pose fire hazards.[16] These systems might potentially be improved by a few seconds through use of even more effective early warning systems that rely on the less-destructive pressure waves (called primary waves, or P-waves) that precede the far more lethal secondary waves, or S-waves. Unlike P-waves, which propagate as a compressive pulse emanating from the focus of an earthquake, S-waves propagate as transverse waves that cause the ground to ripple.[16]

Early warning on a scale of hours to days before an impending major earthquake would allow for more coordinated preparedness and could dramatically decrease injury and loss of life in these events. To date, no such system has been developed. In the past, sudden changes in well water depth, foreshock patterns, and unusual animal behavior have been used on a nonscientific basis to predict earthquakes. These efforts have been met with limited but occasional success. Seismologists predicted the 1975 Haicheng earthquake one day in advance, principally using foreshock data, and they issued a warning to the city of 1 million that limited the loss of life in this area to 10,000.[17,18]

In the weeks preceding the 1989 Loma Prieta earthquake in northern California, and especially in the hours immediately preceding the earthquake, researchers detected by chance marked increases in ultra-low-frequency electromagnetic radiation activity.[19] Since then, this effect has been occasionally recorded before large earthquakes.[17,20] Multiple ultra-low-frequency electromagnetic detectors are currently being installed in earthquake-prone areas for research purposes. One explanation proposed for this unusual phenomenon is that rock layers subjected to extreme compression by sliding fault lines may develop electrical currents that result in emission of the radiation. Although still in the experimental stage, technology exploiting this effect could prove helpful in earthquake prediction in the future.

Individual Preparedness

Until earthquakes become predictable, planning and preparation for earthquakes must be undertaken at a range of levels—from individual to societal—to minimize casualties and devastation. Public health messages in earthquake-prone areas are key to prepare the population to survive an earthquake.

The California Education Code requires all schools in the state to conduct regular earthquake drills, which teach children to "drop, cover, and hold on" in the event of an earthquake.[21] In addition to preparing students for an earthquake while at school, the program teaches the population about the importance of acting immediately to find shelter. Such drills may save lives years later, given that students are likely to retain these principles as adults.[22] General principles of disaster preparedness are also disseminated through the media in earthquake-prone regions, though this service is generally available only in developed nations. Governmental organizations distribute preparedness instructions such as the Los Angeles Fire Department's free *Earthquake Preparedness Handbook*[23] and the California Governor's Office of Emergency Services' *Preparedness Tips*.[24] Information from these sources, if effectively distributed and implemented, can help prepare a population for an earthquake. Examples of important messages include keeping three days' worth of water, food, and supplies to get through the immediate crisis and knowing how to shut off gas and electricity lines to a home. Nongovernmental organizations (NGOs) such as the Red Cross and Red Crescent societies also engage in emergency public health communication about earthquake preparedness in different nations on an individual level as well as on a community-wide scale.[25,26]

Training of the general population in first aid is another important component of preparedness for any disaster. This statement holds particularly true for earthquakes because their unpredictability and potential for massive trauma may cause survivors in the community to be called upon to immediately deliver life-saving first aid medical care. The Federal Emergency Management Agency (FEMA) offers a free 18-hour Community Emergency Response Team (CERT) course to mobilize community members autonomously before rescue workers can arrive at the scene of a disaster.[27] This course is designed on an "all hazards" framework to teach individuals about general disaster response principles.

Community Preparedness

Formulation of a preexisting disaster plan is a critical component in orchestrating an effective large-scale earthquake response. Using the Incident Command System (ICS) and its well-defined division of roles allows disasters to be managed at all scales. A first step in preparing for a coordinated earthquake response is the formation of government offices specifically dedicated to this purpose. To this end, the United States has established the National Earthquake Hazards Reduction Program (NEHRP), principally managed by the National Institute of Standards and Technology in collaboration with the United States Geologic Survey, FEMA, and the National Science Foundation.[28] State and local governments in earthquake-prone areas such as California and Alaska have also developed earthquake plans that outline the chain of command and method of response of fire, ambulance, police, hospitals, transportation, energy, and other agencies in case of an earthquake.[29,30] The Department of Homeland Security's National Incident

Management System (NIMS) is designed to provide a framework for instituting an ICS in the event of an emergency of any type or scale,[28] and many U.S. cities' and states' plans have adopted this framework to organize their response planning.

Coordination with the non-governmental and private sectors is also of critical importance before an earthquake strikes. Governmental agencies are unlikely, for example, to own enough heavy equipment to lift rubble in extrication operations, clear blocked roads, and transport supplies after a major earthquake; for this reason, agreements to utilize private resources such as construction companies to assist with earthquake relief should be in place before such an event occurs. Areas with relatively weak, resource-poor governments can expect to rely heavily upon foreign assistance from both governmental and non-governmental agencies to provide initial and often ongoing relief to the victims of an earthquake. In the 2005 Kashmir earthquake, the government did not have a developed earthquake response plan. Partly because of insufficient preparedness for such an event, the initial government response to the earthquake was delayed and disorganized.[1,23,31]

Military forces are often deployed after a major earthquake to assist in the disaster response. Indeed, deployment after major earthquakes is common for both domestic and international forces.[31] Militaries are the most likely entities to have the means to deliver large-scale human resources and supplies to inaccessible areas in the acute phase of a disaster. It is important for these forces to be prepared for deployment in humanitarian operations, which necessitate use of a different set of tactics and strategies than warfare operations and require a different approach to achieve mission success. Preexisting agreements for operational systems between military and non-military entities should be confirmed beforehand to guarantee clear expectations of responsibilities during collaborative relief efforts.

RESPONSE

Incident Command and Coordination

Individuals collaborating informally to free survivors from hazardous areas and begin first aid will always be part of the first step in earthquake response. The effectiveness of this initial response depends on the preparedness of the community to react to a disaster, as outlined earlier in this chapter.

The first step in the emergency public health response to an earthquake is activation of the ICS. The response to a major earthquake goes far beyond simple delivery of emergency medical care to victims, and multiple government and private entities are required to act in the immediate aftermath of a major earthquake to maximize public safety and welfare. For example, search and rescue departments must mobilize to locate survivors, fire departments must prepare for conflagrations, gas and electricity departments (whether government owned or private) must shut off broken lines, water departments must inspect dams and water lines, transportation departments must clear blocked roads and verify the safety of bridges and airfields, public and private hospitals must prepare for casualties exceeding their capacity, police departments must limit the civil disruption that accompanies disasters, hazardous materials departments must evaluate and contain spills and leaks of toxic materials, and areas with capacity to serve as shelters (e.g., schools, stadiums, shopping centers, and dormitories) should prepare for an influx of the newly displaced.[29] As an example of the need for action by many departments, after the 2008 Sichuan earthquake, 80 tons of liquid ammonia leaked from two damaged chemical plants,[32] a derailed train loaded with petrol tanks derailed and caught fire,[33] hundreds of dams were damaged, hospitals were overwhelmed by hundreds of thousands of injured victims, all highways into the most severely affected county were damaged, landslides caused rivers to become lakes that swallowed villages,[34] and Chengdu Stadium became a tent city for 8,000 refugees.[35]

These complex and interrelated tasks are time critical and must be begun immediately after the event to ensure the greatest degree of public health and safety after an earthquake. Thus a preplanned and functional ICS is essential to act as a central repository for information gathering and distribution of appropriate tasks and delegation of control at each level of response.[31] Another important component of the ICS is the designation of a public information officer to serve as a single point of access in relaying information to the media to avoid dissemination of conflicting messages.

Immediate Medical Response

In terms of providing immediate medical care to the injured after an earthquake, principles of simple triage and rapid treatment are vital to prioritize casualties and ensure the best survival rates. For those persons buried by collapsing buildings, more than half die immediately or within the first few hours.[36] Most of these individuals cannot be saved. In addition, when existing medical resources are not sufficient to meet demand, victims who are not buried but who have sustained massive head or chest injuries and would be unlikely to survive in any context should be passed over in favor of less critically injured patients. The highest priorities are critically injured victims who have a reasonable chance of survival with immediate, rapid interventions. Examples include victims who have a pneumothorax (lung injury) that can be decompressed or a potentially lethal hemorrhage that can be bandaged. Part of the initial medical response may go beyond these rapid interventions to include more complex in-field procedures, depending on the responders' training and resources. For example, those responders with appropriate training, sterile equipment, and an injectable sedative or dissociative drug such as ketamine could conceivably perform field amputations for persons with limbs trapped under rubble.[4] Although the convergence of a trained and adequately supplied operator with an appropriate victim during the critical time window is uncommon, field amputations and chest tube insertions have been successfully performed with ketamine by medics in Afghanistan.[37]

The greatest need for emergent patient care will become apparent within the first two days of an earthquake. One earthquake response operations plan that has been proposed relies on three phases of response.[4] First, in the first hour after the earthquake, pretrained regional volunteers with first-aid backpacks in the trunks of their cars self-deploy to deliver immediate care and transport victims by whatever resources remain available to them.

Second, from hours 1 to 12, disaster medical aid centers are established, each of which is less than one hour's walk from any point in the region. Each site has space for a helicopter to land. In Orange County, California, where this plan was developed, this arrangement comprises 150 sites. Each is staffed by three physicians, who are predesignated to report in the event of a severe earthquake, and each is equipped with green, yellow, and red tarpaulins as signals for helicopters to denote level of urgency of need for transport of victims to a hospital. Such a tarpaulin system will be especially useful to combat the likely disruption in telephone communications and logistical difficulties associated with rapid distribution of two-way radios.

Third, from 12 to 72 hours after the quake, patients and healthcare providers are consolidated into casualty collection points in open areas such as parks, golf courses, and malls located approximately 10 miles apart. For Orange County, this arrangement includes approximately 10 locations. These sites can function like the disaster medical aid centers, but are larger and better supplied. Those victims in need of surgery or intensive care are transported from these casualty collection points to those hospitals that remain functional.

Advantages of a response plan such as this include accessibility throughout the region and a degree of autonomous function during the first chaotic hours after an earthquake.[4] A disadvantage is that such a plan is not a realistic solution in a less developed setting because it is both costly and resource intensive.

Earthquakes bury large numbers of victims, and efforts to find them can be facilitated by the use of search and rescue dogs.[38] Search and rescue robots that can fit into small spaces between rubble have also been developed to locate victims.[39] Victims found by such mechanisms have often been trapped for several days with crush injury and without access to water. They are at risk of kidney failure from dehydration and rhabdomyolysis (muscle breakdown). In the 1995 Kobe earthquake, acute kidney injury (AKI) occurred in 24 patients per every 1,000 deaths; in the 2005 Kashmir earthquake, AKI was found in only 0.8 patient per 1,000 deaths because the large geographic area and poor medical access caused those with AKI to die before they could be treated.[40] A medical system in the aftermath of a major earthquake should be prepared for an increased need to initiate dialysis.

Humanitarian Response

After the first few days, the emergency public health response transitions from the acute phase, which centers on extricating and saving earthquake victims, into a much longer phase of humanitarian response, which must rise to meet the challenges of sudden homelessness, injury, diseases linked to poor sanitation and overcrowding, exposure, disruption of civil society, and food insecurity.

Procurement of shelter for survivors is necessary after a destructive earthquake. After the 1995 earthquake in Kobe, Japan, schools served as shelter and evacuation centers; teachers in Japan routinely receive mandatory disaster human resources management training, which proved crucial after this earthquake.[22] Designating shelter is one of the first steps in preparing for the subacute phase of disaster response. All major public health emergencies transition within days from disaster-specific life-saving operations to more complex, general humanitarian relief operations for the displaced and injured. As this transition occurs, the needed response becomes less specific for earthquakes and more dependent on the scope and characteristics of the population affected, whether the public health emergency that caused the humanitarian crisis was initiated by an earthquake, war, famine, or some other trigger.

Notably, camps of internally displaced persons (IDPs) are frequently required in the aftermath of an earthquake. The 2008 Sichuan earthquake, for example, left approximately 5 million individuals in need of shelter.[41] Common secondary crises that develop in the weeks following any disaster include diseases of overcrowding and poor sanitation, such as gastroenteritis, typhoid, giardiasis, and cholera; violence from breakdown of the rule of law and desperate efforts to obtain scant resources; mass starvation from a surging need for inflow of food along fractured supply channels; and exposure crises such as freezing to death and gangrene. The emergency public health system, through collaboration of disparate aid agencies, must seek to prevent and control these emerging secondary disasters. Each of these factors endangers the emergency public health system response.

In 2005, the United Nations' Office of Coordination of Humanitarian Affairs re-designed its response plan into a cluster-based approach to disaster relief. The cluster strategy was first employed in the wake of the Kashmir earthquake.[1] The plan designated 10 clusters of need, each with its own command center, to streamline the system, provide a structure to organize the myriad of NGO and governmental aid entities, and make the response effort more nimble. The clusters consist of shelter, nutrition, health, water and sanitation, camp management, logistics, protection, education, telecommunications, and early reconstruction planning.[42] The leadership of each cluster is allocated to a particular UN agency. Implementation during the Kashmir earthquake revealed numerous problems with this strategy, as discussed in the "Analysis of Case Study" section later in this chapter.

The emergence of volunteers is part of any disaster response. Volunteers have the capacity to function as a critical component of an earthquake relief effort—but only insofar as they do not become victims themselves and do not put a further strain on already scarce resources such as food, water, latrines, and shelter. The coordinating body for the emergency public health response should be prepared to manage the volunteer response by estimating the number needed for various operations and stratifying volunteers by skill set. Those who are trained in first aid, for example, may assist with the initial medical response. The organizing body must also be prepared to turn away volunteers if necessary to decrease confusion and resource demand. Some volunteer responses are massive, but without careful organization, much goodwill and available energy may be squandered.[2]

Recovery

Recovery after a major earthquake takes years, especially in regions that are less prosperous economically. Over time, the humanitarian response phase becomes integrated with the process of recovery. Rebuilding homes and livelihoods is a difficult process on an individual basis, and restoring normalcy to the public systems of health, education, security, economy, and culture is an equally difficult process on a community basis.

Earthquakes have long-lasting psychological consequences in addition to their economic and human toll. Eight months after the 1999 earthquake in Izmit, Turkey, that killed more than 17,000 people and injured 50,000, the prevalence of post-traumatic stress disorder (PTSD) in camp residents was found to be 43 percent.[43] Treatment for PTSD involving sessions in an earthquake simulator consisting of a furnished room mounted on a foundation that creates controllable tremors has been shown to reduce these mental health effects more than conventional therapy alone.[44]

As recovery operations take place and regions become cleared and prepared for rebuilding, reconstruction should take place under the supervision of government-based agencies that ensure that buildings are constructed with reasonable safeguards against earthquakes, thereby minimizing the devastation of the next earthquake.

Sociopolitical Context

The human impacts of an earthquake depend heavily on the economic status of the region. Economic depression results both from paucity of natural resources and poor governance. A weak socioeconomic situation makes a natural hazard much more likely to develop into a true disaster because the population is not buffered from crisis.[2,45] Earthquake-prone metropolitan areas in the world include economically advanced cities such as San Francisco, Tokyo, and Rome; economically marginal cities such as Mexico City, Jakarta, and Tehran; and economically poor cities such as Pyongyang, Dhaka, and Kabul. Less stable societies with greater poverty typically have less stringent building codes (and poorer compliance with these codes) and less ability to draw upon resources to survive a disaster. Furthermore, the response capability of the public health system is more poorly funded and planned in these regions.[46] Authoritarian influences may breed corruption and lead to unequal delivery of services. After the 2005 Kashmir earthquake, for example, the military-run Federal Relief Commission evolved into the Earthquake Reconstruction and Rehabilitation Authority (ERRA), which is nontransparent in its operation; this agency exerts mandatory control over the activities of local assistance groups and may allow corrupt influences to develop.[46]

MITIGATION

Elimination of poor construction practices is among the top priorities for mitigation of damage by a major earthquake.[2,4] Building codes have been developed to ensure safety of structures in the event of a moderately severe earthquake. These include various components of construction and reinforcement that have been adopted by earthquake-prone areas in developed nations. They also comprise zoning restrictions to avoid building in areas subject to destruction by earthquakes such as known fault lines, landslide-prone areas, and land with soil deposits subject to liquefaction by an earthquake.

Less developed areas have varying degrees of building code law and limited capacity to inspect or enforce structure design. Furthermore, the added cost of building a seismically resistant structure may be prohibitive in many economic climates worldwide.[47] Expertise may also be lacking in earthquake-resistant design. In addition to building codes, the designation of building zones based on earthquake risk is another important component of mitigation—and one that is all too often ignored.

The protective effects of sound construction principles cannot be overemphasized. Over the last 50 years, earthquakes that killed more than 20,000 people have occurred in China, Iran, Pakistan, Peru, Armenia, Guatemala, and India—all less developed nations (Table 19-1). Besides these events, 13 other earthquakes in developing nations killed more people than the most devastating earthquake to strike an industrialized nation in the last half-century: Kobe, Japan, in 1995, which killed 5,000 people.[48] Of the four deadliest U.S. earthquakes over this time period, one killed 128 people and the other three each killed between 60 and 65 individuals (Table 19-2).[48] Although these figures partly reflect random chance as to where and how earthquakes have struck recently, they also strongly reflect mitigation measures that industrialized cities have had the resources to undertake.

Safe building practice is, in large measure, a result of one of the most powerful mitigating factors in any public health crisis: economic development. A wealthier society has the capacity to design safer buildings and implement more comprehensive safeguards and emergency response mechanisms in the event of an earthquake. Technological features of mitigation may also be unavailable to less economically developed regions, such as automated cutoff of gas and electricity lines to prevent

TABLE 19-1	World Earthquakes Causing More Than 20,000 Deaths in the Past Half-Century			
Year	**Location**	**Magnitude**	**Deaths**	**Injuries**
1970	Chimbote, Peru	7.9	70,000	150,000
1976	Motagua Fault, Guatemala	7.5	23,000	76,000
1976	Tangshan, China	7.5	255,000	799,000
1988	Spitak, Armenia	6.8	25,000	19,000
1990	Manjil, Iran	7.4	40,000	60,000
2001	Gujarat, India	7.6	20,000	166,000
2003	Bam, Iran	6.6	31,000	30,000
2004	Sumatra, Indonesia	9.1	228,000	125,000
2005	Muzaffarabad, Pakistan	7.6	86,000	69,000
2008	Sichuan, China	7.9	87,000	375,000

Source: Adapted from U.S. Geologic Survey Data, http://earthquake.usgs.gov/regional/world/historical.php.

TABLE 19-2   Earthquakes in the United States Causing More Than 50 Deaths in the Past Half-Century

Year	Location	Magnitude	Deaths	Injuries
1964	Anchorage, Alaska	9.2	128	Not reported
1971	San Fernando, California	6.7	65	2,000
1989	Loma Prieta, California	6.9	63	3,700
1994	Northridge, California	6.7	60	7,000

Source: Adapted from U.S. Geologic Survey Data, http://earthquake.usgs.gov/regional/states/historical_state.php.

fires, effective warning systems for hazardous material leaks, and judicious risk analysis based on fault lines, soil, construction materials, and human impacts.

ANALYSIS OF CASE STUDY

Emergency Public Health System

In 2005, northeastern Pakistan's public health system was unprepared for a severe earthquake.[2] Building codes were neither heeded nor enforced, resulting in cities and towns made vulnerable to disaster owing to poor construction practices with seismically unsuitable building materials. In response to the 2005 Kashmir earthquake, the Pakistani government established the Federal Relief Commission (FRC) to direct the official national and international response to the earthquake. The FRC worked in conjunction with the United Nations' Office for the Coordination of Humanitarian Affairs (OCHA). In the wake of the disaster, hundreds of organizations, ranging from humanitarian and business organizations within Pakistan to international NGOs to foreign governments and multinational organizations such as the European Union and the North Atlantic Treaty Organization, began to arrive in the region to assist with the response and relief effort.[1] The FRC was under the jurisdiction of the Pakistani military,[46] which is the only organization in Pakistan with the capacity to mount a logistical response to such a large-scale crisis. Moreover, the government of Pakistan is a military regime that spends a large proportion of its gross domestic product (approximately 7 percent) on its armed forces.[46]

Both the national and international responses to the PAK earthquake have been criticized as inadequate in scope and coordination.[1] Although initial pledges of international assistance totaled $2 billion, only $9.5 million had been received by Pakistan after one month. Out of the United Nations' requested $550 million for earthquake relief, only $133 million had been received.[2] Donor fatigue was a significant factor limiting fundraising. The Indian Ocean tsunami of 2004, which had occurred only nine months earlier, had been met with a massive outpouring of international aid that stemmed partly from the scope of that disaster and partly from the highly publicized stories of Westerners who were affected by the tsunami. Furthermore, Hurricane Katrina struck New Orleans six weeks before the earthquake in Kashmir, diverting U.S. attention from the earthquake.[49]

When put into practice, OCHA's cluster approach did spread out jurisdiction over the operations as designed, but the clusters were found to overlap to a large degree. For example, camp management intrinsically incorporates elements of shelter, sanitation, nutrition, and numerous other clusters. This overlap decreased clarity in the lines of authority.[1] Although the cluster system was designed to decrease duplication of efforts, it was largely unsuccessful for this reason. Additionally, the 2005 Kashmir earthquake response was coordinated by both OCHA and the FRC. Although the OCHA health cluster was placed in charge of designating sites for temporary hospitals, the FRC actually chose the sites, often poorly.[1] Weakness of OCHA leadership combined with operating within a sovereign nation led to decreased OCHA effectiveness in coordinating the humanitarian response.[46] Relief workers often operate in the absence of a recognizable state structure, such as in Darfur or Bosnia, and may be unprepared to operate under the auspices of a functioning military regime such as exists in Pakistan.[46]

Immediate Medical Response

Those persons who could have been saved by immediate, intensive trauma care generally did not survive the PAK earthquake because the preexisting health system was already fragile and then was rendered utterly inoperable by the disaster. One exception to this problem, however, came in the form of Islamic militia groups. Many such groups operate secret, illegal camps in PAK. Within the first 24 hours after the earthquake, these militias had mobilized to provide assistance by extricating trapped individuals; providing temporary shelter, food, and blankets; and clearing roads.[3] One Islamic group in particular, Lashkar-e-Taiba, plays a large role in coordinating attacks across the border in India; this group arrived in force to provide a large degree of humanitarian relief long before any federal response could be organized, likely saving many lives of those trapped and garnering much credit among the local populations for being present in their time of need.[3] Militia groups such as these represented the first—and in more remote regions, the only—form of de facto emergency public health response, even though it was not organized by any official agency; in fact, the existence of such groups was outlawed.

Humanitarian Response

The most pressing crisis that developed within the first weeks after the earthquake was lack of shelter. Tents were desperately needed to house the millions of displaced persons who had nowhere to sleep. Most families had to sleep in the open or fashion their own makeshift shelters from the remains of their homes, employing bits from their metal roofs and wooden beams from their walls to keep out the harshest of the elements.[2] The first snow fell in Kashmir just five days after the earthquake. The weather was turning colder, and a worldwide shortage of tents was met with increased foreign tent production. By December, 480,000 tents had been delivered, although approximately 85 percent were inadequately designed for survival in winter conditions. Heated rooms were constructed out of wrecked building materials to shelter groups of villagers through the cold winter.[50] The tent cities that formed were soon plagued by the hazards of overcrowded living with poor sanitation conditions, and by the end of October, infectious respiratory and gastrointestinal diseases were widely prevalent.[1,2]

Higher-altitude regions remained effectively cut off from aid through the winter due to impassable roads and a lack of helicopter landing sites. A dearth of helicopters also hampered relief operations.

After one year, 1.8 million people were still living in temporary shelters, according to aid agency Oxfam International. Less than one fifth of the households had been able to begin constructing a new home from the rubble.[51]

CONCLUSION

Whether in the preparedness, response, or mitigation phases of an earthquake, communities can deploy specific high-yield strategies to improve outcomes in the aftermath of this kind of natural disaster (Table 19-3). The public health system at all levels should undertake preparedness measures that include educating the population about earthquakes and training civilians in first-aid basics. The existence of a general plan that is mapped out before the disaster happens is particularly critical for earthquakes, given their suddenness.[31]

Earthquake response is divided into two phases. First, the immediate medical response revolves around extrication and rescue of victims over the first few days. To be effective, the emergency public health response must involve multiple entities, from fire departments to paramedic units to hospital systems to transportation authorities. It must also be able to spring into action semi-autonomously because communication mechanisms are likely to be disrupted in the wake of an earthquake.

In the second phase, the longer-term humanitarian response becomes the focus of relief operations and encounters the same challenges faced in any large-scale disaster, such as ensuring adequate shelter, nutrition, water, sanitation, and safety of the displaced and otherwise affected victims. Many aid organizations often work in tandem in earthquake response, and it remains a difficult challenge for governments or OCHA to successfully orchestrate and streamline the disparate entities to form a cohesive and efficient system. OCHA's recently developed cluster system to organize functions is still being evaluated and refined.

Mitigation of earthquake damage depends heavily on the sociopolitical milieu and economic status of any given region, because successful mitigation includes potentially costly earthquake-resistant engineering designs and retrofitting. In the majority of (but not all) earthquakes, most people are killed by building collapse; therefore, maximizing building safety has great potential to save lives when an earthquake strikes.

Earthquakes are as yet unpredictable and, therefore, cannot be prepared for individually. Instead, the public health system must be prepared to initiate an emergency response at all times and deal with potentially massive death tolls, casualties, and infrastructure obliteration. However, through effective measures of preparedness, response, and mitigation, public health officials at all levels of governance can provide resilience to their constituencies.

TABLE 19-3 Key Strategies in Earthquake Disaster Phases	
Disaster Phase	**Key Strategies**
Preparedness and Planning	
Warning and prediction	• Funding for development of early warning systems
Individual preparedness	• School and workplace drills • Public health messaging • Stockpiling recommendations • First-aid training of population
Community preparedness	• Community disaster plan formulation • Coordination with fire, police, paramedics, and public health department • Coordination with hospitals, gas and electricity utilities, transportation systems, water departments, merchants, construction entities

(continues)

TABLE 19-3 (*cont.*) Key Strategies in Earthquake Disaster Phases	
Disaster Phase	**Key Strategies**
Response	
Incident command	• Initial uncoordinated individual rescue efforts • Fire: mobilize for multiple fires • Utilities: inspect and shut down breaches • Water: inspect dams and pipes • Transport: clear blocked roads, inspect bridges and tunnels • Airport: evaluate runways and communications • Hospitals: enact disaster plan • Police: maintain social order • Hazardous materials: respond to breaches • Schools, stadiums, malls, parks: convert into shelters • Communications: reestablish phone and data links • Construction entities: mobilize for rescue operations
Immediate medical response	• Simple triage and rapid treatment • Rescuer self-deployment • Hospital conversion to disaster mode • Seek buried survivors
Humanitarian response	• Shelter: designate temporary and internally displaced persons (IDP) camps • Nutrition: ensure food security and supply chain • Health: set up mobile clinics • Water and sanitation: arrange stable systems • Protection: ensure adequate security forces • Education: create interim schools for children, teach adults skills pertinent to recovery • Telecommunications: establish stable links • Reconstruction planning: organize recovery operations • Funding: secure donor and other sources
Recovery	• Rebuilding: ensure safely undertaken • Relocation: empty and remove IDP camps
Mitigation	
	• Building codes: ensure sound rebuilding • Zoning laws: strategize building in high-risk areas • Preparedness and planning: see beginning of this table

INTERNET RESOURCES

Individual Earthquake Preparedness Information

Are You Prepared?: San Francisco-based Web site with earthquake preparedness information designed for the public
www.72hours.org

CDC Earthquake Preparedness Information: Earthquake information for the public as well as for clinicians and disaster preparedness coordinators
www.bt.cdc.gov/disasters/earthquakes

FEMA Earthquake Preparedness Information: General information designed for the public
www.fema.gov/areyouready/earthquakes.shtm

Community Earthquake Preparedness Information

International Federation of Red Cross and Red Crescent (IFRC) Societies, Disaster Management Resources: Provides extensive practical information for community-level disaster response implementation
www.ifrc.org/what/disasters/resources/publications.asp#dmtp

National Earthquake Hazard Reduction Program (NEHRP): U.S. federal research and implementation program with multiple online publications regarding community- and government-level earthquake planning and response
www.nehrp.gov/library/response.htm

Earthquake Data

Office of U.S. Foreign Disaster Assistance (OFDA): Provides information about current and past disasters to which OFDA has responded
www.usaid.gov/our_work/humanitarian_assistance/disaster_assistance

U.S. Geological Survey: Extensive earthquake data source
www.usgs.gov/hazards/earthquakes

NOTES

1. Hicks EK, Pappas G. Coordinating disaster relief after the South Asia Earthquake. *Society*. July/August 2006.
2. Ozerdem A. The mountain tsunami: Afterthoughts on the Kashmir earthquake. *Third World Quarterly*. 2006;27(3):397–419.
3. McGirk J. Kashmir: The politics of an earthquake. *Open Democracy*. October 19, 2005. Available at: http://www.opendemocracy.net. Accessed July 25, 2008.
4. Schultz CH, Koenig KL, Noji EK. A medical disaster response to reduce immediate mortality after an earthquake. *New England Journal of Medicine*. 1996:334(7):438–444.

5. United Nations, Office of Coordination of Humanitarian Affairs. Pakistan: Interview with UN Humanitarian Coordinator, Jan Vandemoortele. *IRIN News.* September 7, 2006. Available at: http://www.irinnews.org/report.aspx?reportid=29402. Accessed July 25, 2008.

6. U.S. Geological Survey Earthquake Hazards Program. Available at: http://earthquake.usgs.gov. Accessed July 25, 2008.

7. Wong E. A Chinese school, shored up by its principal, survived where others fell. *International Herald Tribune.* June 15, 2008. Available at: http://www.iht.com/articles/2008/06/15/asia/quake.php. Accessed July 25, 2008.

8. Sina.*Casualties of the Wenchuan Earthquake.* June 8, 2008. Available at: http://english.sina.com. Accessed July 25, 2008.

9. Hanks TC, Kanamori H. A moment magnitude scale. *Journal of Geophysical Research.* 1979; 84(B5):2348–2350.

10. Bilham R. Urban earthquake fatalities: A safer world, or worse to come? *Seismological Research Letters.* 2004;75:706–712.

11. Bilham R. Earthquakes and urban growth. *Nature.* 1988;336:625–626.

12. Hou JJ, Han MK, Chai BL, Han HY. Geomorphological observations of active faults in the epicentral region of the Huaxian large earthquake in 1556 in Shaanxi Province, China. *Journal of Structural Geology.* 1998;20(5):549–557.

13. Montagne R. Remembering the 1906 San Francisco earthquake. *Morning Edition Report*, National Public Radio. April 11, 2006. Available at: http://www.npr.org/templates/story/story.php?storyId=5334411. Accessed July 25, 2008.

14. 1906 archives. Museum of the City of San Francisco. Available at: http://www.sfmuseum.org/1906.2/arson.html. Accessed July 25, 2008.

15. 1906 archives. Museum of the City of San Francisco. Available at: http://www.sfmuseum.org/1906.2/killproc.html. Accessed July 25, 2008.

16. Allen RM, Kanamori H. The potential for earthquake early warning in Southern California. *Science.* 2003;300(5620):786–789.

17. Shou Z. The Haicheng earthquake and its prediction. *Science and Utopya.* 1999;65:34.

18. Yauck J. Confirming a Chinese earthquake prediction. *Geotimes.* June 26, 2006.

19. Fraser-Smith AC, Bernardi A, McGill PR, Ladd ME, Helliwell RA, Villard OG. Low-frequency magnetic field measurements near the epicenter of the Ms 7.1 Loma Prieta earthquake. *Geophysical Research Letters.* 1990;17(9):1465–1468.

20. Karakelian D, Beroza GC, Klemperer SL, Fraser-Smith AC. Analysis of ultra-low frequency electromagnetic field measurements associated with the 1999 M 7.1 Hector Mine earthquake sequence. *Bulletin of the Seismological Society of America.* 2002;92:1513–1524.

21. California Education Code, Section 35295.

22. Shaw R, Shiwaku K, Kobayashi H, Kobayashi M. Linking experience, education, perception, and earthquake preparedness. *Disaster Prevention and Management.* 2004;13(1):39–49.

23. Los Angeles Fire Department. Emergency preparedness handbook. Available at: http://lafd.org/eqbook.pdf. Accessed July 25, 2008.

24. California Governor's Office of Emergency Services. Preparedness tips. Available at: http://www.oes.ca.gov/WebPage/oeswebsite.nsf/ClientOESFileLibrary/Emergency%20Public%20Information/$file/Family.pdf. Accessed July 25, 2008.

25. American Red Cross. Disaster services: Earthquakes. Available at: http://www.redcross.org/ services/disaster/0,1082,0_583_,00.html. Accessed July 25, 2008.

26. Red Cross focuses on disaster preparedness one year after Gujarat earthquake. *Canadian Red Cross National News Releases.* January 24, 2002. Available at: http://www.redcross.ca/article .asp?id=763&tid=001. Accessed July 25, 2008.

27. Community Emergency Response Team. Available at: www.citizencorps.gov/cert. Accessed July 25, 2008.

28. United States Government National Earthquake Hazards Reduction Program. *Expanding and using knowledge to reduce earthquake losses: Strategic plan 2001–2005.* March 2003.

29. Office of Emergency Services, San Luis Obispo County, California. *County of San Luis Obispo earthquake emergency response plan.* August 2005.

30. Government of Alaska. State of Alaska emergency response plan, 2004. Available at: http:// www.ak-prepared.com/plans/acrobat_docs/Alaska_Emergency_Response_Plan.pdf. Accessed July 25, 2008.

31. Weeks MR. Organizing for disaster: Lessons from the military. *Business Horizons.* 2007;50: 479–489.

32. Chemical plants hit by Chinese earthquake. *Chemweek Business Daily.* May 13, 2008. Available at: http://www.chemweek.com/newsletters/cbd/11886.html. Accessed July 25, 2008.

33. Cargo train derails in NW China after earthquake. *People's Daily.* May 13, 2008. Available at: http://english.people.com.cn/90001/90776/90882/6409388.html. Accessed July 25, 2008.

34. Newsroom new images: Lake formation in the aftermath of magnitude 7.9 earthquake. *NASA Earth Observatory News.* May 19, 2008. Available at: http://earthobservatory.nasa.gov/Newsroom/ NewImages/images.php3?img_id=18034&rc=3. Accessed July 25, 2008.

35. Riminton H. Stadium becomes tent city after quake. *CNN News.* May 21, 2008. Available at: http://edition.cnn.com/2008/WORLD/asiapcf/05/21/china.refugee.center/index.html. Accessed July 25, 2008.

36. de Bruycker M, Greco D, Annino I, et al. The 1980 earthquake in southern Italy: Rescue of trapped victims and mortality. *Bulletin of the World Health Organization.* 1983;61:1021–1025.

37. Halbert RJ, Simon RR, Nasraty Q. Surgical training model for advanced emergency medics in Afghanistan. *Annals of Emergency Medicine.* 1988;17:779–784.

38. Handwerk B. Rescue dogs' work a serious "game." *National Geographic News.* August 15, 2002. Available at: http://news.nationalgeographic.com/news/2002/08/0815_020815_rescuedogs .html. Accessed July 25, 2008.

39. Kamegawa T, Yamasaki T, Igarashi H, Matsuno F. Development of the snake-like rescue robot. *Proceedings of the IEEE International Conference on Robotics and Automation.* 2004;5:5081–5086.

40. Vanholder R, et al. Earthquakes and crush syndrome casualties: Lessons learned from the Kashmir disaster. *Kidney International.* 2007;71:17–23.

41. More than 4.8 million homeless in Sichuan quake: official. *Agence France Presse.* May 16, 2008. Available at: http://www.reliefweb.int/rw/RWB.NSF/db900SID/PANA-7EPG6V?OpenDocument. Accessed July 25, 2008.

42. United Nations, Office of Coordination of Humanitarian Affairs. OCHA in 2006: OCHA at work: Humanitarian response reform. Available at: http://ochaonline.un.org/ocha2006/ chap6_6.htm. Accessed July 26, 2008.

43. Basoglu M, et al. Traumatic stress responses in survivors of earthquake in Turkey. *Journal of Traumatic Stress*. 2002;15:269–276.

44. Basoglu M, et al. Single-session behavioral treatment of earthquake-related posttraumatic stress using an earthquake simulator: A randomized waiting list controlled trial. *Psychological Medicine*. 2007;37:203–213.

45. Alexander D. The study of natural disasters, 1977–1997: Some reflections on a changing field of knowledge. *Disasters*. 1997;21(4):284–304.

46. Bamforth T, Qureshi JH. Political complexities of humanitarian intervention in the Pakistan earthquake. *Journal of Humanitarian Assistance*. January 16, 2007.

47. Lupini L. The South Asia earthquake: Rebuilding lives for survivors. *UN Chronicle Online Edition*. January 4, 2007. Available at: http://www.un.org/Pubs/chronicle/2007/webArticles/010407_saeq.htm. Accessed July 25, 2008.

48. World Health Organization, Collaborating Centre for Research on the Epidemiology of Disasters. EM-DAT emergency events database: Disasters list. Available at: http://www.emdat.be/Database/DisasterList/list.php. Accessed July 25, 2008.

49. Lynch C. Donations slowing as disasters mount worldwide. *Washington Post*. October 16, 2005.

50. McIntyre M. Pakistan: Shelter for earthquake survivors involves more than tents. *Refugees International*. December 20, 2005. Available at: http://www.refugeesinternational.org/content/article/detail/7568. Accessed July 25, 2008.

51. Oxfam International. Anniversary of Pakistan earthquake: Earthquake survivors at risk as Himalayan winter starts early. October 3, 2006. Available at: http://www.oxfam.org/en/news/pressreleases2006/pr061004_pakistan_quake. Accessed July 25, 2008.

CHAPTER 20

Hurricanes, Tsunamis, and Cyclones

Elizabeth DeVos

INTRODUCTION

With increasing development in coastal areas around the world, the threat to human life and health due to hurricanes, cyclones, and tsunamis continues to increase. While prediction models and warning mechanisms have improved, public health initiatives in preparedness, response, and mitigation are still necessary to reduce morbidity and mortality related to these events. Public health preparedness entails an understanding of the hazards that will burden a community affected by these storms, with the goal being to implement physical precautions to limit structural hazards, appropriate coordination of medical services, and, if necessary, evacuation. By utilizing federal, state, and local plans to ensure adequate reserves and mobilization of necessary resources, the need for supplies can be anticipated, and the necessary items can be organized and stockpiled so that they are available in the event of such an occurrence. Planning for healthcare facilities should include not only procedures for operations during a storm, but also those operations needed during an evacuation. Finally, public health officials will need to provide targeted risk communication to educate both the media and the public so as to optimize health outcomes. As local resources are rarely augmented by state or local assistance until three days after the event occurs, community-level organization is essential immediately after the event until later aid can be distributed through coordinated responses.

Response to hurricanes and other tropical storms requires anticipation of increased healthcare needs and at least temporary delivery of services in austere conditions. Frequently, communication, water, and electrical systems are disrupted, creating challenges to delivery of home- and hospital-based health care, recovery efforts, and daily activities. These disruptions, in addition to natural hazards such as flooding and wind-induced injuries, frequently shape the pattern of healthcare requests seen after a hurricane's impact.

Mitigation of future tropical storm–related morbidity and mortality requires learning from previous events. The actions taken to minimize a hurricane's effects on a community include risk communication, development of social support networks, and provision of direct medical care. This chapter explores opportunities to improve future public health efforts based on the strengths and weaknesses of responses to hurricanes, tropical cyclones, and tsunamis in recent history.

Case Study

In U.S. history, no natural disaster has caused more damage and devastation than Hurricane Katrina. This massive storm claimed at least 1,833 lives and caused an estimated $125 billion in damages.[1]

Katrina originated as a tropical depression southeast of the Bahamas on August 23, 2005. Over the next two days, the storm strengthened to a tropical storm and moved through the Bahamas, made landfall as a Category 1 hurricane in Miami, and continued gathering strength as it barreled through the Gulf of Mexico. Katrina eventually reached its maximum intensity as a Category 5 hurricane approximately 250 miles south–southeast of the mouth of the Mississippi River. More than a foot of rain from the storm doused Florida on August 25. Winds reached maximums of 175 miles per hour (mph) and pressures as low as 902 millibars (mb) were recorded. Katrina made its second landfall as a Category 3 hurricane in Plaquemines Parish, Louisiana, with winds of approximately 125 mph just after 6 A.M. on August 29, 2005. Still a Category 3 storm with winds of 120 mph, it struck again at the Louisiana–Mississippi border at 9:45 A.M. Throughout the Gulf Coast, storm surges of 23 to 28 feet were recorded. After breaching of levees and floodwalls, approximately 80 percent of the city of New Orleans, Louisiana, flooded. The storm continued as a hurricane approximately 100 miles inland; its wind speeds did not diminish to the tropical storm level until it reached the Ohio Valley on August 30.[2]

HISTORICAL PERSPECTIVES

Hurricanes plague the Atlantic and Eastern Pacific Oceans, typhoons devastate the Western Pacific, and cyclones occur in areas of the Indian Ocean and Southern Pacific. Known throughout the world by different names, all of these storms arise when low-pressure weather systems lacking a "front" occur. These tropical storms are characterized by a warm core and organized circulation. They originate over ocean waters with temperatures at least 27°C, a depth of approximately 46 m, and, typically, at least 480 km from the equator. These storms also require a quickly cooling atmosphere that is unlikely to support moist convection, a disturbance of the water near the surface, and vertical wind shear values approximately 37 km per hour or less between the surface and the troposphere. When these specific atmospheric conditions are met, devastating storms develop.[3,4]

Hurricanes in the United States and Atlantic Basin

In the United States, hurricane season occurs from June 1 to November 30 each year. In an average season, 11 named storms, 6 hurricanes, and 2 major hurricanes are observed. In 2005, records were broken for number of hurricanes (15 versus 12 in 1969) as well as number reaching Category 5 intensity (Emily, Katrina, Rita, and Wilma). Never since recordkeeping began in 1891 have four Category 5 hurricanes been witnessed in one season. The year 2005 also was notable as the first time in which the Greek alphabet was employed to name storms after the English alphabet was exhausted.[2]

The Saffir-Simpson Hurricane Scale was developed to rate the intensity of a storm and to estimate the conceivable property damage and flooding that may occur due to a hurricane landfall. While wind speed primarily determines the divisions of the scale, the category of the storm also relates to storm surge and a storm's propensity for property damage. As wind speed increases, the destructive capacity increases exponentially. Each of the five categories is summarized in Table 20-1.[5]

In recorded U.S. history, only three Category 5 Hurricanes have made landfall on U.S. soil: the Labor Day Hurricane of 1935, Hurricane Camille (1969), and Hurricane Andrew (1992). The Labor Day Hurricane of 1935 also holds the distinction of producing the lowest observed pressure when it struck the Florida Keys with a pressure of 892 mb. Hurricane Camille, though it took a path similar to that followed by Hurricane Katrina, was more compact and spread only 75 miles (as compared to at least 100 miles for Katrina) from the center, also known as the eye of the storm. Camille, with winds up to 190 mph, caused much more localized damage and storm surges of 25 feet onto the Mississippi Gulf Coast.[1] Prior to Katrina, Hurricane Andrew was the costliest U.S. hurricane. Andrew made landfall in August 1992, just south of Miami, Florida, and caused $43.7 billion in damage in Florida alone. Whereas Katrina struck Florida as a Category 1 storm and then strengthened over the Gulf of Mexico, Andrew remained at hurricane force, though weakening as it passed through the Gulf of Mexico, and made a second landfall in Louisiana as a Category 3 storm.

TABLE 20-1   Characteristics of Hurricanes

Category	Average Wind Speed	Storm Surge	Expected Damages	Flooding Time Before Epicenter Arrival	Flooding at Sea Level and Inland	U.S. Examples
1	74–95 mph	4–5 ft	Negligible building damage. Damage to unanchored mobile homes and vegetation. Minor pier damage and coastal road flooding.	None	None	Hurricane Gaston, 2004
2	96–110 mph	6–8 ft	Roof, door, window damage. Significant mobile home and vegetation damage. Moorings break on unprotected small craft.	2–4 hours	None	Hurricane Frances, 2004; Hurricane Isabel, 2003
3	111–130 mph	9–12 ft	Minor curtainwall failure on smaller buildings. Large trees blown down. Destroyed mobile homes and signage. Flood and floating debris damage.	3–5 hours	Inland floods up to 8 miles for terrain less than 5 ft above sea level.	Hurricane Jeanne, 2004; Hurricane Ivan, 2004
4	131–155 mph	13–18 ft	Roof failure of small buildings. All vegetation and mobile homes blown down.	3–5 hours	Massive evacuation need. Flooding up to 6 miles for terrain less than 10 ft above sea level.	Hurricane Charley, 2004; Hurricane Dennis, 2005
5	>155 mph	>18 ft	Complete roof failure of many industrial buildings and complete building failures. All vegetation blown down. Extensive damage.	3–5 hours	Major damage to buildings less than 15 ft above sea level and less than 500 yd from shore. Massive evacuation required within 5–10 miles of shoreline.	Labor Day Hurricane of 1935; Hurricane Camille, 1969; Hurricane Andrew, 1992

Source: Adapted from National Oceanic and Atmospheric Administration, http://www.nhc.noaa.gov/aboutsshs.shtml.

Hurricanes in succession also cause significant hazards in the United States. In 2004, four noteworthy storms—Charley (August 2004, Category 4), Frances (September 2004, Category 2), Ivan (September 2004, Category 3), and Jeanne (September 2004, Category 3)—pummeled the Florida coastline and contributed to significant death and destruction throughout the United States as a result of flooding and storm surges. The most devastating season, however, occurred in 2005. Hurricane Dennis (July 2005) made landfall along the Florida and Alabama coasts as a Category 3 storm, causing approximately $2 billion in damages (mostly due to wind). When Hurricane Katrina struck the Gulf Coast as a Category 3 storm in August 2005, it had already struck land in Miami as a Category 1 storm. Surges exceeding 25 feet along with the levee failures caused widespread flooding in New Orleans and throughout the region, leading to $125 billion in damages and causing approximately 1,833 deaths, the most since a "major hurricane" in Florida in 1928. Hurricane Rita (September 2005) struck the Texas–Louisiana border and produced significant wind damage and storm surges into the Florida Panhandle region. Damages from this storm approached $17 billion, and the death toll soared to 119 (many related to evacuations). Hurricane Wilma (October 2005) struck southwest Florida as a Category 3 storm after earning the distinction of being the strongest Atlantic tropical storm ever registered, producing the lowest pressure on record (882 mb) prior to its landfall. This storm claimed 35 lives and caused $17.1 billion in damages.[1]

Cyclones

Holland and Neumann help to define cyclones as tropical storms that match the previous description, but are located in the South Pacific and Indian Oceans, and usually seen in the local summer season (between November 1 and April 30 each year).[4] On average, nine cyclones occur in a given season, with approximately half of those reaching at least a Category 3 designation. In review of recent events, it is clear that most frequent and most devastating tropical storms occur in the Americas and Asia; however, they can occur throughout the entire world.[6]

The degree of a storm's effects may vary in both economic and human losses in different parts of the world (Table 20-2). The cyclone with the largest recorded death toll made landfall in what is now Bangladesh in November 1970. Cyclone Bhola is responsible for as many as 500,000 deaths. While the winds from this cyclone reached only Category 3 intensity, the storm surge flooded the Ganges delta and surrounding islands.[7] In August 1975, Nina—a particularly terrible cyclone—devastated the Henan Province of China. In three days, record rainfalls across more than 30 percent of the province caused the collapse of at least 12 reservoirs, leading to floodwaters

TABLE 20-2 Morbidity and Mortality of Tropical Storms by Continent, 2000–2009				
	Hurricane/ Cyclone	Number of Events	Number of People Killed	Total Number of People Affected	Damage (thousands of dollars)
Africa	Tropical	38	1,041	4,171,305	681,431
	Average per event		27	109,771	17,932
Americas	Tropical	181	8,336	25,661,154	290,528,371
	Average per event		46	141,774	1,605,129
Asia	Tropical	234	155,113	192,531,628	79,725,682
	Average per event		663	822,785	340,708
Europe	Extra-tropical	35	81	4,394	16,750,050
	Average per event		2	126	478,573
	Tropical	6	43	62	381,050
	Average per event		7	10	63,508
Oceania	Tropical	42	287	332,635	1,879,806
	Average per event		7	7,920	44,757

reaching 30 feet. Direct economic losses totaled $1.2 billion and almost 100,000 fatalities occurred as a result of the storm. This is just one severe example of the approximately 8.8 cyclones that affect China on an annual basis; China is the country with the most frequent cyclones making landfall each year. The cyclone with the greatest overall impact recorded was Tropical Cyclone Tracy, which struck Darwin, Australia, on December 25, 1974. It caused approximately $2.5 billion in damages, and the town of 45,000 occupants required evacuation by air.[8]

Tsunamis

A tsunami consists of a series of waves created by an abrupt oceanic disturbance such as an earthquake. The movement of the oceanic floor results in a series of waves whose wavelengths, amplitudes, and directionality are influenced by the earth's movement, the degree of ocean floor displacement, and characteristics of the affected coastline. Most tsunamis occur in the Pacific Ocean, due to the shifting of light continental plates over more dense oceanic tectonic plates.

The local tsunami (i.e., the portion of the wave transmitted toward shore) gains amplitude and decreases its wavelength as it nears the coast. A trough in the wave pattern is first to reach shore and is observed as a recession of the tide. Typically, tsunamis do not produce breaking waves but rather a series of powerful surges and quickly moving tides. The run-up, or water level increase versus the standard sea level, first approaches and in some cases produces a vertical wall of water known as a bore. These waves travel much farther inland than typical tides and inflict damage by flooding, development of currents, and transport of debris. The energy of the run-up is then returned into the sea and can create further waves and destruction, often with larger waves than the initial run-up lasting for several hours.[9]

While no one can predict exactly when a tsunami will occur, since 1946 the tsunami warning system has monitored seismic data and coastal tides and sought to issue warnings in case of possible tsunami formation. This system cannot, however, identify the location where a tsunami will strike or the characteristics of arriving waves (the latter are shaped by local harbor and coastline contours). Monitoring of earthquakes and tide levels in addition to new deep-ocean tsunami detectors to collect real-time data in tsunami propagation will help to develop ever-improving systems to forecast tsunamis and guide onshore responses such as evacuations.[9]

A particularly devastating loss of life and destruction of property occurred in the Indian Ocean when an earthquake with a momentary magnitude of 9.0 occurred approximately 160 km from Sumatra, on Indonesia's western coast.[10] More than 230,000 deaths occurred throughout Indonesia, Sri Lanka, South India, and Thailand as a result of the massive Sumatra–Andaman Islands earthquake.[11] Waves as high as 15 m hit the region, contributing to the large number of deaths and massive destruction. Children and women were less likely to withstand the strong waves; most survivors presented acutely for extremity injuries, soft-tissue wounds, fractures, and respiratory complaints. One important medical complaint seen by rescue health workers was "tsunami lung": aspiration pneumonia induced by the inhalation of the debris-laden sea water. Medical teams also reported tetanus exacerbated by low underlying vaccination rates and worldwide shortage of immunoglobulin for treatment when recovery-associated injuries occurred.[12] In one study, nearly one fourth of patients presenting to post-tsunami outpatient departments reported at least four of seven depression/post-traumatic stress disorder (PTSD) symptoms in a questionnaire, although only 1.4 percent were formally diagnosed with mental health problems.[13] These figures highlight the need for public health workers to increase their expectations of mental distress after these events and the need for psychological first aid to augment other public health and medical services provided in the aftermath of these natural disasters.

Analysis of recent Asian disasters has shown that foreign assistance is generous but often untimely or inappropriate. Mobile hospitals often arrive too late to provide primary trauma care, foreign medical providers may not add to logistical support, and donations are frequently inappropriate, leading to additional costs for destruction of these goods. However well intentioned, the private agendas of governments, organizations, or individuals can hinder progress if not aligned with and adapted to the receiving community. While the economic costs of the Asian tsunami disaster (estimated at $9.9 billion) were far lower than the $13.5 billion collected in international aid, lack of evidence-based decision making, needs assessment, and coordination of care led to a hindrance rather than support of a return to normalcy for the health system in many of the tsunami-affected nations.[14] For example, reports have documented Achenese physicians and medical students choosing not to return to work when they discovered that they could earn better daily wages while translating for international humanitarian and aid agencies that arrived to respond to the disaster rather than providing direct medical care. This loss of trained healthcare professionals slowed the reinstatement of the local health system and encouraged dependence on outside relief.[15]

PREPAREDNESS AND PLANNING

Advances in meteorology have improved forecasting of hurricanes over the last 25 years.[16] Computer-based models, statistical methods, and prediction rules have improved seasonal forecasting ability significantly; however, little progress has been achieved in the ability to predict the birth and path of a specific storm. While warning systems and satellite tracking technology have clearly improved the ability of local emergency managers to make provisions and to warn residents of impending impacts, the warning is valid only on the order of days at best. Further, engineering has improved the ability to prevent damage from storms, including the enhancement of structures in hurricane-prone areas to withstand high winds and floodwater management systems such as levees. Additional preparations such as covering windows, trimming vegetation, and securing items such as furniture and boats likely to become projectiles in a hurricane can further assist in readying a community for the onslaught of a hurricane.

Hazards expected in a hurricane include storm surge, high winds, tornados, and inland flooding. Storm surge refers to water forced ashore by the powerful hurricane-strength winds. Such surges have an additive effect upon normal tides and increase the mean water level, often resulting in severe coastal flooding. While wind speeds influence storm surges, the slope of the continental shelf is also an important factor. Typically, the more shallow the slope of the continental shelf and the closer a community is to the right-front quadrant of the hurricane, the greater the potential for damage and the larger the area that must be evacuated. In recent years, significant population growth and building development have occurred along the Atlantic and Gulf coastlines of the United States in areas less than 10 feet above mean sea level; all of these communities are at especially high risk for surges with perilous water levels. Emergency public health planners have been advised to assume that a storm one category higher than that forecast will occur when determining evacuation thresholds. When an evacuation is ordered, citizens should follow predetermined evacuation routes, follow instructions on the National Oceanic and Atmospheric Administration (NOAA) weather radios, and expect congestion in traffic.

In addition to flooding, the surge currents created by these now-inland tides can erode roads and building foundations that initially withstood the impact of a hurricane. Further, the presence of saltwater flooding can upset natural habitats and send animals, such as snakes, into urban areas, where they can pose additional hazards to humans.

High winds are another hazard related to hurricanes. The winds associated with a Category 4 storm are expected to cause 100 times the damages of the winds of a Category 1 storm.[17] Even at sub-hurricane levels, tropical storm-force winds can be dangerous to those who have not sought appropriate shelter. Poorly constructed buildings, unsecured structures such as mobile homes, signs, blown-out windows, and trees and shrubbery are all expected to be disrupted by hurricane-force winds. Care to avoid projectiles such as signs and branches propelled by the storm is essential. Furthermore, hurricane-force winds tend to increase with increasing height; thus those persons sheltered in high-rise buildings should stay below the tenth floor while maintaining adequate elevation to avoid flooding. Similar to storm surge, hurricane-force winds are usually strongest on the right side of the storm's "eyewall." These winds decrease significantly within the first 12 hours following the storm's landfall but can cause significant destruction far inland. For example, in 1989, Charlotte, North Carolina. suffered wind gusts of up to 100 mph from Hurricane Hugo; the city was located 175 miles inland from the hurricane's landfall.[17]

While models to approximate inland wind patterns exist, they rely on forecasts that only become accurate at times close to the tropical storm's landfall. Covering windows, reinforcing garage doors, and trimming vegetation are all essential steps to minimize damage from these high winds. Meeting building codes and identifying "safe rooms" prior to any storm are other essential preventive measures to help residents endure these high winds.

Like the other perilous weather elements of hurricanes, tornados are most likely to occur in the right-front quadrant of a hurricane, though they are frequently seen throughout the storm. More than half of all hurricanes produce at least one tornado. Usually tornado development is a result of remaining low-pressure circulation after the landfall of a hurricane; this weather pattern may persist for a few days after a hurricane's landfall. Although the tornados associated with hurricanes are typically not as strong as those produced in the Great Plains region of the United States, they are unlikely to be accompanied by hail and lightning storms—which serve as warning signs for non-hurricane-related tornados.[18] Preparation is crucial for these events: Even with Doppler radar technology, a warning is rarely available more than 30 minutes before a tornado strikes. Preparedness for tornados includes assuring access to a pre-identified safe structure in an interior room away from windows and access to a NOAA weather radio for instructions and warnings.

According to Ed Rappaport of the National Hurricane Center, between 1970 and 1999, inland flooding caused more deaths associated with tropical cyclones than any other hazard.[19,20] The degree of rainfall associated with a hurricane has less to do with wind speed and more to do with the progression of a storm's tropical air mass. Storms that stall over an area can produce significant flooding in a short time span, threatening communities hundreds of miles from the site of the hurricane's landfall. For example, Hurricane Camille dropped 27 inches of rain on Virginia in 8 hours in 1969, directly causing 112 deaths.[1,20] Freshwater flooding caused 59 percent of all U.S. tropical cyclone deaths between 1970 and 1999; nearly 25 percent of those deaths were the result of drowning associated with motor vehicles.[19,20] Essentials of preparedness include knowledge of potential flood zones and public education to warn motorists to avoid attempts to drive across any flowing water. Knowledge of one's insurance coverage is also useful, as most homeowners' insurance policies do not include flood damage, though the federally backed National Flood Insurance Program allows pre-disaster mitigation and protection.

In the United States, business leaders and public health workers have formally collaborated to assure that resources will be available, when necessary, to distribute national caches of emergency supplies known as the Strategic National Stockpile. In addition to providing supplies, businesses may be able to offer storage space, distribution and communication systems, transportation, and personnel with expertise to assist in the event of a public health emergency. In Georgia, model exercises for dispensing resources have been met with great interest and have highlighted strengths and weaknesses of the system prior to its activation so that continual improvements in planning may occur.[21] This effort meets a community desire for involvement while providing much needed resources to often strained public health systems.

In addition to experiencing the direct threats posed by the previously discussed hazards, residents of hurricane-prone areas are at risk for medical problems related to loss of electricity or disruption of services related to evacuations. The Centers for Disease Control and Prevention (CDC) has recommended that everyone download from the CDC Web site a "Keep It with You" medical record form that can serve as a temporary medical record to facilitate replacements and refills of daily medications and to assist with ongoing medical care if it must be arranged away from home.[22] Other challenges associated with managing chronic medical conditions in the aftermath of a tropical storm include maintenance of a cold chain for insulin, availability of power for hemodialysis, and provision of mechanical ventilation in situations where electricity is intermittent or unavailable. While injuries will cause many initial requests for care, public health professionals will need to plan for chronic medical care resulting in a significant number of healthcare visits. During Hurricane Katrina, for example, several off-site triage and shelter or other off-site primary care clinics provided services for evacuees and attempted to alleviate the surge in emergency departments (ED) across the affected regions.[23–26]

One review of collaborative emergency management strategies following the four hurricanes that struck Florida in 2004 emphasized the essential nature of coordinating community resources to ensure appropriate public preparedness. Because a lack of access to information may occur if electricity outages limit access to outlets such as radio and Internet communication, the public must be well aware of risks before a disaster occurs. Recommendations must be consistent and transparent if appropriate action is to occur. Further attempts to balance the number of warnings and recommendations associated with true threats so as to limit the number of "false alarms" must be taken for citizens to heed warnings. Finally, behavioral research has shown that humans will minimize risks when they believe that the recommendations for response seem unachievable; thus empowering residents to take actions in stepwise manners may help to ensure that preparedness activities are carried out.[24]

Further, risk communication directed to patients could decrease post-hurricane ED visits by ensuring appropriate tetanus booster vaccination coverage prior to the event, communicating that the vaccine is not compulsory after disasters, and encouraging residents to maintain emergency medical kits with supplies of critical medications. Community education emphasizing injury prevention for evacuees and relief workers as well as inclusion of prescriptions for refills and a supply of critical medications as a part of an evacuation kit can also improve public health outcomes. Moreover, specific hazards should be reviewed prior to allowing residents to reenter an evacuated area.[25]

Another important consideration regarding risk communication is the importance of media education prior to a public health emergency, so as to avoid perpetuating myths, inciting undue panic, or possibly wasting precious resources. For those persons who are trapped at home, newscasts may be the primary source of information regarding a disaster. Infectious disease epidemics are frequently broadcast as major concerns; in reality, diseases that are not endemic in a community by principles of epidemiology do not produce an outbreak risk. Thus, in the United States, typhoid and cholera are not concerns following a tropical storm. Human remains present low risk for disease transmission and can actually decrease the burden of infectious disease in a population as the carriers are eliminated.[27,28] Appropriate media education prior to a hurricane allows anticipation and debunking of common myths, thereby ensuring the efficient delivery of useful information to those most in need of instruction following such an event.[28]

Public health preparedness is also an excellent time for the formation of public–private partnerships to enhance response capability. As with any disaster, appropriate effective communication is repeatedly noted as an important factor in preparedness, response, and mitigation for hurricanes and other tropical storms. Coordination of response and communication through an emergency response center allows the most effective use of all resources—human and material—and ensures a unified message to the community. Through this organization, prior to hurricane season, resources and information can be shared to capitalize on lessons from prior experiences and to develop public- and private-sector leadership and plans built via consensus to bolster resiliency in the community.[29] As the Florida Division of Emergency Management has stated, "Achieving and maintaining citizen and community preparedness reduces the immediate demands on response organizations."[30]

According to the Federal Emergency Management Agency (FEMA), a Disaster Medical Assistance Team (DMAT) is a group of volunteers from a state or region who serve as a medical response team under the guidance of the national disaster medical system or similar local authority. Because they may be deployed to federally declared disaster areas, these medical teams represent another important component of preparedness for hurricanes and other such events.[31] Within this structure, medical and nonmedical personnel participate in ongoing disaster response and management training, maintain caches of supplies, and can be activated in the event of a public health emergency to augment local resources for health care, often within hours of a call. An analysis of DMAT deployments between 1985 and 2002 revealed 50 deployments in the United

States, with the majority related to "water disasters"—namely, hurricanes and floods. As these events have represented two-thirds of all natural disasters for which DMAT teams have been deployed, preparedness for these types of events should be specifically emphasized in annual training sessions and supplies for teams.[32]

RESPONSE

In Mississippi, three counties (Hancock, Harrison, and Jackson) experienced significant disruption of public infrastructure following the onslaught of Hurricane Katrina. In fact, the Hancock County Emergency Operations Center experienced a storm surge of approximately 27 feet. Consequently, many hospitals and clinics in the area were inoperable or destroyed following the storm's impact. At the request of the Mississippi Department of Health, active surveillance of acute healthcare visits in the three counties with the greatest damage from Hurricane Katrina occurred in emergency departments, federal DMAT operation sites, and outpatient healthcare facilities. Daily reports of patient visits from September 5 to 11, 2005, resulted in collection of data for 11,424 patient visits. One facility saw 183.6 percent more visits in the ED during the study week as compared to the week prior to the hurricane. Approximately 4 percent of patients were admitted and 0.05 percent died. While the largest proportion of visits (38 percent) were for injuries (30 percent of those persons were given tetanus immunization) and 36 percent were for other medical problems, another 21 percent of visits were for prescription refills only. Most illnesses were not critical; they included gastrointestinal, respiratory, and skin infections. As the week progressed, visits for prescription refills decreased and visits for injuries such as sprains and lacerations increased. Five cases of carbon monoxide poisoning were also diagnosed.[33]

Periodic surveillance continued from September 12 to October 11, 2005. During this span, another 27,135 visits were recorded. The greatest proportion of the visits (21.8 percent) was for injuries, with 91.6 percent of those being minor. Upper respiratory infections (6.5 percent), bites and stings along with rashes (4.5 percent), and lower respiratory infections (2.8 percent) were the next most common reasons for patient visits. Approximately 2.5 percent of visits dealt with mental health concerns. (Not every site reported for each data collection point.[33])

One particular hazard during hurricane response is carbon monoxide (CO) poisoning, and the potential to affect entire families due to the nature of this hazard makes the threat of CO poisoning of particular public health importance. After an interruption of electricity, citizens often use generators to assist cleanup and, especially in the summer months in warm climates, to power fans and air conditioners. While the extent of generator use in the Gulf states in the wake of Hurricane Katrina is unknown, in one study 17.5 percent of Florida residents affected by the 2004 hurricane season used portable generators, 5 percent of them indoors.[34] In the Gulf states, 51 cases of CO poisoning were reported from hyperbaric facilities between August 29 and September 24, 2005. Approximately 75 percent of the reported Katrina-associated CO poisonings occurred within the first week following the hurricane's landfall. Thirty-seven patients required hyperbaric oxygen (HBO) therapy; five patients (not treated with HBO) died. Almost all of these incidents were related to improper portable generator placement, although one case report of CO poisoning associated with use of a pressure-washer was recorded.[34] Given that CO poisoning can have nonspecific symptoms (e.g., headache, weakness, nausea and vomiting, and confusion), a clinician must maintain a high index of suspicion for this life-threatening diagnosis and initiate high-flow oxygen therapy immediately to produce a good outcome.

In Orlando, Florida, an area affected by three hurricanes (Charley, Frances, and Jeanne) during the 2004 season, analysis of ED attendance corroborated prior evidence showing that there are fewer visits on the day of an acute storm, but that visits to the ED spike in the following week. Platz and colleagues attempted to identify patterns relating to the succession of storms within 6 weeks in one region. Trends in presentations were similar to those noted in prior studies, including a 112.5 percent increase in patient census in the Level I trauma hospital and a 121.3 percent increase in visits to the community hospital as compared with the prior year. Significant increases were noted in visits for neurosurgical trauma, blunt trauma and lacerations, CO intoxication and problems related to lack of electricity, or other medical needs such as oxygen or hemodialysis. Interestingly, fewer visits were made to these facilities following the second and third storms (Frances and Jeanne) than occurred after the first hurricane (Charley). Perhaps this decline was related to the establishment of field hospitals and shelter clinics, but the authors also postulated that residents became better prepared for the subsequent inland storms.[35] In this case, the recent storms may have reinforced better behavioral outcomes in both preparedness and mitigation of risks.

In response to hurricanes, difficult decisions must be made by hospital administrators and public health planners regarding evacuation of hospitals. For Hurricane Katrina, evacuation orders exempted hospitals in the city. During the storm, New Orleans hospitals housed more than 9,400 people, patients, staff, families, and others seeking refuge.[36] In preparation for the storm, many hospitals discharged ambulatory and stable patients, but there was no city or statewide plan that covered the evacuation of multiple patients from the region's institutions at risk. This omission may be related to hospitals' role as evacuation sites for nursing homes and other such facilities during major storms, reflecting the enhanced resources available at hospitals. Also, patients requiring critical care may be safest inside a hospital during a storm. If evacuation of a hospital becomes necessary, however, difficulties in securing transportation and receiving facilities increase as the storm nears. This relationship underscores the need to balance the risk to already critical patients in transport and transfer with the danger of sheltering in place if resources such as power and supply chains are lost. One New Orleans suburban hospital did, in fact, decide to evacuate all of its patients; most weathered the onslaught of Katrina in a special needs shelter when their buses could not navigate through gridlocked traffic.[36]

While evacuations are both expensive and arduous, the Katrina experience emphasizes the need for disaster protocols that address the placement and transport of human and material resources to care for patients in the event that evacuation becomes necessary. Establishment of a predefined plan for the order of evacuation of patients may prevent disagreements on evacuation triage, such as occurred during the Katrina disaster. Other lessons learned from the Katrina experience include the need to facilitate both transfer of medical records and a tracking system for evacuated patients to ensure the ability to reunite those patients who are unable to speak for themselves with relatives when it becomes appropriate. Hospitals in New Orleans housed family members of staff and patients as well as their pets during Hurricane Katrina; specific plans for the housing and evacuation of these parties should be considered in future policy as well. Attention to security needs during public health emergencies also can improve this situation.

While the availability of crucial medications, consumables, and durable medical equipment is necessary to provide an effective medical response to a disaster such as a hurricane or tsunami, both the Boxing Day Tsunami of 2004 and the Hurricane Katrina disaster highlighted the need for appropriate and coordinated response in the aftermath of such events. Well-intentioned donations that are not useful to or culturally appropriate for the affected population create unnecessary strain on the delivery system, for example. Essential items that should be included among the initial supplies include appropriate antibiotics for skin infections and respiratory complaints as well as supplies of single-agent medications to control chronic conditions such as diabetes and hypertension. Suction tubing, oxygen, nebulizers, wound care supplies, and hemodialysis are also essential initial concerns. Later, as the response continues, caches should be tailored to meet the specific needs of the affected community.[37]

Another vital component of the public health response highlighted especially by the Boxing Day Tsunami of 2004 is mental health. In Thailand, the Department of Mental Health mobilized teams to assess mental health situations and provide emergency support within 72 hours of the tsunami's impact.[38] Aid teams during the response phase focused on comprehension of disaster-induced stress and grief reactions with assistance to return to activities of daily living. In the post-impact phase of the disaster (two weeks to three months), the efforts focused on those persons who were most intensely exposed to the event, but also included other groups at risk for psychosocial distress including the elderly, bereaved persons, children, and individuals with underlying psychiatric conditions.[39] Other studies have shown rescue and aid workers also to be particularly at risk for mental health problems following a natural disaster.[40]

MITIGATION

While no amount of human effort can eliminate the health hazards posed by the arrival of a hurricane, lessons learned from the outcomes of prior storms can help to reduce this burden upon a community. Development of community health clinics where prescription refills can be written and managing low-acuity and primary-care patients away from the emergency department reduces both hospital surge and patient inconvenience. Community education campaigns in the wake of a storm, such as the one instituted in New Orleans to remind residents of proper use of portable generators, can help to avoid unnecessary morbidity and mortality. Indeed, the CDC distributed information in New Orleans through the mayor's office as well as in collaboration with generator providers and other community organizations to ensure wide distribution of CO poisoning prevention information.[34]

Capacity building for mental health has been shown to be a necessity for improvement in the management of public health in disasters. By training specialized cadres of mental health workers who are well versed in the psychosocial needs of public health emergency victims, responders can be employed early, and those at risk can be screened as a routine component of disaster outreach services. Provision of psychological first aid, including management of expectations, and provisions of comfort and assistance in locating family members can reduce stress and thus the psychological impact of an event.

Research conducted during Hurricane Katrina also explored the use of informal networks of faith-based organizations (FBOs) to provide shelter and other services outside of the official National Disaster Response Plan. Investigations revealed that this sector provided approximately 50 percent of shelters that remained open in the third week following Katrina's impact. Some advantages associated with these care providers were that they were administered by one person or small boards, so decisions could be made quickly with little bureaucratic difficulty, and they catered directly to local needs. Several FBOs had the ability to draw on key connections such as national organizations of a religious denomination, which allowed for supplies from private donations among the church's connections. Also, at the local level, the shelters worked together to distribute surplus supplies to areas where they were most needed. Most of these shelters provided for vital immediate needs but required assistance for sustainability; thus these FBO-run shelters provided appropriate local response while awaiting the mobilization of state and federal disaster resources to arrive, which may take 24–72 and 48–72 hours, respectively. Of the studied FBO-run shelters, 75 percent became American Red Cross affiliates throughout their course of existence, which allowed for resources—including financial, material, and human assistance—to be used to ensure the continued sustainability of the shelters.[40] Most of the involved FBOs had no formal disaster training and few disaster plans in place.[40] While they have provided vital services, the role of these FBOs could be enhanced with dedicated planning and earlier inclusion into the formal disaster planning of a region as well.

In the United States, public health systems often must battle for their share of limited funds and suffer from a lack of practitioners. To mitigate the effects of public health emergencies such as hurricanes, focus of attention on developing public health networks that address these problems, particularly for vulnerable groups, will help to improve overall health in the wake of these disasters. Socioeconomically disadvantaged populations have been shown to be disproportionately affected by environmental changes because they have only limited resources with which to make both protective and responsive adaptations. In the case of Hurricane Katrina, many of those persons who remained in New Orleans were unable to evacuate due to financial constraints. In one study, perceived and real financial constraints guided decisions for evacuation, and respondents waiting for month-end paychecks made statements such as the following: "The hurricane came at the wrong time. We were waiting for our payday," and "No money for gas," and "Money was hard to come by at the time."[41]

Public health programs that incorporate services directed at the medically indigent, including such persons who require mental health care, can help to limit these kinds of ill effects of a hurricane.[42] One response is to utilize mobile clinics to visit isolated vulnerable groups to assure that they are receiving adequate medical care.[43] Programs to enable structural changes such as updating construction and shuttering windows have been enacted by faith-based groups as well, in an effort to improve the baseline living conditions and resiliency of communities unable to afford such measures for future hurricanes.[44]

One author suggests that dispatch of public health personnel to distribution sites for generators may also improve morbidity related to carbon monoxide poisioning.[45] Ensuring that warning signs and verbal instructions about proper use are provided in appropriate languages, for example, can limit the risk of CO exposure for consumers.

Moreover, CO detectors, whether engineered into the machine or available as stand-alone items, could help to warn users when CO levels become dangerously high. Finally, a reminder to hospitals and others providing health care, such as clinics and DMAT teams, at the time of a storm could help to raise awareness and early detection of CO intoxication due to its nonspecific presentation.[45]

ANALYSIS OF CASE STUDY

During Hurricane Katrina, medical professionals joined together to support the health of communities in the aftermath of one of the worst natural disasters in U.S. history. While the presence of a levee system indicates that some level of civil engineering planning and preparedness has occurred in a community, that system may not prove sufficient to eliminate all risks, as this event proved. Hurricane Katrina presented many unexpected challenges that affected citizens of the Gulf Coast. Evacuations, though ordered, were limited by resources and gridlocked traffic. Even some hospital patients were forced to shelter en route to their evacuation destinations when the storm struck. When unexpected amounts of flooding crippled the generators located in the basement of Charity Hospital in New Orleans, a facility that was planned to be a refuge for nursing home and chronic needs patients became another site requiring evacuation.

In the response to the hurricane, delays in providing the needed aid highlighted the essential need for coordination of assistance efforts. DMAT teams, humanitarian organizations, and even international donors wanted to assist the victims of Katrina, yet difficulties in moving supplies and personnel to those most in need persisted. As evacuees were eventually moved throughout the region, reunification points for families, triage stations for medical concerns, and gateways to social services were established. Published accounts by healthcare workers emphasized the importance of having a system to track transported patients and their medical records, availability of medications for chronic conditions, and communication of appropriate expectations to residents.

CONCLUSION

Where hurricanes and tsunamis are concerned, the planning and preparedness phases are perhaps the most important parts of the disaster cycle. Advances in technology allow the construction of safer buildings and communities and have led to enhanced prediction and early warning schemes. Citizens at risk must learn how to respond to best protect themselves and must have adequate resources to do so, however. When these public health emergencies occur, as they inevitably do, well-orchestrated responses drawing upon the experience and resources of governmental, private, and community infrastructures to distribute supplies and human resources for meeting the essential needs of everyday life while rebuilding the community are critical. Evidence from prior storms can guide decisions about the initial supplies and expertise necessary to begin recovery; surveillance of local needs should guide the continuing response. Throughout this phase, the community should be reminded of injury prevention mechanisms and provided with access to primary care and psychological support to limit both physical and mental health consequences.

Based on the outcomes of a specific event, communities can take actions to mitigate future hurricanes' impacts. Increasing community training for disasters and utilizing public–private partnerships as well as informal networks accessible to FBOs and other community organizations to augment current disaster response systems, will provide for additional resiliency in the face of a natural disaster. Paying particular attention to vulnerable populations to assist in preparedness and to reach isolated populations during response will ensure the best outcomes for the entire community. Establishing clinics to assist with first aid, access to medication, and primary care will enable functioning emergency departments to focus on the most critical patients.

INTERNET RESOURCES

Hurricanes

National Climatic Data Center: http://www.ncdc.noaa.gov/oa/reports/billionz.html
http://www.ncdc.noaa.gov/oa/climate/severeweather/hurricanes.html

National Hurricane Center: http://www.nhc.noaa.gov/pastall.shtml

U.S. Army: http://chppm-www.apgea.army.mil/news/HurricaneResources.asp

U.S. Department of Health and Human Services:
http://www.hhs.gov/disasters/discussion/planners/playbook/hurricane/index.html
http://www.hhs.gov/disasters/discussion/planners/playbook/hurricane/actionsteps.html

U.S. Federal Emergency Management Agency, Emergency Management Institute:
http://training.fema.gov/IS/

Tsunamis

National Oceanic and Atmospheric Administration (NOAA):
http://www.tsunami.noaa.gov/basics.html
http://nctr.pmel.noaa.gov/

United Nations Educational, Scientific, and Cultural Organization (UNESCO),
Intergovernmental Oceanographic Commission: http://www.ioc-tsunami.org/

University of Southern California Tsunami Research Center:
http://www.usc.edu/dept/tsunamis/2005/index.php

U.S. Geological Survey: http://walrus.wr.usgs.gov/tsunami/basics.html

NOTES

1. Ross N, Lott T. Billion dollar US weather disasters. National Climactic Data Center. Available at: http://www.ncdc.noaa.gov/oa/reports/billionz.html. Accessed July 25, 2008.
2. National Weather Service National Hurricane Center. Tropical Weather summary—2005 Web final. Available at: http://www.nhc.noaa.gov/archive/2005/tws/MIATWSAT_nov_final.shtml. Accessed July 25, 2008.
3. Elsner JB, Kara AB. *Hurricanes of the North Atlantic: Climate and society.* New York: Oxford University Press; 1999. Available at: http://www.nhc.noaa.gov/aboutgloss.shtml. Accessed August 1, 2009.
4. Landsea C. Climate variability of tropical cyclones: Past, present and future. In Pielke R, Pielke R (Eds.), *Storms.* New York: Routledge; 2000, pp. 220–241. Available at: http://www.aoml.noaa.gov/hrd/Landsea/climvari/index.html. Accessed August 7, 2009.
5. National Weather Service National Hurricane Center. The Saffir-Simpson hurricane scale. Available at: http://www.nhc.noaa.gov/aboutsshs.shtml. Accessed July 25, 2008.
6. EM-DAT: The OFDA/CRED international disaster database. Data version v12.07. Université Catholique de Louvain, Brussels, Belgium. Available at: http://www.em-dat.net. Accessed August 7, 2009.
7. Kabir M, Saha B, Hye J. Cyclonic storm surge modelling for design of coastal polder. Institute of Water Modelling. Available at: http://www.iwmbd.org/html/PUBS/publications/P024.PDF. Accessed August 7, 2009.
8. Weyman J, Anderson-Berry L. Societal impacts of tropical cyclones. Fifth International Workshop on Tropical Cyclones. RSMC Honolulu James Cook University Center for Disaster Studies. Available at: http://www.aoml.noaa.gov/hrd/iwtc/AndersonBerry5-1.html. Accessed August 7, 2009.
9. National Oceanic and Atmospheric Administration. The tsunami story. Available at: http://www.tsunami.noaa.gov/tsunami_story.html. Accessed July 31, 2008.
10. Schiermeier Q. On the trail of destruction. *Nature.* 2005; 433:350-353.
11. State University of New York University at Buffalo Libraries. Indian Ocean tsunami disaster December 26, 2004 and aftermath. Available at: http://library.buffalo.edu/libraries/asl/guides/indian-ocean-disaster.html. Accessed July 31, 2008.
12. Bridgewater F, et al. Team Echo: Observations and lessons learned in the recovery phase of the 2004 Asian tsunami. *Prehospital and Disaster Medicine.* 2006;21(1):s20–s25.
13. Redwood-Campbell L, Riddez L. Post-tsunami medical care: Health problems encountered in the International Committee of the Red Cross Hospital in Banda Aceh, Indonesia. *Prehospital and Disaster Medicine.* 2006;21(1):s1–s7.
14. deVille de Goyet C. Health lessons learned from the recent earthquakes and tsunami in Asia. *Prehospital and Disaster Medicine.* 2007;22(1):15–21.
15. Zoraster R. Barriers to disaster coordination: Health sector coordination in Banda Aceh following the South Asia tsunami. *Prehospital and Disaster Medicine.* 2006;21(1):s13–s18.

16. Lehmiller G, Kimberlain T, Elsner J. Seasonal prediction models for North Atlantic Basin hurricane location. *Monthly Weather Review.* 1997;125:1780–1791.

17. National Hurricane Center. Hurricane preparedness: High winds. Available at: http://www.nhc.noaa.gov/HAW2/english/high_winds.shtml. Accessed July 23, 2008.

18. National Hurricane Center. Hurricane preparedness: Tornados. Available at: http://www.nhc.noaa.gov/HAW2/english/tornadoes.shtml. Accessed July 23, 2008.

19. National Hurricane Center. Leading causes of tropical cyclone deaths in the U.S. 1970–1999. Available at: http://www.nhc.noaa.gov/HAW2/english/images/cyclone_deaths.gif. Accessed July 23, 2008.

20. National Hurricane Center. Hurricane preparedness: Inland flooding. Available at: http://www.nhc.noaa.gov/HAW2/english/inland_flood.shtml. Accessed July 23, 2008.

21. Buehler J, Whitney E, Berkelman R. Business and public health collaboration for emergency preparedness in Georgia: A case study. *BMC Public Health* [serial online]. 2006;6:285. Available at: http://www.biomedcentral.com/1471-2458/6/285. Accessed July 11, 2008.

22. Centers for Disease Control and Prevention. Keep it with you: Personal medical information form. Available at: http://www.bt.cdc.gov/disasters/hurricanes/katrina/kiwy.asp. Accessed July 20, 2008.

23. Currier M, King D, Wofford M, Daniel B, deShazo R. A Katrina experience: Lessons learned. *American Journal of Medicine.* 2005;119:986–992.

24. Gavagan T, et al. Hurricane Katrina: Medical response at the Houston Astrodome/Reliant Center Complex. *Southern Medical Journal.* 2006;99(9):933–939.

25. Irvin C, Atas J. Management of evacuee surge from a disaster area: Solutions to avoid non-emergent, emergency department visits. *Prehospital and Disaster Medicine.* 2007;22(3):220–223.

26. Ridenour M, Cummings K, Sinclair J, Bixler D. Displacement of the underserved: Medical needs of Hurricane Katrina evacuees in West Virginia. *Journal of Health Care for the Poor and Underserved.* 2007;18:369–381.

27. deVille de Goyet C. Stop propagating disaster myths [editorial]. *Prehospital and Disaster Medicine.* 1999;14(4):9–10.

28. Arnold J. Disaster myths and Hurricane Katrina 2005: Can public officials and the media learn to provide responsible crisis communication during disasters? [editorial]. *Prehospital and Disaster Medicine.* 2005;21(1):1–3.

29. Kapucu N. Collaborative emergency management: Better community organising, better public preparedness and response. *Disasters.* 2008;32(2):239–262.

30. Florida Division of Emergency Management. The State of Florida comprehensive emergency management plan 2004. Available at: http://floridadisaster.org/documents/CEMP/floridaCEMP.htm. Accessed July 25, 2008.

31. Federal Emergency Management Agency. Resource: Disaster Medical Assistance Team (DMAT)—Basic. Available at: http://www.nimsonline.com/resource_typing/Disaster%20Medical%20Assistance%20Team%20(DMAT)%96Basic.htm. Accessed July 23, 2008.

32. Mace S, Jones J, Bern A. An analysis of Disaster Medical Assistance Team (DMAT) deployments in the United States. *Prehospital Emergency Care.* 2007;11(1):30–35.

33. Centers for Disease Control and Prevention. Surveillance for illness and injury after Hurricane Katrina—three counties, Mississippi, September 5–-October 11, 2005. *Morbidity and Mortality Weekly Report.* 2006; 55(9):231–234. Available at: http://www.cdc.gov/mmwr/preview/mmwrhtml/mm5526a3.htm. Accessed July 20, 2008.

34. Centers for Disease Control and Prevention. Carbon monoxide poisoning after Hurricane Katrina—Alabama, Louisiana, and Mississippi, August–September 2005. *Morbidity and Mortality Weekly Report.* 2005;54(39):996–998. Available at: http://www.cdc.gov/mmwr/preview/mmwrhtml/mm5439a7.htm. Accessed July 20, 2008.

35. Platz E, Cooper H, Silvestri S, Siebert C. The impact of a series of hurricanes on the visits to two central Florida emergency departments. *Journal of Emergency Medicine.* 2007; 33(1):39–46.

36. Gray B, Hebert K. Hospitals in Hurricane Katrina: Challenges facing custodial institutions in a disaster. *Journal of Health Care for the Poor and Underserved.* 2007;18:283–298.

37. Howe E, Victor D, Price E. Chief complaints, diagnoses and medications prescribed seven weeks post-Katrina in New Orleans. *Prehospital and Disaster Medicine.* 2008;23(1):41–47.

38. Chakrabhand S, Panyayong B, Sirivech P. Mental health and psychosocial support after the tsunami in Thailand. *International Review of Psychiatry.* 2006;18(6):599–605.

39. Benedek D, Fullerton C, Ursano R. First responders: Mental health consequences of natural and human-made disasters for public health and public safety workers. *Annual Review of Public Health.* 2007;28:55–68.

40. Pant A, Kirsch T, Subbarao I, Hsieh Y, Vu A. Faith-based organizations and sustainable sheltering operations in Mississippi after Hurricane Katrina: Implications for informal network utilization. *Prehospital and Disaster Medicine.* 2008;23(1):54.

41. Elder, K, Xirasagar S, Miller N, Bowen SA, Glover S, Piper C. African Americans' decisions not to evacuate New Orleans before Hurricane Katrina: A qualitative study. *American Journal of Public Health.* 2007;97(1):S124–129.

42. Walker B, Warren R. Katrina perspectives. *Journal of Health Care for the Poor and Underserved.* 2007;18:233–240.

43. Krol D, Redlener M, Shapiro A, Wajnberg A. A mobile medical care approach targeting underserved populations in post–Hurricane Katrina Mississippi. *Journal of Health Care for the Poor and Underserved.* 2007;18:331–340.

44. Florida interfaith networking in disaster: Mitigation "best practices." Available at: http://www.findflorida.org/files/2004MitigationBestPractices.pdf. Accessed July 28, 2008.

45. Cukor J, Restuccia M. Carbon monoxide poisoning during natural disasters: The Hurricane Rita experience. *Journal of Emergency Medicine.* 2007;33(3):261–264.

CHAPTER 21

Extreme Temperature Emergencies: Heat Waves and Cold Storms

Joy Crook and Alexander Vu

INTRODUCTION

The extremes of temperature produce environments that are hazardous public health emergencies, and they can have a major effect on the morbidity and mortality of a population. Cold weather is responsible for the greatest number of weather-related deaths in the United States, followed by hot weather as a distant second. Despite these numbers, hot weather has a more clearly identifiable direct impact on mortality from both primary heat illnesses and the secondary effects of heat on other diseases such as heart and lung disease and neurological strokes. Easily identifiable physical and social risk factors place certain individuals at a higher risk of suffering from extreme temperature-related illnesses. These factors include age, especially age greater than 65 years; living alone; low socioeconomic status; lack of access to air conditioning; taking multiple medications; and having multiple comorbid medical conditions.

The predictable nature of these extreme temperature events makes it possible to establish early warning systems that use locally identified threshold temperatures above and below which mortality rates dramatically increase. The urban heat island—which is a result of concrete, asphalt, and building development that leads to elevated temperatures within cities—plays a role in these local variations. For public health personnel, the risks and benefits of connecting particular meteorological conditions to a tiered response mechanism should be weighed. The need to inform the population with accurate helpful prevention messages must be balanced against the concerns for the consequences of false alarms. There are multiple areas that lend themselves to appropriate public health education campaigns including the use of air conditioning in extreme heat and the dangers of carbon monoxide poisoning when using heaters, generators, or charcoal briquettes inside. Mitigation efforts can focus on long-term risk reduction and may involve legislation to provide warning labels on generators and to encourage smart urban growth and planning to reduce the heat island effects. Extreme temperature weather patterns may not be avoidable; however, effective ways to manage the risk and prevent adverse outcomes exist.

Case Study

In July 1995, a heat wave struck the middle of the United States and claimed the lives of an estimated 830 people throughout the country. The Midwest took the brunt of the impact of the weather, with the majority of the heat-related deaths occurring in Chicago, followed by Milwaukee. On July 11, temperatures and humidity soared, with heat index calculations reaching the 120 degree Fahrenheit (120°F) range. The heat index is a measure of apparent temperature, or how hot it actually feels, when combining humidity values with the ambient air temperature.[1] Coupled with relatively little cloud cover and virtually no wind, the weather conditions persisted for five days.[2] During the three days from July 13 to July 15, 70 daily maximum temperature records were set in areas from the middle of the United States to the East Coast.[3]

The minimum daily temperatures recorded in Chicago during this time period were also markedly elevated (Figure 21-1) and likely contributed to the significant morbidity and mortality rates during this time span. The Chicago city government was slow to respond and did not declare a heat emergency until July 15, despite a marked increase in deaths and hospitalizations seen by July 14.[4] The weather forecasts predicting the high levels of heat and humidity were accurate and issued between 36 and 48 hours in advance of the heat wave.[3,4] An initial heat advisory was issued on July 12 at 3:30 P.M. by the National Weather Service, but did not include any "call to action statements" that use the same terminology used in other dangerous weather events such as "advisory," "watch," or "warning."[3]

By July 13, a massive influx of patients to hospitals in the Chicago metropolitan area was apparent. There were not enough ambulances to take patients to the hospital for evaluation; indeed, in some instances, fire trucks were used for transport.[4] Around the middle of the heat wave, 18 Chicago area hospitals were on bypass and had no more inpatient hospital beds available to take new patients.[3] Energy consumption increased to record levels on July 14, which ultimately resulted in a power outage that left 40,000 people without electricity for one night and approximately 8,000 people without power into the following

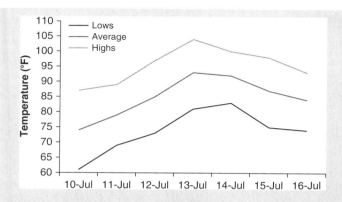

FIGURE 21-1   "High, Low, and Average Temperatures for Chicago, Illinois, Mid-July 1995"
Source: Adapted from NOAA Natural Disaster Survey Report: July 1995 Heat Wave.

day.[4] Subsequently, the local power company began instituting rolling blackouts in suburban areas to help sustain power to the southern, densely populated areas of Chicago.

The impact of the heat wave had more than a human toll, however: It also caused economic impacts in the Midwest beyond the expected increases in electric bills. Roadways and railroads buckled in the heat, which ultimately led to a train accident in Ohio that was blamed on heat-induced movement of the tracks.[4] Work productivity declined throughout the region. Herds of cattle and entire flocks of chickens were killed in the heat. Dairy production slowed as much as 25 percent in Wisconsin during this time.[4]

The deaths attributed to the heat wave followed similar patterns as in prior heat waves studied in the twentieth century. There was lag time between the date on which the extreme heat indexes were noted, on July 11, and the date when the first deaths and hospital admissions due to heat were seen, on July 13.[5,6] Death rates were higher among African Americans.[7] Seventy-three percent of the persons who died were older than the age of 65 years.[4] Persons with preexisting medical problems, those confined to bed, and anyone requiring external assistance to complete daily activities such as visiting home health nurses or aides, housekeepers, and "Meals on Wheels" recipients were all at increased risk of death from heat as a primary or contributing cause.[5] Other social considerations, such as living alone, lack of adequate ventilation in the home, and an unwillingness to open windows, also contributed to death from heat-related illness.[4,5] Common protective factors included the presence of a functioning air conditioner in the home, visiting an air-conditioned building during the daytime hours, having access to transportation, and being visited by a social worker who educated people on the dangers of the heat.[5]

Beyond the increased mortality seen in the heat wave, morbidity rates also increased, as seen in elevated hospital admission rates. Semenza et al. analyzed all hospital admissions from the 47 non–Veterans Affairs (VA) medical centers in Cook County, Illinois, for the weeks surrounding the heat wave in 1995 and compared them to the same weeks in 1994. The researchers noted an 11 percent increase in overall hospital admissions and 35 percent more admissions than expected among the group aged 65 years and older.[6] More than half of these admissions were for dehydration, heat exhaustion, and heat stroke. People with a history of cardiovascular or cerebrovascular disease were at an increased risk for both death and hospitalization during the heat wave.[5,6]

HISTORICAL PERSPECTIVES AND EPIDEMIOLOGY

Severe weather systems are not uncommon and engender much media attention when they occur. Especially in light of recent severe storms, much of the focus on weather-related emergencies tends to be on hurricanes and floods. In reality, in terms of lives lost, excessive cold and heat have exacted the largest human toll in the United States.[8] From 1979 to 2004, almost 11,000 deaths were attributable to cold and another 5,300 deaths to heat. Collectively, this mortality rate represents three times more deaths from the extremes of temperature than deaths from all other natural events in the United States combined.[8] Alaska has the highest state death rate for cold-related deaths (14.5 deaths per 1 million people), followed by Montana and New Mexico. African Americans and men experience higher death rates from extreme cold, as do people older than age of 85 years. The states of Arizona, Missouri, and Arkansas experience the highest crude death rates related to heat. African American men, women, and those older than 85 years of age also have higher death rates from heat-related causes when compared to members of other race, gender, and age categories.[8]

There is extensive and ongoing concern that the climate changes the world is currently experiencing will result in more frequent and more intense weather phenomena. A rise in the mean daily temperature of a location, accompanied by changes in rain patterns, wind, and air quality, will certainly alter local weather patterns. Although it is unclear how these changes will be manifested, the overall increases in air temperatures will most likely result in warmer summers and winters and more significant precipitation.[9,10] For every increase of 2–3°C in mean temperatures, the number of extremely hot days experienced in the summer months will double.[11] Scientists have modeled systems showing marked increases in summertime mortality that may be seen as early as the next decade and will likely be larger than any decline seen in wintertime mortality as a result of warmer temperatures during cold seasons.[9]

Multiple challenges exist when studying variables such as temperature extremes and morbidity or mortality. The first such challenge is that the best indicator of the temperature impact on health remains the subject of debate.[12] "Maximum temperature, minimum temperature, relative humidity, HI [heat index], and duration of exposure are currently used to estimate exposure to heat . . . and more information is needed about which parameters are important in the relationship between weather and health."[12]

The heat index is often used in mortality studies; more importantly, it is a widely publicized measure that is given daily in weather reports. The heat index is a measure of apparent, or perceived, temperature that is based on a combination of temperature and humidity readings. The National Weather Service has created color-coded charts to help people determine which heat index levels could be dangerous (Figure 21-2).[13]

Temperature (°F)

Relative Humidity (%)	80	82	84	86	88	90	92	94	96	98	100	102	104	106	108	110
40	80	81	83	85	88	91	94	97	101	105	109	114	119	124	130	136
45	80	82	84	87	89	93	96	100	104	109	114	119	124	130	137	
50	81	83	85	88	91	95	99	103	108	113	118	124	131	137		
55	81	84	86	89	93	97	101	106	112	117	124	130	137			
60	82	84	88	91	95	100	105	110	116	123	129	137				
65	82	85	89	93	98	103	108	114	121	128	136					
70	83	86	90	95	100	105	112	119	126	134						
75	84	88	92	97	103	109	116	124	132							
80	84	89	94	100	106	113	121	129								
85	85	90	96	102	110	117	126	135								
90	86	91	98	105	113	122	131									
95	86	93	100	108	117	127										
100	87	95	103	112	121	132										

Likelihood of Heat Disorders with Prolonged Exposure or Strenuous Activity
■ Caution ■ Extreme Caution ■ Danger ■ Extreme Danger

FIGURE 21-2 NOAA's National Weather Service Heat Index Chart
Reprinted from http://www.weather.gov/om/heat/index.shtml

Nevertheless, individual susceptibilities to heat and humidity differ, meaning that these charts are only a rough guide and should not be taken as a concrete rule. Regional and local differences occur not only in temperature and weather patterns, but also in the population's vulnerability to temperature extremes. These variables make it virtually impossible to have a single definition for a heat wave or extreme cold.

Studies that look at relationships between weather extremes and morbidity, mortality, or hospitalizations are often limited by the death certifications or discharge diagnoses in primary heat- or cold-related deaths or injuries such as heat stroke, hypothermia, or frostbite. Although many disease processes are secondarily affected and often accelerated by extreme weather conditions, these outcomes may be difficult to distinguish from other diagnoses.[14] As a result, many studies look at increases in all-cause mortality or excess mortality instead of cause-specific deaths. Furthermore, the actual numbers of deaths and injuries related to temperature extremes is far higher than reported.[15]

Multiple studies over the past 20 years have shown that significant all-cause mortality increases from both cold and hot temperatures.[4,5,7,9–11,14–18] One study revealed that typically cold cities, or cities where the average weather is cooler in both the winter and the summer, have increased death rates from both extreme hot and cold temperatures; in contrast, temperature extremes have relatively little effect on cities that have typically hot weather.[16] The vulnerability of people living in generally cooler climates has been seen in recent heat waves involving the upper midwestern United States and northern France and may be explained by poor physiologic acclimatization, a lack of behavioral modifications to the heat, and housing that is not equipped with good ventilation or air conditioning.[17]

A temporal relationship is also seen when comparing death rates to extreme temperatures. The mortality effect of heat lags a few days behind the excessively high temperatures, but returns to baseline almost immediately after temperatures drop; in contrast, the cold effect persists for several days even after the temperature has normalized.[16,19,20] Harvesting—that is, the phenomenon of accelerating the death of people who were likely to die anyway in the near future—is seen with heat waves but not cold temperatures.[16] Thus, although there is increased mortality *during* a heat wave, below-average mortality rates are likely to be observed in the days to weeks *following* the heat wave.

Epidemiological studies have shown that there are "temperature thresholds," or temperatures above and below when excess mortality in the population occurs.[14,15] The study by Kalkstein and Davis, in which they determined these threshold temperatures for 48 U.S. cities, also found that variability between cities existed even within

a particular geographic region.[14] However, no significant variation of these temperature thresholds occurred within a given city, even when age and race were taken into
account.[14] These findings have important implications for issuing heat and cold advisories. After the 2003 heat wave in Europe, "cutoff" temperatures for each department (county) in France were determined. These data were used to activate and
deactivate heat alerts and were based on threshold temperatures above which mortality increases by 1.5 to 2 times while trying to minimize the number of false alerts
that would be issued.[21] Departments immediately adjacent to each other can vary in
their cutoff temperature values by as much as 4°C.[21]

Local and regional variations in temperatures are affected by the topography of
the land, as well as by both geologic and human-made structures. As mentioned earlier, cities tend to produce an effect known as the urban heat island.[15,22] In this phenomenon, concrete, brick buildings, and asphalt all retain heat efficiently and do not
let go of it easily. This tendency, coupled with heat generated from electrical appli-
ances of all sizes, changes in wind patterns owing to buildings, and a lack of shade,
acts synergistically to increase the maximum daily temperatures within cities. Perhaps
more importantly, these factors also antagonize the natural cooling effects of night-
time and increase the minimum temperatures achieved at night.[14] This effect increases the physiologic stress of heat and puts urban dwellers at increased risk for
heat-related illnesses. A study after the 1995 Chicago heat wave, for example, demonstrated that temperatures varied widely from the city to the suburbs to rural areas.[4]
Often, for convenience, the official temperatures used to issue advisories are taken at
airports, but these temperatures may not be an accurate reflection of actual temperatures within a city.[4]

Heating and Cooling Mechanisms

Certain evidence indicates that the duration of exposure to extreme temperatures—
and not the intensity (i.e., how high or low the temperature is)—determines health
outcomes.[14] These data reinforce the concept that individual variations in physiology
and behavior affect how one person will react to extreme temperatures. In addition,
acclimatization plays a role in temperature-related deaths. Notably, heat waves that
occur in the early summer are more deadly than those that occur late in the summer.[14]

The human body produces heat as a by-product of metabolism. Thus the body must
lose heat in an effort to maintain homeostasis. Four main processes work to achieve this
heat loss: conduction, convection, radiation, and evaporation (Table 21-1).[23, 25] The efficiency and effectiveness of these four mechanisms depend on the air temperature and

TABLE 21-1	Mechanisms of Human Heat Loss
	Mechanism
Conduction	Transfer of heat from warmer objects to cooler ones; an especially important mechanism under water.
Convection	Loss of heat to the surrounding air. Minimized if clothing insulation is present; accelerated in high winds.
Radiation	Transfer of heat via electromagnetic waves. Primary mechanism for how the body loses heat if the air temperature is less than body temperature; can also gain heat this way.
Evaporation	Loss of heat as liquid is converted to a gas. Sweat is the primary mechanism; sweating is hampered when humidity levels are high.

humidity, wind speed, and clothing insulation.[23, 24] When these mechanisms are overwhelmed, the body has a net heat gain; when conditions exist where they are too efficient, such as under water or in high winds, then the body has a net heat loss.

Heat gain is a more difficult process for the human body, which has fewer and less efficient mechanisms to accomplish this rise in core temperature. Peripheral vasoconstriction, which shunts warm blood to the core vital organs, and shivering are the most visible processes of heat generation.[26] The body can also increase the metabolic rate in an effort to generate heat. The most effective mechanism, however, is behavior. Increasing the external insulation (e.g., via clothing, shelter) or leaving the environment has the greatest impact on the body's ability to generate heat.

Risk Factors for Heat-Related Illnesses

Multiple physical and social risk factors increase a person's susceptibility to heat and development of heat-related illnesses. Age is a primary risk factor, with the elderly being at highest risk. The source of this risk is multifactorial in nature. The normal aging process reduces the ability to perceive heat, and the body's thirst and perspiration mechanisms can be delayed.[22] Members of the older population are more likely to suffer from multiple medical problems, particularly cardiovascular disease, respiratory disease, and diabetes—all of which can affect thermoregulation. In addition, elderly individuals tend to have lower cardiovascular fitness at baseline—a capacity that is needed for vasodilation and cooling.[27] Furthermore, medications (especially psychotropic medicines, heart medications, and alcohol) can increase sensitivity to heat.[24] Psychiatric illness is a risk factor and significantly contributed to the heat-related deaths of persons younger than age 65 during the 1999 heat waves in Chicago and Cincinnati.[28]

Young children may also be at increased risk of heat-related illnesses, as their surface area-to-mass ratio is larger than that in adults, conferring more environmental heat gains.[12,22] Of note, there were no pediatric deaths in the 1999 Chicago heat wave, though that outcome may be a result of less social isolation of this age group and greater access to air-conditioned buildings.[28]

Heat stress also serves as a direct accelerant in certain disease processes. Heat alters blood viscosity and can accelerate clotting, which in turn may lead to increases in myocardial infarctions and cerebrovascular accidents.[16,29] Respiratory deaths also increase in the heat, an effect that can be seen in both emphysema and pneumonia, although this mechanism is not well understood.[12,16,29] Hospital admissions and emergency department visits also increase during heat waves for both primary and secondary heat-related illnesses.[6,12]

From a social perspective, living in an urban area, living alone, being bedridden, and being socially isolated all confer an increased risk for heat-related illnesses.[5,7,15,24,27] Housing characteristics, such as living on the top floor and having no access to air conditioning, have perhaps the most important roles in contributing to such illnesses.[27] These characteristics all serve as opportunities for intervention and prevention when it comes to reducing the impact of heat.

As previously mentioned, the most important protective factor is access to air conditioning, particularly in the home.[4,27,28] Fans have not been shown to have the same protective effect and can be harmful if the ambient air temperature is higher than body temperature.[28,29] Circulating extremely hot air may actually add to heat stress. Cooling centers are protective in theory; however, it is unclear how extensively they are utilized in an actual heat emergency.[28] Their use requires knowledge of the center and its hours, means of transportation, and the physical ability to get there. For many members of the most at-risk populations, these barriers may be too much to overcome.

Primary heat-related illnesses include heat cramps, heat syncope, heat exhaustion, and heat stroke (Table 21-2).[25,29] These illnesses range from the benign to deadly, and progression to death may occur quickly.[27,28] All persons exposed to heat who show physical symptoms should be evaluated by a medical professional.

Risk Factors for Cold-Related Illnesses

Winter-related storms, including extreme cold temperatures, blizzards, and ice storms, do not garner as much media and research attention as other causes of morbidity and

TABLE 21-2   Primary Heat-Related Illnesses

Illness	Description and Symptoms	Physiology and Treatment
Heat cramps	Painful, involuntary muscle cramps, usually involving the large muscle groups of the calves, thighs, or shoulders.	Caused by relative deficiencies of sodium and potassium at the cellular level.
		Self-limited. Person may be well acclimatized to the heat and able to lose significant volume and electrolytes in the sweat.
		Requires rest until the symptoms have subsided.
		Person needs to be removed from the environment and receive oral rehydration and electrolyte replacement.
		Severe cases may need IV hydration.
		Salt tablets alone are not recommended.
Heat syncope	Sudden loss of consciousness in a heat-affected person.	Result of volume losses and peripheral vasodilation in the heat.
		More common in a non-acclimatized person.
		Person recovers quickly.
		Person needs to be removed from the environment, and often needs oral or IV rehydration and rest.
		Common in the elderly.
		May require further medical evaluation if the history is not clear or the physical exam is abnormal.
Heat exhaustion	Patients may have systemic complaints including fatigue, weakness, dizziness, nausea, vomiting, headache, and myalgias.	Result of significant volume depletion.
	Vital signs may be abnormal—elevated heart rate, low blood pressure, mildly elevated temperature.	Person needs to be removed from the environment. Should be treated with oral or IV hydration, electrolyte replacement, and rest.
	Mental status should remain normal.	May progress to heat stroke.
Heat stroke	No standardized diagnostic criteria.	Medical emergency.
	In general, elevated core temperature, altered mental status, and anhidrosis (i.e., lack of sweating).	Person needs rapid cooling and immediate transport to a hospital.
	Abnormal vital signs and elevated liver enzymes may be present. Person may exhibit multisystem organ dysfunction.	

mortality. Nevertheless, they are responsible for more weather-related deaths than any other phenomena in the United States.[8] Traumatic injuries, whether from accidents, falling debris, burns, and (snow or ice) cleanup efforts, play a major role in direct morbidity, and at times mortality, from these storms.[30,31]

One public health emergency that is unique to cold weather storms is unintentional carbon monoxide poisoning. Carbon monoxide (CO) is an odorless gas that is produced when carbon-containing fuels are burned without enough oxygen.[32] This by-product binds to hemoglobin with greater affinity than oxygen and decreases oxygen's availability to tissues that require it for metabolic processes.[33] Most commonly, CO is produced when cars have exhaust systems that are obstructed with snow, kerosene or propane heaters or gasoline-powered generators are used indoors, or charcoal briquettes are used to cook food indoors.[32,34] A disproportionately high percentage of CO victims do not speak or read English; thus they would not be targets for posted warning labels on charcoal briquettes or public educational campaigns.[34,35] CO poisonings occur—somewhat predictably—two to three days after a storm when the population becomes exposed to CO from indoor charcoal or generator use.[34] All of these characteristics lend themselves to public health and education interventions.

Overall, mortality increases in the winter months, but the relationship between temperature and mortality during extreme cold periods is less clear than that seen in heat waves.[12,14] Some of this "fuzziness" may be due to infectious disease outbreaks such as influenza, respiratory syncytial virus (RSV), and diarrhea that are typically seen during the winter months, but not necessarily related to temperature variations. Some experts hypothesize that global temperature increases will lead to lower mortality rates in the winter, likely as a result of less indoor gathering and more time spent outside.[12] Studies looking at morbidity and mortality during extreme cold and ice storms have shown increases in deaths from cardiovascular disease and myocardial infarctions, as well as increased hospital visits for lower respiratory complaints and chest pain.[16,36] These trends are most consistent among elderly populations.[37] Again, there is no evidence of harvesting in cold weather–related mortality, as is seen in the summer months.[16]

In the United States, primary cold-related illnesses can be seen in the typically cold climates of mountainous areas and the Northeast; however, they can also be found in the typically warmer climates of the South.[12] People in warmer areas lack the experience and behavioral modifications needed to prevent cold-related illnesses. These illnesses include hypothermia (i.e., lowering of the core body temperature) as well as isolated cold injuries including chilblains, trench foot, frostnip, and frostbite (Table 21-3).[26,37,38] Just as with heat-related illnesses, anyone who has an abnormal physical exam after cold exposure should be evaluated by medical personnel. It is imperative to remove the person from the environment and prevent refreezing of the person or extremity.

TABLE 21-3   Primary Cold-Related Illnesses

Illness		Symptoms	Treatment
Hypothermia (core temperatures)	Mild (32–35°C)	Increased metabolism and shivering to try to generate heat.	Passive external rewarming: remove the person from the environment and increase insulation.
	Moderate (30–32°C)	Body slows down, shivering stops, decrease in heart and respiratory rates. Mental slowing.	Active external rewarming: focus heat on the truncal areas, sparing limbs (warmed blankets, warm water immersion, radiant heat).
	Severe (< 30°C)	At risk for spontaneous dysrhythmias. Obtundation of the central nervous system. Bronchorrhea.	Active core rewarming: warmed IV fluids, warmed and humidified oxygen, chest/peritoneal/bladder lavage with warmed fluids, extracorpreal warming or bypass.
Trench foot	Nonfreezing, cold water immersion injury	Tingling, numbness, painful ambulation. Blisters, edema.	Remove wet clothing, warm the extremity in a warm water bath, and keep the extremity dry and elevated until symptoms resolve.
Chilblains	Nonfreezing, dry injury	Itching, burning, nodules and edema may be present.	Remove wet clothing, warm the extremity in a warm water bath, and keep the extremity dry and elevated until symptoms resolve.
Frostnip	Superficial, reversible freezing injury of the skin	Painful, pale or white in color. Symptoms resolve upon rewarming.	Rewarm the extremity in a warm water bath of 40°C. Keep the area clean and dry; may use topical aloe vera.
Frostbite	Deep, irreversible freezing of the skin and deep tissues	Area will be pale, frozen, and hard to the touch. Blisters may form.	Do not thaw the area until there is no chance of refreezing. 40°C rewarming bath, ibuprofen, pain control. Leave blisters intact. Separate fingers and toes; cover skin with topical aloe vera. Provide immediate transport to a medical facility.

PREPAREDNESS AND RESPONSE

As a result of many recent heat and cold storms, as well as the concern that weather patterns are shifting because of climate change, increased emphasis has been placed on public health preparedness to prevent poor outcomes from these weather phenomena. These public health efforts include disaster response plans, early warning systems, and public education campaigns. Local, national, and regional governments as well as health entities such as the World Health Organization (WHO) have recognized that these activities are valuable and worth investments of time, resources, and funds.

Although public health emergencies from severe weather events cannot be prevented, policies can be initiated to prepare populations for them. Early warning systems, similar to those used for hurricanes, have been developed in the United States and internationally to predict the timing and intensity of heat and cold storms. Ebi and Schmier have identified four components as critical parts of such a system:[39]

- Identification and forecasting of the event
- Prediction of the possible health outcomes
- Effective and timely response plan
- Ongoing evaluation of the system and its components

Defining the event and establishing threshold criteria to activate the warning system should be done as close to the local level as possible, where variations in the criteria become more meaningful.[27,39] If possible, use of consistent terminology throughout a region or country will aid in public understanding and provide for a more uniform response. Surveillance mechanisms also must be sensitive enough to detect changes in baseline mortality data so that the response can be designed to fit the crisis—something that did not happen early on during the 2003 heat wave in France.[21,39]

Most response plans are tiered such that limited resources are not used inappropriately.[21,27] When increasing levels of meteorological or epidemiological parameters are met, the response scales up. It is critical to establish leadership and assign roles and responsibilities within the plan prior to an event happening.[40] Importantly, predefined threshold criteria should be consistent with local weather patterns known to increase mortality. Specific components of the response plan may include targeted outreach to high-risk groups, general public awareness campaigns via mass media, lobbying electric and water companies to prevent service shutoffs during these events, and education regarding the dangers of carbon monoxide poisoning and ways to prevent it.[27,34,40] Although expensive and time consuming, a door-to door approach may be necessary to check on elderly high-risk persons; such a system was implemented in Philadelphia during a heat wave, for example.[27]

Medical response capabilities should also be designed to meet the perceived demands of the event. Although these resources are fixed in the short term, reciprocal agreements with neighboring locations may be established to borrow vehicles for transport or road-clearing machinery to assist medical personnel with their work. Hospitals and emergency departments should be notified immediately of potentially dangerous weather, particularly if the forecast calls for multiple days of such weather.

Many warnings are issued 48 hours in advance, which offers enough time to saturate the media with education campaigns about the risks of extreme hot or cold temperatures. To deliver these messages, multiple modalities, including print, television, radio, and the Internet, as well as social and religious networks that may catch high-risk persons who will not see or understand mass media, should be used. It is important to consider the at-risk groups when determining whether messages should be distributed in languages other than English.[35]

Evaluating the effectiveness of an early warning system and corresponding response capabilities can be difficult. Many factors may play a role in decreased morbidity or mortality related to a given weather event other than effective planning and implementation of the response. Nevertheless, public health officials need to review individual components, such as weather forecasting or penetration of public education campaigns, to see how accurate and effective they were. Quality improvement in this realm should be a continuous process.

MITIGATION

Public health professionals should take the opportunity to affect behavior change as well as educate the public before an extreme temperature event actually occurs. Some measures, such as lobbying manufacturers to put warning labels on portable space heaters and generators regarding the dangers of CO poisoning, require significant lead time. Public health officials may need to make necessary arrangements with utility companies not to shut down services during a public health emergency in advance of the emergency itself. Implementing community watch patrols or buddy systems to have people check on one another during times of extreme heat or cold is a resource-laden undertaking and one that is not likely to happen in the immediate aftermath of a disaster. Reciprocal agreements involving other municipalities or states should all be forged in the mitigation phase, in an effort to prevent potential problems from being realized.

One major problem surrounding extreme hot temperatures is the issue of the urban heat island. Buildings, asphalt, and concrete all work together to increase the average temperatures in cities by 1–3°C.[41] The U.S. Environmental Protection

Agency (EPA) has launched a "Heat Island Reduction Initiative" that aims to reduce the urban heat island effect using four main strategies:[41]

- Planting more vegetation
- Installing "green" roofs or roof-top gardens
- Installing reflective roofs
- Using "cool" or permeable pavements

When implemented on a widespread basis, these measures may reduce ambient air temperature, improve air quality, and reduce energy consumption.[41] Furthermore, these initiatives have the potential to decrease heat-related mortality by as much as 25 percent in an area like the Los Angeles Basin.[42] The combination of reforesting, land-use planning, "smart growth" strategies, passive solar systems, and increased surface albedo (i.e., the amount of electromagnetic radiation reflected from Earth back into space) may lead to a modest decline in average temperatures and dew points, yet have a major overall effect.[42]

ANALYSIS OF CASE STUDY

Much has been written about the 1995 Midwest heat wave, and comparisons have been made to subsequent heat waves in the same cities to see if behaviors and responses have changed. Furthermore, the massive heat wave that hit Europe in 2003 and resulted in almost 15,000 excess deaths in France alone reinforced the need for public health measures to prevent excess deaths and improve morbidity related to extreme heat weather events.[19] Risk factors as identified from case-control analysis consistently show that air conditioning is the greatest protective factor to prevent heat-related or heat-assisted death. Social living factors and medical comorbidities play the greatest role in increasing morbidity and mortality from these events.[2,4,5,7]

After the 1995 heat wave, the cities of Chicago and Milwaukee refined their heat-related city-wide response plans. In Chicago, this effort included education programs targeted to those persons at greatest risk for heat-related injuries and death, including the elderly; the Commission on Extreme Weather Conditions was also formed in the aftermath of the 1995 event.[28] For Milwaukee, public health steps included designating multijurisdictional leadership, ensuring more significant involvement of the Milwaukee Health Department, indexing the plan to the National Weather Service advisory criteria, and implementing a system of tiered responses.[18] Both cities' efforts appeared to make a difference in subsequent outcomes: When another heat wave hit the area in the summer of 1999, it resulted in significantly lower death rates in both cities and heat-related emergency medical services (EMS) transports in Milwaukee.[18,28]

Although comparing the two events given the different durations and intensities of heat is extremely difficult, important similarities and differences did occur in outcomes between the two heat waves. In Chicago, people with cardiovascular disease and psychiatric illness were found to be at increased risk for death, as were people who lived on the top floor of a building and those who had lower income levels.[28] In 1999, more than half of the deaths occurred in persons younger than 65 years old—a significant increase in that age group compared to 1995, suggesting that targeted interventions to the elderly were effective.[28] The percentages of deaths in poor and extremely poor neighborhoods both declined in Milwaukee during the 1999 heat wave and heat advisories were issued earlier compared to 1995.[18] Targeted education campaigns, better integrated city planning, and more aggressive warning systems (i.e., lowering the threshold to issue a warning) resulted in better outcomes in 1999.

Mortality related to heat waves is as much a social problem as a medical one. The very people who are at greatest risk during a heat wave are the ones who may not have access to warning systems that would help to educate them about the dangers of extremely hot temperatures. Furthermore, they may not have the physical, social, or economic means to gain access to the single most important protective mechanism: air conditioning.

CONCLUSION

Extremes of temperature result from very common weather patterns and produce a greater death toll than all other weather-related events combined. The populations at greatest risk for both cold- and heat-related events are similar and include persons at the extremes of age, particularly the elderly. Persons with multiple medical problems (especially cardiovascular disease, respiratory disease, and psychiatric illness) and those who are socially isolated are also at higher risk. Because most severe weather conditions can be predicted with at least one to two days of lead time, a significant opportunity exists to engage in public health prevention and education campaigns. Early warning systems should be implemented with appropriate local trigger values and a tiered approach to increase response activities when worsening meteorological or epidemiological conditions are met. Although these weather systems are unavoidable, public health professionals can help decrease their negative impact and improve the overall health outcomes of the populations affected.

INTERNET RESOURCES

American Red Cross, heat emergencies:
http://www.redcross.org/images/pdfs/code/Heat_Emergencies.pdf

U.S. Centers for Disease Control and Prevention, extreme heat emergencies:
http://www.bt.cdc.gov/disasters/extremeheat/

U.S. Centers for Disease Control and Prevention, winter weather:
http://www.bt.cdc.gov/disasters/winter/

U.S. Environmental Protection Agency, extreme heat:
http://www.epa.gov/naturalevents/extremeheat.html

U.S. Federal Emergency Management Agency, extreme heat:
http://www.fema.gov/hazard/heat/index.shtm

U.S. National Oceanic and Atmospheric Administration (NOAA), National Weather Service:
http://www.nws.noaa.gov/

U.S. National Oceanic and Atmospheric Administration (NOAA), winter storms:
http://www.nws.noaa.gov/om/brochures/wintstm.htm

NOTES

1. U.S. National Oceanic and Atmospheric Administration (NOAA), National Weather Service. Heat index. 2009. Available at: http://www.crh.noaa.gov/jkl/?n=heat_index_calculator. Accessed April 26, 2009.
2. Klinenberg E. Denaturalizing disaster: A social autopsy of the 1995 Chicago heat wave. *Theory and Society.* 1999;28:239–295.
3. U.S. National Oceanic and Atmospheric Administration (NOAA). Natural disaster survey report: July 1995 heat wave. Silver Spring, MD: National Weather Service; 1995, p. 74.
4. Changnon S, Kunkel K, Reinke B. Impacts and responses to the 1995 heat wave: A call to action. *Bulletin of the American Meteorological Society.* 1996;77(7):1497–1506.
5. Semenza J, Rubin C, Falter K, et al. Heat-related deaths during the July 1995 heat wave in Chicago. *New England Journal of Medicine.* 1996;335(2):84–90.
6. Semenza J, McCullough J, Flanders W, McGeehin M, Lumpkin J. Excess hospital admissions during the July 1995 heat wave in Chicago. *American Journal of Preventative Medicine.* 1999; 16(4):269–277.
7. Kaiser R, Tertre AL, Schwartz J, Gotway C, Daley W, Rubin C. The effect of the 1995 heat wave in Chicago on all-cause and cause-specific mortality. *American Journal of Public Health.* 2007;97(S1):S158–S162.
8. Thacker M, Lee R, Sabogal R, Henderson A. Overview of deaths associated with natural events, United States, 1974–2004. *Disasters.* 2008;32(2):303–315.
9. Kalkstein L, Greene J. An evaluation of climate/mortality relationships in large U.S. cities and the possible impacts of a climate change. *Environmental Health Perspectives.* 1997;105(1):84–93.
10. Greenough G, McGeehin M, Bernard S, Trtanj J, Riad J, Engelberg D. The potential impacts of climate variability and change on health impacts of extreme weather events in the United States. *Environmental Health Perspectives.* 2001;109(suppl 2):191–198.
11. Curriero F, Heiner K, Samet J, Zeger S, Strug L, Patz J. Temperature and mortality in 11 cities in the eastern United States. *American Journal of Epidemiology.* 2002;155(1):80–87.

12. McGeehin M, Mirabelli M. The potential impacts of climate variability and change on temperature-related morbidity and mortality in the United States. *Environmental Health Perspectives.* 2001;109(suppl 2):185–189, p. 188.

13. U.S. National Oceanic and Atmospheric Administration (NOAA). NOAA's National Weather Service heat index chart. 2009. Available at: http://www.weather.gov/om/heat/index.shtml. Accessed April 7, 2009.

14. Kalkstein L, Davis R. Weather and human mortality: An evaluation of demographic and interregional responses in the United States. *Annals of the Association of American Geographers.* 1989;79(1):44–64.

15. Basu R, Samet J. Relation between elevated ambient temperature and mortality: A review of the epidemiologic evidence. *Epidemiologic Reviews.* 2002;24(2):190–202.

16. Braga A, Zanobetti A, Schwartz J. The effect of weather on respiratory and cardiovascular deaths in 12 U.S. cities. *Environmental Health Perspectives.* 2002;110(9):859–863.

17. Kavats R, Ebi K. Heatwaves and public health in Europe. *European Journal of Public Health.* 2006;16(6):592–599.

18. Weisskopf M, Anderson H, Foldy S, et al. Heat wave morbidity and mortality, Milwaukee, Wisconsin, 1999 vs 1995: An improved response? *American Journal of Public Health.* 2002; 92(5):830–833.

19. Vandentorren S, Suzan F, Medina S, et al. Mortality in 13 French cities during the August 2003 heat wave. *American Journal of Public Health.* 2004;94(9):1518–1520.

20. Conti S, Meli P, Minelli G, et al. Epidemiologic study of mortality during the summer 2003 heat wave in Italy. *Environmental Research.* 2004;98:390–399.

21. Michelon T, Magne P, Simon-Delavelle F. Lessons of the 2003 heat-wave in France and action taken to limit the effects of future heat-waves. In: Kirch W, Menne B, Bertollini R (Eds.), *Extreme weather events and public health responses, Vol 1.* Heidelberg, Germany: World Health Organization Regional Office for Europe; 2005, pp. 131–140.

22. Blum L, Bresolin L, Williams M. Heat-related illness during extreme weather emergencies. *Journal of the American Medical Association.* 1998;279(19):1514.

23. Walker J, Chamales M. Heat wave disasters. In: Hogan D, Burstein J (Eds.), *Disaster medicine.* Philadelphia: Lippincott Williams & Wilkins; 2002, pp. 212–221.

24. Havenith G. Temperature regulation, heat balance, and climatic stress. In: Kirch W, Menne B, Bertollini R (Eds.), *Extreme weather events and public health responses, Vol 1.* Heidelberg, Germany: World Health Organization Regional Office for Europe; 2005, pp. 69–80.

25. Walker J, Hogan D. Heat emergencies. In: Tintinalli J, Kelen G, Stapczynski J (Eds.), *Emergency medicine: A comprehensive study guide, Vol. 1.* New York: McGraw-Hill; 2004, pp. 1183–1189.

26. Bessen H. Hypothermia. In: Tintinalli J, Kelen G, Stapczynski J (Eds.), *Emergency medicine: a comprehensive study guide, Vol. 1.* New York: McGraw-Hill; 2004, pp. 1179–1183.

27. Kovats R, Ebi K. Heatwaves and public health in Europe. *European Journal of Public Health.* 2006;16(6):592–599.

28. Naughton M, Henderson A, Mirabelli M, et al. Heat-related mortality during a 1999 heat wave in Chicago. *American Journal of Preventative Medicine.* 2002;22(4):221–227.

29. Kilbourne E. Heat waves and hot environments. In: Noji E (Ed.), *The public health consequences of disasters.* New York: Oxford University Press; 1997, pp. 245–269.

30. Broder J, Mehrotra A, Tintinalli J. Injuries from the 2002 North Carolina ice storm and strategies for prevention. *International Journal of the Care of the Injured.* 2005;36:21–26.

31. Hartling L, Pickett W, Brison R. The injury experience observed in two emergency departments in Kingston, Ontario during "Ice Storm 98." *Canadian Journal of Public Health.* 1999; 90(2):95–98.

32. Hartling L, Brison R, Pickett W. Cluster of unintentional carbon monoxide poisonings presenting to the emergency departments in Kingston, Ontario during "Ice Storm 98." *Canadian Journal of Public Health.* 1998;89(6):388–390.

33. VanMeter K. Carbon monoxide poisoning. In: Tintinalli J, Kelen G, Stapczynski J (Eds.), *Emergency medicine: A comprehensive study guide, Vol. 1.* New York: McGraw-Hill; 2004, pp. 1238–1241.

34. Hampson N, Stock A. Storm-related carbon monoxide poisoning: Lessons learned from recent epidemics. *Undersea and Hyperbaric Medicine Journal.* 2006;33(4):257–263.

35. Wrenn K, Conners G. Carbon monoxide poisoning during ice storms: A tale of two cities. *Journal of Emergency Medicine.* 1997;15(4):465–467.

36. Community needs assessment and morbidity surveillance following an ice storm—Maine, Janurary 1998. *Morbidity and Mortality Weekly Report.* 1998;47(17):351–354.

37. Kilbourne E. Cold environments. In: Noji E (Ed.), *The public health consequences of disasters, Vol. 1.* New York: Oxford University Press; 1997, pp. 270–286.

38. Rabold M. Frostbite and other localized cold-related injuries. In: Tintinalli J, Kelen G, Stapczynski J (Eds.), *Emergency medicine: A comprehensive study guide, Vol. 1.* New York: McGraw-Hill; 2004, pp. 1175–1179.

39. Ebi K, Schmier J. A stitch in time: Improving public health early warning systems for extreme weather events. *Epidemiologic Reviews.* 2005;27:115–121.

40. Bernard S, MCGeehin M. Municipal heat wave response plans. *American Journal of Public Health.* 2004;94(9):1520–1522.

41. Urban heat island mitigation. 2009. Available at: http://www.epa.gov/heatisland/mitigation/index.htm. Accessed April 28, 2009.

42. Taha H, Kalkstein L, Sheridan S, Wong E. The potential of urban environmental control in alleviating heat-wave health effects in five U.S. regions. *16th Symposium on Biometeorology and Aerobiology.* Vol. Paper J4.3. Vancouver, BC: American Meteorological Society; 2004, pp. 1–8.

SECTION 7

Industrial Emergencies

CHAPTER 22

Hazardous Materials

Terry Mulligan

INTRODUCTION

Hazardous materials (hazmats) are defined as "any item or agent (biological, chemical, physical), which has the potential to cause harm to humans, animals, or the environment, either by itself or through interaction with other factors."[1] If not stored, handled, or transported correctly, hazardous materials can cause harm to workers, members of the public, property, and the environment due to their physical, chemical, and biological properties. Hazardous materials can cause adverse health effects by direct physiologic and chemical properties, including mild to severe poisoning, asthma, skin rashes, allergic reactions, allergic sensitization, burns, cancer, metabolic and electrolyte disturbances, and many other long-term (chronic) diseases from exposure to substances. In addition, many hazardous materials are associated with traumatic injuries from hazardous materials–related fires, explosions, release of hazardous gases, and corrosion.[2] Table 22-1 lists some sources of hazardous materials.

TABLE 22-1 Common Sources of Hazardous Materials	
• Paints	• Herbicides
• Drugs	• Pesticides
• Cosmetics	• Diesel fuel
• Cleaning chemicals	• Petrol
• Degreasers	• Liquefied petroleum gas
• Detergents	• Welding fumes
• Gas cylinders	

Source: Modified from http://www.deir.qld.gov.au/workplace/subjects/hazardousmaterials/definition/example/index.htm.

TABLE 22-2   Definitions of Hazardous Materials

U.S. Agency	Definition of Hazardous Materials

U.S. Occupational Safety and Health Administration (OSHA)	Any substance or chemical that is a "health hazard" or "physical hazard," including:
	
	• Chemicals that are:
	  ▪ Carcinogens
	  ▪ Toxic agents
	  ▪ Irritants, corrosives
	  ▪ Sensitizers
	• Agents that act on the hematopoietic system
	• Agents that damage the lungs, skin, eyes, or mucous membranes
	• Chemicals that are combustible, explosive, flammable, oxidizers, pyrophorics, unstable-reactive or water-reactive
	• Chemicals that, in the course of normal handling, use, or storage, may produce or release dusts, gases, fumes, vapors, mists, or smoke that may have any of the previously mentioned characteristics.
	
	[Full definitions can be found at 29 Code of Federal Regulations (CFR) 1910.1200.]

U.S. Environmental Protection Agency (EPA)	Incorporates the OSHA definition, and adds any item or chemical that: • Can cause harm to people, plants, or animals • When released by spilling, leaking, pumping, pouring, emitting, emptying, discharging, injecting, escaping, leaching, dumping, or disposing into the environment. [40 CFR 355 contains a list of more than 350 hazardous and extremely hazardous substances.]
U.S. Department of Transportation (DOT)	• Any item or chemical that, when being transported or moved, poses a risk to public safety or the environment • Any item or chemical that is regulated as such under the Hazardous Materials Regulations [(49 CFR 100–180); International Maritime Dangerous Goods Code; Dangerous Goods Regulations of the International Air Transport Association; Technical Instructions of the International Civil Aviation Organization; U.S. Air Force Joint Manual, Preparing Hazardous Materials for Military Air Shipments.]
U.S. Nuclear Regulatory Commission (NRC)	Regulates items or chemicals that are "special nuclear sources" or by-product materials or radioactive substances [See 10 CFR 20.]

Source: Data from the Institute of Hazardous Materials Management (IHMM), http://www.ihmm.org/dspWhat IsHazMat.cfm.

Hazardous materials are defined and regulated in the United States primarily by laws and regulations administered by several distinct, but related agencies. Each has its own definition of a "hazardous material" (Table 22-2).

Case Study

Wednesday, August 6, 1997, 2 P.M.
Highway I-94
Michigan City, Indiana

An auto carrier truck slammed into the back of a tanker truck stopped in congested traffic on the eastbound lane of Interstate 94 (I-94). The tanker truck was carrying sodium hydroxide (50 percent solution), and 3,000 to 4,000 gallons of the corrosive chemical spilled from the tanker as a result of the accident. The auto carrier truck veered to the right after the collision, crashed through a guard rail, overturned, and burst into flames. Firefighters came from three neighboring township volunteer fire departments. The driver of the auto carrier died of multiple injuries. The sodium hydroxide, which will burn skin on contact, affected three people, who received minor burns when some of the chemical spilled on them.

All six lanes of the highway were closed, starting a little after 2 P.M., along a nine-mile stretch between Chesterton and Michigan City. The three westbound lanes were reopened on Wednesday, August 6, around 5:30 P.M. At 11 P.M. on Wednesday, the center and left lanes of the eastbound side were reopened; the right-hand lane was still closed well into Thursday.

Approximately 500 to 1,000 gallons of sodium hydroxide remained in the tanker after the accident and was transferred to another tanker. Cleanup of the accident included removing all contaminated soil along the side of the interstate. Two tractor-trailer loads of soil had already been removed by 3:30 P.M., and the cleanup was still under way. Water samples were also taken from a small creek to check for any contamination. OSI Environmental conducted the cleanup, and the local Porter County Hazardous Materials Team and the Indiana Department of Environmental Management oversaw the cleanup. The tank truck company reportedly was responsible for the payment of the cleanup.[3]

HISTORICAL PERSPECTIVES

The U.S. Department of Transportation (DOT) has defined nine classes of hazardous materials, which are distinguished according to their comparative risk during transportation (Table 22-3). All DOT-classified hazardous materials are listed in the DOT's Hazardous Material Table.[4]

TABLE 22-3 Risk Classification System for Hazardous Substances	
Hazard Class	**Materials**

Hazard Class 1: Explosives	1.1 Mass explosion hazard
	1.2 Projectile hazard
	1.3 Minor blast/projectile/fire
	    (These items have the potential for mass detonation.)
	
	1.4 Minor blast
	1.5 Insensitive explosives
	1.6 Very insensitive explosives
	    (These items have characteristics that make mass
	    detonation unlikely.)

Hazard Class 2: Compressed Gases	2.1 Flammable gases 2.2 Nonflammable compressed gases 2.3 Poisonous gases
Hazard Class 3: Flammable Liquids	3.1 Flammable (flash point below 141 °F) 3.2 Combustible (flash point 141–200 °F)
Hazard Class 4: Flammable Solids	4.1 Flammable solids 4.2 Spontaneously combustible materials 4.3 dangerous when wet
Hazard Class 5: Oxidizers and Organic Peroxides	5.1 Oxidizers 5.2 Organic peroxide
Hazard Class 6: Toxic Materials	6.1 Poisonous materials 6.2 Infectious agents
Hazard Class 7: Radioactive Materials	7.1 Radioactive I 7.2 Radioactive II 7.3 Radioactive III
Hazard Class 8: Corrosive Materials	8.1 Destruction of the human skin 8.2 Materials that corrode steel at a rate of 0.25 inch per year
Hazard Class 9: Miscellaneous Dangerous Goods	Any material that presents a hazard during shipment but does not meet the definition of the other classes

Source: Modified from U.S. Department of Transportation, Pipeline and Hazardous Materials Safety Administration, http://www.phmsa.dot.gov/.

Hazardous Materials Incidents and Hazardous Substances Events

In 1990, the U.S. Department of Health and Human Services' Agency for Toxic Substances and Disease Registry (ATSDR) established the Hazardous Substances Emergency Events Surveillance (HSEES) system to collect and analyze information related to incidents involving hazardous materials. Information reported to the HSEES system includes sudden uncontrolled or illegal releases of hazardous substances (excluding releases involving only petroleum products) that require cleanup or neutralization according to federal, state, or local law. In addition, the system identifies threatened releases that result in public health action, such as evacuation. The HSEES system aims to reduce the number of injuries and deaths among first responders, employees, and the general public that result from releases of hazardous substances. It is the only federal database designed specifically to address the public health effects from releases of hazardous substances, and it is one of many that provides resources and information about hazardous substance events.[5] Examples of hazardous material incidents include the following:

- Fire or explosion at a chemical refinery
- Motor vehicle accident of a transport truck with spillage of hazardous substance
- Field workers exposed to pesticides
- Chemical leaks at a factory
- Natural gas leaks
- Random discovery of a container that may contain a hazardous substance
- Intentional or accidental release of biological agents or any type of radiation

Many U.S. states use information from the HSEES system to develop strategies for reducing injuries and deaths from these types of incidents. Appropriate prevention outreach activities can provide industry, responders, and the general public with the knowledge needed to prevent chemical releases and to reduce injuries and death when such releases occur (Table 22-4). Researchers and other government agencies, for example, often request HSEES data for their prevention activities.

Hazardous Materials Transportation

Hazardous materials transportation is a process that involves people performing functions related to handling, packaging, storing, moving, loading, and unloading of hazardous materials, and responding to emergency situations while such materials are in the midst of transportation. A variety of employees may be responsible for the safe transportation of hazardous material. Hazardous materials professionals are properly trained and qualified to handle, transport, and manage such materials. Their responsibilities

TABLE 22-4   Descriptive Data About Previous Hazardous Substance Events

What the Hazardous Substances Emergency Events Surveillance (HSEES) system information has shown about hazardous substance events in the United States:

- The most commonly used poisoning database, PoisIndex, currently lists more than 700,000 potentially toxic compounds, chemicals, and hazardous materials.[6]
- Approximately 9,000 hazardous substances releases occur annually in the 15 states reporting data to HSEES.
- Releases at facilities account for 70 to 75 percent of reported events, and transportation-associated releases account for 25 to 30 percent of reported events.
- Most releases occur on weekdays between 6 A.M. and 6 P.M.
- Releases tend to increase in spring and summer when more shipments of pesticides and fertilizers for agricultural activities take place.
- Equipment failure and human error cause most releases at facilities.
- Human error and equipment failure cause most releases during transport.
- More than 90 percent of events involve the release or threatened release of only one hazardous substance.
- Releases of hazardous substances most often injure employees, followed by the general public and—less frequently—first responders and school children.
- Respiratory irritation and eye irritation are the most commonly reported symptoms or injuries.
- Approximately 50 percent of people who report developing symptoms or injuries from a HSEES event are treated at a hospital and released.
- In the 10 to 30 percent of hazardous substance events that involve victims, trauma is the most common problem.[7,8]
- 65 percent of fatalities following a hazardous materials incident result from trauma, 22 percent from burns, and 10 percent from respiratory compromise.
- Most nontraumatic injuries and deaths are associated with exposures to chlorine, ammonia, nitrogen, fertilizer, or hydrochloric acid. Other commonly involved chemicals include petroleum products, pesticides, corrosives, metals, and volatile organics.[9]
- 80 percent of hazardous substance events occur at fixed facilities, 20 percent are transportation related, and more than 10 percent occur within hospitals.
- More than 40 percent of victims from the general public and more than 20 percent of victims who are exposed at the workplace are decontaminated at hospital emergency departments.

Source: Modified from U.S. Department of Health and Human Services, Agency for Toxic Substances and Disease Registry (ATSDR). *Hazardous Substance Emergency Events Surveillance (HSEES): CDC fact sheet.* Available at: http://www.atsdr.cdc.gov/hs/hsees/hsees_about-factsheet.html.

include advising other professionals on such items at any point in their life cycle, from process planning and development of new products; through manufacture, distribution, and use; to disposal, cleanup, and remediation. The transportation process also incorporates functions to design, manufacture, fabricate, inspect, mark, maintain, recondition, repair, or test a package, container, or packaging component used in

TABLE 22-5   Human Errors Resulting in Hazardous Materials Transportation Incidents

Sources of Human Error

- Lack of knowledge leading to the mishandling of hazardous material
- Lack of knowledge leading to undeclared shipments
- Lack of awareness that hazardous material is present
- Failure to follow established safety procedures
- Lack of understanding of one's role during an incident should such an event occur
- Lack of knowledge on how to respond to an incident if one occurs

Source: Adapted from U.S. Department of Transportation, Pipeline and Hazardous Materials Safety Administration. Available at: https://hazmatonline.phmsa.dot.gov/services/publication_documents/Guide%20to%20 Developing%20a%20Hazardous%20Materials%20Training%20Program.pdf.

TABLE 22-6   Accidental Deaths in the United States, 1999–2003

Type	Five-Year Average	General Population Risk per Year	Risk Based on Exposure or Other Measures
Motor vehicle	36,676	1 out of 7,700	1.3 deaths per 100 million vehicle miles
Poisoning	15,206	1 out of 18,700	
Work related	5,800	1 out of 49,000	4.3 deaths per 100,000 workers
Large trucks	5,150	1 out of 55,000	2.5 deaths per 100 million vehicle miles
Pedestrian	4,846	1 out of 58,000	
Drowning	3,409	1 out of 83,500	
Fires	3,312	1 out of 86,000	
Motorcycles	3,112	1 out of 91,500	31.3 deaths per 100 million vehicle miles
Railroads	931	1 out of 306,000	1.3 deaths per 1 million train miles
Firearms	779	1 out of 366,000	
Recreational boating	714	1 out of 399,000	5.6 deaths per 100,000 registered boats
Bicycles	695	1 out of 410,000	
Electric current	410	1 out of 695,000	
Air carriers	138	1 out of 2,067,000	1.9 deaths per 100 million aircraft miles
Flood	58	1 out of 4,928,000	
Tornado	57	1 out of 5,015,000	
Lightning	47	1 out of 6,061,000	
Hazardous material transportation	12	1 out of 23,350,000	4.2 deaths per 100 million shipments

Source: Modified from U.S. Department of Transportation, Pipeline and Hazardous Materials Safety Administration. Available at: http://www.phmsa.dot.gov/portal/site/PHMSA/menuitem.ebdc7a8a7e39f2e55cf2031050248a0c/?vgnextoid= 8524adbb3c60d110VgnVCM1000009ed07898RCRD&vgnextchannel=c442adbb3c60d110VgnVCM1000009ed07898 RCRD&vgnextfmt=print.

transporting hazardous materials.[2] Given the high complexity of this process, it is perhaps not surprising that the DOT has identified human error as a contributing cause for most hazardous material transportation incidents (Table 22-5), though fatalities from such incidents remain rare (Table 22-6).

PREPAREDNESS AND PLANNING

Hazardous materials event emergency plans describe duties, responsibilities, relationships, and related decisions that must be addressed before an incident occurs. During the acute phase of an emergency, very little time is available to resolve such issues or to practice and refine roles and responsibilities. The complex analysis and preparation required to establish an effective response to a hazardous materials event must be completed in advance so that public officials, healthcare professionals, and response personnel can act quickly and decisively to control dangerous situations and protect the public.

Given this rationale, an emergency plan must be more than just a document (Table 22-7). To be effective, all personnel who will participate in a hazardous materials event incident response must know their roles and responsibilities and be competent in the tasks they will perform. This goal is greatly enhanced by participation of the necessary organizations in an integrated planning process, including exercising the plan and periodically revising the plan as needed.[10]

The Planning Process

There is no single correct way to write a hazardous materials event emergency plan. Each entity must plan according to its own circumstances, based on many varying local factors, such as types of hazards, populations at risk, geographic area, resources and other finances, and other levels of preparedness. Jurisdictions and facilities should assess and survey their local circumstances and environments to choose the most appropriate elements and details of the plan. However, every community and industry needs to evaluate its preparedness for hazardous materials incidents and plan accordingly.[10]

Many teaching materials and other resources are available in the literature that provide in-depth explanations of the planning process:

- *Guide for All-Hazard Emergency Operations Planning* (FEMA SLG 101)
- *Hazardous Materials Emergency Planning Guide* (NRT-1)
- *Technical Guidance for Hazards Analysis* (EPA/FEMA/DOT)
- *Handbook of Chemical Hazard Analysis Procedures* (FEMA/DOT/EPA)
- *Emergency Management Guide for Business & Industry* (FEMA 141)

TABLE 22-7   Definition and Elements of an Emergency Operations Plan

What Is an Emergency Operations Plan?

According to the Federal Emergency Management Agency (FEMA), an emergency operations plan (EOP) is a document that fulfills the following requirements:

- Assigns responsibility to organizations and individuals for carrying out specific actions at projected times and locations in an emergency
- Sets forth lines of authority and organizational relationships, and shows how all actions will be coordinated
- Describes how people and property will be protected in emergencies and disasters
- Identifies personnel, equipment, facilities, supplies, and other resources available for use during response and recovery operations
- Identifies steps to address mitigation concerns during response and recovery activities
- The elements covered in a hazardous materials or terrorist incident response plan and the approach to planning will vary, depending on the jurisdiction's or facility's unique needs.

What Should the EOP for a Hazardous Materials Event Response Plan Include?

- An analysis of the emergencies likely to occur
- An assessment of available resources and existing capabilities
- Detailed response operations strategies and assignments that address notification, command and control, life safety, and other functional requirements
- Identification of prevention measures that can mitigate the seriousness of an emergency or prevent it from occurring

The level of detail contained in the plan will also vary, but must be adequate to allow tasked organizations and individuals to develop comprehensive standard operating procedures in their assigned areas.

Source: Modified from U.S. Fire Association, Federal Emergency Management Agency (FEMA). *Hazardous materials and terrorist incident response planning curriculum guidelines.* Available at: http://www.usfa.dhs.gov/downloads/pdf/publications/hmep9-1801planning.pdf.

An extensive and thorough review of these documents and approaches to hazardous materials event planning are included in the U.S. Fire Association, Federal Emergency Management Association (FEMA) document entitled "Hazardous Materials and Terrorist Incident Response Planning Curriculum Guidelines" (http://www.usfa.dhs.gov/downloads/pdf/publications/hmep9-1801planning.pdf).

Whichever model is adopted for the planning process, a team approach is strongly recommended. The best mechanism for incorporating the various experts and types of expertise necessary in planning, building consensus among organizations and individuals affected by the plan, and promoting professional relationships and understanding among responders is formation of a planning team. Team members can also help ensure that plans are adequately implemented, evaluated, and maintained, and that the proper training and tools are delivered to personnel so that they can achieve and maintain competency in their assigned roles and responsibilities. No specific format is mandated for the results of hazardous materials planning; any format is considered "good" if users understand it, are comfortable with it, and can extract the information they need.

The approach taken in these guidelines identifies two fundamental planning products, both of which are derived from a common hazards analysis and capability assessment base:

- An emergency operations plan that addresses preparedness for, response to, and short-term recovery from hazardous materials events
- A prevention/mitigation section of the plan that addresses measures designed to eliminate or reduce the effects of potential emergencies

In hazardous materials events, the importance of pre-response planning cannot be overstated. In addition to obvious details concerning responsibilities, duties, and tasks related to the actual event, pre-response planning provides the following benefits:

- It provides a mechanism for evaluating operational strategies, defining roles and procedures, communicating organizational assignments, and assessing the adequacy of responder training.
- The integrated team planning process fosters trust and cooperation among individuals and organizations that must work together during an incident.
- Planning leads to effective mitigation and prevention measures, thereby providing communities and facilities with an opportunity to eliminate or reduce the costly and tragic effects of hazardous materials incidents before they occur.

Effective response and prevention planning is directly related to the competency of the personnel assigned responsibility for performing related tasks—public- and private-sector officials, agency and program managers, planners, technical experts, and many others.[10]

Training

Hazardous materials events are often complex and involve the coordinated and timely actions of many different persons, often under stressful conditions. The skill and training of individual responders are only one aspect of safe and effective emergency operations. Indeed, the quality of this coordination, which includes criteria such as clearly defined lines of authority, adequate communication systems, and the availability of resources,

TABLE 22-8	Criteria for Assessing State and Local Hazardous Materials Event Preparedness
Hazards analysis	Identification of potential hazards, determination of the vulnerability of an area as a result of the existing hazards, and assessment of the risk of a hazardous materials event.
Authority	Statutory authorities or other legal authorities vested in any personnel, organizations, agencies, or other entities in responding to or being prepared for responding to hazardous materials events.
Organizational structure	The organizational structure in place for responding to emergencies. There are two basic types of organizations involved in emergency response operations: • The first is involved in the planning and policy decision processes. • The second is the operational response group that functions within the precepts set forth in the state or local plan. • These structures will vary considerably from state to state and from locality to locality.
Communications	Any means of exchanging information or ideas for emergency response with other entities, either internal or external to the existing organizational structure. Communication involves the following elements: • Coordination • Information exchange • Information dissemination • Information sources and database sharing • Notification procedures • Clearinghouse functions
Resources	The personnel, training, equipment, facilities, and other sources available for use in responding to hazardous materials emergencies.
Emergency planning	The emergency plan relates to many of the previously described criteria and stands alone as a means to assess preparedness at the state and local levels of government, and in the private sector. It is not enough to ask if a plan exists; it is important to determine whether the existing plan adequately addresses the needs of the community or entity for which the plan was developed.

Source: Adapted from National Response Team, U.S. Environmental Protection Agency. Hazardous materials emergency planning guide. Available at: http://www.epa.gov/oem/docs/chem/cleanNRT10_12_distiller_complete.pdf.

may play a more important role than individual responder training in minimizing injuries and maximizing control of the emergency.[10]

Assessing State and Local Preparedness

Certain specific criteria can be used to evaluate state and local preparedness for a potential hazardous materials event; these criteria reflect the basic elements judged to be important for a successful emergency preparedness program (Table 22-8). They may be used for assessing the emergency plan as well as the emergency preparedness program in general. It must be recognized, however, that few state or local governments will have the need or capability to address all these issues and meet all these criteria to the fullest extent. Inevitably, resource limitations and the results of the hazards analysis will strongly influence the necessary degree of planning and preparedness. Those governmental units that do not have adequate resources are encouraged to seek assistance and take advantage of all resources that are available.

RESPONSE

A good hazardous materials event emergency response plan will consist of several phases, each with distinct elements, all of which must be coordinated to maintain a continuum of high-quality care and safety for affected patients and health professionals (Table 22-9).

TABLE 22-9   Elements of a Hazardous Materials Event Emergency Plan for Emergency Departments

- Pre-notification criteria
- Prehospital decontamination procedures and equipment
- In-hospital decontamination procedures and equipment
- Personal protective equipment appropriate to predetermined high-likelihood events
- Triage amendments and modifications when necessary
- Plans for possible modifications to normal registration, medical records, and other data collection practices
- Treatment processes, equipment, medications, and other necessary elements for medical care of affected patients
- Instructions for return to normal functioning and operations, including re-equipping of emergency materials
- A post-event assessment and evaluation, including data collection, post-event evaluations, and possible psychological ramifications for health professionals

Source: Adapted from U.S. Fire Association, Federal Emergency Management Agency (FEMA). Hazardous materials and terrorist incident response planning curriculum guidelines. Available at: http://www.usfa.dhs .gov/downloads/pdf/publications/hmep9-1801planning.pdf.

Pre-notification

If the nature of the hazardous materials event allows pre-notification of hospital personnel, the following steps should occur to prepare the emergency department for the arrival of patients:

- Communication with prehospital providers regarding the following issues:
  - The type of incident
  - The type of hazardous material
  - The number of patients
  - Signs, symptoms, and clinical conditions of patients
  - Type of decontamination if performed
  - Estimated time of arrival
- Consideration of activation of emergency department and hospital hazardous materials response plans and disaster plans
- Preparation of decontamination areas, equipment, and personnel
- Preparation of medications, equipment, and antidotes required for clinical care
- Further pre-notification of other individuals to be involved:
  - Poison control centers
  - Medical toxicologists and clinical pharmacologists
  - Industrial hygienists
  - Institutional occupational physicians
  - Hospital safety officers, radiation safety officer, and security personnel
  - Hospital administrator
  - Media relations representative

Access and Retrieval of Hazardous Materials Information

The hazardous materials response plan for the institution should explain how to obtain detailed information about involved hazardous materials when their identities or types are known. Many 24-hour telephone and Internet resources exist that can provide this type of information on an immediate basis, some of which are listed in a section at the end of this chapter.

Material Safety Data Sheets

A material safety data sheet (MSDS) is a document containing important information about a particular hazardous material (which may be classified as a hazardous substance or dangerous good). It provides the following data:

- The hazardous substance's product name
- The chemical and generic name of certain ingredients
- The chemical and physical properties of the hazardous substance
- Health hazard information
- Precautions for safe use and handling
- The manufacturer's or importer's name, address, and telephone number
- Basic first-aid procedures (sometimes outlined; advanced medical information is usually not included)

The MSDS provides employers, self-employed persons, workers, and other health and safety representatives with the necessary information to safely manage the risk from hazardous substance exposure. It is important that everyone in the workplace knows how to read and interpret the MSDS.[11] Access to a MSDS can be provided in several ways:

- Paper and microfiche copy collections of MSDS with microfiche readers open to use by all workers
- Computerized and Internet MSDS databases
- Work sites, employees and employers, and safety officers
- Poison centers
- Commercially available computer databases and other resources, including Chemtrec, NRC, and Dolphin[11]

MSDSs do not exist for all 700,000 hazardous materials and possible scenarios. Nevertheless, they remain an important source of summary information for many hazardous materials and detail approaches to these substances' decontamination, treatment, and removal/cleanup.

On-Scene Decontamination

Whenever possible, decontamination of patients should occur at or around the scene of the exposure, before contaminated patients are placed in transport vehicles and taken to hospitals or other care facilities (Table 22-10). Ideally, all decontamination should occur at the scene and outside of the hospital and the immediate vicinity of the emergency department (Table 22-11). In reality, this approach is utilized with only a small minority of decontaminated patients due to issues related to resources, training, and simple logistics of hazardous material incidents: Most of the "walking wounded" patients typically transport themselves to the nearest hospital's emergency department.

TABLE 22-10   Safety Precautions for On-Scene Management of Hazardous Materials Events

1. Approach cautiously from upwind.
   - If the wind direction allows, consider approaching the incident from uphill.
   - Resist the urge to rush in; others cannot be helped until the situation has been fully assessed.
2. Secure the scene.
   - Without entering the immediate hazard area, isolate the area and ensure the safety of people and the environment, keeping people away from the scene and outside the safety perimeter.
   - Allow enough room to move and remove your own equipment.
3. Identify the hazards.
   - Obtain or otherwise locate any available placards, container labels, shipping documents, material safety data sheets, rail car and road trailer identification charts, and/or knowledgeable persons on the scene.
   - Evaluate all available information and consult the recommended guides to reduce immediate risks.
     - Additional information, as provided by the shipper or obtained from another authoritative source, may change some of the emphasis or details found in the guide.
   - Remember—the guide provides only the most important, worst-case scenario information for the initial response in relation to a family or class of dangerous goods. As more material-specific information becomes available, the response should be tailored to the situation.
4. Assess the situation.
   - Consider the following issues:
     - Is there a fire, a spill, or a leak?
     - What are the weather conditions?
     - What is the terrain like?
     - Who or what is at risk: people, property, or the environment?
     - Which actions should be taken: Is an evacuation necessary? Is diking necessary? Which resources (human and equipment) are required and are readily available?
     - What can be done immediately?
5. Obtain help.
   - Advise your headquarters to notify the responsible agencies and call for assistance from qualified personnel.
6. Decide on site entry.
   - Any efforts made to rescue persons and to protect property or the environment must be weighed against the personal safety and health risks for responders.
   - Enter the area only when wearing appropriate personal protective equipment.
7. Respond.
   - Respond in an appropriate manner.
   - Establish a command post and lines of communication.
   - Rescue casualties where possible and evacuate if necessary.
   - Maintain control of the site.
   - Continually reassess the situation and modify the response accordingly.
   - The first duty is to consider the safety of people in the immediate area, including your own.

Source: Modified from U.S. Department of Transportation, Pipeline and Hazardous Materials Safety Administration. Emergency response guidebook: A guidebook for first responders during the initial phase of a dangerous goods/hazardous materials transportation incident. Available at: http://phmsa.dot.gov/staticfiles/PHMSA/DownloadableFiles/Files/erg2008_eng.pdf.

TABLE 22-11   Decontamination Zones

Hot Zone
- This is the area of contamination.
- Entrance requires proper training, appropriate protective equipment, and use of "the buddy system."
- Removal of exposed patients and care starts here.
- Remember that these patients may have traumatic injuries as well as exposure to toxic substances.
- **Never forget ABCs of BLS, ACLS, and ATLS.**

Warm Zone
- Area surrounding the hot zone.
- Serves as a safety buffer and is the area of initial decontamination.
- ABCs during decontamination:
  1. Airway
  2. Breathing
  3. Circulation/cervical spine stabilization
  4. Decontamination
  5. Evaluation for systemic toxicity.
  6. Full spine immobilization/backboard if needed
  7. Oxygen supplementation
  8. Limited invasive procedures→IVs
  9. CPR as needed

Cold Zone
- Safe area, isolated from contamination.
- Should be situated uphill, upwind, upstream, with safe and easy access.
- This is where EMS equipment and transport vehicles will be kept.
- "Clean" patients are triaged, checked for adequate decontamination, and transported to medical care providers as needed.

Personal Protection Equipment

Personal protective equipment (PPE) includes equipment that is used and worn by first responders, healthcare workers, and emergency personnel. The main function of PPE is to protect emergency and rescue personnel from contamination and injury during their rescue and response activities in contaminated environments or with contaminated patients. Many types of PPE are available, and each hazardous materials incident calls for different types of PPE (Table 22-12).

Decontamination Process

The goal of decontamination is to decrease the dose or amount of hazardous materials exposure to the patient. Complete disrobing of exposed clothing and thorough washing

TABLE 22-12 Types of Personal Protective Equipment

Protective Respiratory Devices

Self-Contained Breathing Apparatus (SCBA)

SCBA consists of a full face piece connected by a hose to a portable source of compressed air. It provides clean air under positive pressure from a cylinder; the air is then exhaled into the environment. SCBA provides the highest level of respiratory protection.

Supplied-Air Respirator

SAR consists of a full face piece connected to an air source away from the contaminated area via an airline. Because SARs are less bulky than SCBA, they can be used for longer periods. These devices are also easier for most hospital personnel to use.

Air-Purifying Respirator

An APR consists of a face piece worn over the mouth and nose with a filter element that filters ambient air before inhalation. Three basic types of APRs are available:

- **Powered air-purifying respirators (PAPRs):** Deliver filtered air under positive pressure to a face piece mask, helmet, or hood, which provides respiratory and ocular protection.
- **Disposable APRs:** Are usually half-masks, which do not provide adequate eye protection. This type of APR depends on a filter, which traps particulates.
- **Chemical cartridge:** The use of a high-efficiency particulate air (HEPA) filter or its use in combination with a chemical cartridge enhances disposable APRs.

High-Efficiency Particulate Air Filter

HEPA filters are incorporated into various protective respiratory devices including PAPRs. This type of filtration is required when caring for a patient infected with a disease requiring "airborne precautions."

Surgical Mask

Surgical masks are designed to protect the sterile field of the patient from contaminants generated by the wearer. Although surgical masks filter out large-size particulates, they offer no respiratory protection against chemical vapors.

Protective Clothing

Most protective clothing is aimed at protection against chemicals and chemical warfare agents (CWAs).

Chemical-Protective Clothing

Chemical-protective clothing (CPC) consists of multilayered garments made out of materials that protect against various hazards. Because no single material can protect against all chemicals, several layers of various materials are usually used to increase the degree of protection.

Barrier Gown and Latex Gloves

Barrier gowns are waterproof and protect against exposure to biological materials, including body fluids, but do not provide adequate skin or mucous membrane protection against chemicals. Latex gloves also protect wearers from biological materials but are inadequate against most chemicals. Barrier gowns, latex gloves, and leg and/or shoe covers together satisfy requirements for "contact precautions."

Source: Huebner KD, Lavonas EJ, Arnold JL. CBRNE: Personal protective equipment. June 16, 2008. Available at: http://emedicine.medscape.com/article/831240-overview.

with water by decontamination personnel in the warm and cold zones is essential to ensure removal of the hazardous material. If decontamination is performed at or inside the hospital, specially designated areas outside the building or outside from the main patient areas must be used for this operation to avoid turning the emergency department into a second "hot zone" and exposing other patients to the hazardous materials.

Whether decontamination is performed at the scene or at the hospital, the following general rules should be followed:

- Dry, particulate matter should be brushed off clothing and skin by use of a gloved hand or in another fashion. Care should be taken not to use water for removing dry material, given the risk of chemical reactions and thermal and chemical burns that can occur with exposure of some dry hazardous materials to water (e.g., metals such as lithium, potassium, and sodium).
- Clothing with dry particulate matter and clothing potentially exposed to radioactive hazardous material should be taken off carefully to avoid further exposure of surface material to the patient.
- All clothing should be separated, bagged, and removed from the scene to avoid further risk of exposure and contamination.
- Whole-body decontamination should then take place using copious amounts of water and a mild shampoo, and should take place where the effluents do not cause risk to other patients.

The hospital can be considered a part of the "cold zone," so efforts should be made to prevent secondary decontamination inside this facility. After rescue, life support, triage, thorough decontamination, and other initial stabilizing care are given at the scene, transport of victims to the hospital emergency department in protected vehicles can proceed. Further decontamination at the hospital emergency department can be done in a separate contained area designated as a decontamination area with water hoses and other decontamination equipment. Many hospitals now have separate "Hazmat Decon" areas.

Triage

Despite advances in training, pre-notification systems, and hazardous materials incident plans, very often real-life hazardous incidents do not follow the life cycle outlined in textbooks. Notably, patients invariably arrive at healthcare facilities in various states of contamination and by various means of transportation. Nevertheless, triage of contaminated patients should occur according to the standard principles of all triage systems—namely, determining the *priority of care* for multiple contaminated patients. One cardinal rule is that *no contaminated patients should be allowed to enter the emergency department.* Potential contamination of this previously "cold zone" can render it contaminated and affect the health of other patients and healthcare personnel. All personnel who enter the hospital should be wearing appropriate PPE as well.

Ideally, an appropriately trained and attired triage officer should meet the incoming prehospital personnel involved in a hazardous materials incident at a staging and receiving area located outside the normal triage area. Determinations of exposure and appropriate and adequate levels of decontamination should be made at this point, especially for acutely injured or sick patients whose high acuity and instability may have meant that their decontamination procedures were either inadequate or skipped altogether. Because the contamination of the hospital can adversely affect the care of all patients and other healthcare personnel, decontamination of acutely ill patients before bringing them into the facility should be a high priority.

Treatment and Toxidromes

General points regarding definitive treatment of toxicities and associated trauma and injuries can be addressed in the emergency department after decontamination and triage. The appropriate treatments and antidotes depend on the substance involved, and the primary goal for healthcare providers should be identification of the contaminating material (Table 22-13).

After decontamination and triage that includes assessment of the patient's stability and a primary survey, a secondary survey should be undertaken to consider the possibility of toxic syndromes (toxidromes). Similar to toxic exposures to medications, recreational drugs, and other substances, toxic exposures to hazardous materials can produce recognizable toxidromes. These toxidromes should be suspected, looked for, and evaluated in all possible hazardous materials incidents because their presence or absence can both lead healthcare personnel to suspect an exposure to hazardous materials in patients with unknown exposure history and point to the class or type of hazardous material to which the patient was potentially exposed. As with all toxidromes, however, the presence or absence of these familiar classes of toxic syndromes should not be considered definitive proof of exposure (or lack thereof); instead, they should be used as guidelines to be taken into account with all other relevant clinical information.

Some common toxidromes involve the following signs and symptoms:

- Nausea and vomiting
  - These symptoms may indicate toxic ingestion with resultant gastrointestinal (GI) effects.
  - They can suggest systemic toxic exposure or a toxic effect.

TABLE 22-13   Resources for Identification of Hazardous Materials

Resources at the Hazardous Material Site

U.S. Department of Transportation (DOT) placards (used with the DOT *Emergency Response Guidebook* [ERG])[12]: diamond-shaped placards on tank trucks or rail cars

United Nations classification numbering system on vehicles

Waybill and shipping papers (maintained by the driver or train conductor)

National Fire Protection Association (NFPA) 704 marking system labels on containers (at fixed facilities)

Material safety data sheet (MSDS)

Company records or company safety officer CAS number: unique number assigned to specific chemical or mixture (http://chemfinder.cambridgesoft.com/)

Resources at Remote Sites

Regional Poison Control Center: 800-222-1222

Chemtrec: 24-hour assistance to emergency responders regarding chemicals spills: 800-262-8200; www.chemtrec.com

ATSDR emergency response 24-hour hotline: 404-639-0615

EPA environmental response hotline: 201-321-6660

National Response Center: 800-424-8802

Centers for Disease Control and Prevention (CDC): 404-639-3311

National Pesticide Telecommunication Network: 800-858-7378

Computer databases: PoisIndex, Dolphin, Tomes Plus, ToxNet

- In some cases, the vomitus itself may contain hazardous materials; thus it should be treated as contaminated.
- A small number of hazardous materials can react with the acidic environment of the stomach to produce additional toxic substances, including toxic gases such as cyanide.
- Administration of activated charcoal should generally be avoided due to the associated risk of aspiration, and emesis should not be induced.
- Cough, shortness of breath, or other airway compromise
  - These symptoms can indicate any degree of inhalation exposure to many different hazardous materials that can cause direct pulmonary irritation.

- Significant systemic absorption can also occur via inhalation.
- Inhalation injuries can lead to direct orotracheal, pharyngeal, and pulmonary damage from chemical effects, which may then lead to pulmonary edema and respiratory compromise.
- Thermal inhalation injuries should also be suspected, regardless of the type or class of hazardous material involved.
- Decreased or altered mental status
  - Altered mentation can indicate serious and life-threatening systemic exposure to inhaled, ingested, or absorbed hazardous materials, such as cyanide.
  - This condition can also be a sign of hypoxia and hypoxemia from any number of causes.
  - Head injury, trauma, and other causes of shock must not be overlooked.
  - Children are at greater risk of developing methemoglobinemia.
- Cutaneous skin irritation or burns
  - These signs can indicate exposure to caustics, acids, or other irritating substances, or could be caused by other (traumatic) mechanisms.
  - Regardless of its source, altered skin integrity from any cause (i.e., traumatic abrasion or lacerations) can facilitate increased systemic absorption of hazardous materials.
  - Children are more susceptible to skin absorption due to several factors, and are more susceptible to developing hypothermia from wet skin.
  - Some systemically absorbed toxins can have significantly delayed presentations (more than 24 hours after exposure) and require admission for monitoring and observation.

MITIGATION

Because most hazardous materials accidents are caused by human activities, communities and employers can diminish the probability of incidents and the magnitude of their effects by emphasizing prevention in hazardous materials emergency management. Prevention can be defined as a "proactive attitude, effort, and process for eliminating or reducing the effects of hazardous materials events in advance of occurrence." In other words, prevention focuses on helping communities and citizens avoid becoming disaster victims in the first place and reducing the impact of incidents when they occur.[10]

Hazardous materials prevention includes efforts to eliminate or reduce risk due to either accidental releases of hazardous materials or exposure to toxic substances. Basic prevention strategies can be broadly summarized as follows:

- Improve methods and procedures for storing, transporting, handling, and processing hazardous materials.
- Promote compliance with safety codes, regulations, and statutes.
- Develop and enforce land-use plans that regulate the location of sites with hazardous chemicals.
- Increase public and community awareness and support for prevention.[10]

Hazardous materials incidents caused by human error can be reduced through the implementation of an effective training program (Table 22-14). An effective training program comprises a systematic method for providing training, which includes tests and quizzes. It may consist of materials such as handouts, overheads, videos, and exercises, as well as interactive computer-based training, tests, and quizzes. The training program may be a tutored or self-study course. The training provider may be the employer or an independent training agent.

In recent years, both government and industry have made significant strides in hazardous materials prevention. Even so, more must be done to encourage a change from the traditional focus on disaster preparedness and response to a new emphasis on accident prevention. This shift in perspective by business leaders and emergency management professionals will require adjustments in corporate and community attitudes about prevention, improvements in safety management methods and technologies, better access to information and research, and stronger cooperation between government agencies and hazardous materials end users.

One of the most effective ways of promoting this transition is through prevention training and education programs (Table 22-15). Training helps employees understand

---

TABLE 22-14   Impact of Hazardous Materials Mitigation Training

- Develops a strong safety culture
- Heightens employee safety by helping employees protect themselves
- Improves a company's effectiveness, efficiency, and productivity
- Increases employee skills
- May prevent regulatory sanctions
- Aids in ensuring safe and secure shipments of hazardous materials
- Reduces the likelihood of a catastrophic event such as a fire
- Provides employees with understanding of why compliance and safety are necessary

Source: Adapted from U.S. Department of Transportation (DOT), Pipeline and Hazardous Materials Safety Administration. A guide to developing a hazardous materials training program. Available at: https://hazmatonline .phmsa.dot.gov/services/publication_documents/Guide%20to%20Developing%20a%20Hazardous%20Materials %20Training%20Program.pdf.

TABLE 22-15 Sample Hazardous Materials Incident Mitigation Training Scheme			
Audience	**Prerequisites**	**Training**	**Refresher**
Hospital emergency department personnel who may coordinate or provide treatment to patients who have been exposed to or contaminated by hazardous materials. Moderate class size promotes better interaction and discussion.	None, beyond professional competencies associated with the individual's role in the hospital emergency department.	Competencies: • Knowledge of contamination hazards, decontamination procedures, patient flow, health treatment procedures, roles and responsibilities • Ability to implement decontamination, use of reference materials, and use of personal protective equipment Classroom and lab instruction with simulated emergencies, hands-on psychomotor skill training.	1. Technical updates 2. Updates on changes in hospital protocols and procedures 3. Renewal of skills in decontamination, patient treatment, and use of personal protective equipment

Source: Adapted from U.S. Fire Administration, Federal Emergency Management Agency (FEMA). Hazardous materials and terrorist incident response planning: Curriculum guidelines. Available at: http://www.usfa.dhs.gov/downloads/pdf/publications/hmep9-1801planning.pdf.

the nature and causes of potential safety problems, apply safe work practices and procedures, and participate in the design of effective prevention programs. For this reason, federal and state agencies have consistently identified training as a critical component in all prevention activities.[10]

CASE STUDY ANALYSIS

In the case study, as with most hazardous material incidents, the overall costs and impact extended far past those associated with more typical public health and medical incidents (Table 22-16). The proper response to this and many hazardous material incidents, regardless of scope and material, requires the full cooperation of many different aspects of both the private and public sectors:

- Fire, police, and ambulance services
- Local, regional, national, and sometimes international governments
- Medical, legal, environmental, engineering, and transportation sectors
- Public- and private-sector cooperation
- Extensive education, training, and dissemination of information

TABLE 22-16   Estimated Costs Associated with Case Study Incident (Michigan City, Indiana)

	Field	Value
Hazardous materials information	Commodity	Sodium hydroxide solution
	Class	Corrosive material
	Quantity spilled	3,000–4,000 gallons (13,200–17,600 liters)
Accident information	Location	Mile marker 29 on highway I-94, Michigan City, La Porte County, Indiana
	Fatalities	1 person: $2,800,000
	Injuries	3 people with minor injuries: $12,000
	Evacuation	0
Damages	Product loss	$35,000
	Carrier damage	$107,000
	Public/private property damage	$2,300
	Other damage	$11,940
	Decontamination/cleanup	$13,500
	Incident delay	$83,025
	Environmental damage	$3,063
Total estimated cost		$3,067,828

Source: Comparative risks of hazardous materials and non-hazardous materials truck shipment accidents/incidents. Prepared for the Federal Motor Carrier Safety Administration, March 2001. Available at: http://www.phmsa.dot.gov/staticfiles/PHMSA/DownloadableFiles/Files/hazmatriskfinalreport.pdf.

• Establishment of national and international accepted standards of labeling, identification, transport, and regulation

CONCLUSION

Hazardous materials are a ubiquitous part of modern society, and thorough knowledge of hazardous materials, classes, preparedness and planning, response, and mitigation are necessary to ensure the proper treatment of patients and the safety and security of the larger public health population in an incident involving these substances. A multidisciplinary approach is required to ensure proper labeling, handling, manufacture, planning, response, mitigation, and treatment in relation to hazardous materials. Hazardous materials and their study provide an illustrative example of the need for public health oversight, planning, and integration into multiple facets of society to ensure the overall best welfare of the public.

INTERNET RESOURCES

U.S. Agency for Toxic Substances and Disease Registry, Hazardous Substances Emergency Events Surveillance: http://www.atsdr.cdc.gov/hs/hsees/

U.S. Department of Transportation, Pipeline and Hazardous Materials Safety Administration: http://www.phmsa.dot.gov/hazmat

U.S. Environmental Protection Agency, *Addressing Toxics, Hazardous Materials, and Waste:* http://www.epa.gov/international/toxics/index.htm

U.S. National Response Center: www.nrc.uscg.mil/

U.S. Occupational Safety and Health Administration, *Hazardous and Toxic Substances:* http://www.osha.gov/SLTC/hazardoustoxicsubstances/index.html

NOTES

1. Institute of Hazardous Materials Management (IHMM). Available at: www.ihmm.org, http://www.ihmm.org/dspWhatIsHazMat.cfm.
2. Department of Justice and Attorney-General, Workplace Health and Safety, Queensland Government, Australia. National Occupational Health and Safety Commission. Approved criteria for classifying hazardous substances. Available at: http://www.deir.qld.gov.au/workplace/subjects/hazardousmaterials/definition/example/index.htm.
3. Comparative risks of hazardous materials and non-hazardous materials truck shipment accidents/incidents. Prepared for the Federal Motor Carrier Safety Administration, March 2001. Available at: http://www.phmsa.dot.gov/staticfiles/PHMSA/DownloadableFiles/Files/hazardous material riskfinalreport.pdf.
4. U.S. Department of Transportation. Hazardous material table. Available at: http://ecfr.gpoaccess.gov/cgi/t/text/text-idx?c=ecfr&sid=5b0f467f91a98f9cf6833dbda89429af&rgn=div6&view=text&node=49:2.1.1.3.7.2&idno=49.
5. U.S. Department of Health and Human Services, Agency for Toxic Substances and Disease Registry (ATSDR). Fact sheet. Available at: http://www.atsdr.cdc.gov/hs/hsees/hsees_about-factsheet.html.
6. PoisIndex. Available at: http://www.micromedex.com/products/poisindex/.
7. Kales SN, Polyhronpoulos GN, Castro MJ, et al. Injuries caused by hazardous materials accidents. *Annals of Emergency Medicine.* 1997;30(5):598.
8. Hall HI, Dhara VR, Price-Green PA, Kaye WE. Surveillance for emergency events involving hazardous substances: United States, 1990–1992. *Morbidity and Mortality Weekly Report.* 1994; 43(2):1.

9. Phelps AM, Morris P, Giguere M. Emergency events involving hazardous substances in North Carolina, 1993–1994. *North Carolina Medical Journal.* 1998;9(2):120.

10. U.S. Fire Administration, Federal Emergency Management Agency. Hazardous materials and terrorist incident response planning: Curriculum guidelines. Available at: http://www.usfa.dhs.gov/downloads/pdf/publications/hmep9-1801planning.pdf.

11. Department of Justice and Attorney-General, Workplace Health and Safety, Queensland Government, Australia. National Occupational Health and Safety Commission. Material safety data sheets. Available at: http://www.deir.qld.gov.au/workplace/subjects/hazardousmaterials/definition/msds/index.htm.

12. U.S. Department of Transportation. *Emergency response guidebook 2000.* (Obtain by calling 800-327-6868)

CHAPTER 23

Nuclear Energy Reactors

Y. Veronica Pei and Angela Lee

INTRODUCTION

Currently 436 nuclear power plants operate worldwide,[1] with 104 nuclear power plants operating in the United States alone.[2] Between 1944 and 1995, approximately 382 major radiation accidents occurred worldwide, highlighting the need for emergency public health preparedness related to these events. The largest nuclear accident to date took place on April 26, 1986, at the Chernobyl nuclear power plant in Ukraine; it resulted in hundreds of cases of acute radiation sickness, 30 deaths, and potentially long-term adverse effects to almost 6 million people.[3] In the United States, the most significant nuclear power plant incident occurred at Three Mile Island, Pennsylvania, on March 28, 1979. In contrast to the Chernobyl incident, no identifiable health impacts resulted from the Three Mile Island incident.[2]

The Three Mile Island incident uncovered multiple areas of weakness in the preparedness and response to nuclear reactor accidents and served as a catalyst for significant reform in areas of nuclear power plant operations, regulations, and protocols. Additionally, it led to expanded U.S. government involvement in the oversight, planning, and preparedness process as well as more stringent protocols and regulations. The incident at Chernobyl highlights the complexity of a nuclear power plant incident on both the national and international levels, as well as the potential devastation to the surrounding area from such an incident, both immediately and for years to come. Minimization of the public health risk from a nuclear power plant radiation release requires continuous and active engagement of the government, regulatory agencies, and public health officials in all phases of the public health emergency life cycle: planning and preparedness, response, and mitigation.

Case Study

On March 28, 1979, the most significant nuclear power plant accident in the United States occurred at Three Mile Island, a facility located 10 miles downstream from Pennsylvania's capital city of Harrisburg.[4] An unclear causal event led to increased pressure in the primary reactor and the loss of cooling water to the reactor core. A combination of factors, including equipment failure, poor instrument representation, and operator errors, eventually led to a partial nuclear core meltdown.[5] Super-heated water and steam reacted with zirconium alloy surrounding the fuel, causing an explosion in the reactor building. Fortunately, the walls of the containment building were not breached, so very little radiation was released into the environment. Contaminated water was pumped into a storage tank next door in the auxiliary building and quickly filled the tank. Radioactive gases dissolved in the reactor's coolant water escaped into the air but were not released to the outside environment, owing to the action of the exhaust system, which contained iodine and particulate filters. After nearly 16 hours, circulation to the reactor core was reestablished and the situation was brought under control. By then, one third of the nuclear core had melted and radioactivity had escaped into the environment.

Within 5 hours of the accident, the U.S. Nuclear Regulatory Commission (NRC) and the White House (the Jimmy Carter administration) were notified of the incident and response teams dispatched. Non-essential personnel began evacuating the premises at 11 A.M. Throughout the course of the event, infield measurements were performed to track the plume. On March 30, the governor of Pennsylvania, Richard L. Thornburgh, issued an advisory for all pregnant women and preschool-age children within a 5-mile radius of the nuclear plant to evacuate the area. On March 31, a new crisis emerged when concerns arose about the potential explosion of a large hydrogen bubble that had formed in the reactor. This fear was quickly allayed when experts determined the bubble could not explode due to a lack of oxygen within the system and, therefore, posed minimal danger.[5-7]

After the accident was brought under control, environmental sampling was performed. The NRC released a statement regarding the decontamination and disposal of radioactive waste, estimating that the cleanup would take 5 to 9 years.[5] The cleanup operation was divided into four separate operational stages:

1. Stabilizing the plant
2. Waste management

3. Decontamination
4. Defueling

This operation was carefully monitored; after its completion, it was cited as one of the top engineering achievements in the United States by the National Society of Professional Engineers.[5] Officially, no deaths or injuries to plant workers or in the nearby community were attributed to either the accident or the ensuing cleanup. As mentioned earlier, this incident subsequently inspired major changes in nuclear plant operations, regulation, and safety protocols in the United States.

In contrast, the Chernobyl accident, which took place on April 26, 1986, in Unit 4 of the facility, resulted in explosions that cracked the reactor vessel, started fires that lasted 10 days, and led to the release of significant amounts of radioactive particles into the environment. Nearly 1 million people were exposed to doses of radiation exceeding 50 millisieverts (mSv), some of whom died due to their initial radiation exposure; another 5 million people were exposed to 10 to 20 mSv of radiation.[8] More than 4,000 cases of childhood/adolescent thyroid cancer were eventually detected in children who were exposed to radiation during the accident, and monitoring for other health consequences of this radiation exposure continues.[9] Continued radiation contamination threat from the Chrnobyl accident persists because the nuclear reactor site was temporarily contained by an imperfect, decaying structure and nuclear waste was quickly and inappropriately disposed of during the incident. Appropriate decontamination/containment and waste disposal have yet to be undertaken.[8]

HISTORICAL PERSPECTIVES

Nuclear power was considered to be a source of clean, inexpensive energy. "The reaction is self-sustaining, the curve is exponential," announced Enrico Fermi as the nuclear age began in 1942.[5] Nuclear power refers to the process of extracting energy from atomic nuclei through controlled nuclear reactions. While several nuclear reactions can release energy, the only method in use today is nuclear fission, whereby the nucleus of an atom splits into smaller components, releasing energy in the process. The greatest advantage in developing nuclear power is that it is not dependent on the world's limited supply of fossil fuels. Storage, transportation, and disposal of nuclear waste safely are all challenging, however, and potentially pose major environmental hazards. Additionally, malfunctions in the control of the nuclear reactors that tightly control the fission process can evolve into catastrophic incidents if a large amount of radiation is released into the environment.

In 1954, the Obninsk nuclear power plant in USSR became the world's first nuclear power plant to generate electricity. Soon after, the United States brought the Shipping-port power plant online in 1958. Currently, 104 nuclear power plants are operational in the United States, accounting for nearly 20 percent of the country's total energy consumption.[10] With 436 nuclear power plants operating worldwide, and 382 major radiation accidents occurring from 1944 to 1995, nuclear power plant safety remains both a domestic and international concern.[3,11] The major public health concern with respect to these accidents is radiation release. Radiation exposure takes place primarily through inhalation of airborne radioactive contamination and ingestion of food and liquid contaminated with radioactive material.[2] The general public is routinely exposed to varying amounts of radiation from background cosmic radiation (higher levels when flying in airplanes), medical diagnostic and treatment applications, and occupational exposures, but these levels are all carefully monitored.

Three conventional measurements for radiation exist: (1) emitted radiation, (2) radiation dose absorbed, and (3) biological risk from radiation (Table 23-1). Emitted radiation is the amount of radiation emitted or released into the environment and is represented by the conventional unit of the curie (Ci) or the Système Internationale (SI; Internal System of Units) unit known as the becquerel (Bq). Radiation absorbed refers to the amount of energy deposited per unit of human tissue, represented by the conventional unit of the rad or the SI unit known as the gray (Gy). Biological risk refers to the risk of health effects related to radiation exposure and is measured by the conventional unit of the rem or the SI unit known as the sievert (Sv).

The average person living in the United States receives approximately 3 mSv or 200 mrem per year of background radiation from naturally occurring radioactive materials and cosmic radiation.[12] In comparison, a person having a chest x-ray receives

TABLE 23-1   Radiation Measurements

Measurement	Conventional Units	SI Units	Conversion Factor
Emitted radiation: amount of radioactivity released	Ci	Bq	1 Ci = 37 billion Bq
Radiation dose: amount of energy deposited per unit weight of human tissue	rad	Gy	1 Gy = 100 rad
Biological risk: risk of health effects to individuals exposed to radiation	rem	Sv	1 Sv = 100 rem

approximately 10 mrem or 0.1 mSv of radiation; a person having a body computed tomography (CT) scan receives approximately 1 rem or 10 mSv. A variety of factors affect radiation dose exposure on international flights, with exposures ranging from 3 msv to 9.7 mSv per flight.[13]

Prior to 1975, the regulation and licensing of nuclear facilities in the United States was under the control of the Atomic Energy Commission (AEC), an agency established after World War II to promote and regulate peacetime efforts to develop atomic technology. With the development of commercial nuclear power, the U.S. Congress designated responsibility for both the promotion and the regulation of nuclear power to the AEC. However, the inherent conflict of interest in encouraging the growth of the nuclear industry and enforcing stringent requirements to ensure public safety led to growing controversy over the AEC's role. In 1974, President Gerald Ford signed into legislation the Energy Reorganizing Act, which divided the responsibilities of nuclear technology promotion and regulation into two agencies. The Nuclear Regulatory Commission (NRC) was identified as the responsible agency for regulatory functions; the promotional function of the nuclear industry was placed under the Emergency Research and Development Administration, which later became a part of the Department of Energy.

Today, the NRC's primary function is to protect the public and the environment from nuclear hazards through strict regulations that control the possession, use, and disposal of nuclear materials. Its area of control includes the licensing, inspection, and oversight of nuclear reactors as well as development of emergency preparedness plans in case of a radiological emergency. Additionally, the NRC works in conjunction with a number of other federal agencies, including the Department of Homeland Security (DHS) and the Federal Emergency Management Agency (FEMA), in emergency preparedness.

On an international level, after the Chernobyl disaster, it was recognized that international efforts and inputs were critical to ensure nuclear safety on a worldwide basis. In 1987, the World Health Organization (WHO) established the Radiation Emergency Medical Preparedness and Assistance Network (REMPAN) to provide emergency medical and public health assistance, follow up on accident victims, facilitate long-term care, and conduct relevant research, acceding to the international conventions defined by the document known as *Early Notification and Assistance in the Case of a Nuclear Accident or Radiological Emergency*.[14] The international response focuses on the preparedness and planning phase as well as the response phase (rather than mitigation). Activities include engaging in emergency medical preparedness and response, improving public health advice, studying radiation emergencies, and making recommendations for long-term follow-up.[3]

While nuclear reactors have multiple inherent safety mechanisms, the possibility of a potential major accident was recognized early on in their development. In 1955, the

AEC sponsored the first study entitled *Theoretical Possibilities and Consequences of Major Accidents in Large Nuclear Power Plants* ("The Brookhaven Report") that estimated the possible effects of a nuclear accident. This study concluded that if a nuclear reactor had no containment, there would be 3,400 deaths, 43,000 injuries and property damage of $7 billion from a major accident at such a facility.[15] It also estimated that the chance of a major nuclear accident was between 1 in 100,000 and 1 in 1 billion. Over the years, the NRC has attempted to improve the nuclear accident risk assessment via a number of studies. Currently, this agency is in the process of developing a state-of-the-art computer model to estimate the radiological consequences of a severe nuclear accident, referred to as State-of-the-Art Reactor Consequence Analyses (SOARCA) project.[16]

PREPAREDNESS AND PLANNING

Preparedness and planning refers to activities that occur prior to an actual disaster and includes planning, drills, supply stockpiles, and response plans. The incident at Three Mile Island underscored the need for emergency preparedness planning in relation to nuclear incidents.

Government Oversight

The U.S. federal government maintains oversight of nuclear power plants through two agencies, the NRC and FEMA. Federal law requires all nuclear power plants to have an emergency response plan in place in the event of an accident prior to receiving a license to bring the facility online. The NRC is responsible for licensing nuclear power reactors, ensuring on-site preparedness, reviewing on-site plans and training, and overseeing FEMA's nuclear planning and response efforts. FEMA reviews and assesses off-site planning and response as well as assists state and local governments prepare for such an event. The NRC has the authority to take action to ensure public health and safety.[2]

Emergency Response Plan

Each nuclear power plant must meet minimum governmental safety requirements. All nuclear power plants are required to have an emergency plan, and they must engage in regular drills and exercises to monitor and improve their emergency responses. All nuclear power plants must conduct joint response exercises with the NRC, FEMA, and off-site authorities at least once every two years.

In the event of a nuclear accident, two specific emergency planning zones (EPZ) are designated based on radial distance around the plant. The plume exposure pathway comprises a 10-mile radius around the facility; populations within this pathway during the incident are at greatest risk of inhalation or airborne radioactive contamination. These individuals may require potassium iodide (KI) tablets to reduce the risk of thyroid cancer in those who are exposed to radioactive iodide. The second zone, the ingestion pathway zone, encompasses a 50-mile radius around the site; in this area, the greatest risk arises from ingestion of radioactively contaminated food and liquid.

During an incident, events are classified by level of risk to the public, which helps determine the level of response and actions to be taken. There are four levels of risk:[11]

1. *Notification of unusual events:* Events are in process or have occurred, but no release of radioactive material has occurred that would require an off-site response or monitoring.
2. *Alert:* Events are in process or have occurred, and actual or potential substantial degradation to the safety of the plant has occurred. Radioactive release, if any, is a fraction of the amount listed in the EPA action guides.
3. *Site area emergency:* Events are in process of occurring that involve actual or likely failures of plant function needed for protection of the public. With this level of risk, radioactive material release should not exceed EPA Protective Action Guides (PAGs), except at the site boundary.
4. *General emergency:* Events have led to actual or imminent core damage, melting of reactor fuel, and potential loss of containment integrity.

Multiple levels of monitoring and communications exist for nuclear reactor safety. Nuclear power plant personnel must monitor and report plant conditions, including elevating risk, as appropriate, and must make recommendations to state and local government agencies for protecting populations. State or local government agencies make decisions on actions to protect the public and also relay this information to the public. Personnel and government agencies must make decisions regarding protective actions that may include evacuation, sheltering, and potassium iodide supplementation. In general, evacuations take place in a "keyhole" pattern, consisting of a 2-mile ring around the plant to be evacuated plus the zone downwind of the projected path within 5 miles.[11]

Medical Response Preparedness

As part of emergency response planning, emphasis must be placed upon population monitoring after exposure. On an international level, Radiation Emergency Medical Preparedness and Assistance (REMPAN) functions to strengthen emergency preparedness, treat and monitor exposed populations, improve public health advice, mitigate long-term effects of radiation exposure, and improve long-term follow-up and preparedness.[14] In the event of radiation release, it is imperative that those persons who are at risk of exposure be notified as soon as possible not only about their risk, but about ways to minimize their risk. To perform these notifications, methods and plans must be in place to identify exposed and at-risk populations, along with methods for communication and tracking these populations so as to monitor their future health over an extended length of time.

Administration of potassium iodide within 4 hours of radiation exposure and no more than 12 hours after exposure is critical. The iodide in these tablets will become attached to thyroid binding sites such that all subsequently inhaled or ingested iodide (i.e., the radioactive isotope), having no place to bind, will be eliminated from the body. Children and teenagers are at the greatest risk of developing thyroid cancer after exposure. Planning for the stockpile and delivery of this treatment is a vital component of preparedness in high-risk areas.

Thus preparedness and planning for a nuclear plant incident requires extensive collaboration among government officials, individual nuclear power plants, and first responders. All of these entities need training, regular drills, appropriate stockpile of supplies, and close monitoring to ensure that the plans function to ensure maximal public safety.

RESPONSE

The response phase of a nuclear incident includes all activities from immediate response to relief activities and then to rehabilitation and reconstruction. The response to a nuclear plant accident is complex and multifaceted. It involves coordinated actions between the plant facility, local responders, and a variety of state and federal agencies. Response to nuclear accidents can be divided into the following components:[17]

1. Notifying appropriate authorities
2. Securing the source of radioactivity and preventing further release
3. Monitoring and tracking radioactivity released into the environment
4. Monitoring and tracking radioactivity in the affected area
5. Providing information about the accident to the public and appropriate agencies to diminish health consequences
6. Securing and remediating the area affected by the incident
7. Treating plant personnel and civilians affected by the accident

It is imperative that each power plant facility become familiar with the emergency classifications of plant conditions as outlined by NRC regulations so that it will be prepared to initiate the proper protective actions in the event of a nuclear incident.[11] Familiarity with the procedures for alerting the appropriate federal, state, and local agencies that will respond to a nuclear accident is also vital to the disaster response. Once informed about an incident, a number of government and civilian agencies can be mobilized to provide technical and personnel support in response to the disaster (Table 23-2). These organizations can assist in monitoring and tracking of regions affected by the radioactive materials released.[18–26]

Disaster planning at local health facilities is also important. Local health professionals should have training in the management of exposure to radioactive materials, including training in decontamination procedures and prophylactic use of pharmacological agents such as potassium iodide. Currently, only 21 of the 34 states with reactors have obtained sufficient supplies of potassium iodide to cover their populations within the 10-mile emergency planning zone. As alternatives to potassium iodide administration, sheltering and evacuating the public can be implemented as measures to prevent potential exposure to radioactive material. Sheltering includes keeping the public indoors, which helps to minimize further exposure. Complete evacuation of the 10-mile EPZ is not always necessary. Given that the spread of radioactive material released from a reactor usually follows the prevailing wind direction, the zone of evacuation is mapped in accordance with the path of release. In general, the evacuation area consists of a minimum of a 2-mile radius around the nuclear power plant plus a 5-mile zone downwind from the projected path of release—a scheme referred to as the "keyhole" pattern.[11]

A variety of government and civilian agencies are available to assist with the response to a nuclear plant incident. During a nuclear or radiological incidenct of national significance, the Department of Homeland Security is responsible for the overall coordination of incident response. For incidents of lesser significance, the responsible agency is the designated coordinating agency—"that Federal agency which owns, has custody of, authorizes, regulates, or is otherwise deemed responsible for the radiological facility or activity involved in the incident."[27] For example, the NRC is the coordinating agency for all nuclear incidents occurring at its licensed facilities. The Department of Defense or Department of Energy is the designated coordinating agency for incidents occurring at facilities under their jurisdiction. The Environmental Protection Agency is the coordinating agency for nuclear incidents at facilities not licensed by a federal agency. During a response to an incidenct of national significance, the coordinating agency provides technical expertise, personnel, and equipment in support of the actions taken by the Department of Homeland Security, which in turn is responsible for overall coordination of the response. A detailed list of coordinating agencies can be found in the Nuclear Radiological Incident Annex: National Response Plan.[27]

TABLE 23-2   Summary of Major U.S. Nuclear/Radiological Response Assets and Functions

Responding Organization	Main Objectives	Oversight Authority		Expertise and/or Resources
Air Force Radiation Assessment Team (AFRAT)	On-site detection, identification, and measurement of any radiation hazard.	U.S. Department of Defense	U.S. Air Force	Expertise in areas of health physics, environmental monitoring, and radiation measurement. Handheld radiological monitoring equipment, air sampling equipment, and laptop plume modeling software.
Medical Radiobiology Advisory Team (MRAT), http://www.afrri.usuhs.mil/outreach/meir/mrat.htm	Provides health physics, medical, and radiobiological advice to military and civilian commands in a nuclear incident.		Armed Forces Radiobiology Research Institute (AFRRI)	2 to 20 personnel who are experts in chemical, biological, radiological, nuclear, and explosives matters.
National Guard Weapons of Mass Destruction—Civil Support Team (WMD-CST)	Supports local and state authorities at responding to domestic incidents.			Acts as first military responders to initiate the response process and pave the way for other state and federal assets. Provides mobile laboratory and field communications to assist in initial threat assessment and provide technical assistance.
Radiological Advisory Medical Team (RAMT)	Works with local medical personnel to provide assistance in mass-exposure screening, decontamination, and casualty treatment.		U.S. Army	Personnel with expertise in health physics, radiation medicine, and mental health. Provides a variety of radiation detectors for mass screening.
Aerial Measuring System (AMS), http://nnsa.energy.gov/emergency_ops/1713.htm	Provides rapid survey of radiation contamination following a radiological incident.	U.S. Department of Energy	National Nuclear Security Administration (NNSA)	Aircraft equipped to detect and measure radioactive materials in the air and on the ground.
Accident Response Group (ARG), http://nnsa.energy.gov/emergency_ops/1715.htm	Responds to nuclear weapon accidents.		NNSA	Technical support for responding to nuclear weapon accidents, including nuclear weapons recovery, stabilization, transport, disposal, and safety.

Federal Radiological Monitoring and Assessment Center (FRMAC), http://nnsa.energy.gov/emergency_ops/1711.htm	Coordinates and manages radiological incident response using federal assets.	NNSA	Supports field operations through radiation monitoring and analysis as well as medical support. A Phase I response team can arrive within 6 to 10 hours at any location within the United States.
National Atmospheric Release Advisory Center (NARAC), http://nnsa.energy.gov/emergency_ops/1712.htm	Real-time predictions of atmospheric spread of radioactive material.	NNSA	Provides computer modeling of potential spread of radioactive contamination to aid in determining the impact of the event.
Radiological Assistance Program (RAP), http://nnsa.energy.gov/emergency_ops/1709.htm	Provides first response assistance to ensure the safety of the public and the environment. Assists other agencies in detection, identification, and analysis of radioactive materials.	NNSA	Provides telephone consultation as well as on-site guidance. Covers nine geographic regions, with a minimum of three teams stationed in each region. Offers technical assistance as part of the initial response. Provides a mobile laboratory, personal protective equipment, detection, monitoring, identification, and decontamination equipment and expertise.
Radiation Emergency Assistance Center/Training Site (REAC/TS), http://nnsa.energy.gov/emergency_ops/1714.htm	Provides medical expertise in support of a radiological emergency.	NNSA	Provides telephone consultation as well as on-site medical care. Also provides care at the REAC/TS medical facility. Provides training in treatment of radiation exposure to healthcare professionals.
Nuclear Regulatory Commission (NRC)	Acts as the response coordinating agency.		Provides technical assistance to calculate plume dispersion and dose assessment.

Source: Adapted from Maiello ML, Groves, KL. Resources for nuclear and radiation disaster response. *Nuclear News.* September 2006: 29–34.

MITIGATION

Mitigation refers to those actions taken to prevent and reduce the effects of reactor failure associated with the release of radioactive materials. Mitigation activities focus on pre-disaster assessment, prevention of an incident, training, safety regulations, and reactor design and construction.

The NRC has adopted stringent regulations dealing with the safety of both plant design and emergency planning. Today's nuclear power plants are built with multiple layers of physical barriers and redundant safety mechanisms to prevent release of radioactive material. The NRC requires that each plant facility develop and submit an emergency plan as well as conduct periodic drills to prepare for implementation of the emergency plan during a genuine emergency. Plant personnel must meet qualification requirements and are required to follow strict training programs.

Nuclear Power Plant

Both the Chernobyl accident and the accident at Three Mile Island reinforced the importance of physical plant design and operator proficiency in preventing the release of radioactive materials during an incident. Today, nuclear power plants are physically designed to have multiple layers of containment technology aimed at preventing the release of radioactive materials. Redundant safety mechanisms and cooling systems allow the plant to shut down automatically if necessary. Lessons learned from the Three Mile Island incident led to improved instrumentation designs and stricter monitoring of radiation levels. Building maintenance and inspections must now take place regularly. Recently, however, concerns have arisen regarding the longevity of nuclear power plants in terms of their construction, particularly with respect to water pipes and corrosion.

Plant Security

Following the terrorist attacks that occurred in the United States on September 11, 2001, security experts drew attention to the fact that nuclear power plants are potential targets for terrorist attacks and raised concerns about the vulnerability of nuclear power plants. In response, the NRC adopted new plant security requirements and enhanced coordination between federal, state, and local response organizations.[28] The Energy Policy Act of 2005 required the NRC to tighten its security requirements and mandated background checks on all nuclear power plant employees. Public education in targeted geographical areas near nuclear plants can help to prevent mass panic during heightened security alerts about possible terrorist attacks. It is especially important that the communities surrounding nuclear power plants become familiar with the emergency response as well as the evacuation procedures to be followed in the event of a nuclear accident.

ANALYSIS OF CASE STUDY

Historically, the most significant incident in the history of U.S. commercial nuclear reactors was the accident at Three Mile Island in 1979. While a combination of equipment failure and plant operator error eventually led to a partial core meltdown and the release of a small amount of radioactive material, the incident caused no injuries, deaths, or long-term health effects. However, the event drew attention to flaws in nuclear plant designs and operator training as well as inadequacies in local, regional, and national planning and response to a potential nuclear power plant crisis.

The Kemeny Commission concluded that the Three Mile Island accident was a result of "human, institutional, and mechanical failures."[7] The accident was triggered by equipment failure, which led to a series of additional plant failures that were not recognized by the plant operators due to insufficient training. The control room at the power plant was poorly designed and could not detect the equipment malfunction in a clear manner. As a result, more than 100 alarms went off during the early stage of the accident, and the operators were not able to identify key indicators of the problem. There also were no instruments designed to follow the course of the event. Overall, the intrinsic flaws in plant design and inadequate operator training exacerbated the accident. The Kemeny Commission recommended improved equipment design to allow key plant safety indicators to be grouped in a single panel and distinct warning signals. Furthermore, it recommended that the nuclear industry establish standards for operator training and accreditation.[7]

Although the Three Mile Island incident did not result in the release of large amounts of radioactive material, this event revealed a lack of planning for nuclear emergency preparedness and response at the federal, state, and local levels. The high confidence at the NRC in the intrinsic safety features built into the power plants, as well as a desire to avoid raising public concern, led to a lack of emphasis on emergency planning at the NRC. While the NRC required the plant to have an emergency plan covering the 2-mile radius surrounding the plant, there was no requirement for a municipal, county, or state emergency plan. Communication was poor among the various parties involved in the response, and no clear delineation of roles for the governing bodies at each level existed, including at the NRC.

In the aftermath of the Three Mile Island event, the NRC adopted more stringent requirements for nuclear facility licensing, including mandatory FEMA-approved local and state level emergency planning that specifies the response-related responsibilities of both the facility and government agencies. Each plant facility is also required to exercise its emergency plan in coordination with off-site agencies at least once every two years. In addition, the NRC established EPZs and an emergency classification system for plant conditions to be used during emergency planning.

No major health consequences were reported as a result of the Three Mile Island incident.[29] However, public health preparedness at that time was clearly lacking. In 1979, the NRC did not require obligatory notification of state or local health authorities in the event of a nuclear incident. The state health department did not have sufficient resources to respond to radiological emergencies. No coordinated evacuation plan had been put in place for the hospitals located near the power plant. The health professionals there as well as the on-site physicians at the power plant were ill prepared to deal with medical care relating to radiological emergencies. Although the use of blocking agents such as potassium iodide for the protection of the thyroid gland against radioiodine was widely known at the time of the accident, sufficient supplies of potassium iodide were not available commercially to treat the population within a 20-mile radius of the reactor. To overcome these shortcomings, the Kemeny Commission recommended better cooperation with the local, state, and national health authorities in planning for a response to radiological emergencies. Public health preparedness should include increased surveillance and monitoring to determine the consequences of radiation exposure and enhanced educational programs for health professionals relating to radiological emergencies.

In contrast to the relatively benign outcome of the Three Mile Island accident, the 1986 Chernobyl nuclear reactor accident was considered to be the worst nuclear power plant incident in history. A combination of operator error and poor plant safety design led to an explosion that destroyed the reactor, which in turn led to the release of massive amounts of radioactive materials into the surroundings. Twenty-eight reactor staff and emergency workers died within 4 months of the accident as a result of acute radiation syndrome.[30] There was widespread contamination of the surrounding areas, including Belarus, the Russian Federation, and Ukraine. Following the accident, delays in evacuation and insufficient public communication further increased the number of individuals exposed to harmful levels of radiation. According to the Chernobyl Forum Report from 2005 and other studies, approximately 4,000 cases of thyroid cancer were diagnosed among exposed individuals who were children and adolescents at the time of the accident.[8,31] While there was no evidence to suggest increased incidence of leukemia and other cancers, there was an increase in the rate of mental illness in persons exposed to the fallout from the plant.[8]

CONCLUSION

With 104 commercial nuclear power plants located in 34 states in the United States, the potential for a nuclear power plant accident is real. As exemplified by the Chernobyl incident, poorly managed containment and response can have devastating consequences for the surrounding environment and population. While the Three Mile Island incident did not result in significant environmental or health damage, it highlighted significant inadequacies in the planning and response to a nuclear power plant accident.

Experiences from Three Mile Island outlined the need for more stringent government oversight of the licensing requirements for both nuclear power plants and the workers at those facilities. Establishing an emergency plan and conducting regular drills and exercises are critical to the success of a coordinated response in the setting of a radiological accident. Coordination and frequent communication among local, state, and federal agencies and health authorities is essential in disaster preparedness, response, and mitigation (Table 23-3).

TABLE 23-3	Summary of Radiological Emergency Preparedness, Response, and Mitigation
Preparedness and planning	• Stringent licensing requirements • Mandatory disaster planning and regular drills • Collaborative efforts among local, state, and federal authorities • Determination of the at-risk population • Identification of potential shelters • Local hospital disaster planning • Potassium iodide stockpile
Response	• Alerting appropriate agencies • Securing the source of radioactivity to prevent further release • Monitoring and tracking of radioactivity released • Monitoring and tracking of exposed population • Public communication • Shelter and evacuation • Medical treatment and potassium iodide distribution
Mitigation	• Safe power plant design • Stringent education and training protocols for plant employees • Enhanced power plant security • Stringent safety regulations • Public education • Health professional education

Public health authorities should be closely integrated into the planning and response to a radiological emergency. Their role in disaster preparedness should include surveillance and monitoring in case of radiation exposure and enhanced health professional education in the management of radiation exposure. In addition, public health authorities should be prepared to assist local healthcare facilities in the radiological disaster response and the coordination of the dispensing of potassium iodide from stockpiles if an event occurs.

INTERNET RESOURCES

Centers for Disease Control and Prevention, radiation emergencies:
http://emergency.cdc.gov/radiation/

International Atomic Energy Agency, incidents and emergencies:
http://www-ns.iaea.org/tech-areas/emergency/default.htm

U.S. Federal Emergency Management Agency, Radiological Emergency Preparedness Program:
http://www.fema.gov/about/divisions/thd_repp.shtm

U.S. Nuclear Regulatory Commission, emergency preparedness and response:
http://www.nrc.gov/about-nrc/emerg-preparedness.html

World Health Organization, radiation accidents and emergencies:
http://www.who.int/ionizing_radiation/a_e/en/

NOTES

1. European Nuclear Society. Nuclear power plants worldwide. Available at: http://www.euronuclear.org/info/encyclopedia/n/nuclear-power-plant-world-wide.htm. Accessed April 29, 2009.
2. U.S. Nuclear Regulatory Commission (NRC). Backgrounder on emergency preparedness at nuclear power plants. January 2009. Available at: http://www.nrc.gov/reading-rm/doc-collections/fact-sheets/emerg-plan-prep-nuc-power-bg.html. Accessed September 8, 2009.
3. Souchkevitch GN, Tsyb AI (Eds.). *Health consequences of the Chernobyl accident: Scientific report.* Geneva: World Health Organization; 1996, pp. 248–250.
4. U.S. Nuclear Regulatory Commission (NRC). Fact sheet on the Three Mile Island accident. August 2009. Available at: http://www.nrc.gov/reading-rm/doc-collections/fact-sheets/3mile-isle.html. Accessed September 1, 2009.
5. Miller KS. Radiologic history exhibit: The nuclear reactor accident at Three Mile Island. *Radiographics.*1994:215–224.
6. Wing S. Objectivity and ethics in environmental health science. *Environmental Health Perspectives.* 2003;111(14):1809–1818.
7. Kemeny JG, et al. *President's Commission: The need for change: The legacy of TMI.* Washington, DC: U.S. Government Printing Office; 1979. Available at: http://www.threemileisland.org/downloads//188.pdf. Accessed September 1, 2008.

8. The Chernobyl Forum. Chernobyl's legacy: Health, environmental and socio-economic impacts and recommendations to the governments of Belarus, the Russian Federation and Ukraine. Available at: http://www.iaea.org/Publications/Booklets/Chernobyl/chernobyl.pdf. Accessed September 8, 2008.

9. U.S. Department of Health and Human Services, Food and Drug Administration, Center for Drug Evaluation and Research. Guidance: Potassium iodide as a thyroid blocking agent in radiation emergencies. December 2001. Available at: http://www.fda.gov/downloads/Drugs/GuidanceComplianceRegulatoryInformation/Guidances/ucm080542.pdf. Accessed September 8, 2008.

10. U.S. Energy Information Administration. Annual energy review 2008. June 2009. Available at: http://www.eia.doe.gov/emeu/aer/pdf/pages/sec9.pdf. Accessed September 23, 2009.

11. U.S. Nuclear Regulatory Commission (NRC). Emergency preparedness at the nuclear power plants. January 2009. Available at: http://www.nrc.gov/reading-rm/doc-collections/fact-sheets/emerg-plan-prep-nuc-power-bg.html. Accessed September 8, 2009.

12. Centers for Disease Control and Prevention. Radiation emergencies: Fact sheet. August 2004. Available at: http://emergency.cdc.gov/radiation/measurement.asp. Accessed September 1, 2008.

13. Bottolier-Dupois JF, Chau Q, Buisset P, et al. Assessing exposure to cosmic radiation during long-haul flights. *Radiation Research.* 2000;153(5):526–532.

14. Souchkevitch G. The World Health Organization Network for Radiation Emergency Medical Preparedness and Assistance (REMPAN). *Environmental Health Perspectives.* 1997;105(6): 1589–1593.

15. U.S. Atomic Energy Commission (AEC). *Theoretical possibilities and consequences of major accidents in large nuclear power plants.* 1957. Available at: http://www.dissident-media.org/infonucleaire/wash740.pdf. Accessed September 23, 2009.

16. U.S. Nuclear Regulatory Commission (NRC). Overview of state-of-the-art reactor consequence analyses (SOARCA). June 2009. Available at: http://www.nrc.gov/about-nrc/regulatory/research/soar/overview.html#1. Accessed September 23, 2009.

17. Maiello ML, Groves, KL. Resources for nuclear and radiation disaster response. *Nuclear News.* September 2006: 29–34. Available at: http://hps.org/hsc/documents/Sep06NNResources.pdf. Accessed September 19, 2008.

18. Scott R. *Air Force medical service concept of operations for Air Force Radiation Assessment Team Nuclear Incident Response Force 1 and 2 (FFRA1 and FFRA2).* Brookside Press; 1999. Available at: http://www.brooksidepress.org/Products/OperationalMedicine/DATA/operationalmed/Operational Settings/Air%20Force/AFMSCONOPs.htm. Accessed September 24, 2008.

19. Armed Forces Radiobiology Research Institute, Uniformed Services University of the Health Science. Medical Radiobiology Advisory Team. Available at: http://www.afrri.usuhs.mil/outreach/emergency_response.htm. Accessed January 26, 2010.

20. Mercier J. *Mission and capabilities of the U.S. Army Radiological Assistance Medical Team (RAMT).* Washington, DC: Health Physics Office, Walter Reed Army Medical Center. Available at: http://irpa11.irpa.net/pdfs/7g13.pdf. Accessed September 24, 2008.

21. U.S. Department of Energy, National Nuclear Security Administration. Aerial Measuring System. Available at: http://nnsa.energy.gov/emergency_ops/1713.htm. Accessed September 24, 2008.

22. U.S. Department of Energy, National Nuclear Security Administration. Accident Response Group. Available at: http://nnsa.energy.gov/emergency_ops/1715.htm. Accessed September 24, 2008.

23. U.S. Department of Energy, National Nuclear Security Administration. Federal Radiological Monitoring and Assessment Center. Available at: http://nnsa.energy.gov/emergency_ops/1711.htm. Accessed September 24, 2008.

24. U.S. Department of Energy, National Nuclear Security Administration. National Atmospheric Release Advisory Center. Available at: http://nnsa.energy.gov/emergency_ops/1712.htm. Accessed September 24, 2008.

25. U.S. Department of Energy, National Nuclear Security Administration. Radiological Assistance Program. Available at: http://nnsa.energy.gov/emergency_ops/1709.htm. Accessed September 24, 2008.

26. U.S. Department of Energy, National Nuclear Security Administration. Radiation Emergency Assistance Center/Training Site. Available at: http://nnsa.energy.gov/emergency_ops/1714.htm. Accessed September 24, 2008.

27. U.S. Department of Homeland Security. National response plan: Nuclear/radiological incident annex. 2004. Available at: http://hps.org/documents/ NRPNuclearAnnex.pdf. Accessed September 3, 2008.

28. Holt M, Andrews A. CRS report for Congress: Nuclear power plant security and vulnerabilities. 2008. Available at: http://www.fas.org/sgp/crs/homesec/RL34331.pdf. Accessed September 3, 2008.

29. BehLing UH, Hildebrand JE. Radiation and health effects: A report on the TMI-2 accident and related health studies. Middletown, PA: General Public Utilities Nuclear Corporation; 1996. Available at: http://www.threemileisland.org/downloads//224.pdf. Accessed April 30, 2009.

30. U.S. Nuclear Regulatory Commission (NRC). Backgrounder on Chernobyl nuclear power plant accident. April 2009. Available at: http://www.nrc.gov/reading-rm/doc-collections/fact-sheets/chernobyl-bg.html. Accessed April 29, 2009.

31. Stsjazhko VA, Tsyb AF, Tronko ND, Souchkevitch G, Baverstock K. Childhood thyroid cancer since accident at Chernobyl. *British Medical Journal.* 1995;310:801.

SECTION 8

Special Populations and Issues

Mental Health Emergencies and Post-traumatic Stress Disorder

Siddharth Ashvin Shah

INTRODUCTION

From a public health perspective, complex emergencies and large-scale disasters produce enormous and multifaceted mental health morbidity.[1] Individuals will encounter symptoms of emotional distress that are primarily nonpathologic (in contrast to psychiatric illness) but, at the same time, worthy of emergency attention. Nevertheless, much of the suffering that is deemed "mental" is missed, overlooked, or deferred indefinitely due to a focus on physical injuries.

Within psychiatry, the American Psychiatric Association's *Diagnostic and Statistical Manual*, fourth edition, text revision (*DSM-IV-TR*) defines a traumatic event as one in which a person is confronted with a significant threat and the person's response to that threat involves "intense fear, helplessness or horror."[2] A broader, working definition of "trauma" is a stressor that overwhelms an individual's capacity to respond and cope adaptively. In Western societies, although wide consensus exists about post-traumatic stress disorder (PTSD) being the most identifiable post-traumatic sequela, the health professional evaluating traumatized populations should have a differential diagnosis breadth that includes the following mental health morbidities: generalized anxiety disorder, panic disorder, major depression, complicated grief, acute stress disorder (thought to have predictive power of long-term morbidity), substance abuse, somatoform disorders, poor physical health, multiple idiopathic physical symptoms (or "MUS," medically unexplained symptoms), arrest or regression of childhood developmental progression, behavioral changes, and work and relationship disturbances, including family conflict.[3–21] This chapter provides a "best practices" framework for selecting and applying mental health interventions for public health emergencies. It outlines the preparedness, intervention, and mitigation strategies for proactive and systematic emergency mental health response.

Case Study

On December 26, 2004, the Asian tsunami caused catastrophic and overwhelming traumatic events in socioeconomically vulnerable populations across multiple nations. At least 5 million people were affected, 1 million were displaced, and 280,000 were killed; all of these outcomes involved layers of mental suffering. In the days immediately following the tsunami, countless oceanside fishing communities were in shock: grieving the loss of family, neighbors, property, and livelihood.

Many practitioners responding to this incident encountered diverse biopsychosocial complaints. Studies later revealed the specific syndromes that became prevalent following the tsunami. However, in real time immediately after the initial event, fieldworkers reported that some of the most common complaints cited by the affected population were "We are not sleeping" and "We are worried about more tsunami" (anticipatory apprehension due to rumors of further tsunami and reports of aftershocks).[22,23] These two complaints were connected: People were averse to sleep so that they could take evasive actions in case of future tsunami waves.

FRAMEWORK

To promote effective recovery from mental trauma and to mitigate harm, a framework that helps determine best practices, flags harmful practices, and streamlines interagency activities should be in place on a "pre-event" basis.[1] During a public health emergency, important differences and specific needs can be easily missed in favor of "just getting through it" minimalism. The problem with minimalism is that interventions are arbitrarily chosen, opportunities are lost, and outcomes suffer.[1] The solution is to systematize the mental health approach and engage in "best practices." Figure 24-1 depicts a simple framework by which public health officials and healthcare workers can meet a best practices standard for mental health interventions.

Situation, phase, population and patient (SPPP) are the four fundamental parameters for calibrating mental health interventions in public health emergencies. To be effective, emergency responders must have a familiarity with ways to discern the SPPP parameters and implement interventions accordingly. Each parameter can be better understood by asking a specific question about the major issue at hand.

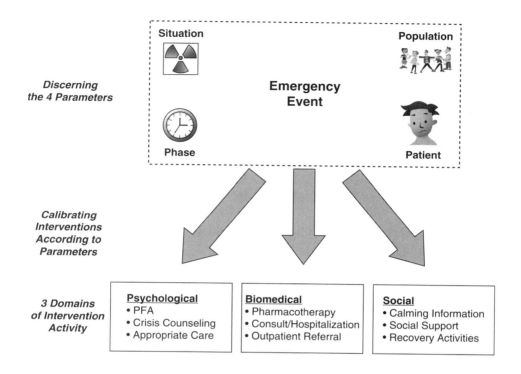

FIGURE 24-1   Framework for Emergency Mental Health Interventions

Situation-specific parameters: What is it about this event that overwhelms the capacity to respond and cope adaptively?

Large-scale public health emergencies are characterized by situational factors that make for a highly emotional and stressful environment: the injurious event itself, confused reactions to limited information, maladaptive coping mechanisms (e.g., rumors, aggression), and evacuation trauma.[24] For example, psychological stresses specific to a radiological disaster are complex owing to the following facts: the invisible, odorless, and unfelt nature of radiation; its unfamiliarity; fear of sterility/impotence; fear of malformed offspring; fear of malignancy; and possible social stigma associated with a perceived or real exposure.[25]

Phase-sensitive parameters: Which concerns, symptoms, and syndromes are paramount at this point in time after the event (or as the event unfolds)?

The time elapsed since the traumatic event determines the extent to which signs and symptoms are "expected and normal" as opposed to signs and symptoms that are pathological and deserve special attention. The demarcations of *impact*, *acute*, and *post-acute* are frequently used phases; however, their exact onset/resolution are subject to systemic factors and clinical judgment.

- *Impact:* The impact spans the period from the initiation of the traumatic event up to the first 24 to 48 hours after the termination of the event. During this phase, a community's "fight, flight, or freeze" responses are at their peak. Confusion, insomnia, intense emotions, heroism, disorganized behavior, and shock are to be expected. Other than psychosis and harm to self or others, most reactions are normal responses to trauma; however, if the reactions cause a person to become emotionally inflexible and nonfunctional, then professional attention is warranted.
- *Acute:* Extending for two months after the event, the acute phase consists of processing, or "taking stock of," the trauma. Communities and families attempt to understand their losses while the brains of individuals are transitioning from fear responses to goal-directed thinking. Rapid shifts in mood and arousal are pervasive.
- *Post-acute:* After two months and beyond, the community establishes a "new normal" in which a routine has been established and stress levels are close to their pre-event levels. Psychiatric syndromes (anxiety disorders, PTSD, depression) in response to the event will be more discernable during this time.

This chapter focuses on the impact and early acute phases (collectively called "early intervention" in some of the literature) when emergency response is most active.

Population-based parameters: What is known about the people needing assistance? Which barriers prevent healthcare professionals from reaching those persons who may not present themselves for assistance?

The interventions and protocols used in public health emergencies should be appropriate to the affected population. Demographics and risk factors are important to understand in this regard. Social and political history also may play into how the population reacts. Thus a well-honed understanding of the situation-specific parameters and expertise in lowering the barriers to mental health assistance for subgroups that are marginalized or self-isolating will improve the efforts of public health professionals.

Patient-centered parameters: What interventions would assist this particular individual to cope adaptively and reduce morbidity?

To be patient centered means to choose interventions that are effective based on an individual's past history, pre-event emotional stresses, and cognitive style. In such a case, assessment is focused not simply on PTSD, but also on the range of post-traumatic morbidity relevant to an individual.[26] Those patients with pre-event histories of mental illness should be assessed for exacerbations of psychosis/mania, impulses to self-harm, or the interruption of medications.[27,28]

Interventions should be chosen to promote health and healing in a way that emotionally and cognitively engages the individual in the process. During a public health emergency surge, patient-centered parameters may be the most difficult to follow. However, even after the post-acute phase, emergency department personnel, primary care systems, and public health professionals should assess for exposure and coping skills in a trauma-exposed population: Studies show that survivors will seek help in large numbers for medical problems, such as cardiovascular disease, and these medical visits offer an opportunity to simultaneously conduct mental health screenings.[29–31]

PREPAREDNESS AND PLANNING

Regarding the systems in play during a public health emergency, the emergency medicine literature increasingly recommends that emergency medical services (EMS) systems coordinate with government and other agencies through the hazard management concept known as the Incident Command System (ICS).[32–34] The ICS operates to exchange information and coordinate multiple agencies in an effort to improve the response and prevent counterproductive activities.

Individual agencies, such as hospitals, must have designated personnel who are fluent in the ICS and who can forge relationships with the local-, regional-, and national-level response systems as well as with the many voluntary organizations that become active in disasters. According to the U.S. government, these designated personnel provide 1 of 15 Emergency Support Functions (ESF) within the National Response Framework. For example, ESF 8 is "Public Health and Medical Services"; at the level of a hospital, ESF personnel are responsible for coordinating services, providers, facilities, equipment, training, materials, and supplies needed for emergency and disaster operations.

The National Response Framework recognizes that mental health concerns are integral to a public emergency response. In addition to maintaining print and multi-media psycho-educational materials ready for the affected community, ESF requires regular updates of the database of interventions to be used by providers. Especially during an emergency, protecting the mental health of a population requires that ESF has maintained pre-event linkages that include plans, procedures, arrangements, and agreements to identify, acquire, and mobilize services and resources (Table 24-1).[35–40]

Surge capacity is an important metric for healthcare institutions that has recently come under intense scrutiny.[41–44] According to Hick et al., surge capacity describes "the

TABLE 24-1   Linkages with Mental Health Services and Resources
1. Psychiatric, psychological and social work services within one's own institution ("in-house")
2. Relief agencies—international, governmental, nongovernmental (e.g., federal/central government, United Nations, United Nations High Commissioner for Refugees [UNHCR], Centers for Disease Control and Prevention [CDC], Substance Abuse and Mental Health Services Administration [SAMHSA], U.S. Department of Health and Human Services, state and county departments of social services, regional behavioral health authorities, Red Crescent/Red Cross, World Vision, Save the Children, regional associations of psychologists/psychiatrists/social workers)
3. Neighboring academic medical centers
4. Community-based mental health practitioners and agencies that connect patients (e.g., Mental Health Association hotline, 800-LIFE-NET)
5. Faith-based institutions and spiritual care practitioners
6. Schools and other means of contact with youth

ability of a health care system to respond to a sudden increase in patient care demands."[45] Mental health concerns are more likely to be neglected when a surge overwhelms personnel, resources, and physical facilities (referenced elsewhere as "staff, stuff, and structure"). The adage "All disasters are local" emphasizes the necessity of developing the community's capacity, because state, federal, and other relief groups often cannot respond to these needs in a short time frame.

Formulated in conjunction with ESF coordinators, standardized roles and processes should be practiced by institutions during non-surge times. Maintaining and continuing standardized roles and processes during overwhelming situations minimizes institutional anxiety, arbitrariness, panic, and fear. The aforementioned linkages and pre-event coordination are part of this institutional resilience, but no amount of confidence or linkages can override the need for institutions to establish plans and standards of care for professionals to adhere to during the course of a surge.

INTERVENTIONS

Emergency interventions to safeguard a population's mental health involve activities from three interlocking domains: psychological, biomedical, and social.[46–48] When calibrated by the SPPP parameters, the following intervention activities serve a broad range of needs.

Psychological Interventions

Psychological First Aid

In the United States and other countries, psychological first aid (PFA) is gaining acceptance as the set of early interventions with the best evidence base and least potential for harm. While the terminology of PFA may differ slightly from one source to another, interventions should include the following measures:

- Provide a human presence for those who are highly distressed
- Enhance ongoing safety and comfort; shielding survivors from further harm or unnecessary triggers or reminders
- Reduce physiologic arousal and teach calming techniques
- Impart information to minimize uncertainty
- Facilitate reunion with loved ones and utilize social support systems

PFA has been described in several excellent publications, including the National Institutes for Health (NIH) publication titled *Mental Health and Mass Violence: Evidence-Based Early Psychological Intervention for Victims/Survivors of Mass Violence* and the National Child Traumatic Stress Network and National Center for PTSD publication titled *Psychological First Aid: Field Operations Guide* (which includes handouts for providers and survivors).[49] PFA also supports the religious/spiritual views of survivors. If a survivor clearly finds strength using religious or spiritual terminology and the assigned member of the healthcare team is not comfortable with such usage, then the public health professional should transfer the survivor to another member for appropriate care.

Crisis Counseling

Naturally, some proportion of survivors will actively seek out human interactions for the release of their traumatic experience and memories. These interactions then take on elements of crisis counseling—an intervention that cannot be provided on a large scale in the impact phase of a public health emergency because of the limited supply of trained professionals available. If feasible, referral to outpatient counseling is most practical.

Debate exists over what constitutes "debriefing" and its benefits. Studies and meta-analyses suggest that single sessions of psychological debriefing (in which subjects are asked to recount or discuss their traumatic experience soon after the event) have little or no benefit in preventing PTSD and may induce worse outcomes in the general population.[50–55] "Debriefing" can also be taken to mean critical incident stress debriefing

(CISD), which is one component of a larger program called critical incident stress management (CISM).[56–58] Research shows that CISM is effective for emergency service workers (e.g., firefighters, police, humanitarian workers) who, in preparing to be in harm's way, are oriented to CISM as part of their job training and team culture.[59–61] Thus, when traumatic experiences occur, these CISM-trained emergency workers anticipate CISD to follow. Single sessions of debriefing are against CISM protocol.

If crisis counseling is indicated (because a patient feels pressure to speak about his or her experiences and that communication cannot be deferred until after the impact phase), careful attention should be paid to whether the recounting of trauma is associated with problematic physiologic arousal or dissociation. When problematic reactions occur, a reversion to PFA interventions is important to prevent further harm. If signs of decompensation occur, then psychiatric evaluation is likely indicated and hospitalization may potentially be necessary.

Delivery of Appropriate Care to Vulnerable Populations

A vulnerable population is a group of people who are prone to being overlooked or underserved, even before a public health emergency occurs. Several studies show poorer mental health outcomes in vulnerable subpopulations such as persons of lower socioeconomic status (SES), younger children, and minorities. Other vulnerable groups, for whom sufficient outcomes data are not available, include the elderly, disabled persons, and immigrants.[19,62–65] Generally speaking, vulnerable groups are less able to cope with unfolding emergencies for a variety of reasons. Notably, these groups may manifest significant variations in traumatic effects and help-seeking behavior. They are often disenfranchised and marginalized and, therefore, have limited access to mainstream resources for assistance.

Although it is important not to over-generalize, awareness of specific factors characterizing different groups allows public health professionals to target outreach to those groups whose members might otherwise fail to seek assistance. Once these individuals are enrolled in aid programs, assessment and interventions must be appropriately adapted to address the life circumstances of vulnerable members. For example, assisting children involves an evaluation of families as a system, given that a child's reactions are significantly shaped by parental reactions. Modifying parental responses (e.g., via psycho-education) may significantly diminish post-traumatic morbidity and support natural resilience of children. Additionally, interventions are most effective when they are developmentally appropriate for the reactions of infants, preschool-aged children, school-aged children, and adolescents.[66,67]

Biomedical Interventions

Pharmacologic Agents

Medical professionals should strive for clarity and consistency regarding the intention behind prescribing medications for emergency mental health concerns. Arbitrary practices and biases in emergency medical care may, for example, lead to either over-treatment or under-treatment.[36,68] In the emerging field of neuro-ethics, there is concern that over-treatment might preempt an individual's opportunity to form memories of the event or impede what is known as post-traumatic growth.[69–71] On balance, in the impact and early acute phase of a public health emergency, the acceptable indications for medications are to alleviate overwhelming distress by reducing symptom burden and to improve functioning.

In a training session offered by Disaster Psychiatry Outreach ("Early Therapeutic Interventions Post-Disaster: Psychopharmacology" lecture, March 2008, National Voluntary Organizations Active in Disaster), it was noted that "Despite the limited evidence base for acute pharmacotherapy, the judicious use of short term medications appears to be humane and helpful." In the spirit of promoting rational and humanitarian practices for emergency medical care by nonpsychiatrists, a basic and conservative framework for pharmacological interventions is advocated here. For example, concern over insomnia may warrant pharmacotherapy. Hyperarousal may include severe insomnia for two nights or more, and the ensuing exhaustion and cognitive impairment may significantly hinder an individual's ability to take positive steps toward self-care and recovery. In another example, signs of moderate agitation in a parent may warrant pharmacotherapy; without treatment, the parent's apprehension and disorganization may create a ripple effect, thereby impairing a whole family unit.

Best practices for addressing such agitation and hyperarousal symptoms include a short-term pharmacologic regimen (2 to 5 days) chosen in a patient-centered manner—that is, following a review of the patient's current medications, medical and psychiatric history, allergies, and social support resources. If the agitation presents with significant signs of autonomic hyperarousal, a single dose of propranolol might prove beneficial in reducing the hyper-adrenergic state in the short term. For acute agitation, a single dose of a fast-acting anxiolytic (e.g., lorazepam, diazepam, alprazolam) may be appropriate. For residual agitation, a slow- and long-acting agent such as clonazepam given over 2 to 5 days may be beneficial.

For insomnia, hypnotics such as zolpidem and zaleplon are frequently used. A more conservative choice for insomnia, often used with children, is diphenhydramine.

Psychiatrists routinely prescribe a range of other agents for sleep induction, including trazodone, lorazepam, clonazepam, and quetiapine.

For more serious mental health dysfunction (i.e., decompensation related to psychosis or mood disorders with agitated features), useful agents include antipsychotics such as haloperidol, risperidone or olanzapine.[72] Although rare, adverse effects such as neuroleptic malignant syndrome and sudden cardiac death can occur with even one-time use of antipsychotics; therefore, initial use of these agents should ensure that appropriate support is available should these side effects occur. At very low dose (e.g., risperidone 0.5 mg, olanzapine 2.5 mg), atypical antipsychotics are unlikely to cause severe side effects (extrapyramidal symptoms) and anticholinergic effects (e.g., orthostasis). Importantly, both olanzapine and haloperidol can be administered intramuscularly, which is useful when oral dosing is problematic. As soon as feasible, children and adults who are decompensating should be further evaluated and treated by mental health professionals.

A more speculative area of pharmacologic intervention focuses on prophylaxis (secondary prevention) of PTSD. Recent studies have shown that using propranolol (e.g., 40 mg three or four times per day, with a taper) immediately after a traumatic event in otherwise healthy individuals reduces the chances of developing PTSD.[73–76] Although propranolol and other agents are being examined for PTSD prevention, there is no widespread protocol for prophylaxis for this condition.

There is a combination of strong and weak data supporting the use of antidepressant medications (primarily selective serotonin reuptake inhibitors [SSRIs]) to prevent depression and anxiety disorders (including, but not limited, to PTSD) in the intermediate and long term.[77] Given that these medications can increase feelings of agitation in the initial days of usage, the decision to use them is best left to psychiatrists, who may opt to prescribe a benzodiazepine along with the antidepressant. Several other agents have been under investigation; however, there is not enough evidence that the benefits outweigh the possible adverse effects to recommend their use in this setting.[78,79]

Emergent Mental Health Evaluation and Emergency Hospitalization

The following problems warrant emergent evaluation and a consult by a mental health professional: hallucinations, other psychotic thinking/behavior, severe agitation (unrelenting distress), persistent state of shock (catatonic or frozen), inability to care for self or children, self-destructive impulses, or homicidal thinking. One barrier to mental health care of individuals with these conditions that should be addressed on a "pre-event" basis is that some personnel in the medical center may perceive admitting patients with dangerous mental health concerns as a "resource drain" during a public emergency. This perception is where prior development of an appropriate standard of care during surges is indispensable. Explicit guidelines about the indications for consultation or emergency hospitalization will result in greater efficiency in handling difficult issues without adding to problems due to strained resources.

Outpatient Follow-up

Explicitly arranging follow-up, as opposed to simply advising a patient to "return if there is a problem," can mitigate distress.[17] Pre-event linkages with mental health services and resources (whether available on an in-house basis, at a community-based clinic, or an academic medical center) greatly facilitate patient referral. After initial emergent mental health triage and care, a follow-up outpatient appointment (as well as standard mechanisms to assure that follow-up actually occurs) is indicated in the following cases:

- Patients who warranted evaluation by the mental health team
- Patients who demonstrated intense distress, numerous risk factors, symptoms that might affect daily functioning, or symptoms that might impair executive thinking
- Patients who received antipsychotic agents in the emergency department or have a previously untreated psychiatric disorder
- Patients with severe mental illness who have no longitudinal care or are at risk for medication interruptions

Social Interventions

Providing Calming Information

Information in emergency public health situations can be managed and delivered in multiple, beneficial ways. Accurate and up-to-date information about the unfolding emergency event and relief activities helps to contain anxiety and fears that stem from the unknown. Effective risk communication allows people to comprehend appropriately what harm they have sustained, undertake strategies that safeguard them and their loved ones from further harm, and seek medical necessary countermeasures when indicated.[17,80,81]

Practical information can promote adaptive functioning. Specifically, the public can be educated about typical trauma reactions (palpitations, flashbacks), the difference between normal and pathological reactions, healthy coping techniques (human contact, focusing on breathing), and common maladaptive coping responses (withdrawal, alcohol use). Frequently, persons in crisis experience psychological regression, temporarily losing skills and know-how that would otherwise be automatic. Reminding people to breathe calmly, avoid making major decisions, and seek help can all be done with relative ease through available print and multimedia education. These interventions require surprisingly little effort on the part of public health professionals in comparison with their positive and high-yield impact. In their communications with media and public officials, emergency personnel can impart information, give hope, and make positive recommendations. Studies show that the manner in which a tragic story is managed can either exacerbate or soothe a population's psychological wounding.[82,83] A designated media liaison should be delegated the responsibility of preparing such communications.

Utilizing Social Support Systems

As a key feature of PFA, social support deserves special mention. Emergency responders should facilitate communication that brings families and other primary support persons together for either brief or ongoing contact. Fostering social support includes asking isolated individuals how they might effectively seek support or services once they leave emergency care. Religious or spiritual support systems can also prove calming and organizing for persons who suffer from loss, uncertainty apprehension, or grief.

Involving Survivors in Recovery Activities

Anecdotal evidence from different cultures suggests that survivors feel better when they can participate in constructive, recovery-related activities.[80] Trauma research suggests that the ability to execute purposeful action counteracts the frozen and helpless neurobiological states of trauma.[84] Thus, if a survivor actively seeks to volunteer, emergency staff can point trauma survivors toward organizations that are able to enroll volunteers at a level in keeping with their skills. While some harm-reduction counseling may be appropriate due to the physical and emotional risks to volunteers who engage in recovery activities, as a general rule, trauma-affected persons should not be barred from taking positive action to assist their community during any phase of the public health emergency.

MITIGATION

Many components of preparedness simultaneously serve to mitigate emergency-related mental health consequences. Systems of coordination should be clearly delineated so that agencies and institutions do not clash but rather act synergistically to achieve the best possible outcomes. Often, in the midst of a crisis, the need for PFA or other mental health interventions is shunted to the side or becomes lost. Anticipating this problem of deprioritization and given the evidence on post-traumatic morbidity, mitigation involves mental health advocacy and some degree of automation that ensures interventions are not overlooked.

Resilience is an important capacity to recognize and reinforce in both individuals and communities. Most people exposed to trauma do not develop PTSD or other syndromes. Moreover, communities tend to make heroic recovery efforts and display enormous capacity for hope. Recognizing that recovery and growth are the most common outcomes can help to organize future interventions along a model of health, rather than disease, while leaving room to identify those individuals who require professional care for mental health issues.

A *risk factor* is a characteristic that increases the probability of developing post-traumatic morbidity in persons who have that risk factor as compared to those who do not have the same risk factor. At the intersection of emergency healthcare services and public health, mitigation involves outreach to those members of the community with risk factors. Mitigation efforts for mental health issues can involve secondary and tertiary prevention campaigns directed at those with the following risk factors: female gender, middle age (40 to 60 years old), living in a highly disrupted or traumatized community, prior psychiatric history, prior exposure to trauma or disaster, lack of social supports, ethnic minority status, and having children present in the home. Prevention campaigns may provide education about the extreme stress of emergencies and raise awareness about the need to seek assistance from one's own support system as well as to obtain expert care.

It is important to understand that vulnerable subpopulations (discussed earlier in the "Interventions" section) and subpopulations with risk factors are not necessarily the same groups. For example, being middle-aged (40 to 60 years old) is an individual risk factor for post-traumatic morbidity during disasters, whereas people older than age 60 ("older age") constitute a vulnerable population (i.e., they are prone to being overlooked or underserved). Low SES is both a vulnerability and a risk factor.[85] Finally, certain risk factors cannot be identified on a pre-event basis. Nevertheless, a good mitigation plan will set aside resources for the following groups: those with the highest exposure (dose) to the unfolding emergency and those experiencing forced evacuation, quarantine, or separation from loved ones as a result of the incident.

Another component of mitigation that overlaps with preparedness and planning is cultural adaptation. *Cultural adaptation* refers to educational efforts and practices through which providers become ethno-medically competent and services are appropriately geared toward different cultural groups. Ideally, mental health interventions should not be "one size fits all" measures—that is, taken "off the shelf" from one setting and applied to another, non-identical situation.[65,86–89] A culturally adapted intervention responds to a specific population's patterns of psychological distress and help-seeking behavior.[90,91] For example, similar to ethnic minority populations, low-SES members in the ethnic majority may tend to avoid mainstream mental health care, and they disproportionately rely on primary care services to address their psychological distress. Adaptation can be valuable in any setting and with any population in which the trauma or emergency response is viewed differently.

There is a major opportunity to engage in mitigation and prevention efforts directed toward forestalling mental health problems in first responders (paramedics, police, rescue workers), humanitarian aid workers, medical staff, and mental health providers who become stressed during a public health emergency. PTSD and other psychological morbidity prevalence rates among this population are high, particularly when the emergency involves a human-made or technological disaster.[92,93] For example, 44 percent of the police officers involved in the 1989 Hillsborough football stadium disaster in the United Kingdom, when assessed 1 to 2 years after exposure to this event, were classified with severe symptoms of PTSD, and 44 percent were classified with moderate symptoms.[94] Five months after religious and mob violence affected India in 2002, 100 percent of humanitarian aid workers attributed the onset of at least one new post-trauma symptom (with moderate or severe severity) to their work.[95] After the September 11, 2001, terrorist attacks, 22 percent and 20 percent of disaster workers were found to suffer from PTSD at 2 weeks and 10 to 15 months, respectively.[96]

Perceived physical safety in disaster workers, including emergency staff, has a direct relationship to worker morale and productivity.[38,97] The ongoing psycho-emotional stresses of this type of work calls for pre-event training and during-event support to mitigate vicarious traumatization, also known as secondary traumatic stress. Notably, mental health professionals may be specifically assigned to assist ED staff with their own emotional needs ("caring for the caretaker").[86,98,99] By providing such training and support services, emergency response agencies may not only prevent morbidity in first responders themselves, but also enable those responders to provide better PFA to survivors.

ANALYSIS OF CASE STUDY

Applying the SPPP parameters and intervention guidelines, the sleep disturbances in fishing villages in the aftermath of the Asian tsunami can be analyzed within this framework.

Situation

The suddenness of the tsunami wave, its ability to go inland, and rumors of further earthquakes and waves served to make many on the coast feel exquisitely vulnerable. When asked why they were not sleeping, many individuals stated that they did not want to be caught off-guard by any other act of nature. Others said they tried to sleep but kept remembering the tsunami wave, their terror, and their losses. In the tightly packed shelters at night, individuals often heard neighboring persons cry out or sob. The fact that many human bodies were washed away meant that death rituals could not be performed and that the souls of the dead had no closure.

Phase

Four days after the event, in the acute phase of the emergency, people were deep in grief over sudden losses. They were struggling with vigilance for further trauma on the one hand; and on the other hand, they were considering what it would take to rebuild and move on. Hence, hypervigilance and rapid shifts into sadness were common post-traumatic difficulties.

Population

What was known about fishing communities is that individuals and family units tend to be fiercely independent. They are known to revere the ocean for its power. The tsunami had shaken some of their faith, yet some people wanted to get back to fishing as soon as possible. As to barriers in accessing mainstream services, they were accustomed to managing with minimal health services unless they lived in a metropolis; even there, however, many individuals relied on traditional healers for health care, rather than biomedical professionals. Members of these populations often delayed seeking assistance until a condition handicapped them in their livelihood.[100] Some had contact with nonprofit organizations and nongovernmental organizations (NGOs) in their vicinity.

Patient

Taking sleep as one among many possible concerns, using a patient-specific perspective revealed that different persons complaining of insomnia had different reasons for why they could not sleep. Some individuals wanted to remain awake in case they had to flee another act of nature with very little warning. Some tried to sleep but had flashbacks; others became filled with grief when they heard their neighbors crying.

Finally, some were troubled by thoughts of souls of the dead not having received culturally appropriate death rituals (burials or other rites).

Resumption of decent sleep soon after traumatic experiences is an important facilitator—and indicator—of the recovery process. Severe insomnia is both an effect and a further cause of autonomic arousal that keeps people feeling depleted and unable to focus on executing purposeful actions.

In this case, identifying patient-specific reasons for the insomnia provided clues as to which psychological/social interventions would emotionally and cognitively engage the individual. For example, local NGOs developed a resourceful solution for the many persons who were not sleeping for fear of another emergency. Because survivors were sleeping in close proximity, groups were asked to nominate and rotate individuals to stay awake for a "watch" lasting two hours. That is, individuals agreed to take turns throughout the night keeping watch and sleeping. After several days, feelings of predictability and basic security returned so that this intervention was no longer necessary. This intervention was made up of psychological and social components.[101]

Physicians in the area provided people with medications as sleep aids. This biomedical intervention was particularly useful for those individuals who were in hyperaroused, hyperadrenergic states. After a few days, many felt their minds and bodies "reset themselves," and they were able to move on with rebuilding without further use of sleep aids.[102] Finally, in a social intervention, local clergy and NGOs collaborated to create new rites for a community affected by mass death without bodies to sanctify.

CONCLUSION

The intersections among public health, mental health, and emergency health care represent opportunities to prepare, intervene, and prevent morbidity in the case of traumatic events. Much room exists for further development in this area, however, as awareness continues to increase regarding mental health traumatic events. Communities can suffer greatly if large numbers of people remain overwhelmed, terrorized, and frozen after trauma, leading to increased suffering, reduced productivity, and diminished quality of life.

The SPPP parameters are presented as a model to calibrate interventions in public health emergencies. Institutional preparedness and linkages provide a foundation from which evidence-based responses can be launched and mitigation efforts can be sustained. The tsunami case study illustrates how using the SPPP lens can help bring clarity to a complex situation and assist the emergency public health provider in service delivery during emergency response, a time when confusion and errors are more likely to occur. Protecting and improving the mental health of people affected by an emergency is of paramount importance. In the case of terrorism, experts agree that psychological and social sequelae are likely to be the most enduring, widespread, and socially and fiscally costly of all health effects.

As emphasized by the Inter-Agency Standing Committee (IASC; established by UN resolutions 46/182 and 48/57 as the primary mechanism for interagency coordination of humanitarian assistance), responding to a population's diverse mental health needs requires coordinated action among several governmental and nongovernmental entities. Bringing together all stakeholders—government, healthcare providers, voluntary agencies, and communities—with the concepts in this chapter can serve to yield competent and comprehensive emergency management.

INTERNET RESOURCES

Centers for Disease Control and Prevention (CDC): trauma and disaster mental health resources
http://www.bt.cdc.gov/mentalhealth

Disaster Psychiatry Outreach: a nonprofit organization with direct service components that also provides education and training
http://www.disasterpsych.org

Inter-Agency Standing Committee (IASC): coordinates humanitarian assistance between UN and non-UN agencies and published *IASC Guidelines on Mental Health and Psychosocial Support in Emergency Settings.*
http://www.humanitarianinfo.org/iasc

International Society for Traumatic Stress Studies: a multidisciplinary, professional membership organization that promotes advancement and exchange of knowledge about severe stress and trauma
http://www.istss.org/what/index.cfm

National Child Traumatic Stress Network (NCTSN): a searchable learning center that includes child- and family-focused factsheets and guidelines, a child- and adolescent-focused version of PFA, and a range of trauma-focused training videos/Webinars
www.nctsn.org

National Institute of Mental Health (NIMH): "Mental Health and Mass Violence: Evidence-Based Early Intervention for Victims/Survivors of Mass Violence" (best practices document)
http://www.nimh.nih.gov/health/publications/massviolence.pdf

The Sphere Project: an international effort for Humanitarian Charter and Minimum Standards in Disaster Response
http://www.sphereproject.org/index.php

U.S. Department of Health and Human Services: disasters and emergencies
http://www.phe.gov/preparedness/pages/default.aspx

U.S. Department of Health and Human Services, Substance Abuse and Mental Health Services
Administration: Disaster Technical Assistance Center (DTAC)
http://mentalhealth.samhsa.gov/dtac/default.asp

U.S. Department of Veterans Affairs, National Center for PTSD: maintains information pages
and multiple resources including Published International Literature on Traumatic Stress
(PILOTS), the largest database of publications on PTSD
http://www.ptsd.va.gov

U.S. Department of Veterans Affairs, National Center for PTSD: *Psychological First Aid: Field
Operations Guide*
http://ncptsd.kattare.com/ncmain/ncdocs/manuals/nc_manual_psyfirstaid.html

World Health Organization (WHO): "Mental Health in Emergencies: Mental and Social Aspects
of Health of Populations Exposed to Extreme Stressors"
http://www.who.int/mental_health/media/en/640.pdf

NOTES

1. Mollica RF, Cardozo BL, Osofsky HJ, Raphael B, Ager A, Salama P. Mental health in complex
   emergencies. *Lancet.* 2004;364:2058–2067.
2. *Diagnostic and statistical manual of mental disorders* (4th ed., text rev.). Washington, DC:
   American Psychiatric Association; 2000.
3. Neria Y, Nandi A, Galea S. Post-traumatic stress disorder following disasters: A systematic
   review. *Psychological Medicine.* 2008;38:467–480.
4. Neria Y, Gross R, Olfson M, et al. Posttraumatic stress disorder in primary care one year after
   the 9/11 attacks. *General Hospital Psychiatry.* 2006;28:213–222.
5. Schuster MA, Stein BD, Jaycox LH, et al. A national survey of stress reactions after the
   September 11, 2001 terrorist attacks. *New England Journal of Medicine.* 2001;345:1507–1512.
6. McFarlane AC, Hooff MV, Goodhew F. Anxiety disorders and PTSD. In Neria Y, Galea S,
   Norris FH (Eds.), *Mental health and disasters.* Cambridge, UK: Cambridge University Press;
   2009, pp. 47–66.
7. Maguen S, Neria Y, Conoscenti LM, Litz BT. Depression and prolonged grief in the wake of
   disasters. In Neria Y, Galea S, Norris FH (Eds.), *Mental health and disasters.* Cambridge, UK:
   Cambridge University Press; 2009, pp. 116–130.
8. Staab JP, Grieger TA, Fullerton CS, Ursano RJ. Acute stress disorder, subsequent posttraumatic stress disorder and depression after a series of typhoons. *Anxiety.* 1996;2:219–225.
9. Ehring T, Ehlers A, Cleare AJ, Glucksman E. Do acute psychological and psychobiological
   responses to trauma predict subsequent symptom severities of PTSD and depression? *Psychiatry Research.* 2008;161:67–75.
10. Bryant RA, Creamer M, O'Donnell ML, Silove D, McFarlane AC. A multisite study of the
    capacity of acute stress disorder diagnosis to predict posttraumatic stress disorder. *Journal of
    Clinical Psychiatry.* 2008;69:923–929.

11. Seery MD, Silver RC, Holman EA, Ence WA, Chu TQ. Expressing thoughts and feelings following a collective trauma: Immediate responses to 9/11 predict negative outcomes in a national sample. *Journal of Consulting and Clinical Psychology.* 2008;76:657–667.

12. Lommen MJ, Sanders AJ, Buck N, Arntz A. Psychosocial predictors of chronic post-traumatic stress disorder in Sri Lankan tsunami survivors. *Behavior Research and Therapy.* 2009;47:60–65.

13. van der Velden PG, Kleber RJ. Substance use and misuse after disaster prevalences and correlates. In Neria Y, Galea S, Norris FH (Eds.), *Mental health and disasters.* Cambridge, UK: Cambridge University Press; 2009, pp. 94–115.

14. Schnurr PP, Friedman MJ, Sengupta A, Jankowski MK, Holmes T. PTSD and utilization of medical treatment services among male Vietnam veterans. *Journal of Nervous and Mental Disease.* 2000;188:496–504.

15. Yzermans CJ, van den Berg B, Dirkzwager AJE. Physical health problems after disasters. In Neria Y, Galea S, Norris FH (Eds.), *Mental health and disasters.* Cambridge, UK: Cambridge University Press; 2009, pp. 67–93.

16. Schnurr PP, Jankowski MK. Physical health and post-traumatic stress disorder: Review and synthesis. *Seminars in Clinical Neuropsychiatry.* 1999;4:295–304.

17. Bailer J, Witthöft M, Bayerl C, Rist F. Trauma experience in individuals with idiopathic environmental intolerance and individuals with somatoform disorders. *Journal of Psychosomatic Research.* 2007;63:657–661.

18. Cloitre M, Stolbach BC, Herman JL, et al. A developmental approach to complex PTSD: Childhood and adult cumulative trauma as predictors of symptom complexity. *Journal of Traumatic Stress.* 2009;22:399–408.

19. Hoven CW, Duarte CS, Mandell DJ. Children's mental health after disasters: The impact of the World Trade Center attack. *Current Psychiatry Reports.* 2003;5:101–107.

20. Silver RC, Holman EA, McIntosh DN, Poulin M, Gil-Rivas V. Nationwide longitudinal study of psychological responses to September 11. *Journal of the American Medical Association.* 2002; 288:1235–1244.

21. Maguen S, Stalnaker M, McCaslin S, Litz BT. PTSD subclusters and functional impairment in Kosovo peacekeepers. *Military Medicine.* 2009;174:779–785.

22. Ghodse H, Galea S. Tsunami: Understanding mental health consequences and the unprecedented response. *International Review of Psychiatry.* 2006;18:289–297.

23. Cardozo BL, van Griensven F, Thienkrua W, Panyayong B, Chakkraband MLS, Tantipiwatanaskul P. The mental health impact of the Southeast Asia tsunami. In Neria Y, Galea S, Norris FH (Eds.), *Mental health and disasters.* Cambridge, UK: Cambridge University Press; 2009, pp. 387–395.

24. Norris FH, Rosen CS. Innovations in disaster mental health services and evaluation: National, state, and local responses to hurricane Katrina. *Administration and Policy in Mental Health.* 2009; 36:159–164.

25. Koenig KL, Goans RE, Hatchett RJ, et al. Medical treatment of radiological casualties: Current concepts. *Annals of Emergency Medicine.* 2005;45:643–646.

26. Zatzick DF, Kang SM, Hinton WL, et al. Posttraumatic concerns: A patient-centered approach to outcome assessment after traumatic physical injury. *Medical Care.* 2001;39:327–339.

27. Fullerton CS, Ursano RJ. Mental health intervention and high-risk groups in disasters. *World Psychiatry.* 2002;1:157–158.

28. Pandya A, Katz C, (Eds.). *Disaster psychiatry: Intervening when nightmares come true.* Hillsdale, NJ: Analytic Press; 2004.

29. Beckham JC, Moore SD, Feldman ME, Hertzberg MA, Kirby AC, Fairbank JA. Health status, somatization, and severity of posttraumatic stress disorder in Vietnam combat veterans with posttraumatic stress disorder. *American Journal of Psychiatry.* 1998;155:1565–1569.

30. Schnurr PP, Spiro A 3rd, Paris AH. Physician-diagnosed medical disorders in relation to PTSD symptoms in older male military veterans. *Health Psychology.* 2000;19:91–97.

31. Holman EA, Silver RC, Poulin M, Andersen J, Gil-Rivas V, McIntosh DN. Terrorism, acute stress, and cardiovascular health: A 3-year national study following the September 11th attacks. *Archives of General Psychiatry.* 2008;65:73–80.

32. Barbera JA, Macintyre AG. *A comprehensive functional system description for mass casualty medical and health incident management.* Washington, DC: George Washington University, Institute for Crisis, Disaster, and Risk Management; 2002.

33. *Hospital Incident Command System.* California Emergency Medical Services Authority. Available at: http://www.emsa.ca.gov/HICS/default.asp. Accessed November 8, 2009.

34. *National Incident Management System.* Federal Emergency Management Agency, Department of Homeland Security. Available at: http://www.fema.gov/emergency/nims/index.shtm. Accessed November 8, 2009.

35. Garakani A, Hirschowitz J, Katz CL. General disaster psychiatry. *Psychiatric Clinics of North America.* 2004;27:391–406.

36. Norwood AE, Ursano RJ, Fullerton CS. Disaster psychiatry: principles and practice. *Psychiatric Quarterly.* 2000;71:207–226.

37. de Jong JTVM. Nongovernmental organizations and the role of the mental health professional. In Ursano RJ, Fullerton CS, Weisaeth L, Raphael B (Eds.), *Textbook of disaster psychiatry.* Cambridge, UK: Cambridge University Press; 2007, pp. 206–224.

38. Diaz JO. Integrating psychosocial programs in multisector responses to international disasters. *American Psychology.* 2008;63:820–827.

39. Thara R, Rao K, John S. An assessment of post-tsunami psychosocial training programmes in Tamilnadu, India. *International Journal of Social Psychiatry.* 2008;54:197–205.

40. Berger R, Gelkopf M. School-based intervention for the treatment of tsunami-related distress in children: A quasi-randomized controlled trial. *Psychotherapy and Psychosomatics.* 2009;78: 364–371.

41. Barbisch DF, Koenig KL. Understanding surge capacity: essential elements. *Academic Emergency Medicine.* 2006;13:1098–1102.

42. Kaji A, Koenig KL, Bey T. Surge capacity for healthcare systems: A conceptual framework. *Academic Emergency Medicine.* 2006;13:1157–1159.

43. Shih FY, Koenig KL. Improving surge capacity for biothreats: Experience from Taiwan. *Academic Emergency Medicine.* 2006;13:1114–1117.

44. Schultz CH, Koenig KL. State of research in high-consequence hospital surge capacity. *Academic Emergency Medicine.* 2006;13:1153–1156.

45. Hick JL, Koenig KL, Barbisch D, Bey TA. Surge capacity concepts for health care facilities: The CO-S-TR model for initial incident assessment. *Disaster Medicine and Public Health Preparedness.* 2008;2(suppl 1):S51–S57.

46. Foa EB, Cahill SP, Boscarino JA, Hobfoll SE, Lahad M, McNally RJ, et al. Social, psychological, and psychiatric interventions following terrorist attacks: Recommendations for practice and research. *Neuropsychopharmacology.* 2005;30:1806–1817.

47. van Ommeren M, Saxena S, Saraceno B. Mental and social health during and after acute emergencies: Emerging consensus? *Bulletin of the World Health Organization.* 2005;83:71–76.

48. Hobfoll SE, Watson P, Bell CC, et al. Five essential elements of immediate and mid-term mass trauma intervention: Empirical evidence. *Psychiatry.* 2007;70:283–315.

49. *Mental health and mass violence: Evidence-based early intervention for victims/survivors of mass violence (A workshop to reach consensus on best practices).* National Institutes of Mental Health, NIH Publication No. 02-5138. Washington, DC: U.S. Government Printing Office; 2002.

50. Watson PJ, Friedman MJ, Ruzek JI, Norris F. Managing acute stress response to major trauma. *Current Psychiatry Reports.*2002;4:247–253.

51. Solomon Z, Neria Y, Witztum E. Debriefing with service personnel in war and peace roles: Experience and outcomes. In Raphael B, Wilson JP (Eds.), *Psychological debriefing: Theory, practice and evidence.* Cambridge, UK: Cambridge University Press; 2000, pp. 161–173.

52. Bisson JI, McFarlane AC, Rose S. Psychological debriefing. In Foa EB, Keane TM, Friedman MJ (Eds.), *Effective treatments for PTSD: Practice guidelines from the International Society for Traumatic Stress Studies.* New York: Guilford Press; 2001, pp. 317–319.

53. Rose S, Bisson J, Wessely S. Does brief psychological debriefing help manage psychological distress after trauma and prevent post traumatic stress disorder? In *The Cochrane database of systematic reviews: Evidence update.* Liverpool, UK: Effective Health Care Alliance Programme; 2006.

54. Gist R, Devilly GJ. Post-trauma debriefing: The road too frequently travelled. *Lancet.* 2002; 360:741–742.

55. van Emmerik APA, Kamphuis JH, Hulsbosch AM, Emmelkamp PMG. Single session debriefing after psychological trauma: A meta-analysis. *Lancet.* 2002;360:766–771.

56. Mitchell JT, Everly GS. *Critical incident stress debriefing: An operations manual for the prevention of traumatic stress among emergency services and disaster workers* (2nd ed.). Ellicott City, MD: Chevron; 1996.

57. Devilly, GJ, Cotton P. Psychological debriefing and the workplace: Defining a concept, controversies and guidelines for intervention. *Australian Psychologist.* 2003; 38:144–150.

58. Everly GS, Mitchell JT. The debriefing "controversy" and crisis intervention: A review of lexical and substantive issues. *International Journal of Emergency Mental Health.* 2000;2:211–225.

59. Tuckey MR. Issues in the debriefing debate for the emergency services: Moving research outcomes forward. *Clinical Psychology: Science and Practice.* 2007;14:106–116.

60. Mitchell JT, Everly GS. Critical incident stress management and critical incident stress debriefings: Evolutions, effects and outcomes. In Raphael B, Wilson JP (Eds.), *Psychological debriefing: Theory, practice and evidence.* Cambridge, UK: Cambridge University Press; 2000, pp. 71–90.

61. Robinson R. Debriefing with emergency services: Critical incident stress management. In Raphael B, Wilson JP (Eds.), *Psychological debriefing: Theory, practice and evidence.* Cambridge, UK: Cambridge University Press; 2000, pp. 91–107.

62. Neria Y, Olfson M, Gameroff MJ, et al. The mental health consequences of disaster-related loss: Findings from primary care one year after the 9/11 terrorist attacks. *Psychiatry.* 2008; 71:339–348.

63. Ahern J, Galea S. Social context and depression after a disaster: The role of income inequality. *Journal of Epidemiology and Community Health*. 2006;60:766–770.

64. Fairbank JA, Fairbank DW. Epidemiology of child traumatic stress. *Current Psychiatry Reports*. 2009;11:289–295.

65. Norris FH, Alegría M. Promoting disaster recovery in ethnic-minority individuals and communities. In Richie EC, Watson PJ, Friedman MJ (Eds.), *Interventions following mass violence and disasters: Strategies for mental health practice*. New York: Guilford Press; 2006, pp. 319–342.

66. Chokroverty L, Heath D, Harwitz, D. The kids' corner: A safe haven for children and adults amidst disaster. *Emergency Psychiatry*. 2002;8:49–54.

67. Pynoos RS, Nader K. Psychological first aid and treatment approach to children exposed to community violence: Research implications. *Journal of Traumatic Stress*. 1988;1:445–473.

68. Katz CL, Pellegrino L, Pandya A, Ng A, DeLisi LE. Research on psychiatric outcomes and interventions subsequent to disasters: A review of the literature. *Psychiatry Research*. 2002;110: 201–217.

69. Bell J. Propranolol, post-traumatic stress disorder and narrative identity. *Journal of Medical Ethics*. 2008;34:e23.

70. Bell JA. Preventing post-traumatic stress disorder or pathologizing bad memories? *American Journal of Bioethics*. 2007;7:29–30.

71. Levy N, Clarke S. Neuroethics and psychiatry. *Current Opinion in Psychiatry*. 2008;21:568–571.

72. Stanovic JK, James KA, VanDevere CA. The effectiveness of risperidone on acute stress symptoms in adult burn patients: A preliminary retrospective pilot study. *Journal of Burn Care and Rehabilitation*. 2001;22:210–213.

73. Pitman RK, Delahanty DL. Conceptually driven pharmacologic approaches to acute trauma. *CNS Spectrum*. 2005;10:99–106.

74. Vaiva G, Ducrocq F, Jezequel K, Averland B, Lestavel P, Brunet A, et al. Immediate treatment with propranolol decreases posttraumatic stress disorder two months after trauma. *Biological Psychiatry*. 2003;54:947–949. Erratum in: *Biological Psychiatry*. 2003;54:1471.

75. Stein MB, Kerridge C, Dimsdale JE, Hoyt DB. Pharmacotherapy to prevent PTSD: Results from a randomized controlled proof-of-concept trial in physically injured patients. *Journal of Traumatic Stress*. 2007;20:923–932.

76. Pitman RK, Sanders KM, Zusman RM, et al. Pilot study of secondary prevention of posttraumatic stress disorder with propranolol. *Biological Psychiatry*. 2002;51:189–192.

77. Bennett WRM, Zatzick D, Roy-Byrne P. Can medications prevent PTSD in trauma victims? *Current Psychiatry*. 2007;6:47–55.

78. Cukor J, Spitalnick J, Difede J, Rizzo A, Rothbaum BO. Emerging treatments for PTSD. *Clinical Psychology Review*. 2009;29:715–726.

79. Mello MF, Yeh MS, Barbosa J, et al. A randomized, double-blind, placebo-controlled trial to assess the efficacy of topiramate in the treatment of post-traumatic stress disorder. *BMC Psychiatry*. 2009;9:28.

80. Covello VT. Principles of risk communication. In Brenner GH, Bush DH, Moses J (Eds.), *Creating spiritual and psychological resilience: Integrating care in disaster relief work*. New York: Routledge; 2009, pp. 39–74.

81. DiGiovanni C, Reynolds B, Harwell R, Stonecipher E, Burkle F. Community reaction to bioterrorism: Prospective study of simulated outbreak. *Emerging Infectious Diseases*. 2003;9: 708–712.

82. Bonanno GA, Gupta S. Resilience after disaster. In Neria Y, Galea S, Norris FH (Eds.), *Mental health and disasters*. Cambridge, UK: Cambridge University Press; 2009, pp. 145–160.

83. Otto MW, Henin A, Hirshfeld-Becker DR, Pollack MH, Biederman J, Rosenbaum JF. Posttraumatic stress disorder symptoms following media exposure to tragic events: Impact of 9/11 on children at risk for anxiety disorders. *Journal of Anxiety Disorders*. 2007;21:888–902.

84. van der Kolk BA. Clinical implications of neuroscience research in PTSD. *Annals of the New York Academy of Science*. 2006;1071:277–293.

85. Norris FH, Friedman MJ, Watson PJ, Byrne CM, Diaz E, Kaniasty K. 60,000 disaster victims speak: Part I. An empirical review of the empirical literature, 1981–2001. *Psychiatry*. 2002;65:207–239.

86. Shah SA. To do no harm, spiritual care and ethnomedical competence: Four cases of psychosocial trauma recovery for the 2004 tsunami and 2005 earthquake in South Asia. In Brenner GH, Bush DH, Moses J (Eds.), *Creating spiritual and psychological resilience: Integrating care in disaster relief work*. New York: Routledge; 2009, pp. 157–178.

87. Wessells MG. Do no harm: Toward contextually appropriate psychosocial support in international emergencies. *American Psychologist*. 2009;64:842–854.

88. Wessells MG, Monteiro C. Healing the wounds following protracted conflict in Angola: A community-based approach to assisting war-affected children. In Gielen UP, Fish J, Draguns JG (Eds.), *Handbook of culture, therapy, and healing*. Mahwah, NJ: Erlbaum; 2004, pp. 321–341.

89. Norris FH, Alegria M. Mental health care for ethnic minority individuals and communities in the aftermath of disasters and mass violence. *CNS Spectrum*. 2005;10:132–140.

90. Shah SA. Ethnomedical best practices for international psychosocial efforts in disaster and trauma. In Tang CS, Wilson JP (Eds.), *Cross-cultural assessment of psychological trauma and PTSD*. New York: Springer Verlag; 2007, pp. 51–64.

91. Wessells MG. Culture, power, and community: Intercultural approaches to psychosocial assistance and healing. In Nader K, Dubrow N, Stamm B (Eds.), *Honoring differences: Cultural issues in the treatment of trauma and loss*. New York: Taylor & Francis; 1999, pp. 267–282.

92. Fullerton CS, Ursano RJ, Wang L. Acute stress disorder, posttraumatic stress disorder, and depression in disaster or rescue workers. *American Journal of Psychiatry*. 2004;161:1370–1376.

93. Stellman JM, Smith RP, Katz CL, et al. Enduring mental health morbidity and social function impairment in World Trade Center rescue, recovery, and cleanup workers: The psychological dimension of an environmental health disaster. *Environmental Health Perspectives*. 2008;116:1248–1253.

94. Sims A, Sims D. The phenomenology of posttraumatic stress disorder: A symptomatic study of 70 victims of psychological trauma. *Psychopathology*. 1998;31:96–112.

95. Shah SA, Garland E, Katz C. Secondary traumatic stress: Prevalence for humanitarian aid workers in India. *Traumatology*. 2007;13:59–70.

96. Centers for Disease Control and Prevention. Mental health status of World Trade Center rescue and recovery workers and volunteers—New York City, July 2002–August 2004. *Morbidity and Mortality Weekly Reports*. 2004;53:812–815.

97. Fullerton CS, Ursano RJ, Reeves J, Shigemura J, Grieger T. Perceived safety in disaster workers following 9/11. *Journal of Nervous and Mental Disease*. 2006;194:61–63.

98. Fullerton CS, Ursano RJ. Mental health intervention and high-risk groups in disasters. *World Psychiatry*. 2002;1:157–158.

99. Ursano RJ, Fullerton CS, Kao TC, Bhartiya VR. Longitudinal assessment of posttraumatic stress disorder and depression after exposure to traumatic death. *Journal of Nervous and Mental Disease*. 1995;183:36–42.

100. Carballo M, Heal B, Hernandez M. Psychosocial aspects of the tsunami. *Journal of the Royal Society of Medicine*. 2005;98:396–399.

101. Becker SM. Psychosocial care for women survivors of the tsunami disaster in India. *American Journal of Public Health*. 2009;99:654–658.

102. Rajkumar AP, Premkumar TS, Tharyan P. Coping with the Asian tsunami: Perspectives from Tamil Nadu, India on the determinants of resilience in the face of adversity. *Social Science and Medicine*. 2008;67:844–853.

CHAPTER 25

Children and Public Health Emergencies

Heather Machen

INTRODUCTION

Public health emergencies, both human made and natural, are an unfortunate part of life. While we cannot escape them, how we fare during and after complex emergencies is largely determined by our level of preparedness. The better prepared a community is, the more it can decrease its vulnerability. As a society, we have improved in our emergency planning. Where we have not shown sufficient progress, however, is in planning for disasters involving children. Often, disaster planning committees do not even include anyone with pediatric experience. The Medical Reserve Corps, which coordinates volunteer healthcare professionals during times of disaster, does not require a pediatric expert to be part of the response.[1] This chapter explores some of the key differences in the needs of children and examines the logistical considerations that must be taken into account given that the majority of large-scale emergencies faced by communities will affect children as well as adults. It also offers suggestions as to how we can best address these needs.

Case Study

Hurricane Katrina struck the city of New Orleans on Monday, August 29, 2005. The levees surrounding the city broke the following day, resulting in massive flooding. Eighty percent of the city experienced floodwaters that in some areas reached depths of 20 feet.[2] On Wednesday, August 31, evacuation of the region began, with approximately 373,000 people ultimately being removed from New

Orleans and the Gulf Coast.[3] Included in this number were 25,000 people evacuated from the Superdome in New Orleans to the Reliant Center/Astrodome complex in Houston. Busloads of displaced persons began arriving in Houston after a 12-hour journey. While the area children's hospital in Houston was aware of their arrival, it was not involved in the planning and conduct of this operation. Many of the individuals arriving in Houston had not had food, water, medications, or even dialysis for days. Formula was not available for many of the babies, and some of the breastfeeding mothers were too dehydrated to be able to provide an adequate milk supply.[4]

In an attempt to treat the multitude of evacuees requiring care, a clinic supported by Harris County and the city of Houston was established at the Reliant complex. When it became evident that thousands of children were among the evacuees requesting medical care at this site, local pediatricians left their busy private and hospital practices to volunteer at the clinic. Of the thousands of people who arrived in the first 48 hours, 30 percent were seen in the clinics and 30 percent of these individuals were children.[4]

After the levees broke in New Orleans, hundreds of people sought shelter from the rising water on roofs and were eventually evacuated by helicopter. Due to the high winds and rain, this already difficult task became more dangerous and many additional injuries were sustained in the process. A 10-year-old boy was attempting to climb into a basket to be lifted off the roof of his home when he fell back onto the roof, injuring his feet. On the second attempt, he was successfully pulled into the helicopter. From there, the child was transferred to a bus and made the trip to Houston. His parents were placed on different buses and did not travel with him. On arrival, the lacerations to the boy's feet were treated, but no additional injuries were found on his exam. The patient had a rapid heart rate and was dehydrated. Like many of the individuals arriving in Houston, he had not had anything to drink in three days. He was not speaking, and because he was unaccompanied, no one could provide identification or a medical history.[4]

PREPAREDNESS

Triage

Following a mass-casualty incident (MCI), the needs of the patients are likely to far exceed the available resources. Consequently, triage is a vital aspect of every MCI. Physicians are often not the best triage officers because their instinct is to do everything possible for every patient. Unfortunately, this level of care is not possible in an MCI, because spending a prolonged period of time on one patient may cost the lives of several others who have a better chance of achieving a good outcome. A review of 10 terrorist bombing incidents showed that inappropriate triage was associated with increased morbidity and mortality.[5] The goal in any mass-casualty triage situation is to care for as many people as possible in the least amount of time. At the scene of an MCI, the primary triage should consist of a rapid "once-over" to quickly identify those patients in most urgent need of medical intervention versus those who can wait for further assessment.[6] Effective preparedness for the care of children during public health emergencies will require training and familiarity of the use of pediatric-appropriate triage systems.

Algorithms for adult triage are well established. While they serve as good guidelines, application of some of the principles to pediatric patients may lead to children being over- or under-triaged. For example, a crying child may be inappropriately triaged ahead of one who is quiet but has more serious injuries. Nevertheless, when surveyed, only 19 percent of emergency medical services (EMS) systems reported using a pediatric-specific triage protocol for public health emergencies involving children.[5]

Several triage scores and systems have been established and are in use in different parts of the world: the Pediatric Triage Tape (PTT), Careflight, Simple Triage and Rapid Treatment (START), and JumpSTART. Evidence to support the superiority of one system over another is limited. The most commonly used guideline in pediatric MCI triage in the United States is JumpSTART; in contrast, START is typically used for adults. JumpSTART rules take into consideration the unique physiology and developmental stages of children. Often the age of a patient will be unknown in an MCI. Therefore, any patient who looks like a child should be triaged under JumpSTART rules. If the patient appears to be a young adult, traditional triage guidelines should be applied. A combined algorithm has been developed to accommodate both types of patients (Figure 25-1). Under either the START or JumpSTART system, patients are tagged with the following clinical classifications:[7]

- Red: Immediate treatment
- Yellow: Delayed treatment
- Green: Ambulatory (no acute treatment necessary)
- Black: Deceased/expectant

Under START triage rules, if a patient is not breathing, his or her airway is repositioned. If this action does not result in the return of spontaneous respirations in an adult, the patient is tagged as "expectant" (black, meaning "near death"), and the responder should move on to the next patient without any further intervention. Because the vast majority of pediatric arrests have a respiratory cause, children are managed differently. In pedi-

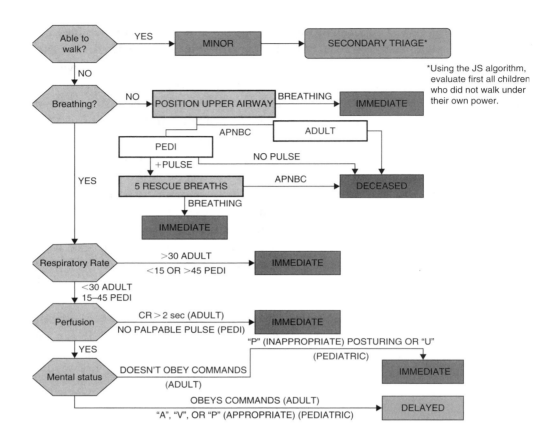

FIGURE 25-1   Combined START/JumpSTART Algorithm
Copied with permission from The JumpSTART Pediatric MCI Triage Tool and START triage developed by Newport Beach Fire Department and Hoag Memorial Hospital Presbyterian.

atric cases, the patient's airway is opened. If the child fails to breathe spontaneously, five rescue breaths are given. If the patient begins to breathe on his or her own, the individual is triaged to receive immediate (red) treatment. If the child is still not breathing, he or she is tagged as "deceased/expectant" (black).[7]

Respiratory rates vary with age, with young children having a higher baseline rate than older children and adults. Adults with a respiratory rate exceeding 30 breaths per minute are triaged to receive immediate treatment. Using this same rate in a small child would result in over-triaging, however, and would place this child ahead of other patients with more immediate needs. For infants and young children, respiratory rates of less than 15 or more than 45 breaths per minute warrant their placement in the immediate treatment group.[7]

In addition, young children may not be able or willing to follow commands when they are frightened or injured. If an adult is unable to follow commands, he or she is triaged to receive immediate treatment; in contrast, this is not a helpful assessment in a small child. Because triage is a dynamic and ongoing process, patients initially tagged as deceased/expectant should be reevaluated as soon as time allows.

Tracking and Reunification

The first goal after a public health emergency is to move people to a safe location as quickly as possible. Unfortunately, this process often leads to confusion and separation of families, and children may end up in shelters far from their parents. This separation of children from parents occurred frequently after Hurricane Katrina, for example, as people were placed on multiple buses in the urgency to evacuate. Clearly, planning and preparedness for effective tracking systems and reunification procedures are essential. When surveyed, only 26.5 percent of EMS agencies reported that their local disaster response plan included guidelines for reunification of children with their families.[5]

Equipment and Personnel

The majority of EMS training and experience is with adult patients. In many areas, less than 10 to 15 percent of EMS calls involve pediatric patients.[4] In fact, training in pediatrics accounts for less than 10 percent of course time in EMS training programs in many regions. In the United States, EMS systems are regulated by state and local governments. Currently, no federal requirements on pediatric equipment and training exist.[8] First responders to a public health emergency may, therefore, have limited experience and comfort in dealing with children. In addition, appropriate resources and supplies for treating children may be limited in the prehospital setting. Establishing pediatric-specific supplies and resources during the preparedness phase will allow for more effective management of children and their injuries during a public health emergency.

After a complex emergency, many people will require medications to treat acute illness and injury as well as maintenance medications that they are unlikely to have with them. Both prescription and over-the-counter medications will be necessary. An estimated 54 percent of all individuals seen at the treatment sites at Houston's Reliant complex were given over-the-counter medications.[3]

The federal Strategic National Stockpile is available to supply states with the antidotes and medications needed following a disaster. The Food and Drug Administration (FDA) has not approved most of these medications for pediatric use, however, and the stockpile does not contain pediatric doses of most medications.[8] Local and regional public health agencies should consider obtaining their own supplies of pediatric medications for treating children. These pharmaceutical stockpiles should include appropriate medications for children, appropriate dosages, and appropriate formulations (such as liquid rather than pill forms for infants and young children).

RESPONSE

Psychosocial Issues

The National Institute of Mental Health defines post-traumatic stress disorder (PTSD) as an anxiety disorder that can develop after exposure to a terrifying event or ordeal in which grave physical harm either occurred or was threatened.[9] Children may express this emotional trauma by not eating, having sleep disturbances, or becoming either aggressive or withdrawn. Studies conducted after Hurricane Katrina indicate that "the New Orleans area . . . lost 89 percent of its psychiatrists and 84 percent of its psychiatric beds" at a time when there was a significant and increasing need for mental health services.[10]

Children and teens can experience the consequences of PTSD for years following an event. Dealing with this emotional trauma can prove challenging under the best of circumstances. Children naturally rely on the emotional stability of their caregivers. Thus their parents' stress will have a negative effect on the emotional state of the children. For this reason, helping the parents cope with their emotions is often the most helpful intervention for children.

Exposure

Chemical or biological exposure can occur through inhalation, ingestion, and physical contact with substances. Children will be affected by exposures differently from adults. Small children touch and put everything in their mouths and are, therefore, far more likely to ingest substances. Pediatric respiratory and heart rates are higher than adult rates, so children will be affected more quickly by air- and blood-borne toxins. Because children are closer to the ground, poisonous aerosolized substances such as chlorine, anthrax, and sarin gas, which are heavier than air and, therefore, present at higher concentrations near the ground, will affect children more quickly than adults.[8]

Children will also suffer from dehydration and extremes of temperature more quickly than adults due to their thinner, less keratinized skin and lower fluid volumes. Protecting children from heat loss, particularly during decontamination procedures, is vital. "Radiant warmers and other re-warming equipment are of greater importance to child disaster victims than adults."[11]

Susceptibility to Abuse

After any emergency, tensions run high and patience is limited. Even uninjured children are likely to be fussier than normal and parents are likely to have less patience than usual. Children are at greater risk of abuse during this time period. According to the World Health Organization (WHO), in the counties affected by Hurricane Floyd in 1999, there was a 500 percent increase in traumatic brain injury due to abuse in children younger than six months of age.[8] Providing support for families can reduce this risk to children. When abuse occurs, appropriate agencies need to be rapidly involved to protect children from further injury.

Injuries

Children are more susceptible to blunt trauma from storm debris than adults because their organs are proportionally larger, closer together, and less well protected than adult organs. In addition, children are less able to protect themselves from external threats.[12] After a disaster, particularly an environmental event, healthcare providers are likely to see an immediate increase in the number of patients with injuries. This increase is likely to persist even after the initial event is over, as people become injured while trying to rebuild their homes, clear debris, negotiate unstable buildings, and cross high water.

During this period, parents are likely to be distracted and may be less vigilant of their children than normal. Children are naturally curious and will want to investigate the changes in their environment and take advantage of their parents' distraction. Schools are often closed, and children's time will likely be less structured than usual. Exploring partially downed trees, downed power lines, bodies of water, and unstable buildings may look like an adventure to a child but can result in serious injury. Because of their lack of understanding of the danger presented by emergency situations, children will often approach and investigate danger instead of fleeing from it. Providing a safe, supervised area for children to play is an essential, but often overlooked, part of any emergency public health response.

Normalization of Routine

Children do better when their lives are organized into routines and they are subject to clear expectations. Disruption of routine, in contrast, leads to uncertainty in the child and may produce disruptive behavior. Post-emergency, caregivers and providers should rapidly return children to as much of their normal daily lives as possible. Following a disaster, homes may be destroyed, parents may be deceased or separated from the child, and children may be forced to live in overcrowded shelters surrounded by strangers. One of the most basic parts of a child's routine is school, and local agencies should make concerted efforts to reopen schools or create temporary school settings as quickly as possible.

Disease Prevention

Following an emergency, food and water supplies may be contaminated or even unavailable. Facilities for personal hygiene are often limited and sanitation may be substandard. Outbreaks of diarrheal disease are common under these conditions and can have devastating outcomes. Children tend to be especially susceptible to diarrheal disease because of their tendency to put everything in their mouths and lack of interest in hand washing. Consequently, a safe water supply and adequate hygiene and sanitation should be among the first priorities when working with victims of a public health emergency.

Vaccinations

Immunization and hand washing are the best tools available to prevent outbreaks of disease. Ensuring that individuals' tetanus vaccinations are up-to-date should be a priority because the risk of sustaining a contaminated wound is high when people are trying to evacuate or rebuild after a public health crisis. Moreover, individuals displaced by a disaster are unlikely to have access to their vaccination records. According to the Centers for Disease Control and Prevention (CDC), if the records are available, children and adults should be vaccinated according to routine schedules; the CDC's recommended schedule of vaccinations can be found at its Web site (http://www.cdc.gov/vaccines/recs/schedules). If records are unavailable, children 10 years of age and younger should be treated as if their vaccinations are up-to-date and should be given the recommended vaccines for their age. Individuals 10 to 18 years should be given Tdap (the adult formulation of tetanus and diphtheria toxoids and the acellular pertussis vaccine). In addition, children 11 to 15 years old should be given the meningococcal vaccine.

Specific recommendations may change for individual events, of course. The CDC will work with disaster relief centers to determine which vaccinations should be provided and help them to secure the necessary products. Additional information can be obtained from the CDC's Web site.[13] Emergency planning and response efforts should include maintaining supplies of pediatric vaccinations in addition to stockpiles of other emergency pediatric medications.

Exacerbation of Chronic Diseases

Any disaster situation will inevitably lead to new injuries and illness. There will also be a significant exacerbation of chronic diseases. Patients may not have access to medications or may simply forget to take maintenance medications. Dietary requirements may often go unmet. The stress of living under crowded conditions can worsen an existing disease such as diabetes or asthma. As part of the public health response, ensuring that patients have access to the resources needed to maintain health is as important as dealing with the issues caused by the immediate event.

CASE STUDY ANALYSIS

Hurricane Katrina was one of the most costly and deadly disasters to strike the United States. It required an enormous concerted effort to deal with the multitude of problems created by this catastrophe. If we can learn from these experiences, we will have a much better chance of minimizing the damage from future large-scale emergencies.

Preparedness Issues

Triage

By caring for people who were not gravely ill at the Reliant complex, less stress was placed on the already-taxed surge capacity of the area hospitals. In 13 days, more than 3,500 pediatric patients were triaged, evaluated, and managed. Fewer than 50 of these patients were transported to hospitals, and no deaths occurred.[4]

Multiple clinics worked independently within the Reliant complex. This pattern of multiple agencies working side by side, but not together, to provide care following an emergency is common but less effective than a coordinated effort. "In complex emergencies, the provision of health care is often less uniform than in stable situations and ensuring comprehensive, coordinated and appropriate care is difficult where multiple organizations are working, different levels of referral services, supply and delivery systems are lacking or insufficient."[14] Good communication between agencies is essential so that limited resources are not wasted on duplicative efforts. Agencies that are working side by side should decide early on how provision of care will be divided. Regular meetings to ensure good communications and allow for the inevitable adjustments that will have to be made to accommodate the changing conditions are essential. Notably, the uncoordinated triaging of the large numbers of patients within a single venue may lead to children not receiving the appropriate resources or care.

Tracking

In the months following Hurricane Katrina, the National Center for Missing and Exploited Children received reports of 5,088 children who were missing or displaced as a result of the storm.[15] In the rush to evacuate New Orleans, hundreds of children became separated from their parents and arrived in strange cities frightened and alone and in some cases orphaned. Some of these children arrived at shelters unaccompanied. Those with injuries or preexisting medical problems were often unable to provide any information that might lead to family reunification. Because of the massive influx of people and the lack of a uniform, rapid tracking system, precise numbers are not available to quantify the extent of this problem.

Because of the large influx of displaced people, tracking was initially very difficult. At the peak of the evacuation to Houston, 9,000 people arrived at the Reliant complex in a 12-hour period.[3] Following Hurricane Katrina, it took 6 months to reunite the last child with her family.[15] After Hurricanes Katrina and Rita, approximately 2,500 of the children separated from their parents were unable to identify themselves or their caregivers to relief workers.[8] If parents write their children's names, phone numbers, addresses, and birth dates in permanent ink on the child's back, a child who is not able to communicate can be easily identified in such a situation.[8] In emergency planning, every attempt should be made to minimize the number of children who are separated from their parents. This will not always be possible, of course, because children may not be with their parents at the time that disaster strikes, family members may have died during the event, and medical needs may require that families are separated. Thus methods for effective tracking and reunification need to be in place before a disaster occurs.

The 350-mile journey from New Orleans to Houston would have been an ideal time to start triaging patients, gathering tracking information, and initiating treatment where possible. Unfortunately, this did not happen. Upon arrival in Houston, information was manually entered into a tracking system as people disembarked from buses. Due to the amount of time required per individual and the large numbers, this system was quickly overwhelmed.[2]

Following Hurricane Katrina, the Regional Hospital Preparedness Council of Houston purchased a patient tracking system. All 120 hospitals and 13 counties in the region have now adopted the system, which allows individuals to be banded with a unique identifier. Handheld devices and keyboards allow a driver's license or other identification to be swiped and automatically enter the individual's demographic information into the system. Once transportation has been arranged, the receiving facility—which may be a shelter, hospital, or morgue—receives notification listing the person, chief complaint, triage criteria, and estimated time of arrival. The system includes a built-in electronic medical record, and information on family members and pets can be attached.[16] If this system were applied on a widespread basis, it would make tracking, treatment, and reunification of families during a public health emergency much easier.

Equipment and Personnel

Most patients seen at the Reliant complex had common complaints, such as minor injuries, rashes, asthma, and psychological issues.[2] However, many of the patients seen during the first 12 to 24 hours that the Reliant clinic was open had more serious conditions, and many more patients required treatment than there were available supplies. "It is estimated that the Astrodome/Reliant Center Complex housed approximately 27,000 evacuees at its peak in operations, with a total of 65,000 evacuees processed there before being sent to other shelters."[3]

Virtually any MCI will involve children. It is, therefore, essential that appropriately sized equipment be available and that individuals with the experience to treat children be involved in the public health response. Modification of adult-sized equipment to fit children is time consuming and often not feasible. Medication dosing in children is weight based, and many children are unable to swallow pills. Compounding pills into liquid form may result in inaccurate dosing and delays in care. Individuals with knowledge of pediatric dosing and access to appropriate medications are essential when dealing with sick or injured children.

Response Issues

Psychosocial Issues

This chapter began by outlining the experiences of one 10-year-old boy. While his case was singled out as an example, it was hardly unique. Countless other children experienced similar situations. The child did not appear to have a medical reason not to be drinking or speaking and was repeatedly encouraged to drink. When it became clear that the impediment was emotional rather than physical, a social worker was found. She spent 8 hours with him; finally, he began drinking well and did not require any additional medical intervention. The stress of his ordeal had led to PTSD and made a normally self-sufficient adolescent unable to communicate or take care of basic needs, even when the facilities to care for these needs were available to him.[4]

An estimated 500,000 Hurricane Katrina victims probably need (or needed) mental health treatment.[10] Post-Katrina data indicate that children and adolescents affected by the hurricane are experiencing behavioral problems, depression, and anxiety at twice the rate of children of the same age who were not affected by the storm.[10] When the unstable situation persists and support systems are disrupted, as was the case for so many Katrina evacuees, regaining a sense of balance and normalcy becomes that much more difficult.

Normalization of Routine

Ten days after evacuees arrived at the Reliant complex, almost all of the children were enrolled in and bused daily to area schools.[3] This practice provided a sense of stability and routine for children living in very tenuous situations. The schools also provided a welcome distraction and safe environment for much of the day and a much needed break for the parents.

Emotional Needs

One of the basic principles in pediatrics states that "Children are not little adults." Anyone who has cared for children well recognizes the truth of this statement. While adults may be able to understand their situations and respond in a rational way, children will process the information differently. Therefore, involving people with expertise in working with children early in the process is vital. Social workers, child life specialists, and counselors should be brought in as soon as possible. "Children are particularly vulnerable in complex emergencies. Addressing their specific needs, including health in complex emergencies, is critical to the success of relief efforts and requires child-specific, effective and coordinated interventions."[14] When possible, a family-centered approach should be taken. The earlier children receive help in dealing with the complex emotions brought on by experiencing trauma, the better their long-term outcome is likely to be.

Disease Prevention

Many children arrived in Houston in the clothing they had been wearing during the hurricane and subsequent flood. In many cases, their clothing was still covered in mud and feces.[4] Perhaps not surprisingly, an outbreak of diarrheal disease occurred among evacuees at the Reliant complex following Hurricane Katrina. Stool samples were tested and the causative agent was determined to be norovirus. More than half of the specimens submitted for analysis via polymerase chain reaction (PCR) tested positive for this infectious agent. It was evident that isolating affected individuals from the rest of the population was the key to preventing the outbreak from reaching epidemic proportions. A 25-bed isolation unit was set up next to the pediatric clinic for patients who required intravenous rehydration therapy. In addition to the rehydration unit, a 400-bed isolation area was established for those evacuees who had diarrhea but did not require medical intervention, as part of an effort to isolate these individuals from the general population. These measures helped to minimize the spread of disease and allowed patient flow within the pediatric clinic to resume.[2] Hand washing and toilet facilities for staff were separated from those being used by evacuees in a further attempt to minimize disease spread. Several days after the buses began arriving at Reliant Center, fresh clothing and shower facilities were provided to the evacuees.

CONCLUSION

We cannot usually predict how and when a public health emergency will occur. We can, however, be certain that one eventually will arise. Planning is, therefore, essential. Because of the unique challenges involved in treating children, individuals with pediatric expertise should be involved in every stage of the planning, response, and post-event review processes. The inclusion of pediatric specialists will ensure that the needs of this vulnerable population are met before, during, and after a crisis. Lessons learned as a result of Hurricane Katrina and other public health crises, if applied correctly, will allow public health professionals to better protect and care for children in future crisis situations.

INTERNET RESOURCES

American Academy of Pediatrics (AAP), children and disasters: http://www.aap.org/disasters/index.cfm

Federal Emergency Management Agency (FEMA), helping children cope with disasters: www.fema.gov/rebuild/recover/cope_child.shtm

National Association of Child Care Resource and Referral Agencies, children and disasters: www.naccrra.org/disaster/

National Commission on Children and Disasters: www.childrenanddisasters.acf.hhs.gov

U.S. Department of Health and Human Services, National Mental Health Information Center, *Reaction of Children to Disasters:* http://mentalhealth.samhsa.gov/publications/allpubs/ken01-0101/

NOTES

1. American Academy of Pediatrics. *Position statement: The pediatrician and disaster preparedness.* 2005.
2. Sirbaugh PE, Gurwitch KD, Macias CG, Ligon BL, Gavagan T, Feigin RD. Creation and implementation of a mobile pediatric emergency response team: Regionalized caring for displaced children after a disaster. *Pediatrics.* May 2006;117:5428–5438.
3. Hamilton DR, Gavagan TF, Smart KT, Upton LA, Havron DA, Weller NF. Houston's medical disaster response to Hurricane Katrina. *Annals of Emergency Medicine.* April 2009;53:505–514.
4. Sirbaugh PE. Personal communication. March 2009.
5. Shirm S, Liggin R, Dick R, Graham J. Prehospital preparedness for pediatric mass-casualty events. *Pediatrics.* 2007;120:756–761.
6. Wallis LA, Carley S. Comparison of paediatric major incident primary triage tools. *Emergency Medicine Journal.* 2006;23:475–478.
7. Romig LE. The JumpSTART pediatric MCI triage tool. Available at: http://www.jumpstart triage.com.
8. Gajdeczka AA. *A makeshift shelter from the storm: An evaluation of pediatric disaster preparedness in Texas.* Prepared for the Children's Hospital Association of Texas (CHAT). June 2007.
9. National Institute of Mental Health. Post traumatic stress disorder. Available at: http://www.nimh.nih.gov/health/topics/post-traumatic-stress-disorder-ptsd/index .shtml.
10. Rowe CL, Liddle HA. When the levee breaks: Treating adolescents and families in the aftermath of Hurricane Katrina. *Journal of Maternal and Family Therapy.* April 2008;34:132–148.
11. Cicero MX, Baum CR. Pediatric disaster preparedness: Best planning for the worst case scenario. *Pediatric Emergency Care.* July 2008;24;478–481.
12. Weiner DL, Manzi SF, Waltzman ML, Morin M, Meginniss A, Fleisher GR. FEMA's organized response with a pediatric subspecialty team: The National Disaster Medical System response: A pediatric perspective. *Pediatrics.* 2006; 117:S405–S411.
13. Centers for Disease Control and Prevention. Interim immunization recommendations for individuals displaced by disaster. Available at: http://www.bt.cdc.gov/disasters/disease/vaccrec displaced.asp.
14. World Health Organization. *Consultation on child health in complex emergencies.* Meeting report, 2004.
15. National Center for Missing and Exploited Children. *Final Report: Katrina/Rita Missing Persons Hotline Update on Calls/Cases, Wednesday 3/22/2006.* Available at: http://www.missingkids.com/ en_US/documents/KatrinaHotlineUpdate.pdf
16. Upton LA. Personal communication. March 2009.

CHAPTER 26

Public Health Emergencies and Substance Abuse

Deborah Podus, Jane Carlisle Maxwell, and M. Douglas Anglin

INTRODUCTION

Emergency public health planning for special populations, particularly those persons with substance abuse problems, is a relatively new development in terms of public health preparedness. Well-developed literature on the topic does not exist, and funding for substance abuse preparedness and response has historically been limited. This chapter discusses the impacts of Hurricanes Katrina and Rita on affected substance abuse treatment systems, provides a brief overview of substance use in the United States, examines the various ways in which substance use may become an issue in terms of emergency settings, and provides examples of how these issues are salient at the different stages of a large-scale emergency. Although the chapter discusses both alcohol and other drug use, the primary focus is on drug abuse and dependence.

Case Study

In August 2005, Hurricane Katrina caused major damage throughout the Gulf Coast region of the United States, with particularly devastating impacts occurring in New Orleans, Louisiana, and along the Mississippi Coast. The storm inflicted loss of life, psychological trauma, extensive property damage, loss of electrical power, disruption of telecommunication systems, shortages of essential supplies, and damage to local healthcare systems; it also led to the dispersal of more than 1 million households from affected communities to other parts of the country. Three weeks later, Hurricane Rita made landfall in eastern Louisiana near the Louisiana–Texas border.

In terms of the substance abuse treatment system, Hurricanes Katrina and Rita led to program closures in the most heavily affected communities and to a surge of displaced patients at some treatment programs in areas where patients were evacuated. In New Orleans, flooding forced all seven of the city's methadone treatment programs, which had served more than 1,000 patients, to close.[1] Residential substance abuse treatment programs were also damaged.[2,3] Based on official reports from Louisiana and Mississippi,[4] it appears that more than one-third of substance abuse treatment capacity in Louisiana was disrupted and 88 percent of the patients in addiction treatment prior to Hurricane Katrina were unable to be located. In Mississippi, 5 out of 15 mental health regions reportedly experienced significant damage to their treatment facilities, including those used for substance abuse treatment, and one region lost all of its treatment facilities.

In east Texas, where many Katrina victims were evacuated, Texas state data indicate that in the first five months after the storm, 369 Katrina evacuees received publicly funded substance abuse treatment; the majority were displaced methadone recipients who were admitted to methadone treatment programs within the first 30 days after the hurricane.[3] Treatment programs in other parts of the region were affected as well. A survey of 90 for-profit and nonprofit methadone treatment programs in 50 counties and parishes in the five Gulf Coast states found that 51 percent reported one or more service delivery problems (e.g., influx of displaced patients, difficulties verifying records for displaced patients) due to the dispersal of individuals in the aftermath of Hurricane Katrina.[5]

The impact of Hurricanes Katrina and Rita on substance use by affected individuals is less clear. Analysis of data from the National Survey on Drug Use and Health collected in the Gulf State areas affected by the two hurricanes found that, compared to the prior year, there were no significant differences in the prevalence of illicit drug use, binge alcohol use, or cigarette use.[6] However, among adults aged 18 or older who were displaced from their homes for two weeks or more, past-month rates of illicit drug use, marijuana use, and cigarette use in the year after the storms were significantly higher than those for individuals from the area who were not displaced. Specifically, the rates for the two groups were 4.9 percent versus 10.5 percent for illicit drug use, 2.9 percent versus 8.1 percent for marijuana use, and 24.9 percent versus 34.1 percent for cigarettes. Other data and anecdotal reports suggest more pronounced effects on substance use among hurricane-affected individuals. For example, in Mississippi the number of liquor cases sold during an approximately two-month period shortly after Hurricane Katrina was somewhat higher than the sales in a comparable period one year before the hurricane; moreover, one year after Katrina came ashore, crisis counselors in Mississippi were reporting increasing use of alcohol as a means of coping with post-disaster chronic stressors and many new cases of substance abuse.[4]

HISTORICAL AND GENERAL PERSPECTIVES _____

The use of tobacco, alcohol, and other drugs is fairly common in U.S. society. Data from the National Survey of Drug Use and Health (NSDUH)—the primary source of information on the use of illicit drugs and alcohol in the civilian, non-institutionalized population of the United States—indicate that in 2008 slightly more than half of Americans aged 12 or older (approximately 129 million people) reported being current drinkers of alcohol. In addition, an estimated 20.1 million Americans (8 percent of the population) reported using an illicit drug in the preceding month. Illicit drugs include marijuana, cocaine, heroin, hallucinogens, inhalants, and prescription-type medications such as painkillers, tranquilizers, stimulants, or sedatives used on a nonmedical basis.

Within the overall population, the prevalence of substance use, the types of substances used, and the method of administration may vary significantly depending on geographical location and on demographic and cultural characteristics including age, race and ethnicity, gender, education, occupation, and other factors. Moreover, trends in drug use change over time. Thus, in planning for emergency preparedness and response for substance use issues, it is important to take local and regional drug use patterns into consideration.

Epidemiology of Substance Use

Data from the 2008 NSDUH indicate that an estimated 22.2 million persons (9 percent of those aged 12 or older) in the United States were diagnosed with substance *dependence* or *abuse* in the past year based on the criteria specified in the *Diagnostic and Statistical Manual of Mental Disorders*, fourth edition, text revision (*DSM-IV-TR*).[7] Of these individuals, 3.1 million were classified with dependence on or abuse of both alcohol and illicit drugs, 3.9 million were dependent on or abused illicit drugs but not alcohol, and 15.2 million were dependent on or abused alcohol but not illicit drugs. Based on the *DSM-IV-TR*, drug dependence is more severe than a diagnosis of drug abuse; the former entails a pattern of repeated substance use that can result in tolerance for the substance, withdrawal symptoms if a person is unable to obtain the substance, and compulsive drug-taking behavior. In 2008, the number of people with past-year dependence on or abuse of marijuana was 4.2 million. For pain relievers, this population numbered 1.7 million; for cocaine, 1.4 million; and for heroin, 282,000. An unknown number of people have historically had a substance use disorder, but have achieved a period of sobriety. For such individuals, the potential for relapse into drug use as a result of an emergency situation is a primary public health concern.

Scientific research indicates that substance dependence is best characterized as a chronic medical illness that affects both the brain and behavior and that has treatment adherence and relapse rates similar to those associated with other chronic diseases such as hypertension, asthma, and type 2 diabetes.[8] Nevertheless, among the general public, there continues to be stigma assigned to persons with a substance abuse disorder. Further research is needed to understand more fully the biological and behavioral origins of addiction and to elucidate how patterns of alcohol and drug use change over the life course. Studies conducted to date have found a connection between stress and substance abuse and between stress and relapse into substance use among individuals who have been treated for addiction and attained abstinence.[9]

Vulnerable Subgroups

Given the association between disasters and stress, from an emergency public health standpoint there are at least four subgroups of users for whom substance use becomes an amplified problem during large-scale crisis situations:

- Patients who are enrolled in an ongoing course of substance abuse treatment at the time of the disaster
- Persons who are in recovery and who as a result of disaster-related stress may have urges to return to substance use
- Current substance users who as a result of disaster-related stress increase their use, leading to increased public safety concerns such as driving under the influence
- Persons who realize they have a substance use problem of which they had not previously been aware

Each of these subgroups requires a different type of disaster planning approach. At the same time, the widespread use of substances in U.S. society and the persistence of stigma toward addiction and toward substance abuse treatment continue to complicate the development of policies to address effectively the problems of this diverse population during a public health emergency. The implications for emergency preparedness and response are discussed more fully in the following section.

PREPAREDNESS AND PLANNING

As noted previously, substance abuse treatment programs are among the many types of healthcare programs whose delivery of services has been disrupted as a result of hurricanes. According to data collected by the National Survey of Substance Abuse Treatment Services (N-SSATS), in 2007 there were more than 13,000 such facilities in the United States, with a total census of more than 1.1 million patients on an average day. Three main types of drug treatment modalities are used:

- Medication-assisted programs
- Inpatient and residential programs
- Outpatient drug-free treatment programs

In addition to these formal treatment system components, a host of mutual-support groups, such as Alcoholics Anonymous and Narcotics Anonymous, provide services for persons in recovery.

Of the three main treatment modalities, medication-assisted treatment— especially methadone maintenance—is particularly vulnerable to public emergencies because disruption in client access to medication can result in significant health problems. Methadone maintenance treatment (MMT), also know as narcotic maintenance treatment, entails the daily use of liquid methadone medication, typically in conjunction with counseling and other services, to treat persons who are addicted to heroin and other opiates. Generally, most methadone recipients must attend their regular treatment program almost every day of the week to be dosed. Because MMT is subject to strict federal and state regulation in the United States, and because lack of patient access to medication results in the onset of aversive withdrawal symptoms, which in turn may lead to drug use relapse, maintaining treatment continuity for patients in the event of a disaster is an important planning concern. Another medication that has been used more recently to treat opiate addiction is buprenorphine (Suboxone, Subutex). In part because of the historical circumstances in which its use has evolved, buprenorphine is less tightly regulated than methadone and may be prescribed by a private, office-based physician who has been specially trained in buprenorphine treatment for opioid addiction or by a methadone clinic. Local public health professionals and substance abuse treatment providers may consider developing measures to ensure adequate supplies of these and other addiction medications for use in emergency settings in consultation with federal and state regulatory authorities.*

Residential programs may also face special challenges because the large number of patients in such programs, coupled with the general social stigma toward persons in substance abuse treatment facilities, may make it difficult for programs to find

---

*Substantial research has been devoted to the development of new medications for addiction over the last two decades. In addition to medications for the treatment of opioid addiction discussed here, medications have been approved to treat alcoholism (e.g., naltrexone [Revial], depo-naltrexone [Vivitrol], and acamprosate [Campral]) and clinical trials are under way for medications to treat addiction to cocaine and other drugs. To the extent that use of medication-assisted treatment expands in the coming years, emergency planners and treatment providers may need to consider planning for a broader array of addiction pharmacotherapies.

shelter for displaced residents if evacuation becomes necessary. In addition, for adolescent residential treatment programs, assistance in establishing communication between patients and their family members in an emergency is an important disaster response concern.

Little information is available about local emergency planning and preparedness activities with respect to substance abuse (see Table 26-1 for a summary of the potential strategies that might be used in this phase of a public health emergency). However, a survey of 90 (of 141) MMTs in the Gulf Coast region[5] suggests that such programs are not well integrated into local emergency planning activities. For example, more than 30 percent of programs reported that they were *not aware* of or only *knew a little* about how local responders such as police, emergency management personnel, health or mental health providers, or the American Red Cross would respond to a disaster in their community. In addition, only 39.3 percent thought it likely that they would receive the help they needed from local agencies in the event of a disaster; 24.7 percent thought it unlikely, and 36 percent did not know whether such help would be forthcoming. Further complicating the integration of MMTs in local emergency planning and preparedness activities is the fact that in many MMTs, the most common way staff update their knowledge of disaster planning is through informal conversation.

Increased Collaborations

While greater outreach on the part of community public health professionals can lead to improved planning and preparedness by local substance abuse treatment programs, the inclusion of substance abuse treatment providers in the planning process can help the community better prepare for disaster-related substance abuse issues. For example, these providers not only have expertise regarding the identification of persons with substance abuse or dependence, but also are a valuable source of information about drug use trends in their local community and, hence, the types of disaster-related substance use problems that may emerge. Moreover, collaboration before a public health emergency occurs can be useful for developing a clearer understanding of how local treatment programs can contribute to community emergency response efforts. For example, some treatment programs may have the capacity to admit new patients after an emergency, while others may not.

Advance planning may also be helpful with respect to establishing appropriate referral procedures for healthcare pain patients who may be experiencing withdrawal from methadone or other opiates. These types of patients proved to be a serious problem after Hurricane Katrina. The Center for Substance Abuse Treatment[1] rec-

TABLE 26-1   Emergencies and Substance Abuse: Preparedness Strategies

Treatment Modality	Preparedness Options
Medication-assisted programs	Programs appoint a disaster planning team and develop a facility-specific disaster plan.
	Program leadership participates in local emergency planning and drills.
	Programs prepare plans to contact patients, local officials, and media about closures and alternative programs that may be open during emergencies. Programs execute written agreements with alternative programs.
	Programs develop emergency plans regarding supply and management of medications in consultation with appropriate federal, state, and local authorities.
	Programs keep backup copies of client records and dosing information at an off-site location that is accessible in an emergency.
Inpatient and residential programs	Programs appoint a disaster planning team and develop a facility-specific disaster plan.
	Program leadership participates in local emergency planning and drills.
	Programs develop contingency locations to transfer patients during evacuation periods and develop written agreements with contingency facilities.
	Programs maintain ongoing communications with local officials about surge capacity to accept additional patients during emergencies.
Outpatient drug-free treatment programs	Programs appoint a disaster planning team and develop a facility-specific disaster plan.
	Program leadership participates in local emergency planning and drills.
	Programs prepare plans to contact patients, local officials, and media about closures and alternative programs that may be open during emergencies. Programs establish written agreements with alternative programs.
	Programs develop linkages with self-help programs to provide support in shelters and in the community.

ommends that such patients be referred to a local physician or pain management specialist. Although MMTs are not precluded from treating substance-dependent patients who also have pain problems, regulatory guidelines are not clear. Clarifying procedures to address such issues with local providers before a large-scale emergency occurs can help to prevent inappropriate referrals and misunderstandings during and after a crisis situation.

RESPONSE

A major problem that has emerged across multiple public health emergencies is the substantial variability in shelter policies with respect to substance abuse patients. In Colorado, for example, the Red Cross would not allow Narcotics Anonymous or Alcoholics Anonymous meetings on-site in shelters set up to receive Katrina evacuees.[10] Interviews with MMT providers in the Gulf Coast states indicate that shelter policies with respect to methadone medication also varied.[3,11] Some disaster shelter operators allowed MMT patients to bring take-home medication doses into the shelter; others did not. Similarly, some allowed programs to dose methadone recipients at the shelter; others did not. In several states, many shelter workers were not trained to recognize opiate withdrawal symptoms. Such symptoms may include diarrhea, stomach cramps, vomiting, muscle aches, and chills.[12] In one Houston shelter, when methadone-dependent patients began to experience withdrawal and developed diarrhea, some shelter staff wanted to quarantine them for fear of an outbreak of disease.[3]

Increased collaboration between substance abuse treatment providers and shelter operators with respect to substance abuse planning and increased involvement of treatment professionals in shelter triage efforts may help to improve relevant shelter policies. Research on the disaster response in the aftermath of Hurricanes Katrina and Rita, for example, indicated that substance abuse treatment staff provided valuable services.[3] Unfortunately, limited public funding to support such activities has meant that, in many cases, treatment providers have borne much of the costs of those efforts.

As with other healthcare services, power outages, disruptions in telecommunication and Internet services, and transportation difficulties—all of which often occur in public health emergencies—hamper the ability of substance abuse treatment providers to maintain continuity of essential services to their clients. Although these difficulties are especially problematic for programs in the areas directly affected by the disaster, they are also a problem for treatment providers outside the disaster impact area that receive displaced patients and are unable to communicate with the originating clinics to verify patient status. Several staff and patients interviewed in the Gulf Coast MMT study commented that it would be helpful to have the operating status of substance

TABLE 26-2 Emergencies and Substance Abuse: Response Strategies	
Responding Entity	**Response Options**
Local government	Institute uniform policies on receiving, maintaining, and dispensing regulated medications for temporary treatment facilities.
	Help coordinate transfer of inpatients between programs during evacuations.
Nongovernmental organizations (e.g., American Red Cross)	Consider allowing and assisting ongoing outpatient drug-free programs and self-help groups within ongoing emergency assistance efforts.
	Help communicate the availability of ongoing medication-assisted and drug-free treatment services.
Shelters	Educate shelter workers about withdrawal signs and symptoms that may appear among evacuees.
	Help coordinate the transfer of substance abuse treatment records along with other medical and mental health records.
	Consider allowing ongoing outpatient drug-free programs and self-help groups to operate within shelters.

abuse treatment clinics publicly announced in radio broadcasts, as is typically done for schools and other community agencies.

Another problem after various disasters has been challenges faced by staff members as they try to access their treatment program and program records if the clinic is inside a restricted area; in many cases, officials managing access control points have not previously been made aware of the clinic's existence and needs.[13] Greater collaboration between emergency planners, emergency responders, and substance abuse programs during the emergency planning and preparedness stage could help to better address these and other issues and enable affected programs to maintain treatment services during the response and recovery phases. Table 26-2 summarizes the response strategies that may be employed by various entities to deal with substance abuse problems in the response phase of a public health emergency.

MITIGATION

Lessons learned from past public health emergencies suggest several measures that can improve the local response to emergency-related substance abuse issues:

- Substance abuse treatment system representatives must be involved in local planning efforts. Increased communication between emergency responders and such providers can foster greater understanding between the two groups and lay the groundwork for more effective collaboration in future disasters.
- Previous experience suggests the need to credential substance abuse treatment staff in advance so that they can participate with local government, the Red Cross, and other voluntary agencies in disaster response efforts.
- Cross-training of staff in emergency response and substance abuse treatment would be useful to improve local preparedness and response.
- Public health and emergency management preparedness plans should incorporate preparedness for substance abuse–related issues.
- Inclusion of treatment program staff in local preparedness activities such as training workshops and tabletop exercises would likely foster relationship building and contribute to improved cooperation with respect to the disaster response.
- Systematic surveillance and monitoring of post-disaster drug use and treatment program issues can serve both to identify emerging problems and to pro-

TABLE 26-3 Emergencies and Substance Abuse: Mitigation Strategies	
Mitigation Entity	**Mitigation Options**
Local government	Institute systematic surveillance and monitoring strategies to track substance abuse patterns during and after emergencies.
	Include substance abuse treatment providers in emergency planning activities.
Nongovernmental organizations (e.g., American Red Cross)	Train substance abuse treatment providers in basic medical response courses such as first aid and CPR.
	Maintain an up-to-date list of treatment programs, which can be used to refer victims during and after emergencies to available resources.
Treatment programs	Allow treatment providers to attend local emergency training programs and drills.
	Develop a consortium of local programs that maintain communication of shared resources during emergencies.
	Consider the various options available and establish written agreements to transition inpatients to outpatient programs during emergencies.

duce a better understanding of the interrelationships between large-scale emergencies and substance use in the future.

Table 26-3 summarizes the various mitigation strategies for substance abuse problems during a public health emergency.

CONCLUSION

The issue of emergency planning as related to substance abuse issues is not a topic that has heretofore received much policy, practice, or research attention. Nevertheless, the widespread prevalence of substance use in U.S. society and the association between substance use and stress suggests that it is an important local, regional, and national emergency public health concern. Multiple modalities of substance abuse treatment exist, each of which has its own set of vulnerabilities in an emergency setting. Research suggests that substance abuse treatment programs have not generally been included in local disaster planning and preparedness activities. In many communities, the stigma attached to substance users and substance abuse treatment programs persists in an emergency and can exacerbate the problems experienced by clients and providers alike. Greater collaboration between public health professionals and substance abuse treatment providers can lead to improved response for affected individuals in this vulnerable population.

ACKNOWLEDGMENT

Deborah Podus's work on this chapter was supported in part by funding from the National Institute on Drug Abuse (NIDA R21 DA023045) and from the Substance Abuse Policy Research Program of the Robert Wood Johnson Foundation (Grant No. 61374). M. Douglas Anglin is also supported by NIDA Senior Research Scientist Award (K05 DA00146).

INTERNET RESOURCES

Clinical Opiate Withdrawal Scale (COWS): http://www.suboxone.com/pdfs/OWR.pdf

State Opioid Treatment Authority, contact information: http://www.nasadad.org/resource.php?doc_id=1947

Substance Abuse and Mental Health Services Administration, Center for Substance Abuse Treatment: http://csat.samhsa.gov/

Substance Abuse and Mental Health Services Administration, Center for Substance Abuse Treatment, Directory of Single State Agencies for Substance Abuse Services: http://www.samhsa.gov/Grants/ssadirectory.pdf

Substance Abuse and Mental Health Services Administration, Substance Abuse Treatment Facility Locator: http://findtreatment.samhsa.gov/

NOTES

1. Substance Abuse and Mental Health Services Administration. Dear Colleague letter. September 9, 2005. Available at: http://www.dpt.samhsa.gov/pdf/dearColleague/GuidanceKatrina_090905.pdf. Accessed December 7, 2009.

2. Toriello P, Morse P, Morse E, Kissinger P, Pedersen-Wasson E. The resuscitation of a New Orleans substance abuse treatment agency after Hurricane Katrina. *Journal of Health Care for the Poor and Underserved* 2007;18:482–486.

3. Maxwell JC, Podus D, Walsh D. Lessons learned from the deadly sisters: Drug and alcohol treatment disruption, and consequences from Hurricanes Katrina and Rita. *Substance Use & Misuse* 2009;44:1681–1694. Available at: http://informahealthcare.com/doi/pdf/10.3109/10826080902962011. Accessed December 7, 2009.

4. McKernan B. Public health arena: Substance abuse needs: Lessons learned from the 2005 hurricane response. Presentation at the 134th Annual Meeting of the American Public Health Association, Boston, MA, November 7, 2006. Available at: http://www.samhsa.gov/csatdisaster recovery/lessons/09-APHA_DisasterSA_11-7-06_CSATCDROM.pdf. Accessed November 1, 2009.

5. Podus D. Disaster planning and opioid treatment programs. *The Dialogue*. 2009. Available at: http://download.ncadi.samhsa.gov/ken/pdf/dtac/DialogueIssue3_09.pdf. Accessed December 7, 2009.

6. Substance Abuse and Mental Health Services Administration. *The NSDUH report: Impact of Hurricanes Katrina and Rita on substance use and mental health*. Rockville, MD: Office of Applied Studies; 2008. Available at: http://www.oas.samhsa.gov/2k8/katrina/katrina.htm. Accessed December 7, 2009.

7. American Psychiatric Association. *Diagnostic and statistical manual of mental disorders*, 4th ed., text rev. Washington, DC: American Psychiatric Association; 2000.

8. McLellan AT, Lewis DC, Obrien CP, Kleber H. Drug dependence, a chronic medical illness: Implications for treatment, insurance and outcome evaluation. *Journal of the American Medical Association*. 2000;284:1689–1695.

9. National Institute on Drug Abuse. Stress and substance abuse: A special report. 2001. Available at: http://www.drugabuse.gov/stressanddrugabuse.html. Accessed November 3, 2009.

10. Substance Abuse and Mental Health Services Administration. *Results from the 2008 National Survey on Drug Use and Health: National findings* (NSDUH Series H-36, HHS Publication No. SMA 09-4434). Rockville, MD: Office of Applied Studies; 2009 Available at: http://www.oas.samhsa.gov/nsduh/2k8nsduh/2k8Results.pdf. Accessed December 7, 2009.

11. Podus D, Maxwell JC, Anglin MD. *Disaster planning and substance abuse stigma with respect to methadone maintenance treatment.* Poster presentation, Addiction Health Services Conference, San Francisco, CA, October 29, 2009.

12. Wesson DR, Ling W. The Clinical Opiate Withdrawal Scale (COWS). *Journal of Psychoactive Drugs.* 2003;35:253–259.

13. Dewart T, Frank B, Schmeidler J. The impact of 9/11 on patients in New York City's substance abuse treatment programs. *American Journal of Drug and Alcohol Abuse.* 2006;32:665–672.

Index

Figures and tables are indicated by f and t following page numbers.

A

AARP, 113
Abuse
 children, susceptibility to, 523
 substance abuse. *See* Public health
  emergencies and substance abuse
Accountability in disaster response, 89, 112
ACIP (Advisory Committee on Immunization
  Practices), 145
Activation of resources/capabilities, 57–60
Active surveillance systems, 23, 178
Acute radiation syndromes (ARS), 368,
  370–371*t*
Administrative law, 38–39
Administrative Procedure Act (1946), 39
Administrative search, 41
Advance response planning, 22
Advisory Committee on Immunization
  Practices (ACIP), 145
Advocacy NGOs, 104, 108
AEC (Atomic Energy Commission), 477, 478
Afghanistan. *See also* Emerging public health
  systems
 Avian influenza in, 75, 136
 mental health system, 71, 418
 mentioning programs in, 77–78
Afghanistan National Development Strategy
  (policy document), 70
Afghan National Army (ANA), 67–68
Afghan National Police (ANP), 67–68

Afghan Public Health Institute (APHI), 70
Aged receptors, 349
Agency for Toxic Substances and Disease
  Registry (ATSDR), 340, 451
Agency preparedness for contagious diseases
  epidemics, 213
Agenda 21 (UN program), 106
Agriculture Department, U.S., 18
AIDS/HIV programs, 76, 86
Air and water quality, 13, 14
Airborne infectious disease transmission, 313,
  313*t*, 327
Air logistics expertise, 98
Alcoholics Anonymous, 535, 538
Alpha particles, 359
Al-Qaeda, 65, 357
American Association of Retired Persons
  (AARP), 113
American Psychiatric Association, 493
American Red Cross
 evacuation centers, 168–172, 538
 founding of, 105
 funding for, 112–114
 Hurricane Katrina and, 86, 126
 National Response Framework and, 116
 personal preparedness guidelines, 293
 U.S. federal government relationship and,
  111
American Society for Microbiology, 261–262
AmeriCares, 108–110

AMRIID (U.S. Army Medical Research Institute for Infectious Diseases), 307
ANA (Afghan National Army), 67–68
ANAB (ANSI-ASQ National Accreditation Board), 293
Annexes, emergency support function, 47–49, 48*f*, 117, 481
ANP (Afghan National Police), 67–68
ANSI-ASQ National Accreditation Board (ANAB), 293
Anthrax, 309–311, 310*t*, 325
Antidotes
  administration of, 340–341
  cyanide kit, 346
  MARK I kit, 341, 349
  stockpiling, 338
APHI (Afghan Public Health Institute), 70
Argus-1, 136
Army Corps of Engineers, 132–133
Army Medical Research Institute for Infectious Diseases (AMRIID), 307
ARS (acute radiation syndromes), 368, 370–371*t*
Articles of Confederation, 37
Asian tsunami (2004)
  government partnerships and, 87
  mental health impacts from, 494, 506–508
  meta-initiatives and, 93
  NGO contribution, 117–118
  overview of, 409–410
  public-private partnerships and, 84–85, 98
  single-company public-private partnerships and, 92
Asphyxiants, 344–347, 345*t*
Association of Public Health Laboratories, 262
Astrodome, Houston, 518, 525–529
Atomic Energy Commission (AEC), 477, 478
ATSDR (Agency for Toxic Substances and Disease Registry), 340, 451
Avian influenza, 75, 136, 143–144

B
Bacillus anthracis (anthrax), 310, 310*t*
Bacterial meningitis, 217–219
Basic health center, Afghanistan (BHC), 70, 74
Basic Package of Health Services, Afghanistan (BPHS), 72, 74
Baton Rouge Area Foundation, 126
Behavioral Risk Factor Surveillance System, 189

Benzodiazapines, 349
Beta particles, 359
BHC (basic health center, Afghanistan), 74
Bhutanese refugees, 173
Bill of Rights, federal, 38, 40
Biological agents, 305–334
  anthrax, 309–311, 310*t*, 325
  biodefense structure, U.S., 325–327
  botulism, 305–306, 311–312
  brucellosis, 318–319
  case study, 305–306, 327–328
  category A agents, 309–318, 310*t*, 313*t*
  category B agents, 318–325
  category C agents, 324–325
  epsilon toxin, 319–320
  food safety threats, 320–321
  glanders, 321
  healthcare institutions and, 261
  healthcare providers, care of, 326*t*, 327
  historical perspectives, 306–309, 308*t*
  melioidosis, 321–322
  mitigation, 325–327
  overview, 305–306
  plague, 313–314, 313*t*
  psittacosis, 322
  Q fever, 322–323
  ricin toxin, 323
  smallpox, 314–315
  staphylococcal enterotoxin B, 324
  tularemia, 315–316
  viral hemorrhagic fevers, 316–318, 317*t*
  water safety threats, 324
Biological risk of radiation exposure, 476, 476*t*
Biological Weapons Convention (UN), 307
Biomedical interventions, 501–503
Biosafety levels, 268
BioSense, 135, 136, 263
Biosurveillance, 135–136
Bioterrorism, 20. *See also* Biological agents
Blanco, Kathleen, 132
Blast injuries, 297
Bombing events, 285–304. *See also specific bombing events*
  case study, 285–287, 300–301
  civilian population, 293, 297, 299–300, 301
  confined-space bombings, 295–296
  government agencies role in, 290–292, 292*t*, 294–295, 294*f*, 298, 299*f*, 300
  health care, 292–293, 295–297, 298–299, 301

historical perspectives, 287–289
mitigation, 298–300, 299*f*
nongovernmental organizations, 293, 297, 299–300, 301
open-air bombings, 295–296
overview, 285–287
preparedness, 289–293, 290*f*
private-sector organizations, 293, 297, 299–300, 301
response, 294–295
structural-collapse bombings, 295–296
Botulism, 305–306, 311–312
Boxing Day Tsunami (2004), 417–418
BPHS (Basic Package of Health Services, Afghanistan), 72, 74
Brazil, Goiania (radiological accident, 1987), 373–374
Bristol-Myers Squibb, 86
"The Brookhaven Report" (Atomic Energy Commission), 478
Brucellosis (*brucellae* species), 318–319
Bubonic plague, 313–314
Burkholderia mallei (glanders), 321
Burkholderia pseudomallei (melioidosis), 321–322
Burns, chemical agents, 342–344, 343*t*
Business Roundtable Partnership for Disaster Response, 98
Business-sector preparedness for pandemic influenza, 236, 236*t*

C
California, earthquakes, 131, 383, 385
California Education Code, 385
California Governor's Office of Emergency Services', 386
Calming information, 503–504
Capabilities
deployment of, 57–60
multisector/multijurisdictional, 8–9
personnel and physical, assessment of, 55–56, 55*f*
Capability-based preparedness, 52–53, 52*f*
Capacity, demands for, 88–89
Capacity building, 17–18, 418
Carbamate insecticides, 349
Carbon monoxide (CO) poisoning
characteristics of, 344–345, 415–416, 435
mitigation efforts, 418, 419–420
Careflight, 519
CARE organization, 90, 106, 120

Carter, Jimmy, 474
Case-control studies, 154*t*, 155
Case law, 39–40
Case-series studies, 153, 154*t*
Category A biological agents, 309–318, 310*t*, 313*t*
Category B biological agents, 318–325
Category C biological agents, 324–325
CDC. *See* Centers for Disease Control and Prevention
Center for Emergency Preparedness and Response (Canada), 179, 272
Center for Strategic and International Studies, 374
Center for Substance Abuse Treatment, 536
Centers for Disease Control and Prevention (CDC)
in Afghanistan, 71
antidote stockpiling, 338
biosurveillance and, 135
bioterrorism agents and diseases, classification of, 308*t*, 309
disease surveillance networks of, 16
food supply safety threats, 320
goals of during emergencies, 18–19, 19*t*
harmful chemicals list, 341
H1N1 vaccine production, 145
International Emerging Infections Program, 272–273
Morbidity and Mortality Weekly Report, 179
National Electronic Disease Surveillance System, 179
notifiable infectious conditions, 211, 211–212*t*
Outbreak Management Program, 136, 137*t*
personal medical records, 413
personal preparedness guidelines, 293
radiological incident, role in, 363
shelter-based surveillance system, 168
smallpox vaccination program, 315
vaccinations, recommended schedules for, 524
World Trade Center, response to, 14
Centralized approach to state responses, 20
Centralized IT architecture, 138–139
CERT (Community Emergency Response Team), 293, 386
Chain of custody, laboratory, 268
CHC (comprehensive health center, Afghanistan), 70, 74

CHE. *See* Complex humanitarian emergency
Chemical agents, 335–356
    asphyxiants, 344–347, 345*t*
    burns, 342–344, 343*t*
    case study, 335–336, 350–351
    historical perspectives, 336–337
    irritant gas syndromes, 341–342, 342*t*
    metabolic poisoning syndromes, 344–347, 345*t*
    mitigation, 350
    organophosphate syndrome, 347–349, 347*t*
    overview, 335–336
    preparedness and planning, 337–338
    response, 339–349, 339*t*
    vesicant syndrome, 342–344, 343*t*
Chemical Weapons Convention (UN 1997), 350
CHEMPACK push packs, 349
Chernobyl, Ukraine (nuclear incident, 1986), 473, 475, 486
Chernobyl Forum Report, 486
Chicago, (heat wave, 1995), 426–428, 427*f*, 439–440
Children and public health emergencies, 517–530
    case study, 517–518, 525–529
    chronic diseases, exacerbation of, 525
    disease prevention, 524, 528–529
    emotional needs, 528
    equipment and personnel, 521–522, 527
    exposure, 522–523
    injuries, 523
    normalization of routine, 524, 528
    overview, 517–518
    preparedness issues, 518–522, 525–527
    psychosocial issues, 522, 527–528
    response issues, 522–525, 527–529
    reunification, 521
    susceptibility to abuse, 523
    tracking, 521, 526–527
    triage, 518–521, 520*f*, 525–526
    vaccinations, 524–525
Children's Health Program (UN), 85
Chiles, Lawton, 46
China, cyclones, 407–408
China, earthquakes
    Haicheng, (1975), 383, 385
    Shaanxi Province, (1556), 383
    Sichuan, (2008), 92–93, 382, 388, 390
    Tangshan, (1976), 382
Chlamydia psittaci (psittacosis), 322

Chlorine, 341–342
Chloroacetophenone (tear gas), 341
Choking agents, 341–342
Cholera outbreak (Zimbabwe, 2008–2009), 177
Chronic diseases, exacerbation of, 525
CIKR (critical infrastructure and key resources), 50
CISD (critical incident stress debriefing), 500
CISM (critical incident stress management), 500
Cities Readiness Initiative, 18
Citizen Corps Program, 338
Civilian populations, role in bombing events, 293, 297, 299–300, 301
Classification system
    bioterrorism agents and diseases, 308*t*, 309
    hazardous materials, 450, 450*t*
    pandemics, 232–233, 232*f*
Climate in Afghanistan, 67
Clostridium botulinum (botulism), 305–306, 311–312
Clostridium perfringens (epsilon toxin), 319–320
Cluster-based approach to disaster relief, 391, 395
Cluster sampling, 191–192
CO. *See* Carbon monoxide (CO) poisoning
Coast Guard, U.S., 18
Coca-Cola, 92–93
Code of conduct, NGOs, 111–112, 113*t*
Code of Federal Regulations, 39
Cohort studies, 154*t*, 155
Cold-related illnesses, 433–436, 436*t*
Cold storms. *See* Temperature extremes, emergencies
Cold War (US-USSR), 313
Collaborations. *See also* Public-private partnerships (PPPs)
    with pediatric professionals, 517, 519
    with substance abuse programs, 536–538
Commission on Extreme Weather Conditions (Chicago), 439
Common good, 36
Common law, 34
Communicable disease cluster program, 70
Communicable Disease Control in Emergencies (WHO), 175
Communications
    during contagious diseases epidemics, 220–222
    electronic reporting, 23–24, 137–138

Hurricane Katrina and, 145–146
information technology and, 134–135
public-private partnerships and, 92
during radiological agent events, 369–372
risk communication strategy, 25, 341,
    413–414
sharing of among actors/agencies, 9, 56–57,
    57f, 59f, 60
technological improvements in, 179–180
telecommunications, 134
telemedicine, 243
World Trade Center and, 9
Community-based organizations, 106
Community Emergency Response Team
    (CERT), 293, 386
Community preparedness for earthquakes,
    386–387
Complex humanitarian emergency (CHE),
    83–84, 87, 96, 97, 118–121
Comprehensive health center (CHC),
    Afghanistan, 70, 74
Concept plans (CONPLANs), 289
Conference on Environment and Development
    (UN 1992), 106
Confined-space bombings, 295–296
Conflict
    post-conflict/disaster, 70–78
    war and, 118–121
Congo, Democratic Republic of, 120, 173
CONPLANs (concept plans), 289
Consequence management, 24–25
Constitution, U.S., 36–38, 40–41
Contagious disease epidemics, 201–226
    agency preparedness, 213
    bacterial meningitis, 217–219
    case study, 203–204, 223
    communications during outbreak, 220–222
    fever patterns and febrile illnesses, 204–205,
        205–206t
    global preparedness, 207–209, 208t, 210f
    historical perspectives, 203–207
    hospital surge capacity, 203–204
    immigration-related illnesses, 205–206
    measles, 202–203, 215–217, 223
    mitigation, 220–223
    notifiable infectious conditions, 211,
        211–212t
    overview, 201–203
    preparedness, 207–213
    response, 213–220

surveillance systems (U.S.), 209–212,
        211–212t
    travel-related illnesses, 203–204, 204t
    tuberculosis, 75–76, 214–215
    under-immunization, 220–223
    viral hepatitis A, 219–220
Cooling mechanisms, 431–432
Corporate social responsibility, 90
Corporation for National and Community
    Service, 116
Country Reports on Terrorism (Department of
    State, 2008), 288
Coxiella burnetii (Q fever), 322–323
Crisis counseling, 499–500
Critical incident stress debriefing (CISD), 500
Critical incident stress management (CISM),
    500
Critical infrastructure and key resources
    (CIKR), 50
Cross-sectional surveys, 153–154, 154t
Cryptosporidium parvum (water contaminant),
    324
Cultural adaptation in mental health emergen-
    cies, 505–506
Culture in Afghanistan, 67
Cumulative sum score (CUSUM), 170
Cyanide, 345–346
Cyclone Bhola (1970), 407
Cyclone Nina (1975), 407
Cyclones. *See* Hurricanes, tsunamis, and
    cyclones
Cyclone Tracy (1974), 407

D
DALY (disability adjusted life-years), 155–156
Darfur, Sudan, 87, 96
Databases, 139–140
Data management, 72–74
Death rate statistics, earthquake, 393, 393–394t
Debriefing, psychological, 499–500
Decentralized approach to state responses, 20
Decontamination
    hazardous materials, 460–462, 461–462t
    procedures, 340, 351, 462–464
    radiological agents, 366–367
Defense Department, U.S., 481
Democratic Republic of Congo, 120, 173
Department of ___. *See specific name of
    department*
Dermal, 348

Deutsche Post World Net, 98
Development Programme (UN), 92
DEWS (Disease Early Warning System, Afghanistan), 70–71
DHHS. *See* Health and Human Services Department, U.S.
DHS. *See* Homeland Security Department, U.S.
Diagnostic and Statistical Manual (DSM-IV-TR), 493, *533*
Diagnostic technology, 143–144
Diagnostic testing, 268
Differential diagnosis of pandemic influenza, 229–231, 231*t*
Direct antigen tests, 144
Directional information systems, 140–141
Dirty bombs, 360–361
Disability adjusted life-years (DALY), 155–156
Disaster Medical Assistance Teams (DMATs), 16, 269, 414
Disaster Psychiatry Outreach, 501
Disaster Resource Network (DRN), 93
Disasters. *See also specific types of disasters*
    declared, 3, 3*f*
    NGOs and, 116–118
    rise in number of, 110–111, 110*f*
Disease Early Warning System, Afghanistan (DEWS), 70–71
Diseases
    chronic, exacerbation of, 525
    contagious. *See* Contagious disease epidemics
    infectious. *See* Emerging/re-emerging infectious diseases
    prevention, 524, 528–529
    profile in surveillance system, 177
Disease surveillance systems, 262
Distributed IT architecture, 139
DMATs (Disaster Medical Assistance Teams), 16, 269, 414
Domestic disasters, 116
DRN (Disaster Resource Network), 93
DSM-IV-TR (Diagnostic and Statistical Manual), 493, *533*

E

Early Aberration Reporting System (EARS), 170
Earth Observing System (EOS), 272
Earthquake Preparedness Handbook (Los Angeles Fire Department), 386

Earthquake Reconstruction and Rehabilitation Authority, Kashmir (ERRA), 392
Earthquakes, 379–402. *See also specific earthquakes*
    case study, 380–382, 394–396
    characteristics of, 383
    community preparedness, 386–387
    death rate statistics, 393, 393–394*t*
    historical perspectives, 382–384
    humanitarian response, 382, 390–391, 396
    incident command and coordination, 387–388
    individual preparedness, 385–386
    medical response, 381–382, 388–390, 395–396
    mitigation, 392–394, 393–394*t*
    overview, 379–382
    phases, strategies in, 396, 397–398*t*
    planning, 384–387
    predictions of, 384–385
    preparedness, 384–387
    recovery from, 391–392
    response to, 387–392
    secondary disasters, 383–384
    sociopolitical context, 392
Ebola virus, 317–318, 317*t*
ECDC (European Centre for Disease Prevention and Control), 179
Economically fragile settings, 86
Economy in Afghanistan, 66
Education in Afghanistan, 66, 68–69, 77–78
Efficiency in disaster response, 89
Electronic laboratory reporting (ELR), 137–138
Electronic reporting, 23–24, 137–138
Electronic Surveillance System for the Early Notification of Community-Based Epidemics (ESSENCE), 136
ELR (Electronic laboratory reporting), 137–138
El Salvador war, 120
EMAC (Emergency Management Assistance Compact), 59
Embassy terrorist bombings, (United States, 1998), 298, 299*f*
Emergencies
    complex humanitarian, 83–84, 87, 96, 97, 118–121
    epidemiology in public health, 156–161, 156–157*t*, 159–161*t*
    public health security and, 3–10, 7*f*
Emergency departments

hazardous materials, 458, 458*t*
infectious disease, 266–268, 272–275
Emergency hospitalization, mental health,
    502–503
EMERGency IDNET (surveillance network),
    271
Emergency information systems, 132
Emergency management, defined, 132
Emergency Management Assistance Compact
    (EMAC), 59
Emergency Management Guide for Business &
    Industry (FEMA), 454
Emergency Medical Treatment and Active
    Labor Act of 1986 (EMTALA), 38
Emergency operation centers (EOCs), 56, 58
Emergency operations plan, 454, 455*t*
Emergency Research and Development
    Administration, 477
Emergency response plans
    advance response planning, 22
    hospital response plans, 259, 260–261*t*,
        266–268, 272–275
    nuclear energy reactors, 478–479
Emergency Support Function (ESF), 291,
    291*t*, 497
    Annexes, 47–49, 48*f*, 117, 481
Emergent evaluation, mental health, 502–503
Emerging public health systems, 63–82
    cast study, 63–64, 64*t*
    challenges for development of, 67–69
    economic issues, 66
    education issues, 66, 68–69, 77–78
    geographic, climate, and culture issues, 67
    governance issues, 66–67, 69
    historical perspectives, 64–65
    infrastructure issues, 65–66, 68
    Kashmir earthquake and, 394–396
    obstacles to development of, 65–67
    overview, 63–64
    post-conflict/disaster systems development,
        70–78
    security issues, 65
    services and interventions, 74–77, 88
    statistics and data management, 72–74
    surveillance system, 70–72
Emerging/re-emerging infectious diseases,
    251–282
    background, 253
    case study, 251–252, 273–275
    defined, 253

diagnostic testing, 268
disease surveillance systems, 262
historical perspectives, 253–257
Hospital Emergency Incident Command
    System, 259, 296
hospital response plans, 259, 260–261*t*,
    272–275
hospital response to, 266–268
inciting factors, 253–254
laboratory capabilities, 259–262
mitigation, 269–273
outbreak containment, 266, 267*t*, 269
outbreak detection, 265–266
outbreak identification, 254–257, 256–257*t*
outbreak reporting, 271–273
overview, 251–252
preparedness, 258–265
response, 265–269
surge capacity, 258–259
syndromic surveillance, 262–264
Emitted radiation, 476, 476*t*
Emotional needs of children, 528
EMTALA (Emergency Medical Treatment and
    Active Labor Act of 1986), 38
Energy Department, U.S., 18, 51, 477, 481
Energy Policy Act (2005), 484
Energy Reorganization Act (1974), 477
England, London (underground bombing,
    2005), 288
Enumerated powers, 37–38, 40
Environmental Protection Agency (EPA)
    air and water quality, 13, 14
    drinking water standards, 324
    Heat Island Reduction Initiative, 438–439
    nuclear incidents and, 481
    public response role, 18
    radiation exposure limits, 374
EOCs (emergency operation centers), 56, 58
EOS (Earth Observing System), 272
EPHS (Essential Package of Hospital Services,
    Afghanistan), 72, 74
EPI (Expanded Programme on Immunization),
    186, 191–192
Epidemic, definition of, 172
Epidemic Intelligence Exchange (Epi-X), 16
Epidemiological studies, 153–166
    action vs. research, 164–165
    case-control studies, 154*t*, 155
    case series studies, 153, 154*t*
    challenges of, 161–164, 163*t*

Epidemiological studies (*cont.*)
  cohort studies, 154*t*, 155
  cross-sectional surveys, 153–154, 154*t*
  defined, 153
  ethics of research, 164–165
  preparedness phase of emergencies, 157, 157*t*
  public health emergencies and, 156–161, 156*t*
  rehabilitation phase of emergencies, 159–161, 161*t*
  response phase of emergencies, 158–159, 160*t*
  retrospective studies, 154–155
  role of, 153–156, 154*t*
Epidemiology
  in public health emergencies, 156–161, 156–157*t*, 159–161*t*
  substance use, 533–534
  temperature extreme emergencies, 428–436, 429*f*
Epi-X (Epidemic Intelligence Exchange), 16
Epsilon toxin, 319–320
Equipment for children in public health emergencies, 521–522, 527
ERRA (Earthquake Reconstruction and Rehabilitation Authority), Kashmir, 392
ESF. *See* Emergency Support Function
ESSENCE (Electronic Surveillance System for the Early Notification of Community-Based Epidemics), 136
Essential Package of Hospital Services, Afghanistan (EPHS), 72, 74
Ethics of research, 164–165
Europe (heat wave, 2003), 439
European Centre for Disease Prevention and Control (ECDC), 179
Eurosurveillance (ECDC journal), 179
Evacuation
  centers, 168–172, 171f, 172
  of children, 517–518, 525–529
  of hospitals, 416–417
  nuclear incidents and, 481
  radiological agents and, 366–367
Expanded Programme on Immunization (EPI), 186, 191–192
Expatriate staffing, 122–123
Exposure
  chemical/biological, 327, 522–523
  radiation, 367, 369, 374, 476, 479–480

F

Faith-based organizations (FBOs), 418–419
Family planning, 114

FBI (Federal Bureau of Investigation), 18
Federal agencies, roles of, 18–20, 19*t*, 25, 26*t*.
  See also specific agencies
Federal Drug Administration (FDA), 13, 18, 320, 346, 522
Federal Emergency Management Agency (FEMA)
  American Red Cross and, 111
  Community Emergency Response Team course, 293
  Department of Homeland Security and, 325
  disaster preparedness cycle, 289, 290*f*
  hazardous materials incident planning, 454–455
  Hurricane Pam exercise, 193
  National Earthquake Hazards Reduction Program, 386
  nuclear energy reactors oversight, 478
  Nuclear Regulatory Commission, 477
  public-private relationships and, 86
  state's request for assistance from, 20, 59
Federal preparedness and response, 15–20
  capacity building, 17–18
  direct services, 18
  finance capability, 15
  information gathering and dissemination, 17
  policy issues, 15
  public health protection, 15–17
  radiological incident responsibilities, 362–363, 362*t*
  roles of federal agencies, 18–20, 19*t*
Federal register, 39
Federal Relief Commission, Pakistan (FRC), 394
Federal Response Plan (FRP), 46–49, 47*f*
FEMA. *See* Federal Emergency Management Agency
Fermi, Enrico, 475
Fever patterns and febrile illnesses, 204–205, 205*t*, 206*t*, 316–318, 317*t*, 322
Fever zones, 241
Financing of public health initiatives, 15, 20
Flu. *See* Pandemic influenza
Foodborne Diseases Active Surveillance System (FoodNet), 212
Foodborne Outbreak Reporting System, 212
FoodNet, 212
Food safety threats, 212, 309, 320–321. *See also* Biological agents
For-profit public-private partnerships, 91–92
Fourth Amendment, 40–41
Francisella tularensis (tularemia), 315–316

FRC (Federal Relief Commission, Pakistan), 394
Fritz Institute, 93
FRP (Federal Response Plan), 46–49, 47*f*
Fuller's Earth, 344

G

GABA receptors, 349
Gamma-rays, 359–360
GAO (Government Accountability Office), 9
GAR (Global Alert and Response) program, 175, 179, 207, 208*t*
GEIS (Global Emerging Infectious Surveillance), 272
Geneva Conference (1923-1925), 350
Geneva Protocol, 350
Geocoding, 144, 146
Geographical information systems (GIS), 140–141, 158
Geography in Afghanistan, 67
Geological Society of America, 146
Geologic Survey (U.S.), 386
GeoSentinel, 178, 272
Glanders, 321
GlaxoSmithKline, 86
Global Alert and Response (GAR) program, 175, 179, 207, 208*t*
Global Compact (UN), 85–86, 90–91, 91*t*, 98
Global Emerging Infectious Surveillance (GEIS), 272
Global Gag Rule, family planning and NGOs, 114
Globalization, 4, 4*f*, 105
Global Outbreak Alert and Response Network (GOARN), 209, 272
Global positioning systems (GPS), 140, 144
Global preparedness for contagious diseases epidemics, 207–209, 208*t*, 210*f*
Global Public Health Intelligence Network (GPHIN), 179, 209, 272
Goiania, Brazil (radiological accident, 1987), 373–374
Goma, Zaire disease outbreak (1994), 173
Google, 180
Governance in Afghanistan, 66–67, 69
Government
    laws and regulations, 5–6, 15. *See also* Public health law
    public-private relationships, 86–87, 91–92, 96–97, 98
    radiological agents and, 362–363, 362*t*

Government Accountability Office (GAO), 9
Government agencies role in bombing events
    mitigation, 298, 299*f*
    Oklahoma City bombing, 300
    preparedness for, 290–292, 292*f*
    response to, 294–295, 294*f*
Government capacity, 13–30
    advance response planning, 22
    capacity building, 17–18
    case study, 14
    consequence management, 24–25
    direct services, 18
    federal agencies, roles of, 18–20, 19*t*
    federal preparedness and response, 15–20
    financing of public health initiatives, 15, 20
    hazard analysis, 21, 457*t*, 458
    information gathering and dissemination, 17
    laboratory analysis, 24
    local preparedness and response, 21–25
    mitigation, 25–27, 26*t*
    overview, 13
    policy basis for public health, 15
    public health protection, 15–17
    state preparedness and response, 20–21
    surveillance, 22–24
Government oversight of nuclear energy reactors, 478
GPHIN (Global Public Health Intelligence Network), 179, 209, 272
GPS (global positioning systems), 140, 144
Grassroots organizations, 106
Guide for All-Hazard Emergency Operations Planning (FEMA), 454
Gujarat, India (earthquake, 2001), 93

H

Haicheng, China (earthquake, 1975), 383, 385
Haiti (earthquake, 2010)
    disease profile in surveillance system, 178
    information technology and, 131, 133, 143
    NGO response to, 108–110, 115
Hancock County Emergency Operations Centers (Mississippi), 415
Handbook of Chemical Hazard Analysis Procedures (FEMA/DOT/EPA), 454
Hantavirus, 325
Hazard, defined, 4
Hazard analysis, 21, 457*t*, 458
Hazard Analysis and Critical Control Point (HACCP), 320

Hazard identification, 298
Hazardous materials, 447–472
    case study, 449, 469–470, 470*t*
    classification system, 450, 450*t*
    decontamination, on-scene, 460–462,
        461–462*t*
    decontamination process, 462–464
    definitions of, 447, 448*t*, 449
    emergency operations plan, 454, 455*t*
    historical perspectives, 450–454, 450*t*
    identification of, 465, 466*t*
    incidents and substances events, 451, 452*t*
    information, access and retrieval of, 459
    material safety data sheets, 459–460
    mitigation, 467–469, 468–469*t*
    overview, 447–449
    personal protection equipment, 462, 463*t*
    planning process, 454–456
    pre-notification, 459
    preparedness, 454–458, 455*t*, 457*t*
    response, 458–467, 458*t*
    sources of, 447, 447*t*
    state and local preparedness, 457*t*, 458
    training and, 456–458, 468–469*t*
    transportation of, 451–454, 453*t*
    treatment and toxidromes, 465–467
    triage, 464–465
"Hazardous Materials and Terrorist Incident
        Response Planning Curriculum
        Guidelines" (FEMA), 455
Hazardous Materials Emergency Planning Guide
        (National Response Team), 454
Hazardous Substances Emergency Events
        Surveillance (HSEES), 451, 452*t*
Health Alert Network (HAN), 16
Health and Human Services Department, U.S.
        (DHHS)
    Agency for Toxic Substances and Disease
        Registry, 340, 451
    epidemics and infectious disease control, 269
    food safety threats, 320
    funding for, 15
    Office of the Assistant Secretary for
        Preparedness and Response, 325
    pandemic influenza strategic plan, 238–240,
        238–239*t*
    radiological incident, role in, 363
Health as a Bridge for Peace (HBP), 119–120
Health care and bombing events
    mitigation for, 298–300
    Oklahoma city bombing, 301

preparedness for, 292–293
    response to, 295–297
Healthcare institutions and biological agents, 261
Healthcare workers, 252, 266, 274–275, 327
Health information exchange (HIE), 138
Health Information Technology for Economic
        and Clinical Health (HITECH) Act
        (2009), 144
Health information technology (HIT) infra-
        structure, 23
Health Management Information System,
        Afghanistan (HMIS), 73
Health Map organization, 180
Health Protection Agency (United Kingdom),
        179
Health Resources Services Administration's
        National Hospital Bioterrorism
        Preparedness Program, 20
Heat index, 426, 429, 429*f*
Heating mechanisms, 431–432, 432*t*
Heat Island Reduction Initiative, 438–439
Heat-related illnesses, 432–433, 434*t*
Heat wave emergency (1995), 426–428, 427*f*,
        439–440. *See also* Temperature extremes,
        emergencies
Henry Schein, Inc., 93
Hepatitis A, 219–220
High Commissioner for Refugees (UN), 87,
        92, 95
High efficiency particulate air filtration, 266
Hillsborough football stadium disaster (United
        Kingdom, 1989), 506
HITECH (Health Information Technology for
        Economic and Clinical Health) Act of
        2009, 144
HIT (health information technology) infra-
        structure, 23
HIV/AIDS programs, 76, 86
HMIS (Health Management Information
        System, Afghanistan), 73
Homeland Security Act (2002), 49
Homeland Security Bill (2003), 337
Homeland Security Department, U.S. (DHS)
    antidote stockpiling, 338
    biological attach response oversight, 18
    biosecurity programs oversight, 325
    National Incident Management System. *See*
        National Incident Management
        System (NIMS)
    National Response Framework document,
        45–46

Nuclear Regulatory Commission, 477
pandemic influenza preparedness, 236, 236*t*
radiological incident, role in, 363
role of, 18, 481
voluntary accreditation standards, 293
Homeland Security Operations Center
    (HSOC), 49
Homeland Security Presidential Directive 5
    (HSPD-5), 49
Homeland Security Presidential Directive 8
    (HSPD-8), 51
Home rule states, 40
H1N1 outbreak (2009), 144–145, 227–228
Hospital Emergency Incident Command
    System (HEICS), 259, 296
Hospital Infection Control Practices Advisory
    Committee (HICPAC), 266
Hospitalization, emergency for mental health
    patients, 502–503
Hospital Preparedness Program, 18
Hospital response plans, 259, 260–261*t*,
    266–268, 272–275
Hospitals, evacuation of, 416–417
Hospital surge capacity, 203–204
Houston, Reliant Center/Astrodome, 518,
    525–529
HSEES (Hazardous Substances Emergency
    Events Surveillance), 451, 452*t*
Humanitarian issues with public-private part-
    nerships, 96–97
Humanitarian organizations coalition (United
    States), 89
Humanitarian reform proposal (UN), 89
Humanitarian response to earthquakes, 382,
    390–391, 396
Hurricane, Labor Day (1935), 405
Hurricane Andrew (1992), 46, 405
Hurricane Camille (1969), 405, 412
Hurricane Charley (2004), 405
Hurricane Dennis (2005), 405
Hurricane Floyd (1999), 523
Hurricane Frances (2004), 405
Hurricane Hugo (1989), 411
Hurricane Ike (2005), 50
Hurricane Ivan (2004), 405
Hurricane Jeanne (2004), 405
Hurricane Katrina (2005)
    children impacted by, 517–518, 525–529
    communications, 145–146
    evacuation centers, 168–172, 169–171*t*
    evacuation of hospitals, 416–417

faith-based organizations and, 418–419
federal and state agency coordination, 86
impact of and NGO involvement, 104–105,
    124–127, 126*t*
logistical planning and coordination, 9
long-term recovery, 115–116
National Response Plan implementation, 50
overview, 420
rapid needs assessments and, 186–187, 195–196
socioeconomically disadvantaged
    population, 419
storm statistics, 404
substance abuse and, 531–532
surveillance in Mississippi counties, 415
technology and, 132–133, 145–146
Hurricane Mitch (1998), 123
Hurricane Pam exercise (FEMA), 193
Hurricane Rita (2005)
    children impacted by, 526, 531–532
    rapid needs assessments and, 195
    storm statistics, 405, 407
    substance abuse and, 531–532
Hurricanes, tsunamis, and cyclones, 403–424
    case study, 420, 464
    category characteristics, 405, 406*t*
    cyclones, 407–408
    historical perspectives, 404–410
    mitigation, 418–420
    morbidity and mortality by continent,
        407, 408*t*
    preparedness and planning, 410–415
    response, 415–418
    tsunamis, 408–410
Hurricane Wilma (2005), 405
Hydrogen sulfide, 345, 347
Hydroxocobalamin, 346

I

IAEA (International Atomic Energy Agency), 372
IBM's Worldwide Crisis Response Team, 88,
    92, 98
ICD-9 (*International Classification of Disease,*
    version 9), 263
ICRC. *See* International Committee for the
    Red Cross
ICS. *See* Incident Command System
ICT (information and communication tech-
    nology), 134–135
IDSA EIN (Infectious Diseases Society of
    America Epidemic Intelligence
    Network), 272

IFA (immunofluorescence assays), 143
IGOs (intergovernmental organizations), 103
IHR. *See* International Health Regulations
IIMG (Interagency Incident Management Group), 49
IMC (International Medical Corp), 108, 120–121
Immigration-related illnesses, 205–206
Immunizations. *See* Vaccinations
Immunofluorescence assays (IFA), 143
Implementing Recommendations of the 9/11 Commission Act (2007), 293
Improvised nuclear device (IND), 360–361
IMSS (Instituto Mexicano del Seguro Social), 227
Incentives for private-sector engagement, 89–90
Incident Annexes, 47, 49, 481
Incident command and coordination for earthquakes, 387–388
Incident Command System (ICS), 116, 259, 294–295, 294*f*, 497
Inciting factors in infectious diseases, 253–254
IND (improvised nuclear device), 360–361
India, Gujarat (earthquake, 2001), 93
Indiana, Michigan City (hazardous materials incident), 449, 469–470, 470*t*
Individual preparedness for earthquakes, 385–386
Infectious diseases. *See* Emerging/re-emerging infectious diseases
Infectious Diseases Society of America Epidemic Intelligence Network (IDSA EIN), 272
Influenza. *See* Pandemic influenza
Information and communication technology (ICT), 134–135
Information retrieval (IR) systems, 132, 140–141
Information sharing
   geographical information systems, 140–141
   government capacity and, 17
   hazardous materials, 459
   health information exchange, 138
   importance of, 9
   information retrieval systems, 140
   National Response Plan, 56–60, 57–59*f*
Information technology (IT)
   application factors, 138–139
   defined, 131

infrastructure, 23–24
   used in Haiti, 2010 earthquake, 131, 133, 143
Infrastructure
   Afghanistan situation, 65–66, 68
   government laws and regulations regarding, 5–6
   information technology, 23–24
   vulnerability assessments of, 50
Infrastructure management, 159
Infrastructure resilience, 298, 299*f*
INGOs (International NGOs), 103, 105
Initial Rapid Assessment (IRA) form, 190–191
Injuries
   acute kidney injury, 390
   blast injuries, 297
   to children in public health emergencies, 523
   traumatic brain injury, 523
Insecticides, 349
Institute of Epidemiological Diagnosis and Reference (Mexico), 246
Institute of Medicine, 23, 253
Instituto Mexicano del Seguro Social (IMSS), 227
InterAction, 112, 115
Interaction (U.S. humanitarian organizations coalition), 89
Interagency Incident Management Group (IIMG), 49
Intergovernmental organization (IGO), 103
International Atomic Energy Agency (IAEA), 372
International Classification of Disease, version 9 (ICD-9), 263
International Committee for the Red Cross (ICRC), 105, 106, 112, 113, 118–119, 121
International Emerging Infections Program of the CDC, 272–273
International Federation of Red Cross and Red Crescent Societies, 112
International Health Regulations (IHR), 6, 175, 207–209, 270
International Medical Corp (IMC), 108, 120–121
International NGOs (INGOs), 103, 105
International Physicians for the Prevention of Nuclear War, 120
International Red Cross and Red Crescent (IRC), 108
International Rescue Committee (IRC), 126
International Society for Disease Surveillance (ISDS), 135
International Society of Infectious Diseases, 272

Interventions in mental health emergencies, 498–504
Intrepid (surveillance network), 272
Iodine for radiation treatment, 479, 480, 481
IRA (Initial Rapid Assessment) form, 190–191
IRC (International Red Cross and Red Crescent), 108
IRC (International Rescue Committee), 126
Irritant gas syndromes, 341–342, 342*t*
IR (information retrieval) systems, 132, 140–141
ISDS (International Society for Disease Surveillance), 135
Isolation procedures, 266–267, 274–275, 529
IT. *See* Information technology
Italian Red Cross, 118
Izmit, Turkey (earthquake, 1999), 391

J
Jacobson, Henning, 41
Jacobson v. Massachusetts, 41
Japan, Kobe (earthquake, 1995), 390
Japan, Tokyo (subway attack, 1995), 335–336, 350–351
Johns Hopkins School of Public Health, 309
Joint Field Office (JFO), 49, 60
JumpSTART, 519, 520*f*
Justice Department, U.S., 18

K
Kabul Medical University, 68–69
Kashmir earthquake (2005)
    acute kidney injury during, 390
    authoritarian influences during, 392
    cluster-based approach to disaster relief, 391, 395
    Earthquake Reconstruction and Rehabilitation Authority, 392
    government response plan, 387, 394
    overview of, 380–382
Keating, Frank, 286
Kemeny Commission of the Accident at Three Mile Island, 484–485
Kenya revolt (1952), 307
Kobe, Japan, earthquake (1995), 390
Kosovar Refugee Registration Project, 92

L
Laboratory analysis, 24
Laboratory capabilities, 259–262

Laboratory chain of custody, 268
Laboratory reporting, electronic, 137–138
Laboratory Response Network (LRN), 261–262
LAN (local area network), 141
Lashkar-e-Taiba, 395
Lassa fever, 317*t*, 318
Laws and regulations, 5–6, 15. *See also* Public health law
Leadership skills development, 17–18
Legionella species (Q fever), 322–323
Legislative body, limitations on power of, 40–41
Licensing boards, 36
Lisbon, Portugal (earthquake, 1755), 383
Local area network (LAN), 141
Local emergency mitigation, 193–194
Localization information systems, 140–141
Local preparedness and response, 21–25
    advance response planning, 22
    consequence management, 24–25
    hazard analysis, 21, 457*t*, 458
    laboratory analysis, 24
    radiological incident responsibilities, 362–363, 362*t*
    role of, 25, 26*t*
    surveillance, 22–24
Logistic Centre (UN), 93
Logistics and supply chain management, 93
Loma Prieta, California (earthquake, 1989), 131, 385
London (underground bombing, 2005), 288
Long-term planning, 97–98
Long-term recovery, 115–116
Long-term solutions, public-private partnerships, 97–98
Los Angeles Fire Department, 386
Louisiana Department of Health and Hospitals, 168–172
Louisiana Emergency Assistance and Disaster Act (1993), 193
Louisiana Office of Homeland Security and Emergency Preparedness (LOHSEP), 193
Louisiana Red Cross, 168–172
LRN (Laboratory Response Network), 261–262

M
Madrid, Spain (subway bombings, 2004), 288, 299
MAN (metro area network), 141
Management Sciences for Health, Afghanistan (MSH), 75

Mandates for emergency intervention, 88
Marburg virus, 317–318, 317*t*
MARK I antidote kit, 341, 349
Martyrs and Disabled ministry (Afghanistan), 68
Mass-casualty incident (MCI), 518–521
Material safety data sheets (MSDS), 459–460
Mau Mau tribe (Kenya), 307
Mayflower Compact, 34
MCI (mass-casualty incident), 518–521
McVeigh, Timothy, 285
Measles, 202–203, 215–217, 223
Medecins sans Frontieres (MSF), 106, 113, 120–121
Media sources for surveillance data collection, 158
Medicaid, 38
Medical Action Network, 93
Medical records, 146, 413
Medical Reserve Corps, 517
Medical response
    during earthquakes, 381–382, 388–390, 395–396
    to radiation exposure, 479–480
Medical supplies for disasters, 17, 25
Medicare, 38
Medication. *See also* Strategic national stockpile (SNS)
    pediatric medications, 522
    radiological exposure, countermeasures for, 367, 369
    for substance abuse, 535*n*1
Melioidosis, 321–322
Meningitis, bacterial, 217–219
Mental Health and Mass Violence (NIH publication), 499
Mental health emergencies, 493–516
    biomedical interventions, 501–503
    case study, 494, 506–508
    crisis counseling, 499–500
    cultural adaptations, 505–506
    framework, 494–497, 495*f*
    interventions, 498–504
    mitigation, 504–506
    overview, 493–494
    preparedness and planning, 497–498, 498*t*
    psychological first aid, 499
    psychological interventions, 499–500
    resilience and, 505
    risk factor, 505
    social interventions, 503–504
    trauma/traumatic event, defined, 493

Mental health system
    Afghanistan, 71, 418
    capacity building for, 418
    post-traumatic stress disorder, 391
Mentioning programs in Afghanistan, 77–78
Mercalli scale, 383
Merck & Co., 85, 86
MERS (Mobile Emergency Response System), 145
Metabolic poisoning syndromes, 344–347, 345*t*
Meta-initiatives, 93
Methadone maintenance treatment (MMT), 535
Metro area network (MAN), 141
Mexican Institute for Social Security, 227, 245
Mexico City Policy, family planning and NGOs, 114
Michigan City, Indiana, hazardous materials incident, 449, 469–470, 470*t*
Microbial Threats to Health: Emergence, Detection and Response (Institute of Medicine), 253
Microsoft, 92, 95
Midwest heat wave (1995), 426–428, 439–440
Military biological warfare program (United States), 307
Millennium Development Goals (UN), 121
Milwaukee heat wave (1995), 426–428, 439–440
Minimum Standards in Disaster Response (Sphere Project), 112
Ministry of Agriculture, Afghanistan (MoA), 75
Ministry of Higher Education, Afghanistan (MoHE), 68
Ministry of Public Health, Afghanistan (MoPH), 67–68
Ministry of Water Resources, China, 92
Mississippi
    evacuation centers, 171*f*, 172
    surveillance after Hurricane Katrina, 415
Mississippi Department of Health (MDH), 172
Mitigation strategies
    biological agents, 325–327
    bombing events, 298–300, 299*f*
    chemical agents, 350
    contagious diseases epidemics, 220–223
    earthquakes, 392–394, 393–394*t*
    government capacity and, 25–27, 26*t*
    hazardous materials, 467–469, 468–469*t*
    hurricanes, tsunamis, and cyclones, 418–420
    infectious diseases, 269–273
    mental health emergencies, 504–506
    NGOs' response to crises and, 123–124

nuclear energy reactors, 484–485
pandemic influenza, 243–245
public-private partnerships, 93–98, 299–300
radiological agents, 372–373
rapid needs assessments, 193–195
substance abuse population, 539–541, 541*t*
technological resources for, 144–145, 298,
      299–300
temperature extreme emergencies, 438–439
MMT (methadone maintenance treatment), 535
MoA (Ministry of Agriculture, Afghanistan), 75
Mobile Emergency Response System (MERS),
      145
Model State Emergency Health Powers Act, 15
MoHE (Ministry of Higher Education,
      Afghanistan), 68
MoPH (Ministry of Public Health,
      Afghanistan), 67–68
Morbidity and Mortality Weekly Report (CDC), 179
Mortuary response teams, 16–17
Motorola Company, 90
MSDS (material safety data sheets), 459–460
MSF (Medecins sans Frontieres), 106, 113,
      120–121
MSH (Management Sciences for Health,
      Afghanistan), 75
Multisector/multijurisdictional capabilities, 8–9
Muscarinic receptors, 347–348
Mustard gas, 337, 342–344
Mutual aid agreements, 58–59, 58*f*
Myanmar, private humanitarian efforts in, 96–97

N

NAMRU-3 (U.S. Naval Medical Research
      Unit), 75
Narcotics Anonymous, 535, 538
NASA's Earth Observing System (EOS), 272
National Center for Missing and Exploited
      Children, 526
National Center for PTSD, 499
National Child Traumatic Stress Network, 499
National Commission on Terrorist Attacks
      Upon the United States (9-11
      Commission), 293, 325
National Counterterrorism Center (NCTC), 57
National Disaster Medical System (NDMS), 269
National Earthquake Hazards Reduction
      Program (NEHRP), 386
National Electronic Disease Surveillance
      System (NEDSS), 16, 179
National Flood Insurance Program (NFIP), 49

National Governors Association, 17
National Guard, 59
National Hurricane Center, 132
National Incident Management System
      (NIMS), 49, 115, 116, 259, 386–387
National Infrastructure Protection Plan
      (NIPP), 50, 51*f*
National Institute for Health (NIH), 499
National Institute for Occupational Safety and
      Health (NIOSH), 309, 326*t*, 327
National Institute of Standards and
      Technology, 386
National Military Command Center
      (NMCC), 57
National Military Strategy to Combat WMD,
      325
National Molecular Subtyping Network for
      Foodborne Disease Surveillance
      (PulseNet), 212–213
National NGOs, 105
National Notifiable Disease Surveillance
      System, 211, 211–212*t*
National Nuclear Security Administration, 372
National Operations Center (NOC), 56
National planning scenarios, 53
National Red Cross organizations, 88
National Response Coordination Center
      (NRCC), 49
National Response Framework (NRF), 45–46,
      116–117, 497
National response guidelines (NRG), 51–56,
      52*f*, 54*f*, 55*f*
National Response Plan (NRP), 45–62
      case study, 46
      Federal Response Plan, 46–49, 47*f*
      historical perspectives, 46–50
      information sharing, 56–60, 57–59*f*
      national preparedness guidelines, 51–56, 52*f*,
            54*f*, 55*f*
      overview, 45–46
      preparedness, 50–56, 52*f*
      response, 56–60
      situational awareness, 56–60, 57–59*f*
      support functions and annexes, 48, 48*f*
National Response Team, 454
National Science Foundation, 386
National Strategy for Homeland Security, 325
National Strategy for Reconstruction (Afghan
      policy document), 70
National Strategy to Combat Weapons of Mass
      Destruction, 325

National Survey of Substance Abuse Treatment Services (N-SSATS), 534
National Survey on Drug Use and Health (NSDUH), 532, 533
National Weather Service, 132
NATO (North Atlantic Treaty Organization), 307, 309
Natural disasters. *See* Disasters; *specific types*
Naval Medical Research Unit (NAMRU-3), 75
NCTC (National Counterterrorism Center), 57
NDMS (National Disaster Medical System), 269
NEDSS (National Electronic Disease Surveillance System), 16, 179
NEHRP (National Earthquake Hazards Reduction Program), 386
Nerve gas, 337, 341
Neupogen, 369
New World arenaviruses, 318
New York City Medics, 93
NFIP (National Flood Insurance Program), 49
NGOs (nongovernmental organizations), defined, 88
Nicotinic receptors, 347–348
NIH (National Institute for Health), 499
NIMS. *See* National Incident Management System
    9-11 attacks. *See* September 11, 2001, terrorist attacks
    9-11 Commission, 293, 325
NIOSH (National Institute for Occupational Safety and Health), 309, 326*t*, 327
Nipah virus, 325
NIPP (National Infrastructure Protection Plan), 50, 51*f*
Nitrogen mustard, 342
NMCC (National Military Command Center), 57
N95 masks, 267, 275, 318
NOC (National Operations Center), 56
Noncommercial public-private partnerships, 91
Nongovernmental organizations' (NGOs) response to crises, 103–130
    during bombing events, 293, 297, 299–300, 301
    case study, 104–105, 124–127, 126*t*
    challenges facing, 121–123
    characteristics of, 108, 109*t*
    code of conduct, 111–112, 113*t*
    complex humanitarian emergencies and, 118–121

defined, 103
disasters and, 116–118
funding, 112–114
historical perspectives, 105–114
mitigation, 123–124
overview, 103–105, 106–111, 107*f*, 109–110*t*
preparedness, response, and recovery, 114–116
Non-pharmaceutical interventions (NPIs), 244–245
Normalization of routine for children in public health emergencies, 524, 528
North Atlantic Treaty Organization (NATO), 307, 309
Notifiable infectious conditions, 211, 211–212*t*
NPIs (Non-pharmaceutical interventions), 244–245
NRC. *See* Nuclear Regulatory Commission
NRCC (National Response Coordination Center), 49
NRF (National Response Framework), 45–46, 116–117, 497
NRG (national response guidelines), 51–56, 52*f*, 54*f*, 55*f*
NRP. *See* National Response Plan
NSDUH (National Survey on Drug Use and Health), 532, 533
N-SSATS (National Survey of Substance Abuse Treatment Services), 534
Nuclear energy reactors, 473–480
    case study, 474–475, 485–486
    emergency response plan, 478–479
    government oversight, 478
    historical perspectives, 475–478
    measurements, 476–477, 476*t*
    medical response preparedness, 479–480
    mitigation, 484–485
    overview, 473–475
    planning, 478–480
    plant security, 484–485
    power plants, 484
    preparedness, 478–480
    radiation assets and functions, 481, 482–483*t*
    radiation measurements, 476–477, 476*t*
    response, 480–483
    risk levels, 479
Nuclear incidence
    Chernobyl, 473, 475, 486
    Three Mile Island, 473–475, 485–486
Nuclear Radiological Incident Annex: National Response Plan, 481

Nuclear Regulatory Commission (NRC)
    coordinating agency for nuclear incidents, 481
    creation of, 477
    nuclear power plants and, 481
    oversight, 478
    radiological agents security, 372
    Three Mile Island incident, 474
Nunn-Lugar-Domenici Amendment (1997), 337
Nutritional surveillance, 174–175

O
Obninsk nuclear power plant (USSR), 476
Office of Coordination of Humanitarian Affairs
    (OCHA), 87, 391, 394–395
Office of Emergency Preparedness (OEP), 269
Office of Emergency Services (California), 386
Office of Inspector General, 22
Office of Public Health, 168
Office of Rural Recovery and Development
    (Afghanistan), 75
Office of the Assistant Secretary for
    Preparedness and Response (DHHS), 325
Oklahoma City (terrorist bombing, 1995),
    285–287, 300–301
Oleoresin capsicum (pepper spray), 341
Open-air bombings, 295–296
Operational NGOs, 103–104, 108
Operations plans (OPLANs), 289
Ordinances, 40
Organophosphate syndrome, 347–349, 347t
Ornithosis, 322
Outbreak containment, 266, 267t, 269
Outbreak control team (OCT), 136
Outbreak detection, 265–266
Outbreak identification, 254–257, 256–257t
Outbreak management, 136–137
Outbreak Management Program, 136, 137t
Outbreak reporting, 271–273
Outpatient follow-up, 503
Oxfam, 106, 113, 118, 120, 126

P
Pakistan-administered Kashmir (PAK). *See*
    Kashmir earthquake (2005)
Pandemic influenza, 227–250. *See also* Avian
    influenza
    background, 229–233, 230t
    business-sector preparedness for, 236, 236t
    case study, 227–228, 245–246
    clinical presentation of, 229–231, 231t

    consequences of, 237–238, 237t
    control measures, 240–242, 240t
    differential diagnosis of, 229–231, 231t
    high-risk groups for complications of, 235, 235t
    mitigation, 243–245
    non-pharmaceutical interventions, 244–245
    overview, 227–228
    phases of, 232–233, 232f
    preparedness, 233–238, 234–237t
    response, 238–242, 238–240t
    strategies plan for, 238–240, 238–239t
PAPR (powered air-purifying respirators),
    268, 318
Parrot fever, 322
Passive surveillance reporting, 23, 178
Patient-centered parameters of mental health
    framework, 496–497, 507–508
Patient-physician relationship, 32–33
PBI (primary blast injuries), 297
PDA (personal digital assistants), 141–143
Pediatric Triage Tape (PTT), 519
Pennsylvania (Three Mile Island nuclear inci-
    dent, 1979), 473–475, 485–486
PEPFAR (President's Emergency Plan for
    AIDS Relief), 86
Pepper spray, 341
Personal digital assistants (PDA), 141–143
Personal protective equipment (PPE)
    during chemical agents incidences, 339,
        339t, 351
    during hazardous materials incidences,
        462, 463t
    during infectious disease incidences, 268
    NIOSH recommendations, 326t, 327
    types of, 462, 463t
PFA (psychological first aid), 499
Pharmaceutical supplies for disasters, 17, 25
Pharmacological agents, 501–502
Phase-sensitive parameters of mental health
    framework, 495–496, 507
PHEP (Public Health Emergency
    Preparedness), 18–19
Phosgene, 341–342
Physicians for Human Rights, 120
Plague, 313–314, 313t
Planning process and strategies
    chemical agents, 337–338
    earthquakes, 384–387
    hazardous materials incidents, 454–456
    hurricanes, tsunamis, and cyclones, 410–415

Planning process and strategies (*cont.*)
  long-term, 97–98
  mental health emergencies, 497–498, 498*t*
  nuclear energy reactors, 478–480
  response planning, advance, 22
  substance abuse population, 534–538, 537*t*
Pneumonic plague, 313–314
Poisoning
  carbon monoxide. *See* Carbon monoxide
    (CO) poisoning
  metabolic syndromes, 344–347, 345*t*
Poisons. *See* Biological agents
Police power, 34–35
Policies, modernization of, 15
Politically fragile settings, 86
Population and Women program (UN), 85
Population-based parameters of mental health
    framework, 496, 507
Population monitoring, radiological agents,
    367–368
Portugal, Lisbon (earthquake, 1755), 383
Post-conflict/disaster public health systems
    development. *See* Emerging public health
    systems
Post-traumatic stress disorder (PTSD), 391,
    502, 506, 522. *See also* Mental health
    emergencies
Powered air-purifying respirators (PAPR), 268, 318
Power plants. *See* Nuclear energy reactors
PPE. *See* Personal protective equipment
PPP. *See* Public-private partnerships
Pralidoxime (2PAM), 349
Predictions of earthquakes, 384–385
Preparedness issues, children and public health
    emergencies, 518–522, 525–527
Preparedness phase in epidemiological study,
    157, 157*t*
Preparedness strategies
  biological agents, category A, 309–318, 310*t*,
    313*t*
  biological agents, category B, 318–325
  biological agents, category C, 324–325
  Bioterrorism Preparedness Program, 20
  bombing events, 289–293, 290*f*
  capability-based, 52–53, 52*f*
  chemical agents, 337–338
  children and public health emergencies,
    518–522, 525–527
  contagious diseases epidemics, 207–213,
    208*t*, 210*f*
  disaster preparedness cycle, 289, 290*f*

  earthquakes, 384–387
  federal government capacity, 15–20
  hazardous materials, 454–458, 455*t*, 457*t*
  hurricanes, tsunamis, and cyclones, 410–415
  infectious diseases, emerging and re-
    emerging, 258–265
  local government capacity, 21–25
  mental health emergencies, 497–498, 498*t*
  National Response Plan, 50–56, 52*f*
  NGO response to crises, 114–123
  nuclear energy reactors, 478–480
  pandemic influenza, 233–238, 234–237*t*
  personal preparedness guidelines, 293
  public-private partnerships during
    emergencies, 88–93
  radiological agents, 361–363, 362*t*
  rapid needs assessments, 189–191
  state government capacity. *See* State
    preparedness and response
  substance abuse population, 534–538, 537*t*
  surveillance and monitoring, 176–180
  technology and public health crises, 135–138
  temperature extreme emergencies, 437–438
Preparedness Tips (California Governor's Office
    of Emergency Services'), 386
President's Emergency Plan for AIDS Relief
    (PEPFAR), 86
Primary blast injuries (PBI), 297
Principles for effective assessment, 194–195
Principles of partnerships, 90–93, 91*t*
Private actors in public-private partnerships,
    87–88
Private-sector engagement, 89–90, 95–96
Private-sector organizations, bombing events,
    293, 297, 299–300, 301
Private sector-UN partnerships, 92–93
Private voluntary organizations (PVOs), 106
Private Voluntary Organization Standards
    (InterAction), 112, 115
Procedural due process, 39
Project BioSense, 16
Project Bio-Shield, 327
Project Bio-Surveillance system, 325–326
PROMED (surveillance network), 272
Protecting public's health vs. practice of medi-
    cine, 32–34, 35*t*
Provincial reconstruction teams, Afghanistan
    (PRTs), 76
Proxy measurements, 155
Psittacosis (parrot fever), 322
Psychological first aid (PFA), 499

Psychological First Aid: Field Operations Guide
(publication), 499
Psychological interventions, 499–500
Psychosocial assistance, radiological agents,
369–372
Psychosocial issues for children in public health
emergencies, 522, 527–528
PTSD. *See* Post-traumatic stress disorder
PTT (Pediatric Triage Tape), 519
Public health (generally)
delivery of, 106, 107*f*
protection of, 15–17
Public Health Agency of Canada, Center for
Emergency Preparedness and Response,
179, 272
Public health emergencies and substance abuse,
531–543
case study, 531–532
collaborations, 536–538
historical and general perspectives, 533–534
mitigation, 539–541, 541*t*
overview, 531–532
preparedness and planning, 534–538, 537*t*
response, 538–539, 539*t*
substance use, epidemiology of, 533–534
vulnerable subgroups, 534
Public Health Emergency Preparedness
(PHEP), 18–19
Public health informatics, 134–135, 137*t*
Public Health Information Network, 16
Public health law, 31–44
administrative law, 38–39
case law, 39–40
case study, 31, 41–42
common law, 34
constitutional law, 36–38
historical perspectives, 32
legislative body, limitations on power, 40–41
ordinances, 40
protecting public's health vs. practice of
medicine, 32–34, 35*t*
statutory law, 34–36
tort law, 34
types of laws, 34–40, 35*t*
Public health practitioners, 33
Public Health Preparedness office, 269
Public Health Response and Preparedness for
Bioterrorism Program, 20
Public health security, 3–12
emergencies, 3–5
framework for, 6–9, 7*f*

historical perspectives, 5–6
resilience analysis model, 7–8, 8*t*
systemization capabilities, 8–9
Public Health Security and Bioterrorism
Preparedness and Response Act (2002), 6
Public Health Service, 168
Commissioned Officer Corps, 17
Public Health Threats and Emergencies Act
(2000), 5
Public-private partnerships (PPPs), 83–102
accountability, efficiency, and technical
expertise, 89
capacity and resource demands, 88–89
case study, 85, 98
economical settings, 86
governments, 86–87
historical perspectives, 85–88
humanitarian quandaries, 96–97
long-term solutions, 97–98
mandates, 88
meta-initiatives, 93
mitigation, 93–98, 299–300
overview, 83–85
political settings, 86
preparedness and response, 88–93, 412
principles of partnerships, 90–92, 91*t*
private-sector engagement incentives, 89–90
private-sector quandaries, 95–96
private sector-UN partnerships, 92–93
single-company public-private partnerships, 92
UN institutions, 87–88
PulseNet, 212–213
Pushpacks, 269, 338
PVO (private voluntary organization), 106

Q
Al-Qaeda, 65, 357
Q fever, 322–323
Quarantines, 24

R
Radiation
assets and functions, 481, 482–483*t*
dosage, 476
exposure, 367, 369, 374, 476, 479–480
measurements, 476–477, 476*t*
treatment, 479, 480, 481
Radiation Emergency Medical Preparedness
and Assistance Network (REMPAN),
477, 479–480
Radiation emission device (RED), 360–361

Radiological agents, 357–376
    background, 359–361
    case study, 357–359, 373–374
    communications, 369–372
    decontamination, 366–367
    evacuation, 366–367
    government responsibilities, 362–363
    health effects of, 368–369, 370–371t
    mitigation, 372–373
    overview, 357–359
    physiology of, 359–360
    population monitoring, 367–368
    preparedness, 361–363, 362t
    psychosocial assistance, 369–372
    response phases, 364, 365f
    response strategies, 364–372, 365–366f, 370f
    scene management, 364–366, 366f
    screening, 367–368
    terrorist devices, 360–361
Radiological dispersal device (RDD), 360–361
Rapid influenza diagnostic test (RIDT), 144
Rapid needs assessments (RNA), 185–198
    case study, 186–187, 195–196
    cluster sampling, 191–192
    components of, 190–191
    goal of, 185
    historical perspectives, 188–189, 188t
    local emergency mitigation, 193–194
    mitigation, 193–195
    overview, 185–187
    preparedness, 189–191
    principles for effective assessment, 194–195
    protocols for, 188t, 189
    response, 191–192
Rapid Treatment (START), 519–520, 520f
RDD (radiological dispersal device), 360–361
Reagan, Ronald, 114
Real-time data collection, 158
Real-time Outbreak and Disease Surveillance
    (RODS), 136
Real-time reverse transcriptase-PCR
    (rRT-PCR), 143
Recovery Function Annex, 47, 49
RED (radiation emission device), 360–361
Red Crescent organizations, 88
RedVat, 136
Refugees
    Bhutanese, 173
    High Commissioner for Refugees (UN),
        87, 92, 95
    Rwandan, 173

Regional Hospital Preparedness Council of
    Houston, 527
Rehabilitation phase in epidemiological study,
    159–161, 161t
Reliant Center/Astrodome, Houston, 518,
    525–529
Religious support systems, 504
REMPAN (Radiation Emergency Medical
    Preparedness and Assistance Network),
    477, 479–480
Resilience analysis model, 7–8, 8t
Resilience as mitigation for mental health
    emergencies, 505
Resilience of infrastructure, 298, 299f
Resources
    demands for, 88–89
    deployment of, 57–60
Respiratory isolation, 266–267, 275
Respiratory tract irritants, 341–342, 342t
Responders to disasters, types of, 7–8, 8f
Response issues, children and public health
    emergencies, 522–525, 527–529
Response phase
    epidemiological studies, 158–159, 160t
    radiological agents, 364, 365f
Response planning, advance, 22
Response strategies
    biological agents, category A, 309–318,
        310t, 313t
    biological agents, category B, 318–325
    biological agents, category C, 324–325
    bombing events, 294–295
    chemical agents, 339–349, 339t
    contagious diseases epidemics, 213–220
    earthquakes, 387–392
    federal entities, 15–20
    hazardous materials, 458–467, 458t
    hurricanes, tsunamis, and cyclones, 415–418
    infectious diseases, 265–269
    local entities, 21–25
    national response plan, 56–60
    NGO response to crises, 114–123
    nuclear incidents, 480–483
    pandemic influenza, 238–242, 238–240t
    phase in epidemiological study, 158–159, 160t
    public-private partnerships during
        emergencies, 88–93, 412
    radiological agents, 364–372, 365–366f, 370f
    rapid needs assessments, 191–192
    state entities, 20–21, 25, 26t, 362–363,
        457t, 458

substance abuse population, 538–539, 539t
surveillance and monitoring, 22–24, 176–180
technology and public health crises,
 138–144, 158
temperature extreme emergencies, 437–438
Response systems, components of, 8–9
Retrospective studies, 154–155
Reunification of children in public health
 emergencies, 521
Richter scale, 383
Ricin toxin, 323
Ricinus communis (ricin toxin), 323
Ridge, Tom, 49
RIDT (rapid influenza diagnostic test), 144
Risk communication strategy, 25, 341, 413–414
Risk factors in mental health emergencies, 505
Risk groups for complications of pandemic
 influenza, 235, 235t
Risk levels, nuclear energy, 479
Risk of radiation exposure, 476, 476t
Robert Wood Johnson Foundation, 17
RODS (Real-time Outbreak and Disease
 Surveillance), 136
Routine, normalization of, for children in
 public health emergencies, 524, 528
rRT-PCR (real-time reverse transcriptase-
 PCR), 143
Rwandan refugees, 173

S

Saffir-Simpson Hurricane Scale, 405
Salmonella, 320
San Francisco, California (earthquake, 1906), 383
Sanofi-Aventis, 246
Sarin, 335–336, 337, 350–351
SARS. *See* Severe acute respiratory distress
 syndrome
Save the Children, 106, 120–121
Scene management, radiological agents,
 364–366, 366f
Screening, radiological agents, 367–368
SEB (staphylococcal enterotoxin B), 324
Secondary blast injuries, 297
Secondary disasters of earthquakes, 383–384
Secure Embassy Construction and
 Counterterrorism Act (1999), 298
Secure Wireless Infrastructure System
 (SWIS), 92
Security Council (UN), 87
Security in public health
 Afghanistan situation, 65

emergencies, 3–10, 7f
wireless technology and, 141, 142t
Sentinel surveillance systems, 23, 136, 178
September 11, 2001, terrorist attacks
 communications coordination, 9
 Implementing Recommendations of the
 9/11 Commission Act (2007), 293
 National Commission on Terrorist Attacks
 Upon the United States (9-11
 Commission), 293, 325
 phases of public health response, 14
 post-traumatic stress disorders, 506
Septicemic plague, 313–314
Serological testing, 143
Services
 direct delivery of, 18
 emerging public health systems, 74–77
Severe acute respiratory distress syndrome
 (SARS), 175, 251–252, 266, 273–275
Shaanxi Province, China (earthquake, 1556),
 383
Shelters
 Hurricane Katrina and, 168–172, 169f, 170f,
 171f, 187
 nuclear incidents and, 481
 procurement of, 390
 substance abuse patients and, 538
Shippingport power plant, 476
Sichuan, China (earthquake, 2008), 92–93, 382,
 388, 390
SIMBA (Sistem Informasi Manajemen Bencona
 Aceh, Indonesia), 92
Simple Triage, 519
Single-company engagements, 88
Single-company public-private partnerships, 92
SIOC (Strategic Information and Operations
 Center), 57
Sistem Informasi Manajemen Bencona Aceh,
 Indonesia (SIMBA), 92
Situation, phase, population and patient
 (SPPP), 494–497, 506–508
Situational awareness, 56–57, 57f, 59f, 60
Situation-specific parameters of mental health
 framework, 495
Smallpox, 314–315
SNS. *See* Strategic national stockpile
SOARCA (State-of-the-Art Reactor
 Consequence Analyses) project, 478
Social distancing measures, 245
Social interventions, 503–504
Social responsibility, corporate, 90

Social support systems, 504
Sociopolitical context of earthquakes, 392
Southeast Louisiana Catastrophic Hurricane Functional Plan, 193
Southeast Louisiana Hurricane Evacuation and Sheltering Plan, 194
Spain, Madrid (subway bombings, 2004), 288, 299
Sphere Project, 112, 120
Spiritual support systems, 504
SPPP (situation, phase, population and patient), 494–497, 506–508
Sri Lankan Air Force, 93
Stafford Act declaration, 46, 59
Staphylococcal enterotoxin B (SEB), 324
START (Rapid Treatment), 519–520, 520f
State actors in public-private partnerships, 86–87
State constitutions, 36–38
State Department, U.S., 288
State Health Leadership Initiative, 17
State-of-the-Art Reactor Consequence Analyses (SOARCA) project, 478
State preparedness and response, 20–21, 25, 26t, 362–363, 457t, 458
State request for federal aid, 20–21, 46, 59–60
Statistics and data management, 72–74, 155
Statutory law, 34–36
Stop TB Strategy, 215
Strategic Information and Operations Center (SIOC), 57
Strategic national stockpile (SNS)
    antiviral agents, 235, 243
    pediatric medications, 522
    purpose of, 17
    pushpacks, 269, 349
    state request for, 21
Structural-collapse bombings, 295–296
Substance abuse. *See* Public health emergencies and substance abuse
Sudan, Darfur, 87, 96
Support Annexes, 47–49, 48f, 117, 481
Surge capacity, 203–204, 258–259, 497–498
Surveillance and monitoring, 167–184
    active systems, 23, 178
    biosurveillance, 135–136
    case study, 168–172, 169–171f, 180–181
    definition of, 22–23
    disease profile in surveillance system, 177
    disease surveillance systems, 262
    historical perspectives, 172–176
    overview, 167–172

    preparedness and response, 176–180
    sentinel surveillance systems, 23, 136, 178
    syndromic surveillance, 135–136, 262–264
    systems, 16, 22–24, 135–136, 209–212, 211–212t, 262
Surveillance and public health
    Afghanistan situation, 70–72
    for biologic terrorism events, 22–24
    for disease incidences, 16, 22–24, 117–118
    hazardous materials, 451, 452t
    Hurricane Katrina aftermath, 415
    local preparedness and response, 22–24
    nutritional surveillance, 174–175
    passive reporting systems, 23, 178
    purpose of, 70
Surveillance networks, 271–273
Survivors in recovery activities, 504
Susceptibility to abuse, children, 523
SWIS (Secure Wireless Infrastructure System), 92
Synadenium grantii (poisonous plant), 307
Syndrome Reporting Information System (SYRIS), 136
Syndromic surveillance, 135–136, 262–264

T
Taliban, 63–64, 65
Tangshan, China (earthquake, 1976), 382
Target capabilities list, 53, 54f
TB (tuberculosis), 75–76, 214–215
Tear gas, 341
Technical expertise in disaster response, 89
Technical Guidance for Hazards Analysis (EPA/FEMA/DOT), 454
Technology and public health crises, 131–149
    application factor, 138–139
    biosurveillance, 135–136
    case study, 132–133, 145–146
    databases, 139–140
    diagnostic technology, 143–144
    geographical information systems, 140–141
    global positioning systems, 140, 144
    health information exchange, 138
    historical perspectives, 133–135
    information retrieval systems, 140
    localization and directional systems, 140–141
    mitigation, 144–145, 298, 299–300
    outbreak management, 136–137, 137t
    overview, 131–133
    personal digital assistants, 141–143
    preparedness, 135–138

public health informatics, 134–135, 137*t*
rapid vaccine development, 144–145
response, 138–144, 158
wireless technology, 141, 142*t*
Telecommunication, 134
Telemedicine, 243
Temperature extremes, emergencies, 425–443
case study, 426–428, 427*f*, 439–440
cold-related illnesses, 433–436, 436*t*
epidemiology, 428–436, 429*f*
heating and cooling mechanisms, 431–432, 432*t*
heat-related illnesses, 432–433, 434*t*
historical perspectives, 428–436
mitigation, 438–439
overview, 425–426
preparedness and response, 437–438
Terrorist bombing events, 287–289. *See also specific bombing events*
Terrorist devices, radiological agents, 360–361
Tertiary blast injuries, 297
Texas Health and Safety Code, 36
Thompson, Tommy G., 320
Thornburgh, Richard L., 474
Threat-based assessments, 51
Three Mile Island (nuclear incident, 1979), 473–475, 485–486
Tobacco Free Initiative (WHO), 85
Tokyo, Japan (subway attack, 1995), 335–336, 350–351
Tornados, 412
Tort law, 34
Toxidromes, 465–467
Tracking children in public health emergencies, 521, 526–527
Training, hazardous materials, 456–458, 468–469*t*
Transportation Department, U.S. (DOT), 450, 450*t*
Transportation of hazardous materials, 451–454, 453*t*
Traumatic brain injury, 523
Trauma/traumatic event, defined, 493
Travel-related illnesses, 203–204, 204*t*
Treaties banning chemical warfare agents, 350
Triage
for children, 518–521, 520*f*, 525–526
of contaminated patients, 464–465
levels of, 299
Tsunami Evaluation Coalition, 85

Tsunamis. *See also* Hurricanes, tsunamis, and cyclones
Asian. *See* Asian tsunami (2004)
Boxing Day Tsunami (2004), 417–418
warning system for, 409
Tuberculosis (TB), 75–76, 214–215
Tularemia, 315–316
Turkey, Izmit (earthquake, 1999), 391
Turning Point Initiative, 15
2PAM (pralidoxime), 349
Typhoons. *See* Hurricanes, tsunamis, and cyclones

U
Ukraine, Chernobyl nuclear incident (1986), 473, 475, 486
Under-immunization, 220–223
United Kingdom
Hillsborough (football stadium disaster, 1989), 506
London (underground bombing, 2005), 288
United Kingdom Health Protection Agency, 179
United Nations (UN)
Biological Weapons Convention, 307
Conference on Environment and Development (1992), 106
Development Programme, 92
establishment of, 105
Global Compact, 85–86, 90–91, 91*t*, 98
High Commissioner for Refugees (UNHCR), 87, 92, 95
humanitarian reform proposal, 89
International Atomic Energy Agency, 372
Logistic Centre, 93
Millennium Development Goals, 121
Office of Coordination of Humanitarian Affairs, 87, 391, 394–395
Security Council, 87
UNICEF, 120
United Way, 115
Universal surveillance systems, 178
Universal task list, 53
Urban growth, 4, 4*f*
U.S. Department of ___. *See specific name of department*
USAID REACH program, 73
USSR
Cold War, 313
Obninsk nuclear power plant, 476

V

Vaccinations for public health threats
avian influenza in Afghanistan, 75, 136
children in evacuation centers, 524–525
consequence management and, 24–25
government requirements for, 31–32, 36,
41–42
hepatitis A and, 219–220
influenza and, 235
measles and, 203, 215–216, 223
rapid vaccine development, 144–145
schedules for, 524
smallpox, 314–315
under-immunization, 220–223
Vaccine production, 145, 246
Variola virus, 314–315
Vendor Managed Inventory (VMI), 269
Vesicant syndrome, 342–344, 343*t*
Veterinary response teams, 16
Vibrio cholerae (water contaminant), 324
Viral culture testing, 143
Viral hemorrhagic fevers, 316–318, 317*t*
Viral hepatitis A, 219–220
Vital data registration systems, 176–177
Voluntary Private Sector Preparedness
Accreditation and Certification Program,
293
Volunteer responses, organization of, 391
Vulnerability assessments, 50–51
Vulnerable populations, 500, 505, 534

W

War
Cold War, 313
conflict and, 118–121
Democratic Republic of Congo, 120
El Salvador, 120
Warning systems
earthquakes, 384–385
hurricanes, 410
temperature extreme emergencies, 437–438
tornados, 412
tsunamis, 409
Washington Conference (1921–1922), 350
Water safety threats, 324
Weapons of mass destruction (WMD), 325
Weekly Epidemiologic Record (WHO), 179
West Nile virus, 255, 264, 272

WHO. *See* World Health Organization
Wide area network (WAN), 141
Wireless technology, 141, 142*t*
Working Group on Civilian Biodefense,
309, 311
World Disarmament Conference (1933), 350
World Economic Forum, 93, 98
World Health Assembly (1998), 119–120
World Health Organization (WHO)
classification system for pandemics,
232–233, 232*f*
communicable disease cluster program, 70
Communicable Disease Control in Emergencies,
175
Expanded Programme on Immunization,
185, 191–192
Global Alert and Response program, 175,
179, 207, 208*t*
Global Outbreak Alert and Response
program, 209, 272
International Health Regulations, 6, 175,
207–209, 270
pandemic influenza preparedness, 233–238,
234*t*
pandemic influenza response, 136
partnership programs, 85–86
Radiation Emergency Medical Preparedness
and Assistance Network, 477,
479–480
rapid needs assessment protocols, 188*t*, 189
surveillance activities framework, 175, 176*f*
Tobacco Free Initiative, 85
Weekly Epidemiologic Record, 179
World Trade Center, terrorist attacks. *See*
September 11, 2001, terrorist attacks
World Vision International (WVI), 106, 108, 113
Worldwide Crisis Response Team, IBM, 88

X

X-rays, 359–360

Y

Yersinia pestis (plague), 313–314, 313*t*

Z

Zaire. *See now* Congo, Democratic Republic of
Zimbabwe cholera outbreak 2008–2009, 177
Zoonotic pathogens, 253